To
Mom and **Dad,**
Donn, Joseph, and **Jude**
and to the memory of **Nana**

Thank you for so much —
small words, but filled with meanings and feelings

Preface

New techniques and developments in the medical field have a direct influence on the medical assistant's professional duties and responsibilities. Because the educational standards of each medically oriented professional career continue to escalate, each assumes new functions, roles, and responsibilities. With the increasing demands of modern medical practice on members of the medical profession, physicians are turning more and more to trained medical assistants to help administer their offices and perform routine clinical duties.

The intent of this book is to help medical assistants attain the knowledge and skills required to meet the increasing demands of their profession and enable them to function as major contributing individuals in the health care field.

A textbook should expose the student to new ideas, thoughts, and concepts. It should motivate the student or reader, and above all, it should teach. To achieve these goals, this book presents in a concise, clear, and readable style up-to-date, accurate information about clinical assisting and skills, theory, and related medical information that the medical assistant must understand in order to contribute to quality health care services for patients.

The chief objective is to aid the student and the teacher in the learning/teaching process. I have attempted to create a book that students will want to pick up and enjoy because it stimulates them, and thus a book from which they will learn eagerly and easily. I have also tried to make this book one that will excite teachers and in turn help make their teaching tasks easier (an instructor's manual to accompany the second edition is available).

This book is designed to provide knowledge of effective and efficient techniques in contemporary patient care and assisting for beginning medical assistants who are learning these skills. Moreover, it supplies current reference material for those assistants actively employed in a medical setting and serves as an information source for the principles and techniques underlying clinical assisting for individuals who wish to reenter the employment field. Actively employed medical assistants who have the first edition of this book in their office and/or home library say that they refer to it frequently when performing their daily work duties. Those individuals preparing to take the national certification examination administered by the American Association of Medical Assistants will find this book particularly helpful if they use the objectives at the beginning of each unit and the review questions, performance tests, and checklists given as a study guide at the end of each unit.

The scope of this book meets the growing need for a comprehensive and effective textbook that deals with

- routine clinical skills and assisting techniques with related information required of the medical assistant
- patient procedures that may be performed satisfactorily by the medical assistant
- patient procedures in which the medical assistant may be required to assist the physician
- tests and procedures that the medical assistant must know in order to provide the patient with accurate preparatory information
- information necessary for an understanding of the procedures, the medical techniques and their underlying principles, in addition to the functions of other professionals who provide health care
- quality patient care as the medical assistant's primary goal based on the development of a positive attitude toward individual responsibilities and a commitment to the other members of the health care team
- the most current theoretical information available with an emphasis on practical application

Acquiring clinical skills and assisting techniques is best accomplished when learning experiences are organized and the learner is provided with opportunities to acquire knowledge and to practice with professionals in settings that enhance learning. For example, in a skills laboratory, which is a simulation of a joblike environment, learners can practice their new skills with each other, or in a clinical setting, which is a working experience, the learners may work under direct supervision.

This book also introduces the medical assistant to the nature and purpose of many procedures, both diagnostic and therapeutic, utilized by the various medical specialties and related medical fields, such as the changing and ever-expanding specialties of nuclear medicine, radiology, physical therapy, and laboratory technology, so that the medical assistant can anticipate and prepare the patient for procedures in these fields. Although the medical assistant is only indirectly involved with these specialties, it is essential to become knowledgeable of these fields of medical practice.

The *second edition* of this book has been expanded from ten to sixteen units, including a new unit on Laboratory Orientation (Unit 9), in order to present each subject area as a complete unit. You will find that the depth of the text remains, but every unit incorporates new and the most up-to-date information available on clinical procedures and related theory. Numerous new photographs and illustrations have been added to enhance the student's visualization and understanding of the theory, procedures, and equipment presented, thereby increasing the value of this book in the educational process. A glossary of the vocabulary terms from each unit and new Appendices A, B, C, and D have also been added. These are valuable assets and reference sources for the student. Emphasis is on helping the students learn to perform the tasks, to acquire the skills of their profession, to use the related basic scientific and technical knowledge, and to acquire the capabilities for problem-solving, making reliable decisions related to their tasks and adapting to new situations, and to treat the patient as a whole individual and not merely as a condition or as a diseased body part.

The organization in the units of the second edition remains the same as that of the first edition, as this has proved to be educationally effective for the learning and teaching process. Each unit contains the following:

- cognitive and terminal performance objectives
- vocabulary lists with pronunciation keys
- specific procedures and related information

To help reinforce learning, each unit also includes:

- reviews of the vocabulary (most of which use as examples medical reports)
- thought-provoking review questions relating to both theory and skills mastered, many with practical application to an on-the-job situation
- performance tests
- performance checklists

This is more than just a how-to book, it is also a why, when, where, who, and what book.

A few of the special features included are some explanations of what the physician is actually doing during an examination of a patient or procedure in which the medical assistant is participating. In addition this book contains the following:

- a table of common blood tests with normal values and the significance of the results
- a table of urine examinations with the type of specimen required and the normal values for the results
- tables of x-ray and nuclear medicine procedures, with the time period required for each, an indication of when special patient preparation is required, and samples of patient preparation
- a table of patient conditions that benefit from physical therapy and the common modalities used
- AIDS infection control precautions
- guidelines for assisting with the patient history/interview

- expanded coverage on the health care and examinations for the obstetrical and the hypertensive patient
- actual medical reports, case histories, discharge summaries, and so on to allow the student to see how the vocabulary terms presented in the unit are used in an actual report, how the contents of the unit relate to medical reports, and how health care providers document information obtained about a patient
- a summary of studies used for diagnosing conditions affecting body organs and systems
- performance tests and checklists that may be used by the students and adapted for teacher use in the instructor's manual
- charting examples for the assistant to use when recording the completion and results of procedures and tests

To aid the learning process for beginning students, an indication of the correct pronunciation is included for difficult terms as they are introduced. It will be helpful to the students at this time for the teacher to give the correct pronunciation of the term and then have the students repeat it. This pronunciation key adds to the usefulness of this book.

In the unit on physical therapy, students are given the opportunity to design procedural steps, performance checklists, and instructions to be given to the patient to use at home.

Information offered in each unit is written with the assumption that the medical assistant student has a background in or is currently studying basic anatomy, physiology, and microbiology. Thus, detailed explanations pertaining to these subjects are omitted. The teacher of the class for clinical procedures is encouraged to review the theoretical aspects pertaining to these subjects as they relate to each skill the student will be expected to perform.

All procedures (skills and tasks) are presented in a concise step-by-step format. When necessary, explanations of the physician's role, specific notes on patient care, and notes stressing the rationale behind a step are offered. The procedures are written to assist the student in the learning process. Sometimes the ideas or procedure steps are included in another procedure or unit to reinforce the ideas presented. The student should analyze the facts and try to place them in a meaningful order.

It should be remembered that frequently different methods and techniques may be used in a medical procedure. This book presents one method of performing a procedure. Where there are regional differences of opinion, the teachers are encouraged to teach the skill in the fashion most suitable for their area of practice.

This book is written with procedures that may be

performed by medical assistants nationwide, although because of various state laws some procedures may not be considered a duty of the medical assistant. Nevertheless, it is hoped that the information provided will help medical assistants understand the nature and purpose of all procedures presented.

With all these facets in mind, it is my hope that educators, students, and medical assistants will pick up and use this textbook with the enthusiasm and thirst for knowledge equal to my own as I researched, compiled, and wrote this book. It is also my hope that this book will challenge the student to develop a permanent interest in the medical field and a desire for continued growth and knowledge.

Sharron M. Zakus

Acknowledgments

This book could not have been compiled without the encouragement, support, inspiration, and assistance given by many friends, colleagues, and other specialists in the medical field. I am deeply indebted to each one of them.

The completion of the second edition of this book also gives me the opportunity to thank all the educators and students who responded so positively to the first edition.

My very special gratitude is extended to Donn R. Harris for his unlimited support, understanding, faith, and encouragement throughout the writing of the complete manuscript and for his valuable assistance in various stages of preparation.

With pleasure, I gratefully acknowledge the following practicing professionals who offered special area consultations and reviews. I am deeply indebted to each of them for the time, energy, and knowledge that each one so willingly contributed. In alphabetical order they are

Marlene Bonham, RPT, Physical Therapy, Education Co-ordinator, Pacific Presbyterian Medical Center, San Francisco

Ruth Berry Hanley Bultman, RN, Kaiser Hospital Clinic, San Francisco

William Delameter, MT(ASCP), Children's Hospital of San Francisco, San Francisco

Julia Ender, MT(ASCP), San Francisco

John M. Gunning, Mobile Intensive Care Paramedic, San Francisco

Richard A. Jones, Medico Supply Company, Inc., San Francisco

Elizabeth C. Lee, CRT, San Francisco

Deborah Leeds, Pharm D, Director of Pharmacy Services, Shield Healthcare Center, Berkeley, California

Louisa Lo, RPT, Senior Physical Therapist, Outpatient Services, Pacific Presbyterian Medical Center, San Francisco

Betty J. Mattea, BA RT(R), Chairperson, Radiology Department, City College of San Francisco

Tom McCarthy, Medico Supply Company, Inc., San Francisco

Dennis McDevitt, Mobile Intensive Care Paramedic, San Francisco

William C. McDill, RPT, Director, Physical Therapy Services, San Francisco

Bonnie Miller, BSN, OB-GYN Clinic RN, Children's Hospital of San Francisco, San Francisco

James Mochizuki, CNMT, Nuclear Medicine Technologist, Pacific Presbyterian Medical Center, San Francisco

Robert Navarro, Mobile Intensive Care Paramedic, San Francisco

James Pritchard, MT(ASCP), Laboratory Manager, Presbyterian Hospital of Pacific Medical Center, San Francisco

William B. Wolfe, CRT, San Francisco

I would like to extend my appreciation to the authors and publishers for their kind permission to use some of the illustrations from their books, and gratitude to all the firms and their representatives who cooperated with me in supplying illustrations and descriptive literature of their products. Their names are given appropriate credit throughout the book.

To George Dodson, professional photographer, I am particularly grateful for his work in taking numerous new photographs for this second edition.

A very special thank you and many words of appreciation are extended to my nephew, Kevin Zakus, for his artwork needed in the final stages of production.

Gratitude is also due many physicians, other laboratory, pharmaceutical, and medical personnel, and hospitals who contributed medical reports, provided the facilities for taking many of the photographs, and other special area reference material.

With warm appreciation, I sincerely thank Betty Biles, BS, RRA, Director of the Medical Record Technology Program, City College of San Francisco, Rosemary Clark, BA, MS, Health Science Department, City College of San Francisco, and Doris Huey, for assistance in various other areas.

The typing of the manuscript was done by Brian Mailman. He deserves very special thanks and words of appreciation for his patience, dedication, and excellence in his work with the preparation of the manuscript.

I want to sincerely thank the members of the C. V. Mosby Company for all their assistance in the production of this book, and express special words of appreciation to my excellent editorial team, Richard A. Weimer, Senior Editor, and Susan Lawson, Assistant Editor, for their interest and assistance during this endeavor. A special thanks and words of appreciation also to Lisa G. Cunninghis, Editorial Project Manager, the C. V. Mosby Company, and to Lilliane Chouinard from Editing, Design & Production, Inc., for their excellence in editing and their help in the final stages of production.

Finally, I wish to acknowledge all my past and present students whom I have had the privilege of knowing and working with in the classroom, and to many other colleagues, friends, especially Ann A. Gunderson and Eunice E. Larson, and family for their continued interest and support.

S. M. Z.

To the Student

You are about to enter the professional area of clinical medical assisting, an interesting and challenging field. When you have mastered the knowledge and skills presented in this book, you will be capable of enhancing patient care, in addition to increasing your value to the physician, co-workers, and related health specialists.

Always keep in mind that you are an important member of the medical team, and it is only through dedicated professional teamwork that quality and appropriate medical care can be provided and accomplished. Never underestimate your value in the field of medical care.

Points to keep in mind as you are studying and practicing procedures and assisting the physician include the following:

- the importance of being exact (precise) in all that you do
- the great service that you are rendering to the patient and to the physician/employer
- the influence that your attitude (positive or negative) can have on your performance and subsequent relationship with patients
- the legal implications of your actions
- that the career you are learning can be extremely rewarding and intellectually stimulating when you apply yourself and continually strive for improvement and continuing educational endeavors

For each unit in this book, read and master the objectives and vocabulary listed. Test yourself and a study companion with the review questions and performance checklists provided. When you feel that you can perform a particular skill, have your instructor give you the performance test. Written and oral testing may also be given to you at the discretion of your instructor.

Samples of patients' records are provided for review of the vocabulary in the units and to allow you to see how medical personnel record information for a patient's permanent medical record. These records will stimulate your interest, enhance learning, and help you relate your studies to actual on-the-job experiences. Read each report carefully and relate its contents to the current and previous units of study.

Inherent in the performance of all clinical skills are basic principles that you should recall and integrate:

1. Obtain and prepare the equipment necessary for the procedure. This involves knowledge of the procedure.
2. Thoroughly wash your hands before and after each procedure and patient contact.
3. Prepare and assist the patient both mentally and physically.

Mental preparation involves an adequate but simple explanation of the situation. Patients will be more relaxed and cooperative when they know what to expect during an examination or procedure. For your explanation, remember that you must be knowledgeable of medical terminology and prepared to translate that language into terms that the patient can readily understand. Provide reassurance and support while maintaining a supportive, empathetic (not sympathetic) attitude.

Physical preparation involves positioning the patient correctly for the procedure, draping appropriately, and offering assistance as needed. Always provide for the patient's comfort and safety.

4. Perform or assist the physician with the procedure.
5. Record the procedure and findings accurately.
6. Dispose of waste and used equipment correctly.
7. Clean and ready the treatment room and equipment for reuse.

As you begin your studies, I would like to wish you success and happiness in a most rewarding professional career and share with you a poem that I have shared with many of my former students and graduates. Think about it as you begin this program of study and periodically throughout your new career.

TAKE TIME

Take time to think — thoughts are the source of power.

Take time to play — play is the secret of perpetual youth.

Take time to read — reading is the fountain of wisdom.

Take time to pray — prayer can be a rock of strength in time of trouble.

Take time to love — loving is what makes living worthwhile.

Take time to be friendly — friendships give life a delicious flavor.

Take time to laugh — laughter is the music of the soul.

Take time to give — any day of the year is too short for selfishness.

Take time to do your work well — pride in your work, no matter what it is, nourishes the ego and the spirit.

Take time to show appreciation — "thanks" is the frosting on the cake of life.

Author of the poem unknown

S. M. Z.

Contents

Tables

Unit I

Physical Measurements: Vital Signs, Height, and Weight

COGNITIVE OBJECTIVES

On completion of Unit I, the medical assistant student should be able to apply the following cognitive objectives:

1. Define the terms vital signs, temperature, pulse, apical heartbeat, respiration rate, and blood pressure, and list the normal average values for each.
2. Define and pronounce the listed vocabulary terms that relate to temperature, pulse, respiration, and blood pressure, and state verbally or in writing examples of each.
3. List the required equipment for taking a patient's vital signs and the general care for this equipment.
4. Recall and state the *general* instructions for taking temperature, pulse, respirations, and blood pressure.
5. Describe briefly the methods employed to obtain and record a patient's vital signs.
6. When given hourly recordings of patient's temperatures, determine if these sets indicate normal or abnormal variations in daily body temperature.
7. When given the results of 25 patients' vital signs, state which results fall within normal ranges and which do not. State the reasons for the answers given.
8. List five situations in which taking an oral body temperature should be avoided or delayed.
9. List two situations in which taking a rectal temperature and two situations in which taking an axillary temperature should be avoided.
10. List 10 situations that will cause variations in a person's pulse rate.
11. List and locate the seven arteries in the body from which the pulse rate can be obtained with relative ease.
12. Describe what is meant by the rate, rhythm, and volume of the pulse rate; the rate, rhythm, and depth of respirations.
13. List five situations that would increase a person's

respiratory rate and five that would cause this rate to decrease.
14. List five situations that would increase a person's blood pressure and five that would cause it to decrease.
15. List and explain five factors that determine arterial blood pressure.
16. List five methods that may be used to control high blood pressure.
17. State six reasons for measuring a patient's height and weight.

TERMINAL PERFORMANCE OBJECTIVES

On completion of Unit I, the medical assistant student should be able to do the following performance objectives.

1. Demonstrate the correct procedures for obtaining a patient's oral, axillary, and rectal temperature.
2. Identify and locate pulsations on the seven major arteries used to measure a patient's pulse rate; identify and locate the apical heartbeat.
3. Demonstrate the correct procedure for taking a patient's pulse rate and apical heartbeat.
4. Demonstrate the correct procedure for measuring a patient's respiratory rate.
5. Demonstrate the correct procedure for taking a patient's brachial and popliteal arteries' systolic and diastolic blood pressures.
6. Demonstrate the correct procedure for taking a patient's blood pressure by use of the palpation method.
7. Demonstrate the correct procedure for taking a patient's orthostatic blood pressure.
8. When given 20 temperature results recorded in centigrade degrees, convert each to Fahrenheit degrees, and vice versa.
9. Demonstrate the correct procedures for measuring a patient's weight and height.
10. When given 20 weight and height results re-

corded in kilograms and inches, convert these measurements to pounds and feet (and inches if applicable); convert weights recorded in pounds to kilograms.

11. Demonstrate the proper methods for caring for stethoscopes, sphygmomanometers, and thermometers after use.

The student is expected to perform the above with 100% accuracy. Results obtained for a pulse rate and a respiratory rate are acceptable if within two beats or respirations as determined by the instructor. Results for blood pressures are acceptable if within 2 to 4 mm Hg as determined by the instructor.

Among the medical assistant's most routine clinical duties are the taking and recording of the patient's physical measurements, which include vital signs, height, and weight. It is therefore necessary for the medical assistant to know and understand these measurements and be able to correctly obtain and record the values for each. This unit discusses these six measurements along with procedures and related vocabulary.

It is assumed that the medical assistant student has completed or is currently studying anatomy and physiology. Therefore, detailed explanations of how the vital signs are produced by the body will not be included here.

VITAL SIGNS

Vital signs are measurable, concrete indicators that pertain to and are essential for life. The four vital signs are temperature, pulse, respiration (TPR), and blood pressure (BP). These signs are routinely measured in each physical examination. The purpose for obtaining a patient's vital signs is to provide the physician with information that will help

Determine the patient's condition by comparing the patient's body temperature, pulse, respiration, and blood pressure with normal values.
Determine a diagnosis, the course, and the prognosis of the patient's condition.
Designate the treatment that will be instituted.

TEMPERATURE

Body temperature, the degree of body heat, is a result of the balance maintained between heat produced and heat lost by the body. This is regulated by a central heat-regulating center located in a portion of the brain, the hypothalamus, that initiates the various mechanisms to increase or decrease heat loss.

Heat is produced by oxidation of foods in all body cells, especially those in the skeletal muscles and

liver. The blood and blood vessels distribute it to other parts of the body. Eighty-five percent of body heat is lost through the skin by radiation, convection, and evaporation of perspiration. The remainder is lost through the respiratory tract and mouth and through feces and urine.

A variation from the normal range of a patient's temperature may be the first warning of an illness or a change in the patient's condition. As such, it is an important part of the diagnosis and treatment plan for a patient.

Temperature Vocabulary

constant fever—High fever with a variation not exceeding 1 or 2°F (0.6° or 1.2°C) between morning and evening temperatures.

crisis—Sudden drop of a high temperature to normal or below; generally occurs within 24 hours.

fever—Pyrexia, or elevation of body temperature above normal, 98.6°F (Fahrenheit) or 37°C (centigrade or Celsius) registered orally. Some classify it as

Low	99° to 101°F (37.2° to 38.3°C)
Moderate	101° to 103°F (38.3° to 39.5°C)
High	103° to 105°F (39.5° to 40.6°C)

intermittent fever—Variations with alternate rises and falls, with the lowest measurement often dropping below 98.6°F (37°C). An intermittent fever reaches the normal line at intervals during the course of an illness; for example, AM 98°F, PM 100°F; AM 98.6°F, PM 101°F.

lysis—Gradual decline of a fever.

onset—Beginning of a fever.

remittent fever—Variations in temperature but always above 98.6°F (37°C); a persistent fever that has a daytime variation of 2°F (1.2°C) or more, for example, AM 100°F, PM 103°F; AM 99°F, PM 102.4°F (Fig. 1-1).

Normal Temperature Readings

Body temperature is measured by a thermometer placed under the tongue, in the rectum, or in the axilla, because large blood vessels are near the surface at these points. The normal temperature values for these three sites based on a statistical average are as follows:

Oral	98.6°F (Fahrenheit) or 37°C (centigrade or Celsius)
Rectal	99.6°F or 37.6°C
Axillary	97.6°F or 36.4°C

Accurate rectal temperatures will register approximately 1°F or 0.6°C higher than accurate oral tem-

Fig. 1-1. Temperature graph demonstrating the defined terms.

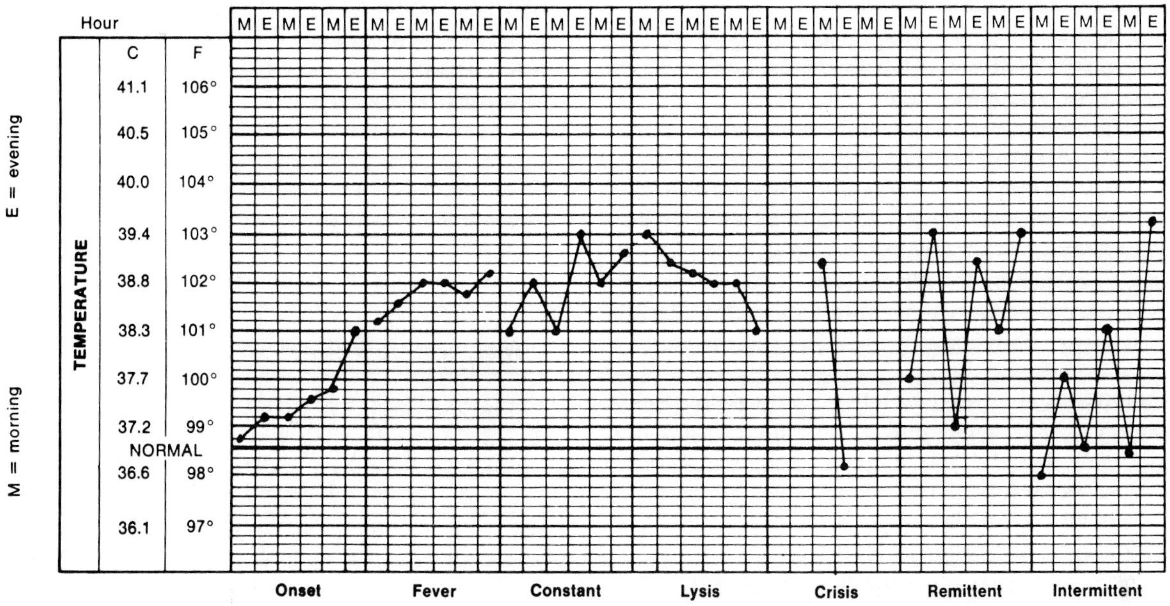

peratures. Accurate axillary temperatures will register approximately 1°F or 0.6°C lower than accurate oral temperatures. The rectal temperature is considered to be the most reliable and accurate reading. The mucous membrane lining of the rectum, with which the thermometer comes into contact, is not exposed to the air, and the conditions do not vary as do those of the mouth or axilla.

Variations in Body Temperature

Normal body temperature varies from person to person and at different times in each person.

- The daily average oral temperature of a healthy person may vary from 97.6° to 99°F (36.4° to 37.3°C).
- The lowest body temperature occurs in the early morning (2 AM to 6 AM).
- The highest body temperature occurs in the evening (5 PM to 8 PM).
- In a woman, body temperature may increase *slightly* during the menstrual cycle at the time of ovulation.
- Body temperature is slightly higher during and immediately after eating, exercise, or emotional excitement.
- Body temperature may vary more and is generally higher in an infant or young child than in an adult.

Abnormal temperatures occur when the body's temperature-regulating system is upset by disease or other physical disturbances.

- Body temperature will *decrease* in some illnesses; if a patient faints, collapses, or hemorrhages; or if the patient is in a fasting state, is dehydrated, or has sustained a central nervous system (CNS) injury. Subnormal temperatures, below 96°F (35.6°C), may occur in cases of collapse.
- Body temperature will *increase* in an infectious process or may increase following a chill. Shivering (chills) is one way the body increases heat production by the muscular activity that occurs; this activity releases heat.

Increases in body temperature are also produced by

Activity
Emotions
Environmental changes
Age (the aged and infants show 1°F higher)
Reactions to certain drugs
The amount and type of food eaten (an increase in metabolic rate increases heat production in the body)

Fever usually accompanies infection and many other disease processes. Fever is present when the oral temperature is 100°F (38.8°C) or higher. Temperatures of 104°F (40°C) or higher are common in serious illnesses.

Thermometers

A thermometer calibrated in Fahrenheit or centigrade (Celsius) degrees is the instrument used to measure body temperature. Various models made of glass or special disposable materials are available. Newer models are electronic. All good thermometers must pass a rigid inspection for proper calibration according to the standards set by the United States National Bureau of Standards.

The frequently used glass thermometers vary in shape. The rounded, short bulb is used when taking rectal temperatures, as it is held better by the rectal muscles. It may also be used when taking an axillary temperature. The slender bulb is considered more effective for oral temperatures. There are also rounded, short bulb thermometers for both oral and rectal use. These are usually color-coded for easy identification; that is, the oral thermometers have a blue identification mark at the end, and rectal thermometers have a red mark. All register the same temperature, although the "normal" temperature arrow will be on the 98.6°F (37°C) mark for the oral thermometer and may be on the 99.6°F (37.6°C) mark for the rectal thermometer (Fig. 1-2).

Safe and easy-to-use, battery-operated electronic thermometers are rapid (within 10 to 45 seconds) and accurately calibrated to within two tenths of a degree. These have disposable covers and interchangeable color-coded probes for both oral and rectal use. The temperature is registered on a dial or on a digital display on the equipment (Fig. 1-3).

How to Read a Glass Thermometer. When reading a thermometer, hold it between your thumb and index finger at the end away from the bulb. Rotate the thermometer until you see the center clear (silver) line of mercury toward the bulb. Follow this line up until it ends. Sometimes you can see this line better by changing the direction of the light source. Fahrenheit thermometers are marked off in degrees, with intermediate marks at two tenths of a degree. Centigrade thermometers are marked off in degrees, with intermediate marks at one tenth of a degree. Centigrade readings can be converted to Fahrenheit readings and Fahrenheit degrees converted to centigrade degrees using the following formulas. Since the metric system is being used more frequently, you should

Fig. 1-2. **A,** three types of thermometers. The slender bulb is best for oral temperatures; the rounded bulb shown in both Fahrenheit and centigrade degrees is best for rectal temperatures and may also be used for axillary temperatures. **B,** one type of disposable thermometer. The last dot to turn dark indicates the temperature reading.

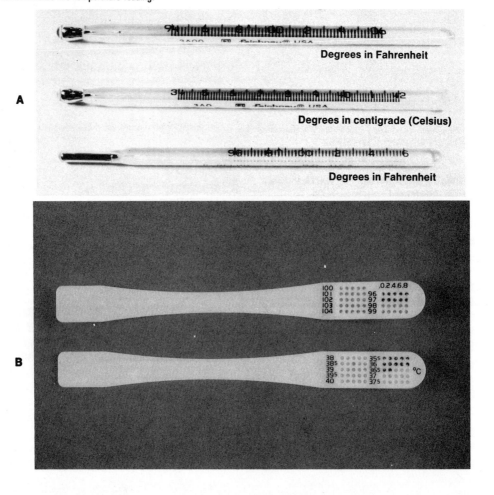

know how to convert Fahrenheit degrees to centigrade degrees. The formula for this is $C° = (F° - 32 \times \frac{5}{9})$. If the Fahrenheit temperature is 98.6°, then:

$$C° = (98.6° - 32) \times \frac{5}{9}$$
$$C° = 66.6° \times \frac{5}{9}$$
$$C° = 333\frac{9}{9}$$
$$C° = 37°$$

To convert centigrade to Fahrenheit degrees, the formula is $F° = (C° \times \frac{9}{5}) + 32$ (Table 1-1).

Table 1-1. Comparison of centigrade and Fahrenheit readings

C	F	C	F
34.0 —	93.2	37.6 —	99.7
34.1 —	93.4	37.7 —	99.9
34.2 —	93.6	37.8 —	100.0
34.3 —	93.7	37.9 —	100.2
34.4 —	93.9	38.0 —	100.4
34.5 —	94.1	38.1 —	100.6
34.6 —	94.3	38.2 —	100.8
34.7 —	94.5	38.3 —	100.9
34.8 —	94.6	38.4 —	101.1
34.9 —	94.8	38.5 —	101.3
35.0 —	95.0	38.6 —	101.5
35.1 —	95.2	38.7 —	101.7
35.2 —	95.4	38.8 —	101.8
35.3 —	95.5	38.9 —	102.0
35.4 —	95.7	39.0 —	102.2
35.5 —	95.9	39.1 —	102.4
35.6 —	96.1	39.2 —	102.6
35.7 —	96.3	39.3 —	102.7
35.8 —	96.4	39.4 —	102.9
35.9 —	96.6	39.5 —	103.1
36.0 —	96.8	39.6 —	103.3
36.1 —	97.0	39.7 —	103.5
36.2 —	97.2	39.8 —	103.6
36.3 —	97.3	39.9 —	103.8
36.4 —	97.5	40.0 —	104.0
36.5 —	97.7	40.1 —	104.2
36.6 —	97.9	40.2 —	104.4
36.7 —	98.1	40.3 —	104.5
36.8 —	98.2	40.4 —	104.7
36.9 —	98.4	40.5 —	104.9
37.0* —	98.6*	40.6 —	105.1
37.1 —	98.8	40.7 —	105.3
37.2 —	98.9	40.8 —	105.4
37.3 —	99.1	40.9 —	105.6
37.4 —	99.3	41.0 —	105.8
37.5 —	99.5	41.1 —	106.0
		41.5 —	106.7
		42.0 —	107.6
		42.5 —	108.5

*Normal oral temperature.

Methods and Procedures for Taking a Temperature

Following these guidelines, determine the correct method of use.

1. *Oral* temperatures should *never* be taken on the following:
   a. Children who are not old enough to know how to hold the thermometer in the mouth (4 years old and younger)
   b. Patients with a nasal obstruction, dyspnea, coughing, weakness, a sore mouth, mouth diseases, or oral surgery
   c. Patients receiving oxygen
   d. Uncooperative, delirious, unconscious, or intoxicated patients
2. *Axillary* temperatures should *never* be taken on the following:
   a. Thin patients who cannot make the hollow under the arm airtight
   b. Perspiring patients whose axilla cannot be kept dry for the required 5 to 10 minutes
3. *Rectal* temperatures should *never* be taken on the following:
   a. Rectal surgery patients
   b. Children or other patients whose body movement cannot be controlled for the required 4 to 5 minutes

Equipment

Thermometer:
   Oral—glass thermometers may be stored in a small container of 70% alcohol solution or other disinfectant solution, with a small pad of cotton in the bottom, and labeled *clean oral thermometers*
   Rectal—glass thermometers may be stored in a small container of alcohol solution or other disinfectant solution, with a small pad of cotton in the bottom, and labeled *clean rectal thermometers*
Box of tissues or small cotton squares
Container for waste
Containers labeled "soiled oral thermometers" or "soiled rectal thermometers" for the ones used
Water-soluble lubricant if a rectal temperature is to be taken, such as K-Y jelly, Vaseline, mineral oil, or baby oil

General Instructions

1. Handle the thermometer with great care, as it is a very delicate instrument.
2. Keep rectal thermometers separate from oral thermometers.
3. Wash your hands before and after handling a thermometer or taking a patient's temperature.

(Text continues on p. 8)

Fig. 1-3. Mark X Electronic Thermometry System, using the latest in electronics and microprocessor technology, is lightweight (about 10 ounces) and is easy to use, maintain, and clean. The 15 second timer can be used for measuring pulse and respiratory rates. Temperature is measured in 30 – 45 seconds. (Courtesy Electromedics, Inc., Englewood, CO)

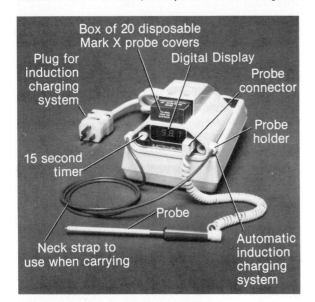

Box of 20 disposable Mark X probe covers

Digital Display

Plug for induction charging system

Probe connector

Probe holder

15 second timer

Neck strap to use when carrying

Probe

Automatic induction charging system

NOTE: The Mark X displays the following letter indications when appropriate:

P = Low battery power, return to charger for a minimum of 4 hours.

H or L = Defective probe, replace with a good probe.

E = Tissue contact lost, eject the probe cover, return the probe to the storage well — repeat all steps for taking patient's temperature.

OPERATING INSTRUCTIONS

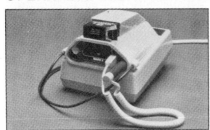

1 Remove the Mark X from the charger base. Select °F or °C (select switch is located on the back of the Mark X).

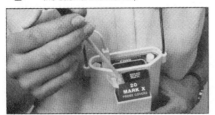

2 Removing the probe from the storage well turns the temperature display, returning the probe to the well shuts off the display. Holding **ONLY** the red or blue collar of the probe, **FIRMLY** insert the probe tip into the probe cover. (Use only HPC-360 probe covers.)

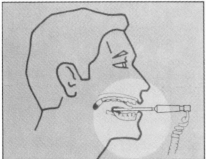

3 For oral temperatures (use blue probe) – Taking 4 to 5 seconds, **SLOWLY** insert the covered probe tip under the patient's tongue into the sublingual pocket.

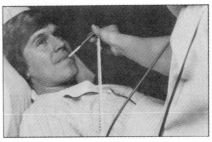

4 Hold probe ensuring good tissue contact until audible tone is heard, record temperature.

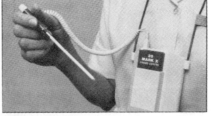

5 DISCARD the probe cover by holding the red or blue collar of the probe between the thumb and fingers while pushing on the white top of the probe with the index finger. Return the probe to the storage well to turn off the display. Also, **ALWAYS** return the Mark X to its charger base when the Mark X is not in use.

Taking Axillary Temperatures – The patients arm should be down against the body 3 minutes prior to **SLOWLY** inserting the covered probe into the axilla. Hold the probe parallel to the trunk of the body until the audible tone is heard.

Taking Rectal Temperatures – Using the (red) rectal probe with probe cover, **SLOWLY** insert probe to depth in accordance with established practice. Slightly tilt probe after insertion, hold the covered probe until the audible tone is heard. Luberication may be used on the tip of the probe cover.

Taking Pulses – Find patient's pulse, push white button on left side of the Mark X front. Count pulses until tone is heard 15 seconds later. Timer may also be used for respiration or I.V. rate. (For best results: **Do Not Use The Timer During** the same moments when taking temperatures.)

Fig. 1-3 *(continued)*

CARE AND PRECAUTIONS

GENERAL CARE AND PRECAUTIONS
- Read complete instructions before using system
- Keep the unit clean and follow established procedures in your office or clinic on clinical usage and cleaning
- Place unit on the charger base when not in use
- Do not use in the presence of flammable anesthetics
- Do not use acetone or similar products to clean unit as the surface could be damaged
- Please review all information in the manufacturer's manual before using the Mark X system

MARK X THERMOMETER
- Always place unit on charger base when not in use to insure that the batteries are fully charged
- Do not steam sterilize
- Read service instructions before attempting repairs or calibrations. Check the calibration of the unit periodically. This can be accomplished by using the calibration plug and verifying that the readout of the Mark X is the temperature indicated on the calibration plug. Should the unit require calibration, there are internal adjustments for fast service
- Do not reuse probe covers and use only Electromedics probe covers
- Replace components with like specification items

CHARGER BASE
Electrical shock hazard. Do not open case. Refer servicing to qualified personnel.
- Connect to properly grounded outlet
- Do not steam sterilize
- Always perform a current leakage test after any repairs

DESCRIPTION OF FRONT AND REAR PANELS

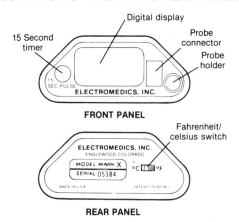

FRONT PANEL

REAR PANEL

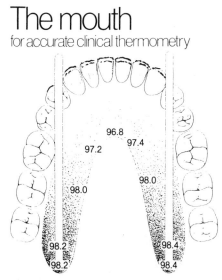

The mouth
for accurate clinical thermometry

The placement of the thermometer probe tip is important for accurate temperature taking since there may be significant differences in temperature over small distances in the mouth.

The diagram shows the hot spots where maximum temperatures are found. These important heat pockets lie at the junction of the base of the tongue and the floor of the mouth on either side of the frenum. If the probe tip is not placed in the heat pocket, temperature readings can vary significantly.

HELPFUL HINTS
THINGS IN GENERAL

The Mark X probes are cleanable. The blue and red sliders on the probes can be removed to allow for cleaning. If you will hold the probe above the slider and pull the slider while turning at the same time, the slider will pull off the probe shaft. You can clean the probe shaft and the slider with any of the cold wipe agents or they may be gas sterilized.

Hold the probe for the patient. Avoid allowing the patient to hold the probe. It is possible that the patient may move the probe out of the sublingual pocket, which would give an incorrect reading of the temperature.

When taking a rectal temperature, have the patient and supplies ready before removing the probe from the probe well and activating the unit. Pre-lube the rectal probe, ready the patient, remove the oral probe, plug the rectal probe into the Mark X, and then follow established procedures for taking the rectal temperature.

IF GETTING INACCURATE TEMPERATURES

Generally, inaccuracy with electronic thermometers is due to placement in the mouth. The map of the mouth shows the different temperature zones. If one is not careful to place the probe in the sublingual pocket, different temperatures will be experienced.

With electronic thermometers being very accurate in measurement, it is possible to vary a tenth or two tenths of a degree. Most of the glass thermometers do not have the ability to read this area as accurately as the electronic units do, so it may lead you to believe you have an accuracy problem. If your thermometers are within the published accuracy specifications and you are getting higher or lower readings, you should suspect measurement technique.

It is recommended that the patient not take anything orally for at least 15 minutes before taking the temperature. It is recommended that you wait for 15 minutes after an enema before taking a rectal temperature. These procedures will allow the tissue to return to the natural temperature and the measurement will be more accurate.

In some cases, you will have performed all of the proper techniques and have different temperature indications. The manufacturer recommends that you check the unit with the calibration key. This will indicate the electronic function and accuracy. You may want to change probes with another unit and see if you have the same readings. It may be helpful to ask the patient if they have taken anything orally or if they have been chewing gum or eating candy before you attempt to measure the temperature.

IF GETTING LOW TEMPERATURES

Low temperatures may be caused by several things. The most common is what is called "The Draw Down Effect." "Draw Down" is the sudden lowering of tissue temperature because of its contact with a probe at a lower temperature. The "Draw Down" occurs within the first few seconds, while recovery may take several minutes. This "Draw Down" effect results from thermal energy flowing from the skin tissue to the probe, until both the probe and the skin tissue are at the same temperature. Recovery then occurs as both tissue and probe temperatures increase to body temperature.

Measurements of "Draw Down" for various probes show that for an initial probe temperature of 75°F and tissue temperature of 98.6°F, the average recovery time of temperature in the local tissue is at least 3 minutes. To avoid the effect of "Draw Down", simply take 4–5 seconds to slowly insert the probe along the gum line. This process will warm the cold probe and not lower the temperature of the sublingual pocket at the base of the tongue.

The second possibility is the failure to insert the probe into the sublingual pocket. As the map of the mouth shows, there are many areas of varying temperatures located in the mouth. The most accurate for this purpose is the sublingual pocket located at the base of the tongue and close to the blood supply from deep within the body. If you are not in the pocket or if you press into the pocket and restrict the blood flow, you may well experience low temperature readings.

The third possibility is the natural temperature variations of humans. It has been found that people have a natural low temperature in the morning hours and a higher temperature in the evenings. If you have applied proper technique and you are experiencing what appears to be low temperature, you may be reading the natural temperature of that person. You may want to check the patient with another unit after about 5 minutes.

4. Read the thermometer with great care to ensure accuracy.
5. Record the reading and indicate if it was other than oral. This notation must be made because of the differences in temperatures when taken in either the axilla or rectum.

Care of Glass Thermometers After Each Use

1. Shake mercury down to below 96°F or 36°C.
2. Wash with soap and cold water, then rinse with cold running water.

3. Place in a disinfectant solution, such as 70% alcohol if it is to be used continuously; then rinse with cold running water and dry with a small piece of cotton before the next use.
4. If the thermometer is not to be reused within 24 hours, follow steps 1 and 2, then dry it and place in a container that has cotton in the bottom to provide protection for the bulb. Before the next use, the thermometer must be soaked for at least 10 minutes in a disinfectant solution and then be rinsed in cold running water and dried with a small piece of cotton.

Oral Temperature

The thermometer is to be placed in the mouth under the tongue. The lips should be closed.

Procedure	Rationale
1. Identify and evaluate the patient. 2. Wash your hands. 3. Assemble equipment.	Defer reading for 15 to 20 minutes if the patient has just finished eating, drinking, or smoking. Patients should not be left alone unless they are absolutely responsible. This is a precaution to avoid any accident or false reading.
4. Instruct the patient to assume a sitting position and explain the procedure. 5. Remove clean thermometer from the container. 6. Rinse with cold running water, and wipe dry from the stem downward to the bulb with a tissue or cotton square. Discard cotton square.	Complete explanations help gain the patient's cooperation and help the patient relax. Provide for the patient's comfort and safety.
7. With a firm hold on the end of the thermometer, shake it down to 96°F (35.5°C) or lower.	This is done by giving the wrist several quick snaps. Be careful to avoid contact with nearby objects.
8. Place the thermometer well under the patient's tongue. 9. Instruct the patient to keep lips closed, breathe through the nose, and not touch the thermometer with the teeth. 10. Leave the thermometer in place for 3 minutes. 11. The pulse and respirations may be taken while the thermometer is registering. 12. Remove the thermometer and wipe it from the top toward the bulb.	Never place pressure on the mercury bulb end of the thermometer.

13. Read the thermometer. Hold it horizontally and rotate it slowly until you see the point at which the mercury column stops.
14. Record the reading at once.
	Charting example:
	   March 2, 19____, 9 AM
	      Oral temp 98.8°F
	      or
	   Temp 98.8°F
	      J. Sublett, CMA

15. Shake the mercury down to 96°F (35.5°C) or below and place the thermometer in the container for used oral thermometers or into a container of cool soap solution.	

Procedure	Rationale

16. If retaking a questionable temperature, the medical assistant should do the following:
 • Check that the thermometer is shaken down to 96°F (35.5°C) or below
  or
 • Use another thermometer
  or
 • Use another method, either rectal or axillary.
17. Wash your hands.
	If the temperature is found to be remarkably high or low and there is no apparent reason for this, take it again.

Axillary Temperature

The thermometer is to be placed in the axilla (armpit).

Procedure	Rationale
1. Perform steps 1 through 7 as for oral temperature technique, using a rounded, short bulb thermometer.	
2. Blot the axillary region dry with tissue or a cotton square.	Avoid rubbing, as friction increases the blood supply in the area, thus increasing the temperature of the skin.
3. Place the bulb end of the thermometer in the hollow of the axillary region with the end of the thermometer slanting toward the patient's chest.	Ensure that the thermometer is in direct contact with the skin surface, not touching clothing or exposed to the air.
4. Have the patient cross the arms over the chest. It may be more comfortable to hold the opposite shoulder.	This prevents as little air as possible from coming into contact with the thermometer. When the patient is unable to put his or her hand on the opposite shoulder, place it there gently and hold it with your own hand or hold the patient's arm close to his or her side. When taking a child's axillary temperature, hold the thermometer in place for the entire time.
5. Leave the thermometer in place for 5 to 10 minutes.	This ensures accurate registration of the temperature.
6. The pulse and respirations may be taken while the thermometer is registering.	
7. Remove and wipe the thermometer from the top toward the bulb, and read it.	Never place pressure on the bulb end of the thermometer.

8. Record reading at once.	Charting example:
	 January 30, 19____, 11 AM
	  Axillary temp 97.6°F
	   or
	 Temp 97.6°F Ⓐ
	  M. Kubiak, CMA

9. Shake the mercury down to 96°F (35.5°C) or below and place the thermometer in the container for used thermometers.	
10. Wash your hands.	

Rectal Temperature

The thermometer is to be carefully inserted approximately 1 inch into the rectum.

Procedure	Rationale
1. Perform steps 1 through 7 as for oral temperature, using a rectal thermometer.	*Never* use an oral thermometer for a rectal temperature.
2. Have the patient turn on the side with the upper leg flexed if possible.	Do not expose the patient unnecessarily.
3. Apply lubricant to the thermometer.	This allows for easier insertion of the thermometer.
4. Separate buttocks so that anus is exposed.	
5. Gently insert thermometer approximately 1 inch into anal canal and instruct the patient to remain still.	Forceful insertion beyond 1 inch may cause damage to the tissues involved. Movement could cause the thermometer to go further into the rectum and possibly cause tissue damage, or the thermometer could slip out of the rectum.
6. *Hold* thermometer in place for 4 to 5 minutes.	*Never leave the patient alone when taking a rectal temperature.*
7. You may take pulse and respiration while the thermometer is registering.	
8. Remove the thermometer, wipe from stem to bulb, and read accurately.	*Never* place pressure on the bulb end of the thermometer. Be certain all fecal material is removed.

9. Record the reading at once.	Charting example:
	May 18, 19_____, 10 AM
	  Rectal temp 99.6°F
	  or
	Temp 99.6°F Ⓡ
	Josh Burns, CMA

10. Shake the mercury down to below 96°F (35.5°C).	
11. Place the thermometer in the container for used rectal thermometers.	Remember to keep used rectal thermometers in a separate container.
12. Wash your hands.	

Taking an Infant's Temperature

1. Lay the infant on the stomach on a firm surface.
2. With your left hand, spread the cheeks of the buttocks so that you can see the rectum.
3. With your right hand, insert the lubricated bulb end of the rectal thermometer into the rectum approximately 1 inch.
4. Place your right hand on the infant's buttocks, hold the buttocks firmly, and pinch the thermometer firmly between your fingers.
5. Place your other hand in the small of the infant's back, and with your arm straight, lean on the infant slightly. This will help hold the infant still (Fig. 1-4).
6. Leave the thermometer in place for 5 minutes.
7. Remove the thermometer, and place it out of reach of the infant.

8. Support the infant.
9. Wipe the thermometer with a tissue, read the temperature registered, and record it promptly.
10. Wash your hands.

Fig. 1-4. Position for holding a thermometer and infant while taking the rectal temperature.

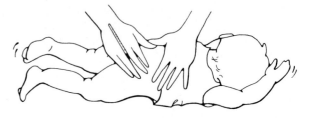

PULSE

The pulse is defined as the beat of the heart as felt through the walls of the arteries. It is the palpable distention or pulsation of the arteries produced by the wave of blood that travels along the arteries with each contraction of the left ventricle of the heart.

The pulse can also be described as a throbbing caused by the alternate expansion and recoil of an artery.

Pulse Variation Vocabulary

abdominal pulse—Abdominal aorta pulse.

acrotism (ak'ro-tism)—Apparent absence of pulse.

alternating pulse—Alternating weak and strong pulsations.

arrhythmia (ă-rith'-mĭ-ă)—Irregularities in pulse or rhythm.

bigeminal (bī-jěm'ĭn-al) **pulse**—Two regular beats followed by a longer pause. It has the same significance as an irregular pulse.

bradycardia (brad-ĭ-kar'dĭ-ă)—Slow heart action; extremely slow pulse, generally below 60 beats per minute.

febrile (feb'rile) **pulse**—A full, bounding pulse at the onset of a fever, becoming feeble and weak when the fever subsides.

formicant (for'mi-kant') **pulse**—A small, feeble pulse.

intermittent pulse—A pulse in which occasional beats are skipped.

irregular pulse—A pulse with variation in force and frequency; may be caused by an excess of tea, coffee, tobacco, or exercise.

pulse deficit—The apical rate is greater than the radial pulse rate.

pulse pressure—The difference between the systolic and the diastolic blood pressure.

> EXAMPLE: If BP is 120/80
>
> 120 = systolic pressure
> − 80 = diastolic pressure
> 40 = pulse pressure

A pulse pressure consistently over 50 points or under 30 points is considered abnormal.

regular pulse—The rhythm of the pulse rate is regular.

slow pulse—A pulse between 40 and 60 beats per minute, often found among the aged and among athletes at rest.

tachycardia (tak"y-kar'di-a)—a pulse of 170 or more beats per minute; abnormal rapidity of heart action.

threadly pulse—A pulse that is very fine and scarcely perceptible, as seen in syncope (fainting).

unequal pulse—A pulse in which some beats are strong and others are weak; pulse in which rates are different in symmetrical arteries.

venous pulse—A pulse in a vein, especially one of the large veins near the heart such as the internal and external jugular. Venous pulse is undulating and scarcely palpable.

Characteristics of the Pulse

When you are taking a pulse, the four important characteristics to note are the rate, rhythm, and volume of the pulse, and the condition of the arterial wall. These characteristics depend on the size and the elasticity of the artery, the strength of contraction of the heart, and the tissues surrounding the artery. The physician will sometimes spend several minutes examining a patient's pulse to obtain information that may reveal abnormalities of the circulation or the heart.

The *rate* (frequency) of the pulse means the number of pulsations (beats) in a given minute. Normal (average) rates are outlined in the following section. Abnormal rates are those above or below the range of norms, and could be described as bradycardia (slow) or tachycardia (rapid).

The *rhythm* of the pulse pertains to the time interval between each pulse. Normal rhythm is described as regular; that is, intervals between pulsations are of equal length. Abnormal rhythm may be described as irregular, arrhythmic, bigeminal, skipping beats, or intermittent. Skipping an occasional beat occurs in all normal individuals, especially during exercise or after ingesting certain stimulants such as coffee. Most of these irregularities go unnoticed but at times may concern a patient sufficiently to seek medical advice. When there are frequent beats skipped or if the beats are highly irregular, the physician should be alerted, because this could be an important sign of heart disease. In such cases, it is sometimes useful to count the radial pulse rate for 1 minute and then to record the apical rate by listening over the heart (see p. 13). If the apical rate is greater, the difference is referred to as the *pulse deficit*. The pulse deficit is important in the examination of the patient with atrial fibrillation, one of the more common causes of a very irregular pulse.

A pulse may vary in intensity in association with irregularities of rhythm. A pulse that varies only in intensity but is otherwise perfectly regular is often a manifestation of heart disease. The *volume* of the pulse pertains to the strength of the pulsations and may be described as full, strong, bounding, weak, feeble, thready, febrile, hard, or soft. It depends on the force of the heartbeat and the condition of the arterial walls.

The *force* of the pulse is an indication of the general condition of the heart and the circulatory system. This intensity may vary from being a weak and feeble beat, as seen in shock, to being a strong and bounding throb, as seen after exercise.

The *condition of the arterial wall* pertains to the texture of the artery that one feels through the skin surface when palpating the pulse. A normal arterial wall is described as soft and elastic; abnormal conditions include hard, ropy, knotty, and wiry.

Common Arteries and Body Locations for Determining Pulse Rate (Fig. 1-5)

radial—Over the inner aspect of the wrist area, on the thumb side. This site is the one most frequently used and accessible in most cases.
facial—Along the lower margin of the mandible.
common carotid—At right and left sides of the neck, at the anterior edge of the sternocleidomastoid muscle.
brachial—Over the inner aspect at the bend of the elbow.
temporal—At the temple, on the side of the forehead.
femoral—The anterior side of the hip bone, in the groin region.
popliteal—At the back of the knee.
dorsalis pedis—On the upper surface of the foot between ankle and toes.

Normal Pulse Rates (Average Number of Pulsations [Beats] in 1 Minute)

At birth	130 to 160 beats per minute
Infants	110 to 130 beats per minute
Children from 1 to 7 years	80 to 120 beats per minute
Children over 7 years	80 to 90 beats per minute
Adults	60 to 80 beats per minute

Variations in Pulse Rate

Individual pulse rates *normally vary* as a result of a person's sex, age, body size, posture, activity level, health status, functions of the nervous system, and the volume and chemical composition of the blood.

In general, the pulse rate is faster in women (70 to 80 beats per minute) than in men (60 to 70 beats per minute) and is usually higher in short people than in tall people. Infants' and children's pulse rates are also more rapid than an adult's. When one is sitting, the rate is more rapid (for example, 70 beats per minute) than when lying down (for example, 66 beats per minute), and increases when standing, walking, or running (for example, 80, 86, and 90 beats per minute respectively). During sleep or rest, the pulse rate may be as low as 45 to 50 beats per minute. In athletes it is not unusual to obtain resting rates as low as 45 to 50 beats per minute. The following list indicates some of the common causes of increases or decreases in the pulse.

Increase

Fear or excitement
Physical activity, exercise
Fever
Certain types of heart disease
Hyperthyroidism
Shock
Pain
Certain drugs
Many infections

Decrease

Mental depression
Certain types of heart disease
Chronic illness
Hypothyroidism
Certain brain injuries that cause pressure
Certain drugs, such as digitalis

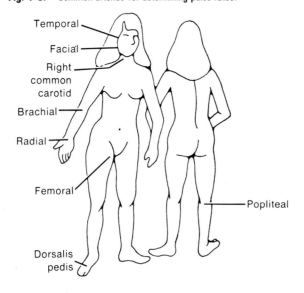

Fig. 1-5. Common arteries for determining pulse rates.

Temporal
Facial
Right common carotid
Brachial
Radial
Femoral
Popliteal
Dorsalis pedis

Procedure for Taking a Radial Pulse

Equipment

Watch with a second hand
Paper or graphic sheet to record pulse
Pen

General Instructions

1. Have the patient assume a comfortable position either sitting or lying down, with the arm supported.
2. Do not take a pulse rate immediately after the patient has been emotionally upset or after exertion, unless so ordered.
3. Never use your thumb to take a pulse, because its own pulse is likely to be confused with the one being taken.
4. Always count any unusual pulse for a full minute, and repeat if uncertain.

Procedure	Rationale
1. Identify the patient and explain the procedure.	Explanations help gain the cooperation and relaxation of the patient.
2. Wash your hands.	
3. Position the patient with the arm supported and at rest.	
4. Taking a firm hold of the patient's wrist, place your first three fingers on the patient's wristbone just over the radial artery, with sufficient pressure to feel the pulsations distinctly. (Pulse rates at other locations previously noted are taken in similar fashion.)	A firm hold will inspire the patient's confidence. Excessive pressure prevents the pulse from being felt. *Never* use your thumb to take a pulse, because your thumb's pulse can be confused with the patient's.
5. Count the pulse for 60 seconds.	This will give the total beats per minute.
6. Note the rate, rhythm, volume, and condition of the arterial wall.	Always report any deviation from normal. If deviations are noted, always count the pulse rate for 1 full minute, and repeat if uncertain.
7. Write the pulse rate down immediately.	Do not trust it to memory.
8. Record accurately on the patient's chart.	Charting example: July 9, 19_____, 2 PM Pulse 78 *or* Radial pulse, right arm — 78 Regular and strong pulsation Rae Evans, CMA

Apical Heartbeat Rate

The apical rate is the rate per minute of the heartbeat as determined by auscultation or feeling the apex of the heart. This is the most accurate pulse site. An apical pulse is taken on all children under 2 years of age and on patients with possible heart problems regardless of age. The normal range is 70 to 90 beats per minute; the average rate is 80 beats per minute.

To count the apical beat, place the chestpiece of a stethoscope over the apex of the heart and count the number of heartbeats for 1 minute.

The apex of the heart is located in the left fifth intercostal space on the midclavicular line, that is, between the fifth and sixth ribs on a line with the midpoint of the left clavicle. This position is usually just below the nipple.

When recording the results, you must indicate that it was the apical rate that was taken. On completion, wipe the earpiece and diaphragm of the stethoscope with an alcohol sponge and return it to the proper storage area.

RESPIRATION

Respiration is the act of breathing and consists of one inspiration or inhalation, which is the taking of air into the lungs, and one expiration or exhalation, which is the expulsion of carbon dioxide from the lungs. More specifically, respiration is the taking in of oxygen (O_2) and its utilization in the tissues, and the giving off of carbon dioxide (CO_2). For this reason, respiration may be classified as external and internal. External respiration is the interchange of gases that takes place in the lungs between the alveoli and blood; internal respiration is the interchange of gases that takes place in the tissues between the body cells and blood.

The autonomic control of breathing is controlled by the respiratory center in the medulla oblongata in the lower portion of the brain stem. A buildup of carbon dioxide in the blood stimulates respirations to occur automatically.

In the human body a relationship exists among the body temperature, pulse, and respiratory rates. The usual ratio of respiration to the pulse is one to four (1:4). Respiration and pulse ordinarily rise proportionally to each degree rise in temperature because of increased metabolism in the tissue cells and the need for more rapid heat dissipation.

Respiration and Respiratory Rate Vocabulary

abdominal respirations—The inspiration and expiration of air by the lungs accomplished primarily by the abdominal muscles and diaphragm.

accelerated respirations—More than 25 respirations per minute, after 15 years of age.

apnea (ap-ne'ah)—Cessation or absence of breathing.

artificial respiration—Artificial methods to restore respiration in cases of suspended breathing.

Biot respiration—Irregularly alternating periods of apnea and hyperpnea; occurs in meningitis and disorders of the brain.

Cheyne-Stokes (chān-stōks) **respiration**—Respirations gradually increasing in rapidity and volume, until they reach a climax, then gradually subsiding and ceasing entirely for from 5 to 50 seconds, when they begin again. These are often a sign of impending death. Cheyne-Stokes respirations *may* be observed in normal persons (especially the aged) during sleep or during visits to higher altitudes.

diaphragmatic respiration—Performed mainly by the diaphragm.

dyspnea (disp-ne'ah)—Labored or difficult breathing.

eupnea (ūp-ne'ah)—Easy or normal respiration.

forced respiration—Voluntary hyperpnea.

hyperpnea (hy"perp-ne'ah)—Increase in rate and depth of breathing.

hyperventilation—Increase of air in the lungs above the normal amount; abnormally prolonged and deep breathing, usually associated with acute anxiety or emotional tensions.

hypoxia (hi-pok'se-ah)—Reduced amounts of oxygen to the body tissues.

labored breathing—Dyspnea or difficult breathing; respiration that involves active participation of accessory inspiratory and expiratory muscles.

orthopnea (or"thop-ne'ah)—Severe dyspnea in which breathing is possible only when the patient sits or stands in an erect position.

rales (rahls)—An abnormal bubbling sound heard on auscultation of the chest; often classified as either moist or crackling and dry.

stertorous (ster'to-rus)—Characterized by a deep snoring sound with each inspiration.

Characteristics of Respirations

When you are taking the respiratory rate of a patient, the three important characteristics to note are the rate, rhythm, and depth.

The *rate* of respirations refers to the number of respirations per minute and is best described as normal, below or above normal, or rapid or slow. In adults, normal rates are between 14 and 20 per minute; subnormal rates are 12 per minute and below and should be considered a serious symptom; above-normal rates are between 34 and 35 per minute; rapid rates are between 36 and 50 per minute. Any rate above 40 should also be considered a serious symptom. Dangerously rapid rates are those that are 60 per minute and above. Usually rapid respirations are also shallow and are seen in some diseases of the lungs. Deep respirations are characteristically slow, dependent on oxygen exchange, and common in conditions affecting brain pressure and in some forms of coma.

The *rhythm* may be described as regular or irregular. Regular breathing or respiration is characterized by inhalations and exhalations that are the same in depth and rate, whereas in irregular breathing, the inhalations and exhalations may vary in the amount of air inhaled and exhaled and in the rate of respirations per minute.

The *depth* of respirations depends on the amount of air inhaled and exhaled and is best described as either shallow or deep. In shallow respirations, small amounts of air are inhaled; they are often rapid. In deep respirations, larger amounts of air are inhaled, as in a "deep breath."

Normal Respiratory Rates

At birth	30 to 60 respirations/minute
Infants	30 to 38 respirations/minute

Children   20 to 26 respirations/minute
Adults   14 to 20 respirations/minute

Variations in the Respiratory Rate

Certain situations, both in health or in diseased states, will cause variations in the normal respiratory rates.

Increased Respiratory Rate

Excitement
Nervousness
Any strong emotion
Increased muscular activity, such as running or exercising
Certain drugs, such as ephedrine
Diseases of the lungs
Diseases of the circulatory system
Fever
Pain
Shock
Hemorrhage
Gas poisoning
High altitudes
Obstruction of the air passages
An increase in the carbon dioxide levels in arterial blood, which in turn stimulates the respiratory center

Decreased Respiratory Rate

Sleep
Certain drugs, such as morphine
Certain diseases of the kidneys in which there is a coma
Diseases and injuries that cause pressure on the brain tissue (for example, a stroke or skull fracture)
Decrease of the carbon dioxide level in arterial blood (causes the respiratory centers to be depressed, causing decreased respiration rates)

Procedure for Taking the Respiratory Rate

Equipment

A watch with a second hand
Paper or graphic sheet to record respiration rate
Pen

General Instructions

1. Have the patient assume a comfortable position.
2. Do not take the respiratory rate immediately after the patient has been emotionally upset or after exertion, unless so ordered.
3. Count any unusual respiratory rate for an additional minute.

Procedure	Rationale
1. Wash your hands.	
2. Do *not* explain procedure to the patient.	The rate of respiration should be counted and its depth, rate, and rhythm studied without the patient's knowledge. The consciousness of being watched will cause an involuntary change in the rate of respiration. A patient can control respirations if he or she wishes to.
3. Place your fingers on the patient's wrist as though counting the pulse.	
4. Count each breathing cycle (inhalation and exhalation) as one breath by watching the rise and fall of the chest or upper abdomen.	When these movements are scarcely perceptible, place the patient's hand, with your fingers remaining on the wrist, gently but firmly on the patient's chest, and count in this manner.
5. Count for 1 full minute.	
6. Record rate on paper immediately.	Do not trust it to memory.
7. Record on patient's chart.	Charting example:
• Note any abnormality if present.	January 15, 19____, 2 PM
• Note any pain associated with breathing.	Respirations 22 and regular
• Note the position the patient assumes, as in some cases it may be significant. Examples include when the patient can breathe easier when sitting up, or when lying on one side or the other.	L. Quarry, CMA

BLOOD PRESSURE

Blood pressure (BP) is the pressure of the blood against the walls of the blood vessels. The pressure results from the pumping action of the heart muscle. This pressure inside the arteries varies with the contracting and the relaxing phases of the heart beat cycle. Systole is the phase when the heart contracts, forcing blood through the arteries, and diastole is the phase when the heart relaxes between contractions. Thus, when you are measuring a person's blood pressure, there are two readings that you will need to take: systolic pressure and diastolic pressure (systole and diastole).

Systolic pressure is measured in the number of millimeters of mercury (mm Hg), representing the force with which blood is pushing against the artery walls when the ventricles of the heart are in a state of contraction. During systole, blood is forced out of the heart into the aorta and pulmonary artery, and the pressure within the arteries is the highest.

Diastolic pressure is the number in millimeters of mercury that represents the force of the blood in the arterial system when the ventricles of the heart are in the state of relaxation. During diastole the two ventricles of the heart are dilated by blood flowing into them, and the pressure within the arteries is at its lowest point.

These measurements provide the physician with valuable information about a patient's cardiovascular system. Systolic pressure provides information about the force of the left ventricular contraction, and the diastolic pressure provides information about the resistance of the blood vessels.

Clinically, diastolic pressure is more important than the systolic pressure because the diastolic pressure indicates the strain or pressure to which the blood vessel walls are constantly subjected. Since diastolic pressure rises or falls with the peripheral resistance, it also reflects the condition of the peripheral vessels. For example, if a patient's arteries are sclerosed, both the peripheral resistance and the diastolic pressure will increase.

Blood pressure is recorded and discussed as the systolic pressure over the diastolic pressure. A typical blood pressure is expressed as 120/80 (mm Hg) *or* 120 over 80. The numerical difference between these two readings (in this case, 40 points) is called the *pulse pressure*, which may indicate the tone of the arterial walls. A normal pulse pressure is about 40; if consistently over 50 points or under 30 points, it is considered abnormal. You may see an increase in pulse pressure in arteriosclerosis mainly because of an increase in the systolic pressure, or in aortic valve insufficiency, the result of both a rise in systolic and a fall in diastolic pressure.

[handwritten margin note: Constant — so its more important]

Blood Pressure Vocabulary

hypertension (hi'per-ten'shun)—High blood pressure; a condition in which a patient has a higher blood pressure than normal for his or her age, (for example, systolic pressure consistently above 160 mm Hg and a diastolic pressure above 90 mm Hg).

hypotension (hi'po-ten'shun)—A decrease of systolic and diastolic blood pressure to below normal (for example, below 90/50 is considered low blood pressure).

benign (be-nīn) **hypertension**—Hypertension of slow onset that is usually without symptoms.

essential hypertension (idiopathic or primary hypertension)—Hypertension that develops in the absence of kidney disease. Its cause is unknown. About 85% to 90% of the cases of hypertension are in this category.

malignant (mah-lig'nant) **hypertension**—Hypertension that differs from other types in that it is a rapidly developing hypertension and may prove fatal if not treated immediately after symptoms develop, before damage is done to the blood vessels. This type occurs most often in persons in their twenties or thirties.

orthostatic (or"tho-stat'ik) **blood pressure**—Blood pressure measured when the patient is in an erect, standing position.

orthostatic hypotension—Hypotension occurring when a patient assumes an erect position.

postural hypotension—Hypotension occurring upon suddenly arising from a recumbent position or when standing still for a long period of time.

renal hypertension—Hypertension resulting from kidney disease.

secondary hypertension—Hypertension that is traceable to known causes such as a pheochromocytoma (tumor of the adrenal gland), hardening of the arteries, kidney disease, or obstructions to kidney blood flow. Approximately 10% to 15% of the cases of hypertension are secondary. Patients with secondary hypertension can often be cured *if* the underlying cause can be eliminated.

Factors that Determine Blood Pressure

A number of factors, acting in dynamic equilibrium and integrated through the central nervous system, determine the arterial blood pressure:

1. *The pumping action of the heart and cardiac output* — How hard the heart pumps the blood, or the force of the heartbeat; how much blood it pumps and how efficiently it does the job.

2. *The volume of blood within the blood vessels* — How much blood the heart pumps into the arterial system.

3. *The peripheral resistance of blood vessels to the flow of blood* — The size of the lumen, the central core of the arteries, directly influences the resistance to the blood flow. When the lumen is narrow, the blood pressure will be higher; with a larger lumen, the blood pressure will be lower.

4. *The elasticity of the walls of the main arteries* — The main arteries leading from the heart have walls with strong elastic fibers capable of expanding and absorbing the pulsations generated by the heart. At each pulsation, the arteries expand and absorb the momentary increase in blood pressure. As the heart relaxes in preparation for another beat, the aortic valves close to prevent blood from flowing back to the heart chambers, and the artery walls spring back, forcing the blood through the body between contractions. In this way the arteries act as dampers on the pulsations and thus provide a steady flow of blood through the blood vessels. This elasticity of the arterial walls lessens with age, and because the arterial wall is resistant, the blood pressure will then be higher.

5. *The blood's viscosity, or thickness* — Blood pressure increases as the viscosity of blood increases. Polycythemia, an increase in red blood cells, will cause this.

The exact contribution of each factor is not known, but it is generally thought that the peripheral resistance and cardiac output have the greatest influence on blood pressure.

Normal Readings and Values for Blood Pressure

At birth the systolic pressure is about 80 mm Hg. *At age 10* (young people), systolic blood pressure varies normally from 100 to 120 mm Hg and diastolic 60 to 80 mm Hg. In *adults* the average BP is 120/80. The *average ranges* are 90 to 140 mm Hg for systolic pressure and 60 to 90 mm Hg for diastolic pressure. In *older people* (around 60 years) the systolic blood pressure normally varies from 140 to about 170 mm Hg, and diastolic varies from 92 to 100 mm Hg, the result of a loss of resilience in the vascular tree and physiological changes of aging.

Variations in Normal Blood Pressure

The blood pressure can vary between the sexes (with women usually having a lower pressure than men), between different age groups, and even between in-

dividuals of the same age and sex. At birth it is the lowest, then continues to increase with age, reaching its peak in advancing age as a rule. Variations are also seen at different times of the day, and the pressure may change with the kind of activity in which a person is engaged. When one is standing or sitting, blood pressure is higher than when one is lying down.

The pressure is normally lowest just before awakening in the morning. There are many other situations that will produce changes in the blood pressure. The following lists indicate some of the common causes of an increase or decrease in a person's pressure.

Increased or Elevated

Exercise
Stress, anxiety, excitement
Conditions in which blood vessels become more rigid and lose some of their elasticity, as seen in old age
Increased peripheral resistance, resulting from vasoconstriction or narrowing of peripheral blood vessels
Endocrine disorders, such as hyperthyroidism and acromegaly
Increased weight
Renal disease and diseases of the liver and heart
In the right arm, it is about 3 to 4 mm Hg higher than in the left arm
Certain drug therapy
Increased intracranial pressure
Increased arterial blood volume

Decreased or Lowered

Weak heart
Massive heart attack
Decreased arterial blood volume (such as in hemorrhage)
Shock and collapse
Dehydration
Drug treatment
Disorders of the nervous system
Adrenal insufficiency
Hypothyroidism
Sleep
Infections, fevers
Cancer
Anemia
Neurasthenia
Approaching death

Abnormal Readings

In children around age 10, upper limits of normal are 140/100, with systolic pressure greater than 140 mm Hg generally recognized as being abnormal. In adults, a systolic pressure consistently above 150 mm Hg and a diastolic pressure consistently above 90 mm Hg are generally recognized as being abnormal. *Hypertension* is systolic pressure over 160 mm Hg or diastolic pressure over 90 mm Hg. If the blood pressure is consistently above this level, it could, if not treated, do damage to the heart, eyes, kidneys, and even the arteries. Diagnosis of hypertension is never based on only one reading. It is based on at least three consecutive daily or weekly blood pressure readings.

Hypotension is systolic pressure consistently under 90 with the diastolic pressure in proportion. In the absence of other signs or symptoms hypotension is generally innocent. An extremely low blood pressure is occasionally a symptom of a serious condition, such as shock, and may be associated with Addison's disease (underfunctioning of the adrenal glands).

A pulse pressure constantly greater than 50 mm Hg or less than 30 mm Hg is considered abnormal.

Detection and Evaluation of High Blood Pressure

Blood Pressure Confirmation

The Joint National Committee on Detection, Evaluation, and Treatment of High Blood Pressure has recommended that all adults with *diastolic* blood pressures of 120 mm Hg or above should be referred promptly to a source of medical care. All persons with blood pressures of 160/95 mm Hg or above should have the blood pressure elevation confirmed within 1 month. All persons *under the age of 50* with a blood pressure between 140/90 mm Hg and 160/95 mm Hg should be checked every 2 to 3 months. All persons *over 50 years* of age with a blood pressure between 140/90 mm Hg and 160/95 mm Hg should be checked every 6 to 9 months. All adults with *diastolic* blood pressures below 90 mm Hg should be advised to have their blood pressure checked yearly.

The *purpose* of the blood pressure recheck is to separate persons with initially elevated blood pressures into (1) those whose diastolic blood pressures have returned to normal and who therefore require only annual blood pressure remeasurement, and (2) those with sustained elevation in pressure that warrants treatment or further diagnostic study.

At each repeat visit, the person's blood pressure should be taken two or more times, and the average pressure obtained should be used as the value for the visit. Blood pressure measurements should be obtained on at least *two* occasions before specific therapy is prescribed unless the initial diastolic blood pressure is greater than 120 mm Hg.

Patient education begins at the same time the blood pressure is initially measured. Without alarming the patient, the person taking the pressure must carefully communicate the importance of following the recommended action.

Recommended Action for Initial Blood Pressure Measurement

Systolic/ Diastolic	Recommended Action
All adults	
Diastolic 120 or higher	Prompt evaluation and treatment
All adults	
160/95 or higher	Confirm blood pressure elevation within 1 month
Under age 50	
140/90 to 160/95	Blood pressure check within 2–3 months
Age 50 or older	
140/90 to 160/95	Check within 6–9 months

Follow-up Recommendations for Referral to Treatment

Average Diastolic Blood Pressure	Recommended Action
120 or higher	Immediate evaluation and treatment indicated
105–119	Treatment indicated
90–104	Individualize treatment
Under 90	Remeasure blood pressure at yearly intervals

Patients not requiring further study or treatment should be reassured, but the importance of an annual blood pressure measurement must be strongly emphasized.

Recommendations for Evaluation

In view of the rarity of the specific recognizable causes of high blood pressure, coupled with both the cost in dollars and the small but real risk to the patient of certain diagnostic procedures, it is recommended that all routine pretreatment workup be limited to defining the severity of the blood pressure and to identifying its complications and associated cardiovascular risk factors. More complex diagnostic procedures designed to discover specific causes of high blood pressure, such as primary aldosteronism (an abnormality of electrolyte metabolism produced by an excessive secretion of aldosterone, a hormone of the adrenal cortex; also called Conn's syndrome), renovascular disease, or pheochromocytoma (tumor in the adrenal gland), can be reasonably reserved for those subjects (1) in whom routine history, physical examination, or the recommended laboratory findings suggest one of the specific recognizable causes; (2) who are under the age of 30, since they have the greatest prevalence of correctable secondary high blood pressure; or (3) in whom drug therapy, as subsequently outlined, proves inadequate or unsatisfactory.

1. **History**
   The medical history should consist of any previous history of high blood pressure or its treatment, the use of birth control pills or other hormones, cardiac or renal disease, stroke, and other cardiovascular risk factors, including diabetes, cigarette smoking, a high salt intake, lipid abnormalities, or family history of high blood pressure or its complications. A history of weakness, muscle cramps, and polyuria suggests further screening for aldosteronism. A history of headaches, palpitations, or excessive sweating suggests further study for pheochromocytoma.

2. **Physical Evaluation**
   In addition to two or more blood pressure measurements (one standing), the pretreatment physical examination should include the items listed below:
   • Height and weight
   • Funduscopic examination of the eyes for hemorrhages, exudates, and papilledema; especially important in persons with diastolic blood pressures of 110 mm Hg or higher
   • Examination of the neck for thyroid enlargement, bruits, and distended veins
   • Auscultation of the lungs
   • Examination of the heart for increased rate, size, precordial heave, murmurs, arrhythmias, and gallops
   • Examination of the abdomen for bruits, large kidneys, or dilation of the aorta
   • Examination of the extremities for edema, peripheral pulses, and neurological deficits associated with stroke

3. **Basic Laboratory Tests**
   Baseline laboratory tests listed below should be obtained before initiating therapy:
   • Hematocrit
   • Urinalysis for protein, blood, and glucose (dipstick)
   • Creatinine and/or blood urea nitrogen
   • Serum potassium
   • Electrocardiogram
   Other tests that may be helpful include a chest x-ray, blood sugar, serum cholesterol, serum uric acid, microscopic urinalysis, and blood count. (Minimal cost to the patient can sometimes be achieved by ordering automated blood chemistries.) Clinical judgment or abnormal findings obtained during the routine evaluation may suggest other tests, such as an intravenous urogram and urinary catecholamines.

4. **Explanation of Findings to the Patient**
   Understanding by the patient of the disease and what actions he or she must take is crucial to high blood pressure control. The patient must be given adequate information and the opportunity to ask questions or discuss points of concern. The patient with high blood pressure must clearly understand the following:
   • The seriousness and lifelong nature of high blood pressure and the possible consequences of not treating it—there is *no* cure; however, hypertension can be controlled
   • The importance of taking medication as directed to maintain blood pressure control
   • The importance of adhering to other methods recommended to control blood pressure such as weight loss, reduced intake of animal fats and foods high in sodium or salt, not smoking, and mild-to-moderate exercise programs as prescribed by the physician—frequently the physician will recommend some combination of the above methods for controlling high blood pressure
   • The asymptomatic nature of the disease—how the patient feels may not reflect the level of blood pressure or the need to continue taking medication
   • The importance of keeping follow-up appointments

Long-Term Maintenance of Control

Management of high blood pressure must be considered a lifelong endeavor, with the levels of blood pressure the criteria of its adequacy. Patients must be periodically monitored to ensure blood pressure control and to overcome a major problem in treatment, specifically poor patient adherence to therapy. After control has been demonstrated and the patient's blood pressure is stable, remeasurement every 3 to 6 months should be adequate for most patients. Physicians should individualize the need for repeat laboratory and baseline tests according to the patient's age, initial severity of blood pressure, and target organ damage.

After normal levels are achieved, it may be possible to reduce drug therapy; however, rarely is it possible to discontinue treatment. This point should be emphasized to the patient. Blood pressures may be measured at home when appropriate in a difficult case or when frequent monitoring is deemed necessary.

Most patients with uncomplicated essential hypertension have few, if any, symptoms related to their hypertension; however, drug therapy may produce unwanted effects about which patients should be forewarned. Every effort should be made to adjust drugs and their dosages to eliminate or minimize such unpleasant effects and, at the same time, to gain patient acceptance of any that remain. Those responsible for monitoring antihypertensive regimens should also be well aware of pharmacologic interactions and adverse effects of antihypertensive agents and should be alert to discover and/or prevent them.

Instruments for Measuring Blood Pressure

Blood pressure is measured with two instruments, a *sphygmomanometer* (sfig"mo-mah-nom'ĕ-ter) and a

stethoscope (steth'-o-skōp). Various models of each and combination kits are available (Fig. 1-6). Two common types of sphygmomanometer (*sphygmo*, pulse; *manos*, slight; *meter*, to measure) are available for general use: the mercury manometer, which uses a column of mercury to measure the blood pressure, and the aneroid (*a*, not; *neroid*, liquid) manometer, which uses compressed air.

Each type has advantages and disadvantages. The mercury manometer offers total reliability, because, once calibrated at the factory, accuracy is assured. However, it may only be used when the column of mercury is in a vertical position, and it is more fragile and larger than the aneroid type. The aneroid manometer, on the other hand, needs periodic adjustment and calibration against a mercury manometer. However, it is smaller, thus offering more convenience and easier portability. Each manometer has four basic parts (Fig. 1-7).

Fig. 1-6. Various types of sphygmomanometers. **A,** Wall mercury sphygmomanometer. **B,** Wall aneroid sphygmomanometer. **C,** Custom Blood Pressure Kit. (**A, B, C,** Courtresy Sybron Corporation, Medical Products Division, Rochester, NY) **D,** Acoustic sphygmomanometer. Wrap cuff around arm in usual way. Make sure microphone is over brachial artery. With cuff in place, raise pressure to approximately 30 mm Hg beyond expected systolic pressure. Watch digital countdown as pressure automatically releases. First systolic then diastolic pressure is displayed, as sphygmomanometer responds to appropriate sounds. When both systolic and diastolic readings are displayed, the touch of a button also lets you read pulse rate.

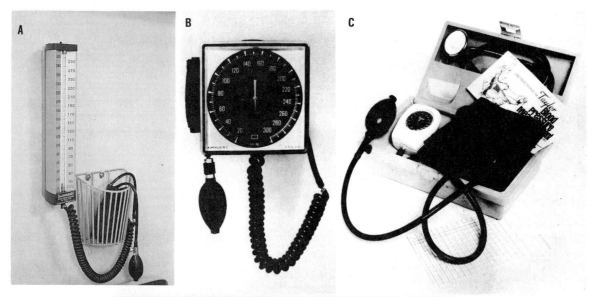

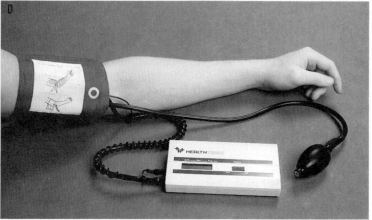

Fig. 1-7. Four basic parts of a sphygmomanometer. (Courtesy Sybron Corporation, Medical Products Division, Rochester, NY)

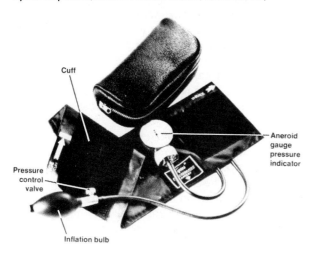

Pressure Indicators. These are the scales used to read the blood pressure. The mercury manometer has a glass tube with numbers on the side to indicate the height of the column of mercury in millimeters. When the cuff is inflated, mercury is forced up into the tube; as the cuff is deflated, the column of mercury will fall. It is at certain points that the level of the column of mercury is noted to provide the blood pressure reading. In the aneroid manometer, an internal gear rotates in response to inflation and deflation of the cuff, which in turn moves a needle across a calibrated dial to provide the blood pressure reading.

Cuff. The compression cuff is a rectangular inflatable rubber bag covered with a nonstretch material. This is wrapped around the patient's arm and secured with Velcro material or with clasps. On older models, the end of the cuff is tucked under one of the turns wrapped around the arm. Various sizes of cuffs are available to ensure a proper fit. Small cuffs are used on children or very thin people; larger cuffs are used on obese people or when taking a pressure reading on the leg (Table 1-2).

Inflation Bulb. This bulb is used to pump air into the cuff through a rubber tube.

Table 1-2. Recommended widths of compression cuffs

Age	Width of Inflatable Bladder
Newborn infants	2.5 cm (1 in.)
Children (1–4 yr)	6 cm (2.3 in.)
Children (4–8 yr)	9 cm (3.5 in.)
Adults	13 cm (5.1 in.)
Obese adults	20 cm (8 in.)

Pressure Control Valve. A valve on the inflation bulb is regulated with a thumbscrew to allow the air in the cuff to escape at different rates as it is opened and closed.

The *second* instrument used to measure blood pressure is the *stethoscope,* a basic diagnostic instrument that amplifies sounds produced by the blood pressure, the heart, and other internal body sounds. The key parts of the stethoscope are shown in Figure 1-8.

chestpiece—Has one, two, or three "heads" consisting of bell-shaped or various diaphragm-type sensors that "pick up" body sounds.

diaphragm—A waferlike sound sensor; its shape and the pressure applied to it determine which sound frequencies, low to high, are picked up.

tubing—Tapered, flexible rubber or plastic tubing through which sound travels from the chestpiece to the binaurals.

binaurals—Rigid metal tubes that connect the tubing to the earpieces.

earpieces—Tips of the stethoscope to be positioned in the examiner's ear.

spring—The external spring that holds the binaural so that the earpiece is firmly positioned in the ear.

Fig. 1-8. Key parts of a stethoscope. (Courtesy Sybron Corporation, Medical Products Division, Rochester, NY)

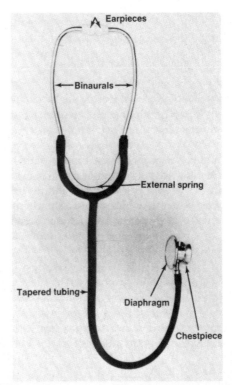

Procedure for Measuring Blood Pressure

Equipment

Sphygmomanometer
Stethoscope
70% isopropyl alcohol
Cotton balls or alcohol sponges
Paper and pencil

Auscultation Method. Auscultation (aws"kul-ta'shun) indicates that you will be listening for sounds representing the pressure inside the arteries. The artery most frequently used is the brachial artery at the antecubital space opposite the elbow. Other locations that may be used are the popliteal artery behind the knee, or less commonly, the pedal artery on the foot.

General Instructions

1. Before taking the patient's blood pressure ask if he or she has been or is currently under treatment for high blood pressure. Anyone under treatment should be encouraged to continue, especially if blood pressure is normal at the time of screening, and should be urged to report an elevated blood pressure to the physician. The potential dangers of discontinuing antihypertensive treatment and the desirability of achieving satisfactory control of blood pressure must be strongly emphasized.
2. Arrangements should ensure as much confidentiality as possible during the recording of the blood pressure.
3. Be sure the patient is relaxed and in a comfortable position. Depending on the physician's orders, the patient may be sitting, standing, or lying.

4. If possible, take all subsequent observations with the patient in the same position and using the same arm.
5. Take readings as quickly as possible, as prolonged pressure affects the accuracy of the readings and is unpleasant for the patient.
6. On all new patients, blood pressure should be taken on both arms. If a discrepancy exists, the arm with the higher pressure is used in future recordings. This discrepancy is to be recorded on the chart.
7. Blood pressure is taken routinely on the following patients, the frequency being determined by their condition:
   - Patients receiving a complete physical examination
   - Patients on hypertensive drugs
   - Patients with a history of heart, kidney, or hypertensive disease
   - New admissions to the hospital
   - Pregnant patients
   - Postpartum patients
   - Preoperative patients
   - Postoperative patients
   - Patients in shock or those who are hemorrhaging
   - All patients with neurological disorders
   - It is also suggested to routinely take the blood pressure on *all* patients as a preventive health measure
8. Check the sphygmomanometer regularly for loss of mercury and for leaks in the tubing, compression bag, and bulb.
9. Before and after each use of the stethoscope, clean the earpieces and the bell or diaphragm with a cotton ball soaked in alcohol or with an alcohol sponge.
10. Handle these instruments gently, as misuse will adversely affect their proper functioning.

Taking Blood Pressure Reading on the Arm

Procedure	Rationale
1. Wash hands and obtain equipment.	
2. Identify patient and explain the procedure.	Explanations help gain the patient's confidence and relaxation.
3. Help the patient assume a comfortable position with the arm extended and supported.	Patient may be sitting, standing, or lying down, depending on the physician's orders.
4. Place a mercury sphygmomanometer on a level surface, in a position in which the scale can be easily read.	Having a mercury manometer at your eye level enables you to take a more accurate reading.
5. Expose the patient's arm well above the elbow.	Clothing should be adjusted to avoid constriction and to prevent rustling of garments.
6. Apply the cuff of the sphygmomanometer over the brachial artery (see Fig. 1-5) 1 to 2 inches above the antecubital space, and wrap the remainder of the cuff around the arm so that each turn covers the previous one (Fig. 1-9). On older model cuffs, tuck the end	The cuff should be applied snugly and neatly. Arm may be flexed slightly after the cuff is applied. Use a child's or infant's cuff for small children or on extremely thin patients, and the larger cuff on obese patients to obtain an accurate reading (see Table 1-2).

Procedure	Rationale
under one of the turns; some cuffs will have clasps or hooks to fasten, and the newer models, with Velcro closures, will adhere to the last turn on the cuff.	
7. Locate the strongest pulsation of the brachial artery in the antecubital space by palpating with your fingers at the bend of the elbow (Fig. 1-10).	
8. Adjust the earpieces of the stethoscope in your ears, place the bell or diaphragm of the stethoscope over the artery pulsation felt, and hold in place (Fig. 1-11).	The bell or diaphragm should always be placed below, not under, the cuff and directly over the strongest pulsation felt of the brachial artery.
9. With your free hand, close the air valve on the hand bulb by turning the thumbscrew in a clockwise direction. Pump air into the cuff of the manometer rapidly until the level of mercury is about 180 to 200 mm Hg or about 20 mm Hg above the palpated systolic pressure (the procedure for taking blood pressure by palpation is explained on p. 25).	Blood is cut off when the cuff is inflated. In order to identify the true systolic pressure, air must be pumped into the cuff rapidly and then the cuff deflated slowly. Inflating the cuff slowly or sending the mercury to a higher level than necessary is very uncomfortable for the patient. To avoid missing the true systolic reading, pressure can initially be taken by the palpation method and then 15 to 30 seconds later the pressure reading can be taken by the auscultation method.
10. Turn the thumbscrew counterclockwise to open the air valve slowly. Allow for a slow release of air to the cuff so that the pressure falls only 2 to 3 mm Hg at a time (Fig. 1-12).	Rapid deflation of the cuff will cause you to miss the exact reading.
11. Listen carefully and read the exact point on the mercury column (or spring gauge if using an aneroid manometer) at which the first distinct sound is heard. Keep this number in mind; this represents the *systolic pressure*.	This sound is caused by an initial spurt of blood into the collapsed artery as deflation of the cuff occurs.
12. Continue to allow the air to escape, thereby letting the cuff deflate slowly. The sounds will get louder, then dull and soft, then fade away (Fig. 1-13).	
13. Read the scale when the sound becomes dull or muffled. Keep this number in mind; it represents the *diastolic pressure*.	The level of mercury at the point where the sound changes from loud to dull or muffled is the *diastolic* pressure, representing the pressure in the arteries during diastole of the heart.
14. Continue to deflate the cuff until the sound disappears. Keep this number in mind, as many physicians request that both numbers be reported for diastolic readings.	
15. Open the valve completely to release all the air from the cuff.	The blood in the veins in the lower arm will not be able to return to the heart if all the air in the cuff is not released. It is harmful for blood to become congested in the veins.
16. If there is any doubt of an accurate reading, wait 15 seconds, then repeat steps 7 through 15. Do not repeat more than twice on the same arm, because the reading will be inaccurate because of blood stasis (blood trapped in the arm).	Between readings, the cuff must be completely deflated. Failure to do so will produce erroneously high readings.

Fig. 1-9. Applying the cuff of the sphygmomanometer above the antecubital space of the right arm.

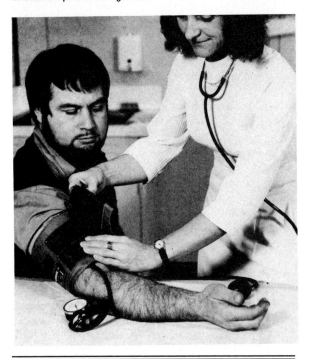

Fig. 1-10. Location of strongest pulsation in the antecubital space.

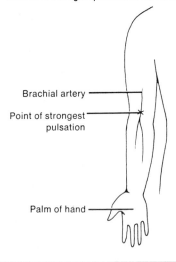

Brachial artery —

Point of strongest pulsation —

Palm of hand —

Fig. 1-11. Adjusting the stethoscope for taking the blood pressure.

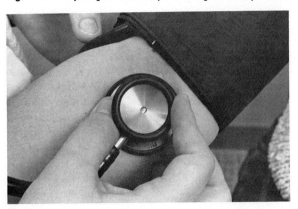

Fig. 1-12. Technique for taking blood pressure using aneroid sphygmomanometer.

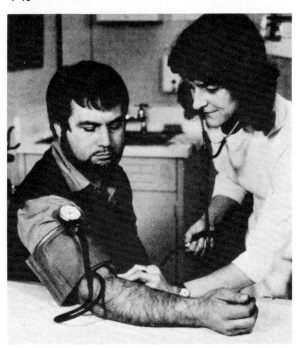

Fig. 1-13. Mercury column descending as air is released from the cuff.

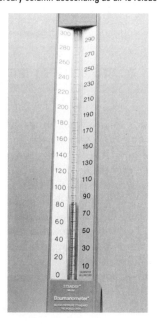

Taking Blood Pressure Reading on the Arm (*continued*)

Procedure	Rationale
17. Write BP down on paper as a mathematical fraction. Depending on your employer's preference, you may inform the patient of the numerical value of the BP.	Do not trust it to memory. Record systolic reading over diastolic reading as a mathematical fraction. For example, 120/80 *or* 120/80–60 (60 indicating where the sounds disappear)
18. Remove the cuff from the patient's arm. **19.** See that the patient is comfortable. **20.** Return equipment to designated area and prepare for storage according to type of apparatus used. Cleanse earpieces and diaphragm of stethoscope with alcohol sponge. **21.** Record BP on the patient's chart.	Charting example: October 1, 19_____, 2 PM BP 118/86 rt arm *or* 118/86–70 Ann Banks, CMA
22. Notify the physician if you have obtained a relatively higher or lower reading than previously recorded.	Further evaluation or only periodic measurement may be needed. Because an initial high reading may reflect only a transient increase, which could be due to anxiety or excitement, the BP should be measured on different days and after the patient has been able to relax for a time.

Taking a Blood Pressure Reading on the Leg

Procedure
1. The procedure is the same as outlined, except that the arterial locations differ. A leg pressure may be taken by either of the following methods: a. Placing the cuff around the thigh and the bell or diaphragm of the stethoscope over the popliteal artery behind the knee (see Fig. 1-5). b. Placing the cuff around the calf of the leg and the bell or diaphragm of the stethoscope over the pedal artery on the foot (see Fig. 1-5). This *is not* a commonly used procedure.

Palpation Method For Measuring Blood Pressure.   This is an alternative method for measuring blood pressure. When the blood pressure is inaudible by stethoscope, you may use this method, but *only* when the physician directs you to use it, as it is generally thought to be an inaccurate method.

The procedure is similar to the auscultation method except that you use your fingers rather than a stethoscope.

1. Place your fingers over the patient's brachial artery.

2. Pump cuff to 200 mm Hg, or at least 10 to 20 mm Hg after pulsation in the artery has ceased.

3. Release the air valve slowly.

4. The *systolic pressure* is read the moment you feel the first pulsation in the artery.

5. The pulse will increase in force and tension and then gradually become softer; it is at this point of change that the *diastolic pressure* is recorded. (Some feel that this is not an accurate diastolic reading, and therefore they do not obtain a diastolic reading for BP taken by the palpation method.)

6. Chart and indicate that the blood pressure was obtained by palpation on the brachial artery.

Measuring Orthostatic Blood Pressure

When a patient is on antihypertensive drug therapy, dehydrated, or suffering from hemorrhagic shock, the blood pressure may take longer than normal to stabilize when the patient is changed from a lying position to a sitting or standing position.

Equipment

Sphygmomanometer
Stethoscope

Procedure	**Rationale**
1. Identify and explain the procedure to the patient.	Explanations help gain the patient's confidence and relaxation.
2. Have the patient assume a recumbent position for 5 minutes, then take the blood pressure and apical pulse.	
3. Instruct the patient to sit up at a 90-degree angle. Take the blood pressure and apical pulse immediately. Ask how the patient feels.	The patient may feel dizzy.
4. Then have the patient stand up at the side of the examining table. Take the blood pressure and apical pulse immediately. Question the patient concerning a change in equilibrium.	The patient may need to rest between the sitting and standing measurements. Standing pressure may be omitted, depending on the physician's order and/or the patient's condition.

5. Chart the blood pressures and apical pulses on the patient's medical record. Indicate which readings were taken when the patient was lying down, sitting, and standing.	Charting example:
	120/80 — lying
	110/80 — sitting
	90/70 — standing
	    August 22, 19_____, 8 AM
	      T. O'Connell, CMA

6. Report the following to the physician: • Any systolic change greater than 10 mm Hg in lying/sitting or lying/standing positions • Any diastolic change greater than 20 mm Hg in lying/sitting or lying/standing positions • Any apical pulse change greater than 20 beats per minute in a lying/sitting or lying/standing position	

PHYSICAL MEASUREMENTS OF HEIGHT AND WEIGHT

The two other important physical or clinical measurements to obtain are the height and weight of the patient. It is common practice to take these measurements as part of a physical examination, as they may provide relevant information for diagnosing, treating, preventing, or evaluating a condition. Height and weight are also measured to determine a child's growth pattern. In addition, the patient's weight is used as a guide for determining the dosage to be administered for certain drugs. There are recommended standards set for the average weight that individuals should be for their height, but it is important to remember that these are only ranges, not absolute standards, with latitude for body types.

Overweight as well as underweight can have serious implications when one is determining the health status of an individual. Frequent complications of overweight include hypertension (high blood pressure), heart disease, and diabetes mellitus. Underweight may indicate malnourishment or metabolic disorders. Either may be the result of psychological problems.

Many patients are very self-conscious of their weight; therefore, it is advisable to have the scales located in an area that ensures privacy. Also to reduce embarrassment, you may have the patient stand with the back to the numbers on the scale. It is important in this procedure, as in all procedures, that you maintain a neutral facial expression to avoid communicating your impressions to the patient.

Be alert, and note any unusual weight gains or losses in established patients and comments regard-ing changes by new patients, either of which may be an important diagnostic aid.

Procedures for Measuring Height and Weight

Equipment

A weight scale with height measuring bar

Procedure	Rationale
1. Wash your hands.	
2. Identify the patient, and explain the procedure.	
3. Place a clean paper towel on the scale foot stand.	This is just one form of expected clean technique. Use a clean towel for each patient.
4. Balance the scale.	Unbalanced scales will result in an inaccurate weight measurement.
5. Have the patient remove shoes and any jacket or heavy outer sweater. In some offices or agencies the patient may be weighed in a patient gown.	The removal of heavy outer clothing provides a more accurate reading.
6. Direct and/or assist the patient onto the scale. NOTE: You may raise the height bar above the patient's estimated height and have it in position before the patient steps onto the scale to avoid moving and manipulating it later.	
7. Ask all patients their usual weight, then move the 50 pound weight to the 50-, 100-, 150-, 200-, or 250-pound mark, ensuring that the weight is resting securely in the weight indicator groove (Fig. 1-14).	Unless the weight is secured correctly in the groove provided, the patient's weight measurement will be off by many pounds.

Fig. 1-14. Obtaining the patient's weight.

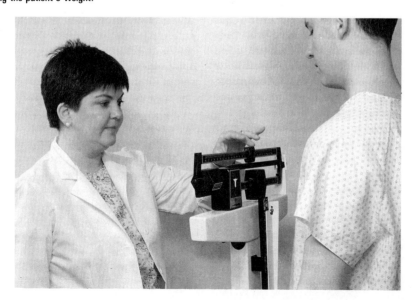

Procedures for Measuring Height and Weight (*continued*)

Procedure	Rationale
8. Gradually move the upper weight across the individual pound register until the arm at the right end of the balance bar rests in a position in the center of the metal frame, not touching either edge of this frame.	
9. Read the weight accurately to the nearest fraction of a pound. NOTE: Pediatric scales will measure weights in pounds and ounces.	
10. Return the weights to zero.	
11. Record the weight on the patient's chart.	When charting, you must indicate if the patient was wearing street clothes or a patient gown.
12. To measure height, have the patient remain on the scale, standing erect, looking straight ahead.	The patient must be standing very straight to obtain the correct height measurement.
13. If the height bar was not raised previously (see step 6), do so now; raise it over the patient's head and extend the hinged arm.	
14. Carefully lower the height bar until it touches the top of the patient's head lightly (Fig. 1-15).	
15. Read the height measurement.	The number (in inches) indicating the patient's height is the last digit or fraction visible at the point where the movable part of the bar enters its stationary holder.
16. Assist the patient off the scale if necessary and return the height bar to the resting position.	
17. Record the height accurately in feet and inches. Use accepted abbreviations.	Charting example: October 27, 19_____, 4 PM Ht. 5'2" Wt. 112 lb in street clothes, s̄ [without] shoes. Annie Fox, CMA

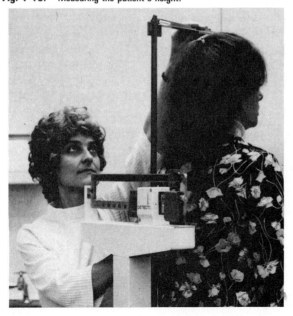

Fig. 1-15. Measuring the patient's height.

Some scales are calibrated in kilograms, and others in pounds. When you wish to convert a weight, use the following formulas:

To convert kilograms to pounds (kg to lb):
  1 kilogram = 2.2 pounds
  Multiply the number of kilograms by 2.2
  EXAMPLE: If a patient weighs 60 kilograms, multiply 60 by 2.2
    60 × 2.2 = 132 pounds
To convert pounds to kilograms (lb to kg):
  1 pound = 0.45 kilograms
  Multiply the number of pounds by 0.45
  EXAMPLE: If a patient weighs 132 pounds, multiply 132 by 0.45
    132 × 0.45 = 59.40 or 59⅖ kilograms.

See Table 1-3 for the conversion of pounds to kilograms and Table 1-4 for the average heights and weights for adults.

Table 1-3. Conversion table: pounds to kilograms*

Pounds	Kilograms	Pounds	Kilograms	Pounds	Kilograms
1	0.45	100	45.36	205	92.99
2.2	1.00	105	47.63	210	95.26
5	2.27	110	49.90	215	97.52
10	4.54	115	52.12	220	99.79
15	6.80	120	54.43	225	102.06
20	9.07	125	56.70	230	104.33
25	11.34	130	58.91	235	106.60
30	13.61	135	61.24	240	108.86
35	15.88	140	63.50	245	111.13
40	18.14	145	65.77	250	113.40
45	20.41	150	68.04	255	115.67
50	22.68	155	70.31	260	117.94
55	24.95	160	72.58	265	120.20
60	27.22	165	74.84	270	122.47
65	29.48	170	77.11	275	124.74
70	31.75	175	79.38	280	127.01
75	34.02	180	81.65	285	129.28
80	36.29	185	83.92	290	131.54
85	38.56	190	86.18	295	133.81
90	40.82	195	88.45	300	136.08
95	43.09	200	90.72		

*To convert:
Pounds to kilograms: multiply number of pounds by 0.45 (0.4536)
Kilograms to pounds: multiply number of kilograms by 2.2 (2.204)

Table 1-4. Desirable weights — ages 25 to 59 based on lowest mortality*

Men				Women†			
Height (in shoes with 1-inch heels)	Small frame	Medium frame	Large frame	Height (in shoes with 1-inch heels)	Small frame	Medium frame	Large frame
Feet / Inches				Feet / Inches			
5 2	128–134	131–141	138–150	4 10	102–111	109–121	118–131
5 3	130–136	133–143	140–153	4 11	103–113	111–123	120–134
5 4	132–138	135–145	142–156	5 0	104–115	113–126	122–137
5 5	134–140	137–148	144–160	5 1	106–118	115–129	125–140
5 6	136–142	139–151	146–164	5 2	108–121	118–132	128–143
5 7	138–145	142–154	149–168	5 3	111–124	121–135	131–147
5 8	140–148	145–157	152–172	5 4	114–127	124–138	134–151
5 9	142–151	148–160	155–176	5 5	117–130	127–141	137–155
5 10	144–154	151–163	158–180	5 6	120–133	130–144	140–159
5 11	146–157	154–166	161–184	5 7	123–136	133–147	143–163
6 0	149–160	157–170	164–188	5 8	126–139	136–150	146–167
6 1	152–164	160–174	168–192	5 9	129–142	139–153	149–170
6 2	155–168	164–178	172–197	5 10	132–145	142–156	152–173
6 3	158–172	167–182	176–202	5 11	135–148	145–159	155–176
6 4	162–176	171–187	181–207	6 0	138–151	148–162	158–179

Courtesy Metropolitan Life Insurance Co., New York, NY
*Weights in pounds according to frame (in indoor clothing weighing 5 pounds for men and 3 pounds for women).
†For women between 18 and 25, subtract 1 pound for each year under 25.

CONCLUSION

You have now completed the unit on Physical Measurements, the most basic clinical procedures that you may be required to perform. When you have practiced these procedures and feel competent in performing them, arrange with your instructor to take the Performance Test. You will be expected to demonstrate accurately your ability to prepare for and take the vital signs and height and weight measurements on individuals assigned to you by your instructor.

REVIEW OF VOCABULARY

This is a sample of how a physician may write up part of a patient's case history. In the following sentences, words that have been defined for you in the unit are used. Read this and define the italicized terms.

Physician's Statement of a Patient's *Vital Signs*

This 40-year-old patient was first seen with the chief complaint of frequent *dyspnea* and *orthopnea* at night.

Consultation Letter to Referring Physician

The following is a sample of a letter received in the physician's office from a consulting physician. After reading this report you should be able to discuss the contents. A dictionary or other reference source may be used as needed.

On examination of the chest, *rales* were heard, and *respirations* were *accelerated* to 30 per minute.

Patient stated that he often *hyperventilated,* especially in stressful situations.

Patient had a *fever* of 103°F, which remained *constant* over the first 24 hours after being seen in my office. The *onset* of this *fever* was apparently 2 days before this examination.

Bigeminal pulse rate, arrhythmia, and *pulse deficit* of at least eight beats—*apical pulse rate* was 130; *radial pulse rate* was 122, approximately. *Venous pulse* in the external jugulars was palpable and also very *irregular.*

BP—systolic, 164; *diastolic,* 128.

Pulse pressure 36. Height 5'6"; weight, 142 lbs.

Family history revealed that this patient's father has *hypertension,* mother has *hypotension,* and sister was diagnosed as having *malignant hypertension* at the age of 29.

For more information on this patient's history, please refer to past notes in the previous chart.

Y. Short, MD

December 15, 19_____

Dr. Y. Short
666 South W Street
Anytown, USA

Dear Dr. Short:

Mrs. Alice Price was seen initially on 9/27/87 at your request because of her progressing nocturnal choking sensations during the past year.

It was of interest to learn that I had seen her sometime before 1969 for a respiratory allergy syndrome that was attributed to dust and other inhalants following some testing procedures.

She indicates that she has been living in the same residence for the past 14 years and has had the same pet, a chihuahua, for the past 12 years. There has been some sputum production without blood with the present illness but no chest pain or peripheral edema. She had retired from her employment as a janitress with the City and County of Anytown 2 years ago.

Past history shows T & A [tonsillectomy and adenoidectomy] age 27, appendectomy and hysterectomy proximate to that date, and a whiplash 3 years ago.

The weight is in the 168 lb. range, and she indicates an allergy to pork and fish, which she believes may precipitate her nocturnal dyspneic events. She has had nocturia three times nightly for the past year; she drinks two cups of coffee and tea per day, uses no cigarettes, and her alcohol intake is moderate. Her medications are limited to the Tri-Pro-Hist prescribed by you for her asthma.

The various laboratory data of 9/10/87 were not remarkable, except for liver enzyme elevation, and it was noted the PME equaled 2% on the differential. Chest x-ray film in 1986 was reportedly negative, and no changes were seen on the 9/27/87 repeat film. Physical signs showed height 66 inches, weight 169 lbs.; the general findings were normal except for blood pressure 160/109.

Vital capacity was 3.0 liters (90% normal) with mild FEV_1 [full expiration volume 1] delay, and EKG showed an intermediate heart with changes suggesting hypocarbia.

It was my belief that Mrs. Alice Price has the following conditions:

1. Arterial hypertension, mild
2. Exogenous obesity, approximately 30 lbs.
3. Paroxysmal nocturnal dyspnea, atopic, possibly associated with food and/or inhalants
4. Hepatic insufficiency, metabolic origin

I advised her of these several entities, prescribed Aldactazide one daily for antihypertensive effect, and suggested that she continue on the antihistamine prescribed by you. When reviewed on 10/3/87, she had had significant diuretic effect, fewer nocturnal events, and blood pressure was 150/92.

I therefore advised her to remain on the Aldactazide daily and supplement the antihistamine with Elixophyllin 0.2 on a prn basis for dyspnea.

She will report back in 1 month, and if there are any unusual circumstances, I shall promptly advise you.

Sincerely yours,

R. G. Lewis, MD

REVIEW QUESTIONS

1. List three purposes for taking a patient's vital signs.
2. For the following situations, indicate if you would normally see an increase or a decrease in each of the following—(1) temperature, (2) pulse rate, (3) respiratory rate, and (4) blood pressure:
   a. A patient who faints
   b. A patient who has a severe infection in her throat
   c. A patient who is hemorrhaging
   d. A patient who has just jogged for 2 miles
   e. A patient who has a brain stem injury
   f. A patient who becomes extremely excited or upset
   g. A patient who is sleeping
   h. A child as compared with an adult
3. List the normal average readings for the following:
   a. Oral temperature in adults
   b. Axillary temperature in adults
   c. Rectal temperature in adults
   d. Pulse rate in adults
   e. Respiratory rate in adults
   f. Blood pressure in adults
4. Convert the following temperatures to centigrade degrees:
   a. 98.6°F   c. 100.4°F
   b. 97.8°F   d. 99.6°F
5. Convert the following temperatures to Fahrenheit degrees:
   a. 39.5°C   c. 38.2
   b. 36°C   d. 37.2°C
6. List and describe the location of the seven most common arteries where a pulse may be felt.
7. If a patient has an extremely sore mouth, how would you take the temperature?
8. What is meant by the pulse rate? The respiratory rate?
9. What is meant by the rhythm of the pulse rate? The rhythm of the respiratory rate?
10. You have just taken a patient's respiratory rate and found it to be 10 respirations per minute. Would you consider this a normal and adequate rate, or as a serious symptom of some physiological change in the body?
11. What action is taking place in the heart during systole? During diastole?
12. Why does blood pressure usually increase in the elderly?
13. If a patient had plaster casts on both arms, where and how would you take the BP?
14. A patient's blood pressure is 130/92. What is the pulse pressure? Is this pulse pressure in the normal range?
15. List four methods that may be used to control high blood pressure.
16. Convert the following body weights to measurements in pounds:
    a. 52 kg   c. 47 kg
    b. 68.5 kg   d. 56 kg
17. Convert the following body weights to measurements in kilograms:
    a. 112 lb   c. 136 lb
    b. 174 lb   d. 155 lb

PERFORMANCE TEST

In a skills laboratory, a simulation of a joblike environment, the medical assistant student is to demonstrate knowledge and skill in performing the following procedures without reference to source materials. For these activities the student will need a watch with a second hand, rectal and oral thermometers, a stethoscope, a sphygmomanometer, alcohol sponges, containers for used thermometers, a scale with height measuring bar, various individuals to play the role of a patient, and patient chart. Time limits and the number of patients to be tested for each procedure are to be assigned by the instructor.

Given an ambulatory patient and the appropriate equipment and supplies, obtain and record accurately*:

Oral temperature
Axillary temperature
Rectal temperature (a model may be used for this procedure)
Pulse rate
Respiratory rate
Blood pressure taken on the brachial artery
Blood pressure taken on the popliteal artery
Apical heartbeat
Orthostatic blood pressure
Height and weight

*Results obtained for the pulse rates and the respiratory rates are acceptable if within two beats or respirations as determined and recorded by the instructor. Results for blood pressure readings are acceptable if within 2 to 4 mm Hg, as determined and recorded by the instructor. The student is expected to attain proficiency in these procedures before progressing to others in this book.

The student is expected to perform the above procedures with 100% accuracy.

Grading systems are flexible in order to meet each instructor's preference. The instructor may wish to use a satisfactory/unsatisfactory grading system, or a pass/fail system, or a point-value system for each step on the checklist. It is recommended that each procedure be assigned a time limit by the instructor.

The following Performance Checklists and Evaluation Chart are examples that may be used by the instructor when evaluating the student's performance of a skill.

In the remaining units of this book, the Performance Checklists are presented in a shorter manner that can be used by students to check their own performance or as a guide to check (evaluate) each other. Performance Tests, Checklists, and Evaluation Charts for the instructor's use when evaluating the student's performance of a skill are provided in the teacher's guide.

PERFORMANCE CHECKLIST

DIRECTIONS: Evaluate student performance of each procedure using the following checklists. When you evaluate "not applicable," "unsatisfactory," or "not observed," please make a comment.

Checklist	S or NA*	U	NO	Comment
Taking a temperature				
1. Identifies and evaluates patient				
2. Washes hands				
3. Obtains appropriate, clean equipment				
4. Positions patient correctly and explains the procedure				
5. Prepares equipment				
a. rinses thermometer with cold water and wipes with a tissue				
b. shakes thermometer down to 96°F or 35.5°C				
c. lubricates bulb of thermometer for a rectal temperature				
6. Places thermometer correctly in patient's				
a. mouth, under tongue, lips closed				
b. axilla, with patient's arm crossed over chest				
c. rectum, inserts approximately 1 inch, holds thermometer in place, and instructs patient to remain still				
7. Leaves thermometer in position for required time				
a. oral—3 minutes				
b. axillary—5 to 10 minutes				
c. rectal—4 to 5 minutes				
8. Removes thermometer from patient, and wipes it from top toward bulb				
9. Reads thermometer for temperature registered				

*S or NA = satisfactory or not applicable; U = unsatisfactory; NO = not observed.

Checklist	S or NA*	U	NO	Comment
10. Records reading on patient's chart				
a. date and time				
b. temperature				
c. route used				
d. signature				
11. Shakes thermometer down to 96°F or below				
12. Places thermometer in appropriate container for used thermometers				
13. Repeats procedure if temperature registered is questionable				
14. Washes hands				
15. Completes each procedure within time limit assigned by the instructor				
Taking a pulse				
1. Identifies patient and explains procedure				
2. Obtains appropriate equipment				
3. Washes hands				
4. Positions patient correctly				
5. Locates arterial pulses with first three fingers				
a. radial				
b. facial				
c. right and left carotid				
d. brachial				
e. temporal				
f. femoral				
g. popliteal				
h. dorsalis pedis				
6. Counts pulse rate correctly for 1 minute (plus or minus two beats differential acceptable)				
7. Records pulse rate accurately on patient's chart				
a. date and time				
b. rate, rhythm, volume, and any abnormality if present				
c. signature				
8. Repeats procedure if any doubt of accuracy				
9. Completes procedure in time limit assigned by the instructor				
Taking a respiratory rate				
1. Washes hands				
2. Obtains appropriate equipment				
3. Identifies patient; *does not* explain procedure				
4. Places first three fingers on patient's wrist as if taking pulse				
5. Counts number of respirations correctly for 1 minute (plus or minus two respirations differential acceptable)				
6. Records respiratory rate accurately on patient's chart				
a. date and time				
b. rate, rhythm, and depth				
c. any noticeable abnormality, such as dyspnea, rates over 22 or under 12				
d. any pain associated with breathing				
e. signature				

*S or NA = satisfactory or not applicable; U = unsatisfactory; NO = not observed.

Checklist	S or NA*	U	NO	Comment
Taking a respiratory rate — continued				
7. Repeats procedure if any doubt of accuracy				
8. Completes procedure in time limit assigned by instructor				
Taking a blood pressure				
1. Washes hands				
2. Obtains appropriate equipment				
3. Identifies patient and explains procedure				
4. Positions patient carefully				
5. Applies cuff properly 1 to 2 inches above the antecubital space				
6. Locates brachial artery, adjusts earpieces of stethoscope in ears, and places bell or diaphragm of stethoscope over brachial artery				
7. Correctly inflates cuff to about 200 mm Hg				
8. Deflates cuff slowly				
9. Correctly reads mercury column for				
a. systolic pressure				
b. diastolic pressure				
(plus or minus 2 to 4 mm Hg differential with instructor's reading acceptable)				
10. Deflates cuff completely				
11. Removes equipment from the patient's arm				
12. Records readings on patient's chart				
a. date and time				
b. systolic pressure over diastolic (as a mathematical fraction)				
c. notation of which arm it was taken on				
d. signature				
13. Cleans earpieces and diaphragm of stethoscope				
14. Prepares equipment for storage according to type of apparatus used				
15. If there is any doubt of an accurate reading, waits 15 seconds, then repeats the procedure				
16. Completes the procedure in time limit assigned by the instructor				
Measuring adult height and weight				
1. Washes hands				
2. Identifies patient and explains procedure				
3. Places a clean paper towel on scale foot stand				
4. Balances scale				
5. Has patient remove shoes and heavy outer clothing				
6. Directs/assists patient onto scale				
7. Varying with preferred technique: raises the height bar above patient's estimated height and extends the hinged arm and then directs or assists patient onto scale				
8. Asks patient usual weight				
9. Moves 50-pound weight; and secures in the correct weight indicator groove				
10. Moves upper weight across individual pound register until the arm balances				
11. Reads the weight correctly				
12. Returns weights to zero				
13. Records weight				

*S or NA = satisfactory or not applicable; U = unsatisfactory; NO = not observed.

Checklist	S or NA*	U	NO	Comment
14. Instructs patient to remain on scale, stand erect, and look straight ahead				
15. If height bar was not raised previously (see No. 7), raises height bar over patient's head, and extends the hinged arm				
16. Carefully lowers the bar until it touches the top of the patient's head lightly				
17. Reads the height measurement				
18. Assists patient off scale when necessary				
19. Returns height bar to resting position				
20. Records the date, time, weight, and height on the patient's chart; signs name				
21. Completes the procedures in time limit assigned by the instructor				

*S or NA = satisfactory or not applicable; U = unsatisfactory; NO = not observed.

Evaluation of student's technique

	Satisfactory*		Unsatisfactory**		
	Very good	**Good**	**Fair**	**Poor**	**Score**
• Temperature	☐	☐	☐	☐	_____
• Pulse rate	☐	☐	☐	☐	_____
• Respiratory rate	☐	☐	☐	☐	_____
• Blood pressure	☐	☐	☐	☐	_____
• Height	☐	☐	☐	☐	_____
• Weight	☐	☐	☐	☐	_____

Very good = Perfect
Good = Sufficient
Fair = Not acceptable; requires more practice
Poor = Totally unacceptable
Pass* = Satisfactory
Fail** = Unsatisfactory

Comments:

Unit II

Health History and Physical Examinations

On completion of Unit II, the medical assistant student should be able to apply the following cognitive objectives:

1. Define and pronounce the vocabulary terms and medical abbreviations listed.
2. List the eight major components of a patient's medical history/record, and describe the information that is recorded in each.
3. List and define the six parts of the patient's medical history.
4. List eight reasons why information gathered during a history and physical examination is valuable to the physician.
5. List and describe six methods of examination employed by the physician when performing a physical examination on a patient, giving an example of when or how each is used.
6. List the essential parts of a physical examination.
7. Differentiate between information obtained in the review of systems and that obtained during the physical examination.
8. Discuss the steps taken by a physician when making a diagnosis.
9. List five forms of treatment.
10. List three reasons for diagnostic studies.

TERMINAL PERFORMANCE OBJECTIVES

On completion of Unit II, the medical assistant student should be able to do the following terminal performance objective.

1. Help take and record a brief medical history or statement of the patient's chief complaint.

The student is to perform the above skill with 100% accuracy 90% of the time (9 out of 10 times).

Vocabulary

health—The state of mental, physical, and social well-being of an individual, and not merely the absence of disease.

positive findings—Evidence of disease or body dysfunction.

prodrome—An early symptom indicating the onset of a disease, such as an achy feeling before having the flu.

prognosis—A statement made by the physician indicating the probable or anticipated outcome of the disease process in a patient; usually stated simply as *good, fair, poor,* or *guarded.*

sign—Sometimes called a *physical sign:* any objective evidence (apparent to the observer) representing disease or body dysfunction. Signs may be observed by others or revealed when the physician performs a physical examination; examples include swollen ankles, a distended rigid abdomen, elevated blood pressure, and decreased sensation.

symptom—Sometimes called a *subjective symptom;* any subjective evidence of disease or body dysfunction; a change in the physical or mental state of the body that is perceptible or apparent only to the individual experiencing the change; examples include anorexia, nausea, headache, pain, itching, and dizziness.

syndrome—A combination of symptoms resulting from one cause or commonly occurring together to present a distinct clinical picture; an example is the dumping syndrome, which consists of nausea, weakness, varying degrees of syncope, sweating, palpitation, and sometimes diarrhea and a feeling of warmth. This may occur immediately after eating in patients who have had a partial gastrectomy.

symmetry—Correspondence in form, size, and arrangement of parts on opposite sides of the body.

In order to provide a basis for decision making and planning for the care of a patient, information of varied types must be gathered, compiled, and maintained in an orderly and confidential manner. Lack of needed information and confidentiality may jeopardize appropriate patient care. Thus there is the need for the patient's confidential medical record, which is a compilation of information concerning the patient, the care provided, progress, and results obtained.

When a physician sees the patient for the first time, identifying information (such as name and address) and all the information necessary for diagnosing the case, prescribing treatment, and planning future care are obtained. Every diagnostic workup has six major components: the history, the physical examination, the summary of positive findings, the interpretation of completed diagnostic studies, the examiner's impression based on all the information gathered, and the care plans including suggested further study.

On subsequent visits the progress or status of the patient's condition is recorded as progress notes. Eventually, when the patient is discharged or the condition has been resolved, the date of discharge and status of the patient at that time are recorded as the discharge summary.

This compilation of information is kept together and called the patient's medical record. These confidential records and reports are arranged in a file folder, binder, or other special type of folder, which is generally referred to as the patient's chart or file.

The medical assistant plays a very important role in obtaining and maintaining data on patients. This responsibility will vary with the preference and specialty of the physician. In some instances the medical assistant is expected to relieve the physician of much of the data collection. In this case, the medical assistant obtains identifying information from the patient, measures the patient's height, weight, temperature, pulse rate, respiration rate, and blood pressure and takes the medical history. In other situations, the medical assistant may only be required to obtain the identifying information from the patient. In addition to recording data, the medical assistant is responsible for preparing the examination room for the examination of the patient, preparing the equipment and supplies needed, preparing the patient both physically and mentally, and assisting the patient, assisting the physician, collecting specimens as requested, and organizing the results of diagnostic studies in the patient's record (see also Unit IX).

This unit discusses the components and related information of a patient's medical record, related vocabulary, medical abbreviations, and the problem-oriented medical record. Unit III presents vocabulary, procedures, and techniques used when preparing for and assisting with various types of physical examinations.

Actual medical reports are cited at the end of the unit in the Review of Vocabulary to help the medical assistant student correlate the contents of this unit with the ways physicians record information about the patient.

HISTORY AND PHYSICAL EXAMINATION

The history and general physical examination are extremely valuable diagnostic tools used by a physician to gather information about the physiological and sometimes psychological condition of a patient. Many people now recognize the value of a regular physical examination as a measure to prevent or treat disease in the early stages. Most authorities recommend that everyone have at least one a year.

Information gathered from a history and general or special physical examination can be used by the physician to determine the following:

- The individual's level of health
- The body's level of physiological functioning
- A tentative diagnosis of a condition or disease
- A confirmed diagnosis of a condition or disease
- The need for additional special examinations or testing
- The type of treatment to be prescribed
- An evaluation of the effectiveness of the prescribed treatment
- Preventive measures to be used

Preventive techniques include educating patients of healthful living habits, administering vaccinations to prevent communicable diseases, using screening procedures such as blood pressure checks and Pap smears, and treating conditions in the early stages to avoid more serious diseases.

The order followed by physicians when taking a history and performing a physical examination may vary somewhat, but the end result is the same, since the same basic areas are covered. One of the two types of forms may be used to record the information obtained. These include a preprinted outline form (see Figure 2-1) or a blank sheet of standard-size paper on which the physician writes out all the information gathered. The preprinted form serves as a reminder so that essential factors will not be overlooked, and it minimizes necessary writing to a narrative record of the abnormal findings.

HISTORY

The history is a record of the information provided by the patient. This includes a series of questions and answers regarding the patient.

Problem areas, either physical or emotional, can be revealed by history taking — not only areas of current problems but also those that may become problems and thus call for preventive care and advice.

Components of History

1. **Chief Complaint.** The chief complaint is a brief statement, made by the patient, describing the nature of the illness and duration of symptoms that led the patient to consult the physician. Chief complaint is abbreviated CC.

(Text continues on p. 44)

Fig. 2-1. Preprinted forms used for patient history and physical examination. **A,** form used for General Practice. **B,** form used for Internal Medicine. **C,** patient questionnaire. (Courtesy of Histacount Corporation, Melville, NY)

GENERAL PRACTICE

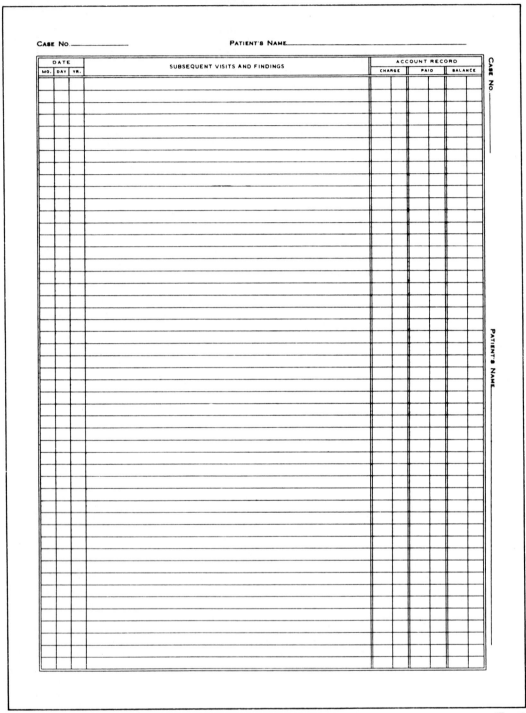

A

(Front)

GENERAL PRACTICE—cont'd

CASE NO.

PATIENT'S NAME

ADDRESS _____ INSURANCE _____ DATE _____

TEL NO _____ REFERRED BY _____ OCCUPATION _____ AGE ____ SEX ____ S.M.W.D.

CASE NO.

FAMILY HISTORY: FATHER _____ MOTHER _____

BROTHERS _____ SISTERS _____

CANCER _____ TUBERCULOSIS _____ INSANITY _____ DIABETES _____ HEART DISEASE _____ RHEUMATISM _____

GOUT _____ GOITER _____ OBESITY _____ NEPHRITIS _____ EPILEPSY _____ OTHER _____

PAST HISTORY: DIPHTHERIA _____ MEASLES _____ MUMPS _____ CHICKEN-POX _____ SCARLET FEVER _____ SMALL POX _____

INFANTILE PARALYSIS _____ TYPHOID _____ MALARIA _____ PNEUMONIA _____ DYSENTERY _____ JAUNDICE _____ BOILS _____

RHEUMATIC FEVER _____ TUBERCULOSIS _____ ASTHMA _____ HEART DISEASE _____ HYPERTENSION _____ DIABETES _____

INFECTIONS _____ GONORRHEA _____ SYPHILIS _____ TONSILLITIS _____ NEPHRITIS _____ OPERATIONS _____

MENSTRUAL: ONSET _____ PERIODICITY _____ TYPE _____ DURATION _____ PAIN _____ L.M.P. _____

MARITAL: MISCARRIAGES _____ ABORTIONS _____ CHILDREN _____ STERILITY _____

HABITS: ALCOHOL _____ TOBACCO _____ DRUGS _____ COFFEE _____ TEA _____ MEALS _____ WATER _____

SLEEP _____ BOWEL MOVEMENTS _____ EXERCISE _____ AMUSEMENTS _____

_____

_____

_____

PRESENT AILMENT: _____

_____

_____

_____

PHYSICAL EXAMINATION: TEMP _____ PULSE _____ RESP _____ B P _____ HT _____ WT _____

GENERAL APPEARANCE _____

SKIN _____ MUCOUS MEMBRANE _____

EYES: VISION _____ PUPIL _____ FUNDUS _____

EARS _____

NOSE _____

THROAT _____ PHARYNX _____ TONSILS _____

CHEST: _____ BREASTS _____

HEART: _____

LUNGS _____

ABDOMEN _____

GENITALIA _____

RECTUM _____

VAGINA: _____

EXTREMITIES _____

LYMPH NODES: NECK _____ AXILLA _____ INGUINAL _____ ABDOMINAL _____

REFLEXES: _____

REMARKS: _____

_____

_____

_____

_____

LABORATORY FINDINGS:

(Urine · Blood · Sputum · Smears · Exudates Transudates · Feces · Gastric Contents · Wassermann Kahn · Chemistry · Pregnancy Tests · X-Ray Fluoroscopy · Schick · Dick · Etc.)

Date

PATIENT'S NAME

DIAGNOSIS _____

_____

TREATMENT _____

_____

SYMBOLS: V NORMAL, _____ ABNORMAL (UNDERLINE WORD)
DEGREE OF ABNORMALITY: X   XX   XXX

(Back)

(Fig. 2-1 continues)

Fig. 2-1 (*continued*)

INTERNAL MEDICINE

INTERNAL MEDICINE

CASE NO. _____

PATIENT'S NAME _____

ADDRESS _____ DATE _____

TEL. NO. _____ REFERRED BY _____ OCCUPATION _____ AGE _____ SEX _____ S.M.W.D. _____

INSURANCE _____

CHIEF COMPLAINT: _____

PRESENT AILMENT: _____

PAST HISTORY (INCLUDING SURGERY) _____

FAMILY HISTORY: _____

SYMPTOM REVIEW

HEAD: Headache Dizziness Fainting	
EYE · EAR NOSE · THROAT:	
RESPIRATORY: Hemoptysis · Cough · Sputum Chest Pain · Night Sweats Chill · Rhinitis · Sinusitis Epistaxis · Post Nasal Discharge	
HEART: Dyspnea · Orthopnea Cyanosis · Pallor · Pain Location · Radiation	
GASTRO-INTESTINAL: Pain · Relation To Food Radiation · Relieved By Med.? Dysphagia · Nausea Anorexia · Flatulence Constipation · Diarrhea Hemorrhoids · Melena · Wt. Loss or Gain	
GENITO-URINARY: Polyuria · Oliguria · Anuria Hematuria · Dysuria · Colic Pain · Frequency · Chills Urgency · Backache	
NEURO-MUSC. SKELETAL:	
VASCULAR	
HEMATOLOGICAL: Bleeding · Anemia	

CASE NO.

PATIENT'S NAME

(*Front*)

B

INTERNAL MEDICINE—cont'd

CASE No._____ PATIENT'S NAME_____

SYMPTOM REVIEW

ENDOCRINE

VENEREAL DISEASE

ALLERGIES

CENTRAL NERVOUS SYSTEM

MENSTRUAL:
Onset · Periodicity · Type
Duration · Pain · L.M.P.

MARITAL:
Miscarriages · Abortions
Children · Sterility

HABITS:
Tobacco · Alcohol · Drugs
Diet · Cathartics · Etc.

REMARKS:

PHYSICAL EXAMINATION: TEMP _____ PULSE _____ RESP. ____ B.P. _____ HT. ____ WT. ____

GENERAL APPEARANCE

SKIN _____ MUCOUS MEMBRANE

EYES: VISION _____ PUPIL _____ FUNDUS

EARS:

NOSE:

THROAT: _____ PHARYNX _____ TONSILS

NECK:

CHEST: _____ BREASTS

HEART:

LUNGS:

ABDOMEN:

GENITALIA:

RECTUM:

VAGINA:

EXTREMITIES:

LYMPH NODES NECK _____ AXILLA _____ INGUINAL _____ ABDOMINAL

REFLEXES:

REMARKS:

LABORATORY FINDINGS:

(Urine · Blood · Sputum · Smears · Exudates Transudates · Feces · Gastric Contents · Wassermann Kahn · Chemistry · Pregnancy Tests · X-Ray Fluoroscopy · Schick · Dick · Etc.)

Date

DIAGNOSIS:

TREATMENT:

DATE			SUBSEQUENT VISITS AND FINDINGS	ACCOUNT RECORD		
MO.	DAY	YR.		CHARGE	PAID	BALANCE

(Back)

(Fig. 2-1 continues)

Fig. 2-1 (*continued*)

PATIENT QUESTIONNAIRE

PATIENT QUESTIONNAIRE

PATIENT'S NAME		BIRTH DATE	SEX	S. M. W. D.
ADDRESS			TEL. NO.	
INSURANCE	REFERRED BY	OCCUPATION		

INSTRUCTIONS: PUT ☑ IN THOSE BOXES APPLICABLE TO YOU AND IN THE "YES" OR "NO" SPACE. IF LINES ARE PROVIDED WRITE IN YOUR ANSWER.

FAMILY HISTORY

	FATHER	MOTHER	BROTHER				SISTER				SPOUSE	CHILDREN					
			1	2	3	4	1	2	3	4		1	2	3	4	5	6
AGE (IF LIVING)																	
HEALTH (G) GOOD (B) BAD																	
CANCER																	
TUBERCULOSIS																	
DIABETES																	
HEART TROUBLE																	
HIGH BLOOD PRESSURE																	
STROKE																	
EPILEPSY																	
NERVOUS BREAKDOWN																	
ASTHMA, HIVES, HAYFEVER																	
BLOOD DISEASE																	
AGE (AT DEATH)																	
CAUSE OF DEATH																	

PERSONAL HISTORY

HAVE YOU EVER HAD . . .	NO	YES	HAVE YOU EVER HAD . . .	NO	YES	HAVE YOU EVER HAD . . .	NO	YES
☐ SCARLET FEVER ☐ SCARLATINA			☐ GONORRHEA ☐ SYPHILIS			ANY ☐ BROKEN ☐ CRACKED BONES		
DIPHTHERIA			ANEMIA			RECURRENT DISLOCATIONS		
SMALLPOX			JAUNDICE			☐ CONCUSSION ☐ HEAD INJURY		
PNEUMONIA			EPILEPSY			EVER BEEN KNOCKED UNCONSCIOUS		
PLEURISY			MIGRAINE HEADACHES			☐ FGOD ☐ CHEMICAL ☐ DRUG POISONING		
UNDULANT FEVER			TUBERCULOSIS			EXPLAIN		
☐ RHEUMATIC FEVER ☐ HEART DISEASE			DIABETES					
ST. VITUS DANCE			CANCER					
☐ ARTHRITIS ☐ RHEUMATISM			☐ HIGH ☐ LOW BLOOD PRESSURE			ANY OTHER DISEASE		
ANY ☐ BONE ☐ JOINT DISEASE			NERVOUS BREAKDOWN			EXPLAIN		
☐ NEURITIS ☐ NEURALGIA			☐ HAY FEVER ☐ ASTHMA					
☐ BURSITIS ☐ SCIATICA ☐ LUMBAGO			☐ HIVES ☐ ECZEMA					
☐ POLIO ☐ MENINGITIS			FREQUENT ☐ COLDS ☐ SORE THROAT			WEIGHT: NOW ONE YR. AGO		
BRIGHT'S DISEASE			FREQUENT ☐ INFECTIONS ☐ BOILS			MAXIMUM WHEN		

ALLERGIES

ARE YOU ALLERGIC TO . . .	NO	YES	ARE YOU ALLERGIC TO . . .	NO	YES	ARE YOU ALLERGIC TO . . .	NO	YES
☐ PENICILLIN ☐ SULFA DRUGS			ANY OTHER DRUGS			ANY FOODS		
☐ ASPIRIN ☐ CODEINE ☐ MORPHINE			EXPLAIN			EXPLAIN		
☐ MYCINS ☐ OTHER ANTIBIOTICS								
☐ TETANUS ☐ ANTITOXIN ☐ SERUMS			ADHESIVE TAPE			☐ NAIL POLISH ☐ OTHER COSMETICS		

SURGERY

HAVE YOU HAD REMOVED . . .	NO	YES	HAVE YOU HAD REMOVED . . .	NO	YES	HAVE YOU . . .	NO	YES
TONSILS			☐ OVARY ☐ OVARIES			HAD HERNIA REPAIRED		
APPENDIX			HEMORRHOIDS			HAD ANY OTHER OPERATIONS		
GALL BLADDER			EVER HAVE A TRANSFUSION . . .			BEEN HOSPITALIZED FOR ANY ILLNESS		
UTERUS			☐ BLOOD ☐ PLASMA			EXPLAIN		

X-RAYS

EVER HAVE X-RAYS OF . . .	NO	YES	DATE	DISEASE PRESENT
CHEST				
☐ STOMACH ☐ COLON				
GALL BLADDER				
EXTREMITIES				
BACK				
OTHER				

C

(*Front*)

PATIENT QUESTIONNAIRE—cont'd

SYSTEMS

DO YOU NOW HAVE OR HAVE YOU EVER HAD . . .	NO	YES	DO YOU NOW HAVE OR HAVE YOU EVER HAD . . .	NO	YES
ANY ☐EYE DISEASE ☐EYE INJURY ☐IMPAIRED SIGHT			KIDNEY ☐DISEASE ☐STONES		
ANY ☐EAR DISEASE ☐EAR INJURY ☐IMPAIRED HEARING			BLADDER DISEASE		
ANY TROUBLE WITH ☐NOSE ☐SINUSES ☐MOUTH ☐THROAT			BLOOD IN URINE		
FAINTING SPELLS			☐ALBUMIN ☐SUGAR ☐PUS ☐ETC. IN URINE		
CONVULSIONS			DIFFICULTY IN URINATION		
PARALYSIS			NARROWED URINARY STREAM		
DIZZINESS			ABNORMAL THIRST		
HEADACHES: ☐FREQUENT ☐SEVERE			PROSTATE TROUBLE		
ENLARGED GLANDS			☐STOMACH TROUBLE ☐ULCER		
THYROID: ☐OVERACTIVE ☐UNDERACTIVE ☐ENLARGED			INDIGESTION		
ENLARGED GOITER			☐GAS ☐BELCHING		
SKIN DISEASE			APPENDICITIS		
COUGH: ☐FREQUENT ☐CHRONIC			☐LIVER DISEASE ☐GALL BLADDER DISEASE		
☐CHEST PAIN ☐ANGINA PECTORIS			☐COLITIS ☐OTHER BOWEL DISEASE		
SPITTING UP BLOOD			☐HEMORRHOIDS ☐RECTAL BLEEDING		
NIGHT SWEATS			BLACK TARRY STOOLS		
SHORTNESS OF BREATH ☐EXERTION ☐AT NIGHT			☐CONSTIPATION ☐DIARRHEA		
☐PALPITATION ☐FLUTTERING HEART			☐PARASITES ☐WORMS		
SWELLING OF ☐HANDS ☐FEET ☐ANKLES			☐ANY CHANGE IN APPETITE ☐EATING HABITS		
VARICOSE VEINS			☐ANY CHANGE IN BOWEL ACTION ☐STOOLS		
EXTREME ☐TIREDNESS ☐WEAKNESS			EXPLAIN		

IMMUNIZATION - EKG

HAVE YOU HAD . . .	NO	YES	HAVE YOU HAD . . .	NO	YES
SMALLPOX VACCINATION (WITHIN LAST 7 YEARS)			POLIO SHOTS (WITHIN LAST 2 YEARS)		
TETANUS SHOT (NOT ANTITOXIN)			AN ELECTROCARDIOGRAM WHEN		

HABITS

DO YOU . . .	NO	YES	DO YOU USE . . .	NEVER	OCC.	FREQ.	DAILY
EXERCISE ADEQUATELY			LAXATIVES				
HOW ?			VITAMINS				
AWAKEN RESTED			SEDATIVES				
SLEEP WELL			TRANQUILIZERS				
AVERAGE 8 HOURS SLEEP (PER NIGHT)			SLEEPING PILLS, ETC.				
HAVE REGULAR BOWEL MOVEMENTS			ASPIRINS, ETC.				
SEX - ENTIRELY SATISFACTORY			CORTISONE				
LIKE YOUR WORK (HOURS PER DAY) ☐INDOORS ☐OUTDOORS			ALCOHOLIC BEVERAGE				
WATCH TELEVISION (HOURS PER DAY)			COFFEE (CUPS PER DAY)				
READ (HOURS PER DAY)			TOBACCO:☐CIGARETTES (PKS PER DAY)				
HAVE A VACATION (WEEKS PER YEAR)			☐CIGARS ☐PIPE ☐CHEWING TOBACCO				
HAVE YOU EVER BEEN TREATED FOR ALCOHOLISM			☐SNUFF				
HAVE YOU EVER BEEN TREATED FOR DRUG ABUSE			APPETITE DEPRESSANTS				
RECREATION: DO YOU PARTICIPATE IN SPORTS OR HAVE			THYROID MEDICATION: ☐NO ☐YES, IN PAST ☐NONE NOW NOW ON GR. DAILY				
HOBBIES WHICH GIVE YOU RELAXATION AT			HAVE YOU EVER TAKEN . . .				
LEAST 3 HOURS A WEEK.			☐INSULIN ☐TABLETS FOR DIABETES ☐HORMONE SHOTS ☐TABLETS ☐NO				

WOMEN ONLY

MENSTRUAL HISTORY . .				NO	YES
AGE AT ONSET			ARE YOU REGULAR: ☐HEAVY ☐MEDIUM ☐LIGHT		
USUAL DURATION OF PERIOD DAYS			DO YOU HAVE ☐TENSON ☐DEPRESSION BEFORE PERIOD		
CYCLE (START TO START) DAYS			DO YOU HAVE ☐CRAMPS ☐PAIN WITH PERIOD		
DATE OF LAST PERIOD			DO YOU HAVE HOT FLASHES		

PREGNANCIES . . .	NO	YES		NO	YES
CHILDREN BORN ALIVE (HOW MANY)			STILL BORN (HOW MANY)		
CESAREAN SECTIONS (HOW MANY)			MISCARRIAGES (HOW MANY)		
PREMATURES (HOW MANY)			ANY COMPLICATIONS		

EMOTIONS

ARE YOU OFTEN . . .	NO	YES	ARE YOU OFTEN . . .	NO	YES
DEPRESSED			JUMPY		
ANXIOUS			JITTERY		
IRRITABLE			IS CONCENTRATION DIFFICULT		

(Back)

2. History of Present Illness.   The history of present illness includes the present illness discussed in detail, the health status of the patient until the onset of the present illness, then the onset of symptoms, the character, duration of each, and any other pertinent facts or relation to other events, such as shortness of breath after exertion. History of present illness is abbreviated HPI (or PI, present illness).

3. Past History.   The past history is a summary of all prior illnesses, allergies, drug sensitivities, childhood diseases, surgical procedures, hospital admissions, and serious injuries and disabilities, including the date of each. For women, the number of pregnancies, live births, and abortions, if any, are also recorded. Past history is abbreviated PH.

4. Family History.   The family history is the health status and age of immediate relatives; if deceased, the date, age at death, and cause are noted. Diseases among relatives that are thought to have a hereditary or familial tendency or cases in which contact may play a role are also recorded. Examples would be cardiovascular, renal, endocrine, metabolic, mental, or infectious diseases, neoplasms or carcinoma, and allergies. Family history is abbreviated FH.

5. Social and Occupational History.   The social and occupational history (may also be referred to as personal history and patient profile) includes information relating to where the patient has lived, occupation(s), and environment. This includes statements about the patient's life-style and habits, any of which may have a bearing on the development of disease, and the patient's general health status and perception of his/her health. These factors may include the following:

• Use of tobacco, alcohol, drugs, coffee, tea
• Diet, sleep, exercise, hobbies, and interests
• Marital history, children, home life; religious convictions; occupation and employment
• Sexual preferences, problems, and attitudes
• Ways of reacting to stress
• Defense mechanisms
• Resources for support and assistance
• Cultural, educational, and environmental factors that may be related to health status

6. Review of Systems.   Review of systems is the last category in the history. The purpose of this systematic review is to reveal subjective symptoms that either the patient forgot to discuss or, at the time, seemed relatively unimportant to the patient. An analysis of the subjective findings, as related by the patient when questioned by the physician, will generally give a clue to the diagnosis and will indicate the nature and extent of the physical examination required. Review of systems is abbreviated ROS.

The following are the major headings in the order in which they appear in the patient's ROS and the items that are usually reviewed by the physician. The physician will question the patient as to the usual or unusual presence or condition and/or occurrence of any of these.

The physician will ask if there has been or is a history of the following conditions and whether as well as what kinds of medications are currently being used for any of the following*:

GENERAL — Chills, fever, sweats, weight gain or loss, fatigue, weakness, nightmares, insomnia, nervousness, loss of memory

HEAD — Headaches, trauma, sinus pain, fainting

EYES — Vision, pain, burning, eyestrain, redness, photophobia, diplopia, blurred vision, excessive tearing, discharge, any eye diseases, prescription glasses, date of last eye examination

EARS — Hearing loss, pain, discharge, tinnitus, dizziness, mastoiditis, trauma, noise exposure, vertigo

NOSE — Smell, head colds, discharge, postnasal drip, epistaxis, pain, obstruction, trauma, allergies

MOUTH — Taste, dryness or excessive salivation, condition of lips, tongue, gums, teeth, dentures

THROAT — Redness, sore throat, tonsillitis, hoarseness, laryngitis, voice changes, speech defects, dysphagia

NECK — Pain, tenderness, swelling, limitation of motion, trauma

RESPIRATORY — Chest pain, cough, expectoration, hemoptysis, asthma, wheezing, dyspnea, orthopnea, hyperventilation, night sweats, recurrent respiratory tract infections

CARDIOVASCULAR (CV) — Chest pain, hypertension, palpitation, tachycardia, bradycardia, peripheral edema, varicosities, cyanosis, dizziness, syncope

GASTROINTESTINAL (GI) — Appetite, anorexia, bulimia, abdominal pain, nausea, vomiting, hematemesis, food intolerance, indigestion, dysphagia, diarrhea, constipation, laxatives, color and form of stools, melena, jaundice, distention, flatus, colic, hemorrhoids, rectal pain, presence of blood, pus, or mucus, pruritus ani, hernia or masses

GENITOURINARY (GU) — Dysuria, oliguria, polyuria, frequency, hesitancy, nocturia, incontinence, enuresis, urgency, retention, hematuria, pyuria, glycosuria, abnormal color or odor, pain, renal colic, stones, pruritus, discharge, sexually transmitted disease(s), sexual habits, potency,

*See Appendix A for definitions and pronunciation keys for many of the terms listed.

prostate disease, testicular masses, history of urinary tract infections

FEMALE REPRODUCTIVE — Leukorrhea, discharge, itching, pain, dyspareunia, date and results of last Pap smear, breast self-examination routine

MENSES (MENSTRUAL PERIODS) — Age at onset, regularity, amount, duration, date of last menstrual period, premenstrual tension, dysmenorrhea, amenorrhea, irregular bleeding, spotting, menopause (age of onset), postmenopausal bleeding, menopausal symptoms

OBSTETRICAL HISTORY — Number of pregnancies, live births and living children, complications during pregnancy and labor, abortions if any

BIRTH CONTROL — Method if used

METABOLIC — Change in weight and appetite

ENDOCRINE — Excessive thirst, goiter, hair distribution, falling hair, change in skin texture or color, temperature intolerance, speech, voice, growth changes, sexual vigor and abnormalities, symptoms of diabetes, hormone therapy

BLOOD — Bruising or bleeding tendencies, blood disorders

SKIN — Allergies, rash, pruritus, moles, sores or ulcers, color change (redness, jaundice, cyanosis, pallor), infections, dryness, sweating, alopecia, past dermatitis

MUSCULOSKELETAL (MS) — Muscle or joint pain, swelling, stiffness, limitation of movement, spasm, tetany, weakness, numbness, coldness, deformities, atrophy, dislocations, fractures, discoloration, varicosities, cramping, edema, thrombophlebitis

NEUROLOGICAL — Headaches, vertigo, fainting, sense of balance, nervousness, sleeping irregularities, tremor, convulsions, loss of consciousness, memory, paralysis, paresthesia, pain

PSYCHIATRIC — Personality type, emotional stability, previous mental illness

Assisting with the Patient History/Interview

At times the medical assistant may be responsible for obtaining some of the information for the patient history. To help guide you in this responsibility, keep the following in mind:

1. Make sure that the environment is as quiet and private as possible. This helps put the patient at ease and will also enhance your own concentration.
2. Introduce yourself and explain to the patient *what* you will be doing and *why* you are doing this interview before the patient sees the physician.
3. Treat the patient the way you would want to be

treated. Successful interviewing begins with your attitude towards the patient. Think of the interview as a *conversation* rather than a preprinted form to be filled out. By doing this, the quality of information that you will get from the patient will be improved. Do not make the interview an interrogation period of blunt questions. Create an atmosphere of mutual respect and trust by showing genuine interest, concern, and empathy. Be calm and take time with the patient. A conversation is a two-way communication. Allow the patient time to complete sentences, even if he/she starts to ramble. You can redirect your questioning as necessary.

4. Encourage the patient to give specific information. This will enable both you and the physician to provide care to meet the patient's needs. Besides medical information, personal information about the patient, such as stressors at home or work, can help to identify factors that may be affecting the patient's health. It is a well-documented fact that stress can lead to a number of physical and emotional problems.
5. Use direct and open-ended questions to ask the patient the reason for the visit to the physician, and when applicable, to describe the chief complaint and symptoms or problems that have been experienced. You may start off simply by asking "How are you feeling?" Most patients will then focus on their chief complaint. The responses given to these questions will help the physician determine the nature and extent of the physical examination required.

When you ask the patient about symptoms you must get specific information but be careful not to influence the patient's answer. You must ask questions that will answer "what," "where," and "when." For example, if the patient is complaining of pain (the "what"), ask the patient to describe the type of pain experienced. Do not ask "Is it a sharp or dull pain?" Ask *where* the pain is and get the patient to show you where the pain is felt. Watch the patient's facial expression and other body language as the pain area is pointed out. Ask *when* the pain first occurred and if there are any special times that it occurs; ask whether anything seems to precipitate the pain and how long the pain lasts. If the patient can't remember when the pain first started, try to pinpoint the time by asking questions such as "Did you have pain on the July 4th holiday?" or similar types of questions.
6. Listen carefully to the patient and pay attention to the sound of the patient's voice. The patient may be anxious, upset, or maybe the pain is so intense that the patient is about to cry. Listen for offhand comments, such as "I probably have this pain because I'm under so much stress. I really shouldn't be here at all." You must reassure the patient that

the right decision was made by coming to see the doctor and encourage the patient to discuss any problems with the physician. Alert the physician of these types of comments. The physician can then ask the patient what is really bothering him or her. It may be that the patient does not wish to disclose an intimate problem to you but may be more willing to discuss it if the physician appears to be receptive and willing to inquire and listen.

7. Summarize the information that you have gathered. Ask the patient if there is anything else that he or she would like to add or if there is anything that you may have left out.

8. Be willing and prepared to answer questions that the patient may have. Respond with interest. If you cannot answer the question, refer it to the physician. Explain that the physician will discuss the answer to the patient's question(s).

PHYSICAL EXAMINATION

After the history is completed, the physician will proceed with the physical examination, often referred to as a physical or a PE. This differs from the history in that it involves a thorough examination of the patient from head to toe for anatomical and physiological functioning.

The key to a physical examination is systematic thoroughness. Generally, a physician will formulate a logical, methodical approach by examining each body system or part, beginning with the head and working down. The information obtained in the history or the chief complaint as stated by the patient will help determine the extent of the examination to be performed. Sometimes a limited or a specific examination of one body part or system may be indicated.

Methods of Physical Examinations

Various methods of physical examinations are used by the physician to learn about the patient's condition. The standard methods follow (Fig. 2-2).

Inspection. Inspection is the visual observation of the body as a whole and of its individual parts. The physician will observe the patient's general appearance, color of the skin, size and shape of the body as a whole and of the individual parts. The physician will also note any rashes, scars, trauma, deformities, swelling, injuries, and nervousness.

In the detailed examination, the physician will use the otoscope to look into the ears and the ophthalmoscope to inspect the eyes. A tongue blade will be of help when inspecting the mouth and throat.

Palpation. Palpation is performed by applying the tips of the fingers, the whole hand, or both hands to the body part. Pressure may be slight or forcible, continuous or intermittent. The physician feels, touches, and sometimes manipulates the external surface of the various parts of the body to determine the physical characteristics of tissues or organs, and also to note if pain or tenderness is present.

Also involved are the physician's senses of temperature, vibration, position, and kinesthesia as the examination is in progress. Some of the organs and parts of the body examined by this method are the breast, chest, abdomen, liver, kidney, bladder, and lymph nodes. In conjunction with external palpation, internal palpation may be done on the uterus, ovaries, and rectum.

Percussion. In medical diagnosis, percussion is done by tapping the body lightly but sharply with the fingers. The physician places one or two fingers of one hand on the part of the body to be examined and then strikes those fingers with the index or middle finger of the other hand.

The purpose of percussion is to determine the density, size, and position of the underlying organs and also to determine the presence of pus or fluid in a cavity. The differing densities of the various parts of the body give off different sounds when struck by the examiner's fingers. The more hollow the part struck, the more drumlike the sound. The sounds that are emitted help the physician make a diagnosis. A solid mass in a hollow organ can be noted because of a change from the normal density. Also, the borders of certain organs such as the heart can be mapped out by comparing the density in the organ with surrounding tissues. Percussion is most commonly used on the chest and back for examination of the heart and lungs, but may also be done on the abdomen, bladder, or bones.

A physician may also use an instrument, the percussion hammer, to check a patient's reflexes by striking the tendon just below the knee and also at the elbow or ankle with this instrument. Failure of the desired reflex gives the physician more information for a diagnosis.

Auscultation. Auscultation is the process of listening to sounds produced in some of the body cavities as the organs perform their functions. A stethoscope is usually used in this method, but it can also be done by placing one's ear directly over a bared or thinly covered body surface. It is used chiefly on the chest to listen to the heart and lungs and also on the abdomen to diagnose an abdominal aneurysm or listen to fetal heart sounds or peristaltic waves. Listening to the sounds produced in these body cavities helps determine the physical condition of the organs.

Fig. 2-2. Methods of physical examinations. **A,** inspection. **B,** palpation. **C,** percussion. **D,** auscultation.

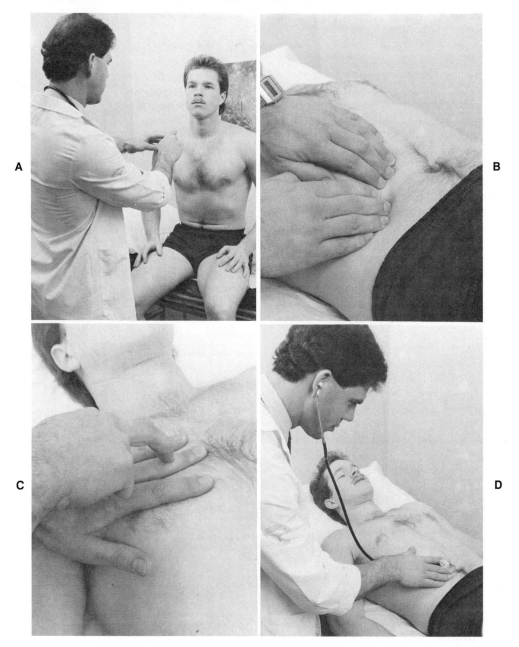

Mensuration. Mensuration is the process of measuring. Clinical measurements include weight, height, temperature, pulse, respirations, and blood pressure. Head circumference is also measured in young children. When recorded and compared with previous measurements, these are extremely important guides for some diagnoses. Chest measurement may also be done to ascertain the amount of expansion and retraction of the two sides accompanying inspiration and expiration. This is important when diagnosing or treating chest conditions such as emphysema, in which there is often a loss of elasticity of the lungs.

Smell. Smell is a much less frequently used method but it is still a relevant method for detecting a disease process. Odors from the breath, sputum, urine, feces, vomitus, or pus can provide valuable information to help the physician make a diagnosis.

Essentials of a Thorough Physical Examination

A complete physical examination report should cover the following as the physician observes, tests, and measures each for normal or abnormal structure and function.

GENERAL INSPECTION — General appearance, nutritional status, apparent age, color, sex, height, weight, attitude, communication

VITAL SIGNS — Temperature, pulse, respiration, blood pressure

SKIN — Color, texture, turgor, warmth, hair distribution, pigmentation, rashes, scars, lesions, moles, warts

HEAD — Position, proportion to rest of body, distribution of hair, masses, evidence of trauma

FACE — Symmetry, size, appearance, facial expression, tenderness

EYES — Visual fields, visual acuity, eyeball movement, conjunctiva, sclera, cornea, iris, pupils, eyelids, ptosis, tearing, discharges

EARS — Hearing, ear canals, tympanic membranes, cerumen, discharge

NOSE — Size, shape, color, deformity, septum, airways, mucosa, discharge, bleeding

MOUTH — Breath, lips, gums, teeth, tongue, mucosa

THROAT — Tonsils, pharynx, larynx

NECK — Suppleness, thyroid gland, lymph nodes, vessels, carotid pulses, position of trachea, tenderness, stiffness, masses

BREASTS — Size, contour, symmetry, nipples, masses, discharge, tenderness

CHEST — Shape, symmetry, expansion, lesions

LUNGS — Rate and quality of respiration, breath sounds, cough, sputum, friction rubs, resonance, fremitus

HEART — Rate, rhythm, point of maximum impulse (PMI), sounds, murmurs, dullness, thrills, gallop

ARTERIES — Pulses, vessel walls, bruits

VEINS — Pulsation, dilation, filling

LYMPH NODES — Enlargement

ABDOMEN — Contour; appearance; liver, kidneys, and spleen (LKS); bladder; scars; peristalsis; tenderness; rigidity; spasm; masses; fluid; hernia

FEMALE GENITALIA — External appearance, Bartholin and Skene glands, discharge, masses; vaginal — bimanual examination of uterus and adnexa, tenderness, masses, Pap smear if required

MALE GENITALIA — Penis, scrotum, scars, lesions, discharge, tenderness, masses, atrophy, enlargement

RECTAL — Sphincter tone, prostate gland, seminal vesicles, fissure, fistula, hemorrhoids, masses, discharge, feces

BACK AND SPINE — Posture, curvature, balance, mobility, gait, tenderness, masses, costovertebral tenderness

EXTREMITIES — Proportion to trunk, range of motion, color, pulses, edema, swelling, deformity, tenderness, ulcers, varicosities

FINGERNAILS — Contour, color

NEUROLOGICAL STATUS — Consciousness, cranial nerves, reflexes, coordination, gait, balance, muscle tone and strength, tactile, pain (deep and superficial), discriminatory sensation

MENTAL STATUS — Orientation to time, place, and person; appearance; behavior; mood and thought content

(See Appendix A.)

Other tests that a physician may have performed as part of the physical examination include a routine urinalysis (UA), a complete blood count (CBC), a chest x-ray film, and electrocardiogram (ECG or EKG). Physical examinations will vary according to the needs or complaints of a patient. Frequently a patient may have a complaint or situation that can be handled in a few minutes or that requires a special type of examination such as a sigmoidoscopy. Other patients may require a complete physical examination. In this case, all of the preceding information will be obtained.

Special Examinations

Certain types of examinations are more specific and restricted. These are local or special examinations, which are confined to specific parts and organs or special functions of the body. They are extensive and detailed and performed to establish complete information of a complex nature. Frequently they are done to examine the interior of body cavities and passages. Some of the local or special examinations are vaginal and obstetrical examinations, proctoscopy, sigmoidoscopy, cystoscopy, bronchoscopy, and skin tests. Other specialized examinations include ultrasound, roentgenological, neurological, ophthalmological, and cardiac studies.

SUMMARY OF POSITIVE FINDINGS

Based on the subjective findings as related by the patient and the objective findings as found by the physician during the physical examination, the physician will sometimes outline a brief summarization of all of the positive findings of the case.

DIAGNOSTIC DATA

The physician arrives at a diagnosis by employing and reviewing multiple factors and information obtained on the patient's condition; that is, the physician uses various studies to arrive at a diagnosis. Three reasons for diagnostic studies are as follows:

- To determine (diagnose) the condition from which the patient is suffering so that treatment may be initiated if feasible.
- To discover disease in its early stage before the patient experiences any signs or symptoms. This is called•screening. Screening for disease often permits the cure of the disease because treatment can be started in the early stages of the disease process (for example, cancer), or early treatment can delay the progression of the disease (for example, hypertension).
- To evaluate past or ongoing treatment received by the patient.

As the field of medical science continues to expand, newer, more accurate, and more sophisticated techniques are made available to help physicians diagnose disease processes. Diagnostic procedures and studies include but are not limited to physical examinations, surgical intervention, and laboratory studies. Laboratory data may include a set of routine laboratory examinations that were performed at the time of the patient's physical examination with the results recorded if the tests have been completed. Other procedures used in diagnosing and treating disease processes may involve the specialized areas of radiology (roentgenology), nuclear medicine, special skin tests, physical medicine, physiotherapy, and electrocardiography. These areas of health care and treatment will be elaborated on in later units of this book.

IMPRESSION

Once all this information has been gathered, the physician will indicate an impression of the patient's condition. This may include any or all of the following:

Diagnosis
Primary diagnosis—a statement that indicates the cause of the patient's current, most important problem/condition.
Secondary diagnosis—a statement that indicates a problem/condition that is less important or urgent than the patient's primary diagnosis.
Tentative or provisional diagnosis—a probable diagnosis. This reflects the physician's impression of the patient's condition, but it is made before any further tests have been completed and a final diagnosis has been reached.
Differential diagnosis—a possible diagnosis. A statement based on comparison of signs and symptoms of two or more similar diseases to determine from which the patient is suffering. Thus, by a process of elimination, the provisional diagnosis may be made.
Rule out (R/O)—a statement that indicates those conditions that the physician believes might be causing the patient's problem/condition. Each condition will be investigated thoroughly and ruled out as a diagnosis, if and when negative testing results are obtained. Again by a process of elimination a diagnosis may be reached. (The current trend is discouraging the use of this term for purposes of more definitive record keeping. In place of *rule out*, the term *possible diagnosis* is used by some.)
Problem list—this is used in the most recent system of recording called the Problem-Oriented System (POS). A problem is any situation, disease, or condition for which the patient needs help or any question that requires a solution. In the problem list, each problem drawn from the data base is numbered, dated, and listed in order of occurrence. (Data base refers to all of the preceding parts of the medical record as discussed.) Problems may be stated in terms of the following:
- Diagnosis
- Symptom or physical findings
- Physiological findings
- Abnormal laboratory results
- Social or personal problems
- Environmental problems
- Behavior factors
- Patient education
Additional explanations of the problem-oriented system and the problem-oriented record will be discussed at the end of this unit.
Prognosis—a statement of the probable or anticipated outcome of the patient's condition.

CARE PLANS AND SUGGESTED FURTHER STUDY

The next part of the medical case record will include the physician's clearly stated plans, which may include one or a combination of the following forms of treatment: drug therapy, physical therapy, diet therapy, surgery, and psychotherapy. In addition, hospitalization will be noted if required. For all of these treatments, patient education should be included. The medical assistant, as a member of the health care team, may be required to do part of the patient teaching. All treatments prescribed and medications ordered are entered on the record in detail.

Suggested further studies will list the laboratory tests, x-ray studies, or any other special tests that the physician deems necessary for the treatment and care of the patient. Instructions for follow-up visits will be stated. Also included may be a statement that the patient has been referred to another physician for consultation or treatment when this is advisable.

After the completion of any special test or consultation, a report is made, which is then incorporated into the patient's medical record.

PROGRESS NOTES

After each future visit, the physician's observations, the status of the patient's condition, and the patient's own report, if it is relevant, are added to the medical record. Any change in treatment or medication is recorded. This is called the progress report or progress note, and each entry must be dated and signed. In a hospital, progress notes are also written by other health care providers, for example, physical therapists.

DISCHARGE SUMMARY

If the patient is discharged, the date and final statement about the patient's health and condition at that time are recorded on the medical record. These may be written at the end of the progress notes or on a separate form.

If death occurs, a statement describing the cause of death is recorded, and the history is marked *"deceased."*

Hospital discharge summaries contain more detailed information; included are

- Admission date, discharge date
- Admitting diagnosis, final diagnosis
- Summary of the history — sex, age, chief complaint, brief history of present illness, pertinent past history
- Pertinent physical findings
- Pertinent laboratory and x-ray findings
- Treatment (operations, drugs, x-ray films, diet, and so on)
- Hospital course (uneventful or list of any complications)
- Condition on discharge
- Prognosis (good, fair, poor, guarded)
- Recommendations on discharge (special orders, follow-up care, medications, and so on)
- Date, hour, and physician's signature

A copy of the patient's hospital discharge summary should be obtained from the hospital for the patient's permanent office record. The summary will be of some importance to the physician for providing continuity of care to the patient on return to the office or clinic for follow-up care or future checkups. Other uses of this form may include research, statistical, insurance, and legal purposes.

PROBLEM-ORIENTED MEDICAL RECORD (POMR)

Over the past years, the problem-oriented medical record has gained great momentum and support from health care providers in a variety of settings. Pioneered by Lawrence L. Weed, MD, of the University of Vermont College of Medicine, the problem-oriented medical record provides a systematic way of recording data pertinent to patient care. Its purpose is to obtain and record in an organized manner all the knowledge needed to accurately diagnose, treat, and provide complete follow-up care for a patient's condition/disease or situation. This record consists of four basic parts, which are as follows:

1. Data base
2. Problem list
3. Plans
4. Progress notes

The *data base* provides the essential data necessary to identify and solve the problem(s). It consists of the patient's medical history, the physical examination, and known laboratory data, all of which were previously described.

The *problem list* results from the information obtained in the data base. All the problems identified are titled, numbered, and dated in order of occurrence. This information is usually placed on the front page of the patient's chart to provide a quick diagnostic profile of the patient. The problems may be stated in various terms as outlined on p. 49.

At subsequent visits any new problems are noted as they arise, dated and numbered consecutively. As problems are resolved, the fact is noted with the date it occurred. The number of a resolved problem is not used again for another problem.

The problem list can be adapted in various ways to accommodate short-term or temporary problems that are seen frequently in the physician's office or clinic. One recommendation is the use of two problem lists: one for short-term or temporary problems, the other for long-term or permanent problems. When a short-term problem persists beyond a reasonable time or recurs frequently, it is added to the long-term or permanent list and removed from the short-term list.

Another recommendation is to use only one problem list, but not to record quickly resolved temporary problems on it. Temporary problems are simply indicated as such in the progress notes and are not numbered.

The *plans* state what will be done to start to solve the problem(s). They are made for each titled and numbered problem. A plan for a problem may be classified as follows:

- Diagnostic, that is evaluative studies, such as laboratory tests and x-ray films, consultations requested, and interviews with the patient's family, all of which help acquire additional information.
- Therapeutic, that is medical, surgical, diet, psychological, and/or physical treatment used to meet the goals of the physician when providing health care.
- Educative, that is, what the patient is told about the therapy and condition, what instructional material, if any, was given to the patient, and what the expectations from the patient are as a partner in the care and treatment plan.

The *progress notes* are added to the record as the plan(s) are carried out. Each progress note is dated, and titled and numbered relating to the problem under discussion. Each problem is evaluated for current status, with a notation of new findings or thoughts, changes in treatment plans, and resolution of the problem.

Each progress note should contain four parts and should be recorded according to the following format:

Number and title of the problem:

S   *Subjective findings* — Statements made by the patient; how the patient feels; other information from the patient's family.

O   *Objective findings* — What is observed or measured by the examiner; specific things done for/on the patient; results of laboratory, x-ray, and other diagnostic reports.

A   *Assessment* — Evaluation and interpretation of the patient's status (S plus O). Assessment may be what the examiner thinks is happening, reasons for changing management of the problem, or significance of the findings; it may be expressed as an impression or as a diagnosis.

P   *Plan* — Diagnostic, therapeutic, and/or educative methods that will be used.

After the data base has been completed and evaluated, the POMR may appear as follows:

Problem list

Nov. 4, 19_____
   Problem No. 1: Hypertension, essential arterial
   Problem No. 2: Obesity, exogenous
   Problem No. 3: Upper abdominal pain — Resolved 11/7/_____

Plan

Nov. 4, 19_____
   Problem No. 1: Aldactazide 50 mg, 1 tab bid; recheck patient in 1 week

   Problem No. 2: 1200 calorie diet; multivitamin ×1 daily: suggested to patient to join a weight watchers club
   Problem No. 3: UGI series; oral cholecystogram

Progress notes

Nov. 4, 19_____
   Problem No. 1: Hypertension, essential arterial
     S — patient states that fatigue and headaches decreasing somewhat
     O — BP ↓ 20 points to 160/84
     A — positive effects from the medication
     P — continue medication for 2 weeks; then to be checked
   Problem No. 2: Obesity
     S — patient has joined a weight watchers club, but states that she hates dieting
     O — wt. down 4 lb to 176
     A — dieting effective
     P — continue 1200 calorie diet and multivitamin ×1 daily
   Problem No. 3: Upper abdominal pain
     S — patient states that the abdominal pain is less severe but persists
     O — UGI and GB series negative; no abdominal distention
     A — deferred until all results complete
     P — abdominal ultrasound

Nov. 11, 19_____
   Problem No. 1: Hypertension
     S — patient states that headaches have stopped, but she still remains fatigued
     O — BP 140/84
     A — medication effective
     P — reduce Aldactazide to 1 tab daily
   Problem No. 2: Obesity
     S — patient states is now adjusting to the diet much better
     O — wt. ↓ 2 lbs to 174
     A — weight loss will benefit problem No. 1
     P — continue 1200 calorie diet
   Problem No. 3: Upper abdominal pain
     S — patient states pain has subsided — 11/7/_____
     O — x-ray results and ultrasound reports negative
     A — temporary condition, resolved 11/7/_____
     P — patient to report if pain recurs and advised that x-ray studies and ultrasound were negative

As you can see, the problem-oriented medical record (POMR) is an orderly method of providing a chronological profile of a patient that helps the physician and other health care providers conduct total patient care. This system provides a quick current reference of the patient's medical case record, including problem management. It greatly reduces the possibility of an oversight, especially for patients receiving long-term care or those with multiple problems.

SPECIAL VOCABULARY

Vocabulary Used to Describe Pain

In performing the complete history and physical examination, the examiner must deal with a variety of terms relating to pain. The following are some of these particular terms, along with an explanation of each term.

Types of Pain

> Superficial or cutaneous
> Deep pain — from muscles, tendons, joints
> Visceral pain — from the viscera (any large interior organ in any great body cavity, especially those in the abdomen)

Adaptation does not exist in the sense of pain. This is especially important, because pain may be a warning signal of danger, and if one became used to it and ignored it, damage to the body would follow.

Terms Relating to Pain

radiating—Diverting from a common central point; for example, gallbladder pain begins in the right upper quadrant of the abdomen, and it is diverted from that central point to the right flank and right scapular area.

stabbing—Deep, sharp, intermittent pain.

intractable—Unmanageable, not controllable with conventional means, that is, rest, heat, medication.

colicky—Acute intermittent abdominal pain usually caused by spasmodic contractions.

excruciating—Torturing, extreme pain, often intractable.

exquisite—Intense pain to which an individual is extremely sensitive.

transient—Fleeting, brief, passing, coming and going.

threshold—The level that must be exceeded for an effect to be produced; the level of pain that an individual can tolerate without external intervention. Threshold is unique to each individual, and the overall physiopsychological makeup of an individual must be considered when evaluating pain.

guarding—A reflex usually related to abdominal pain; the action of muscles tensing, knees

drawn up and/or hand placed over a part to prevent examination and/or protect against increasing pain.

rebound tenderness—A sensation of pain felt when pressure applied on a body part is released.

Vocabulary Used When Recording Physical Findings

The following vocabulary lists *some* of the terms that the examiner may use when recording the *objective* findings of the physical examination of a patient. Each term is presented under the body part or system for which it is used when describing the findings of the physical examination. If the medical assistant student has completed studies in medical terminology, these terms should be familiar; if not, by referring to Appendix A, the medical assistant student should be able to define, pronounce, and become familiar with each term.

Skin

Abrasion	Laceration
Avulsion	Petechiae
Contusion	Purpura
Cyanosis	Turgor
Ecchymosis	Urticaria
Erythema	Ulcer
Jaundice	

Eyes

Acuity	Nystagmus
Adnexa	Papilledema
Arcus senilis	Ptosis
Fundus of the eye	

Ears

Tympanic membranes	Cerumen

Nose

Nares	Nasal septal defect

Neck

Supple	Range of motion
Carotid pulse	

Cardiovascular system (CVS)

Bruit	Ischemia
Congestion	Murmur
Ecchymosis	Petechiae
Engorgement	Purpura
Erythema	Resuscitation
Gallop	Rub
Infarction	Thrill

Respiratory system

Fremitus	Rhonchi
Friction rub	Sputum
Rales	Stridor
Resonance	

Abdomen

Ascites	Hernia
Contour	Protuberant
Distention	Rigidity
Flaccid	Scaphoid

Gastrointestinal system (GI)

Caries	Fistula
Distention	Hemorrhoid
Fissure	Peristalsis

Reproductive system

Adnexa	Introitus
Atrophy	Involution
Gravida	Parous

Genitourinary system (GU)

Introitus	Discharge

Musculoskeletal system (MS) —
  neurological and extremities examination

Claudication	Lordosis
Clubbing	Passive congestion
Crepitation	Protuberance
Edema	Rigidity
Exostosis	Scoliosis
Flaccid	Supple
Gait	Ulcer
Kyphosis	Varicosity

General

Cachexia	Fingerbreadth
Diaphoresis	Lethargic
Dehydration	Patulous
Emaciation	Tenderness

MEDICAL ABBREVIATIONS

In a patient's medical case history, physical examination report, and notes on the chart, you will encounter a variety of abbreviations. The following list includes some of the more common abbreviations. They are grouped together according to general usage. You should recall some of these, while others are new. Pay special attention to when capital letters are used and not used. Prescription abbreviations are given in Unit VII. Others are given in the appropriate units.*

Body systems
  HEENT — head, eyes, ears, nose, and throat
  ENT — ear, nose, and throat
  CR — cardiorespiratory
  CVS — cardiovascular system
  GI — gastrointestinal
  GU — genitourinary

*According to the style of the American Medical Association, medical and pharmaceutical abbreviations are to be written *without* the use of periods. That is, rather than writing a.c. as was done in the past, you will now write ac, and so on.

CNS — central nervous system
MS — musculoskeletal
NS — nervous system
NM — neuromuscular

Patient's history
  CC — chief complaint
  PI *or* HIP — present illness or history of present illness
  PH — past history
  LMD — local medical doctor
  UCHD *or* UCD — usual childhood diseases
  FH — family history
  a & w *or* A & W — alive and well
  ROS — review of systems
  PTA — prior to admission
  c/o — complains of

Physical examination (PE)
  wd — well-developed
  wn — well-nourished
  IPPA — inspection, percussion, palpation, and auscultation
  P & A — percussion and auscultation
  BP — blood pressure
  TPR — temperature, pulse, and respirations
  WNL — within normal limits
  wt — weight
  ht — height

Diagnosis
  Diag *or* Dx — diagnosis
  R/O — rule out
  POS — problem-oriented system

Ears
  TM — tympanic membrane(s)

Eyes
  REM — rapid eye movements
  L & A — light and accommodation
  PERLA — pupils equal and reacting to light and accommodation
  EOM — extraocular movements
  RRE — round, regular, and equal
  OS — left eye
  OD — right eye
  OU — both eyes

Chest (heart and lungs)
  P & A — percussion and auscultation
  PND — paroxysmal nocturnal dyspnea
  SOB — shortness of breath
  PMI — point of maximal intensity (or impulse)
  MCL — midclavicular line
  ICS — intercostal space
  NSR — normal sinus rhythm
  RSR — regular sinus rhythm
  ASHD — arteriosclerotic heart disease
  MI — myocardial infarction
  EKG *or* ECG — electrocardiogram
  AV — arteriovenous, atrioventricular
  CHF — congestive heart failure
  RHD — rheumatic heart disease
  URI — upper respiratory infection

COPD — chronic obstructive pulmonary disease
CHD — coronary heart disease

Abdomen and GI
LKS — liver, kidney, spleen *or* LKKS — liver, kidneys, and spleen
GB — gallbladder
BM — bowel movement

Female reproductive system
BUS — Bartholin, urethral, and Skene glands
LMP — last menstrual period
OB — obstetrics
PID — pelvic inflammatory disease
GYN — gynecology
EDC — expected date of confinement
FHT — fetal heart tones
L & D — labor and delivery
PP — postpartum
IUD — intrauterine device
SAB — spontaneous abortion (miscarriage)

Musculoskeletal system
EMG — electromyogram
MS — multiple sclerosis
LOM — loss of movement or motion
cva — costovertebral angle
DTR — deep tendon reflexes
Fx — fracture
ROM — range of motion

Central nervous system
CSF — cerebrospinal fluid
CVA — cerebrovascular accident
EEG — electroencephalogram
DTR — deep tendon reflexes

Laboratory
CBC — complete blood count
UA — urinalysis
O_2 — oxygen
CO_2 — carbon dioxide
CSF — cerebrospinal fluid
SMA — sequential multiple analysis
HGB *or* HG *or* HB — hemoglobin
Hct — hematocrit
WBC — white blood count
RBC — red blood count
Diff — differential (blood count)
Protime or PT — prothrombin time
pH — hydrogen ion concentration, referring to the degree of acidity or alkalinity of a solution
BUN — blood urea nitrogen
Sedrate — sedimentation rate
Rh — Rhesus blood factor
PKU — phenylketonuria
FBS — fasting blood sugar
PBI — protein-bound iodine
PCV — packed cell volume
RhA — rheumatoid arthritis
STS — serologic test for syphilis

VDRL — Veneral Disease Research Laboratory
C & S — culture and sensitivity
CPK — creatine phosphokinase
LDH — lactic dehydrogenase

X-ray studies
A-P and Lat — anterior, posterior, and lateral
IVP — intravenous pyelogram
GBS — gallbladder series
CT — computed tomography
MRI — magnetic resonance imaging
BE — barium enema
KUB — kidneys, ureter, bladder
UGI — upper gastrointestinal series

Surgical terms
T & A — tonsillectomy and adenoidectomy
D & C — dilation and curettage
I & D — incision and drainage
TUR — transurethral resection
TURP — transurethral resection of the prostate

Hospital departments
ICU — intensive care unit
CCU — coronary care unit
ER — emergency room
OR — operating room
RR *or* PAR — recovery room or postanesthetic room
Lab — laboratory
Path — pathology
OPD — outpatient department
Peds — pediatrics
RT — respiratory therapy

General
Ca *or* CA — cancer or carcinoma
d/c *or* D/C — discontinue
DOA — dead on arrival
OD — overdose
cm — centimeter
lb — pounds
kg or kilos — kilograms
ac — before meals
pc — after meals
stat — immediately
prn — whenever necessary
ad lib — as desired
ASAP — as soon as possible
BR — bed rest
BP — blood pressure
I & O — intake and output
IM — intramuscular
IV — intravenous
sc or SubQ — subcutaneous
LP — lumbar puncture
NPO — nothing by mouth
D/W — dextrose in water
S/W — saline in water
DOB — date of birth
FUO — fever of unknown (or undetermined) origin

GC — gonococcus or gonorrhea
K — potassium
LE — lupus erythematosus
NYD — not yet diagnosed
PM — postmortem
TB — tuberculosis
O_2 — oxygen
CO_2 — carbon dioxide
pt — patient
TLC — tender loving care

Symbols

>— greater than
<— less than
♂— male
♀— female
↑— above, increase
↓— below, decrease
×— times (multiply by)
%— percentage
#— number
=— equals
+— plus
−— minus
ō— none
c̄— with
s̄— without
ā— before
p̄— after

CONCLUSION

You have now completed the unit on Health History and Physical Examinations. You will be expected to discuss the parts and the importance of a patient's health history and other components that make up a medical record. In addition, you should be able to describe the methods used by a physician when performing a physical examination. When you are familiar with the contents of this unit, arrange with your instructor to take a performance test.

REVIEW OF VOCABULARY

The following are samples of a patient's medical history and physical examination. A consultation letter and a hospital discharge summary as dictated by a physician are also included. These are to help familiarize you with the format and contents of medical reports. Read these and be prepared to discuss the contents and define all the medical terms that are used. You should recognize some of the terms; others are new, and you may have to refer to Appendix A or to a medical dictionary for the definitions.

History and Physical Examination

PATIENT: Patrick Nelson
PHYSICIAN: S. Kennedy, MD
DATE: November 12, 19_____

CHIEF COMPLAINT
None

HISTORICAL DATA
This 27-year-old white male enters for a physical evaluation. Actually he has no complaints, but feels that it is wise to have a general physical evaluation.

PAST MEDICAL HISTORY
The patient states that he had the usual childhood diseases. He had the flu in 1984, moderately severe. The patient received all of his immunizations.
Operations: Tonsillectomy as a child.
Injuries: Broken bones and unconsciousness, none.

PERSONAL HISTORY
The patient is single and works with his father.

FAMILY HISTORY
His father and mother are both living, middle-aged, and well. He has an older sister and a younger brother, both in good health.

HABITS
The patient smokes a package to a package and a half of cigarettes per day. Alcoholic intake, about 4 oz per week

MEDICATIONS
None

SYSTEM REVIEW
Head and neck
Eyes: The patient is myopic and wears glasses all the time. He denies headaches or visual disturbances.
Ears, nose, and throat: Not remarkable.
Cardiorespiratory: The patient denies all symptoms in this system, except for being soft. He states that he gets no regular exercise and when he does sudden exercise, he becomes short of breath.
Gastrointestinal: His appetite is excellent. His weight is stable at approximately 160 pounds. Digestion is good. Bowels are regular with use of laxatives. He states that he had some minor hemorrhoid problems in the past.
Genitourinary: The patient denies nocturia. He passes his water several times daily without difficulty. There is no history of kidney stones, bladder infections, or bleeding.
Neuromuscular osseous: The patient recently had a backache from which he has made a satisfactory recovery. Orthopedic consultation at that time was negative.

PHYSICAL EXAMINATION
Height: 72 inches.
Weight: 167 pounds.
Blood pressure: 144/80.
Pulse: 76 and regular.
Temperature: Normal.
Respiration: 16 per minute.
The general impression is that of a well-developed,

well-nourished white male, who appears to be in no acute distress. He is slightly obese, pleasant, and cooperative.

Head and neck:

Eyes: Patient has a positive cover test, with a latent exophoria. He is highly myopic. Funduscopic examination is otherwise not remarkable.

Ear, nose, and throat: Normal. The neck is supple. The trachea is in the midline. The thyroid is not palpable. The neck veins are collapsed.

Chest: Clear to percussion and auscultation. There is good diaphragmatic descent, bilaterally. Breath tones are normal. No adventitious sounds are heard.

Heart: The left border of cardiac tonus is 6 cm from the midsternal line with the point of maximum impulse at the fourth intercostal space. The rhythm is regular. No murmurs or adventitious sounds are heard.

Abdomen: Slightly rotund. The liver, spleen, and kidneys are not palpable. There are no masses or tenderness.

Genitalia: There is a normal male escutcheon. The penis is circumcised. Testes are in the scrotum. The inguinal rings are intact.

Rectal: Examination discloses good sphincter tone. The prostate is small, smooth, and symmetrical. The ampulla is filled with soft, brown stool.

Extremities: There is no evidence of edema, cyanosis, or jaundice. Peripheral pulses are adequate. Most notable is the finding of several small glomus tumors on the fingers. Some of these are painful; others are not.

Neurological: Intact.

Skin: Negative.

Lymphatics: Negative.

IMPRESSIONS

1. Normal, healthy man.
2. Glomus tumors.
3. Latent exophoria.

RECOMMENDATIONS

1. Routine urine and CBC.
2. Chest x-ray film.
3. Lose 10 pounds of weight.
4. Return as needed.
   S. Kennedy, MD

DISCHARGE SUMMARY

HISTORY: The patient is a 36-year-old, juvenile-onset diabetic with multiple problems involving the gastrointestinal, genitourinary, and musculoskeletal systems.

PROBLEM NO. 1 — Diabetes mellitus: onset at age of 15 years, with two episodes of diabetic ketoacidosis at ages 15 and 20, with multiple admissions for hypoglycemic and hyperglycemic symptoms. The patient states he has taken 55 units of Lente in the morning and 15 units of Lente in the evening for 20 years, with slight increases in these periodically, covering himself with regular, 15 units in the AM and 10 units in the PM. The patient is presently on 45 units of Lente and 15 units of regular in the morning, and 15 Lente and 10 regular in the PM, with urines running negative to 2+, with no ketones. The patient states he has not changed his dose or altered his eating habits or skipped a dose in the past 48 hours.

Twelve hours before admission, the patient noted the onset of mild nausea, vomiting, with abdominal distention, bloating and intermittent diarrhea (brown). The patient denies bright red blood per rectum or per mouth, or melena. He denies loss of consciousness or lethargy, fever, chills, night sweats, cough, dysuria, pyuria, but does admit to polydipsia on a chronic basis. Complications from the diabetes include retinopathy, which was first noted in 1986 and treated with lasers; he denies any renal or neurological complications (impotence, bladder, bowel). The patient has also had numerous abscesses in the perianal area and urinary tract infections, including pyelonephritis times one.

PROBLEM NO. 2 — Gastrointestinal complaints: The patient has a greater than 15 year history of peptic ulcer disease, with a history of hematemesis and melena in 1984, for which he had an upper GI series that showed a suggestion of a swollen duodenal bulb, and an endoscopy that read out as a normal examination. The patient also had acid studies done, which showed a basal secretion of 7.86 mEq per hour, going to a post-Histalog stimulation level of 35.7 mEq per hour. The findings were consistent with an ulcerogenic picture. It was elected not to do surgery at that time, because of the lack of anything treatable. The patient was noted to have decreased gastric emptying, which was thought to be due to an inadvertent vagotomy during his hiatal hernia repair in 1985.

The patient presently complains of epigastric pain, worse on lying, with heartburn, relieved by eating and taking antacids. The patient gives a history of melena for 3 days and hematemesis, two episodes in the past 2 months, without recurrence. The patient also takes aspirin for back pain. The patient has a past history of infectious hepatitis, treated in 1980, without recurrence.

PROBLEM NO. 3 — Back pain, chronic: In 1985, the patient suffered trauma to his back, secondary to lifting a heavy object, which resulted in marked decrease in the strength in his lower extremities. The patient was evaluated at that time with an electromyogram [EMG], which was normal, and a myelogram, which showed protrusion of the nucleus pulposus in the L4-5 area. The patient was taken to surgery, where partial hemilaminectomy was done in December 1985. The patient states that he has had no cessation or relief of his back pain secondary to the operation. The patient denies any paresthesia, weakness, or asymmetry in motor-sensory involvement in his lower extremities.

PROBLEM NO. 4 — Chest pain, hypertension: The patient has a history of cardiac "attacks" in 1984 and 1985 times two and in 1986, requiring hospitalization. The patient was told each time that there was no heart damage. The patient describes the pain as substernal, radiating to the neck and back, without associated shortness of breath, palpitations, diaphoresis, but does state that it is precipitated by exercise on occasion or emotional stress. The patient has never had any EKG changes consistent with ischemia and/or infarct. The patient's history of high blood pressure runs in the 140/90 range and has been treated for 1½ years in the past, but he has presently been off medications. The patient states that episodes of chest pain come approximately one to two times per month and only last for seconds. The patient has been treated in the past with nitroglycerin in 1986, but no longer takes the medication.

PROBLEM NO. 5 — Kidney problems: The patient, at the age of 10 years, had pyelonephritis and subsequent recurrent urinary tract infections, which may or may not have included flank pain, fever, and chills. The patient has been treated in the past with antibiotics for his urinary tract infections, the most recent being 7 years ago. The patient has a past history of renal stones in 1986, left-sided, with a normal intravenous pyelogram. The patient was evaluated for calcium, phosphate, and oxalate in his urine, which were all within the normal range. The patient's creatinine in the past has run around 1, with a BUN around 18 in 1986.

PAST MEDICAL HISTORY: Allergies: None. Illness: As above. Surgery: Note above. Habits: 25 years of smoking a pack a day; no alcohol. Medications: Note history of present illness.

SOCIAL HISTORY: The patient lives in Anytown, California, works as a chef, and presently is living with a girlfriend. The patient has been married three times and has one child, who is 14 years old, by his first wife.

FAMILY HISTORY: The family history is positive for diabetes in a maternal uncle and maternal great-grandmother. There is no history of myocardial infarction, high blood pressure, cerebrovascular accident, tuberculosis, rheumatic heart disease, endocrinopathies, or cancer.

REVIEW OF SYSTEMS: This is significant for head, eyes, ears, nose, and throat. He did have a headache in 1986, which was evaluated with an EEG and skull films, all of which were within normal limits; presently without complaint of headache. Lungs: He has been without pneumonia; negative PPD within the last year and a half. Neurological: The patient has a questionable history of psychiatric disease in the past with "rage attacks." The patient has not been evaluated further.

PHYSICAL EXAMINATION: Blood pressure 140/96 lying, with a pulse of 92, going to 140/100 standing up,

with a pulse of 116. Respirations were 20, temperature was 37°C. Generally, a well-developed male, appearing in no acute distress.

Skin: The skin had a midline abdominal scar and an abscess scar on the left medial buttock area. There were ingrown hairs on his anterior and posterior thoracic walls. There was no diaphoresis.

Head, eyes, ears, nose, and throat: Atraumatic; extraocular movements were positive; pupils were equal, round, and reactive to light, without nystagmus. The fundi were remarkable for increased tortuosity of his vessels, with hemorrhages and exudates present in both retinae; his discs were flat. Tympanic membranes showed old scarring, but normal light reflexes. Oropharynx was clear and edentulous.

Neck: Supple, without increase, decrease, or asymmetrical thyroid enlargement; there were no bruits.

Nodes: No cervical, supraclavicular, axillary, or epitrochlear nodes. He did have positive occipital and inguinal nodes, old.

Lungs: Decreased respiratory movements; there was a slight increase in his AP diameter; positive end-inspiratory wheezing, with inspiration: expiration ratio of 1 : 1.2. The patient was without rales; he did have scattered rhonchi. There was no E to A change; no increase or decreased vocal or tactile fremitus was noted.

Cardiovascular examination: The cardiovascular examination showed a point of maximal impulse in the fifth intercostal space, midclavicular line; no heave, thrill, or thrust; no S-3, S-4, or murmur. Pulses were +2 and equal throughout, without bruits. The carotids were good and up bilaterally, without bruits.

Abdomen: The liver was 12 cm by percussion; no spleen, kidney, or bladder palpable; bowel sounds were active, without distention.

Rectal examination: The rectal examination was guaiac-negative; prostate was symmetrically enlarged, without nodularity or mass.

Extremities: There was full range of motion, without cyanosis, clubbing, or edema.

Neurological examination: Oriented times three. Abstract thought, short- and long-term memory were intact. There was no sensory, motor, or cerebellar abnormality in his lower or upper extremities. His cranial nerves II through XII were within normal limits. His reflexes were +1 and equal throughout, except for absent ankle jerks, with downgoing toes. Negative straight-leg raising. No root, grasp, or suck reflexes were noted.

LABORATORY DATA: He had a pH of 7.38, pO_2 of 67, and a PCO_2 of 40 on room air, with a bicarbonate of 24. His glucose was 855. His urinalysis showed +4 glucose, negative ketones. Chest x-ray film was without cardiopulmonary disease, and there was no air under the diaphragm. KUB showed no abnormalities. His sodium was 122, potassium 3.6, bicarbonate 28; BUN was 21 and creatinine was 1.6. His EKG showed normal sinus rhythm, without acute changes.

HOSPITAL COURSE: The patient's hospital course was one of treatment with intravenous insulin and normal saline to correct the abnormalities noted from the hyperosmolar effect of the increased glucose load intravascularly. The patient responded well to rehydration and to IV insulin, receiving 10 units of IV insulin over a 4- to 6-hour period, with a blood glucose drop from 855 to 328. The patient at no time showed any evidence of ketoacidosis, with urines running in the 3 to 4+ range, with negative ketones, and bicarbonate staying in the 28 to 30 range. By morning, the glucose was 106, with negative-negative urine and a bicarbonate of 30. The patient was begun on a normal regimen as he was treated as an outpatient, with 45 units of Lente, 15 of regular in the morning, and 15 of Lente and 10 of regular in the evening. The patient responded well to therapy and is being discharged today for follow-up in my clinic.

The patient's epigastric complaints will be followed on an outpatient basis and worked up accordingly. The patient continued to be guaiac-negative in the hospital for the 2 days.

CHEST PAINS: The patient did have one episode of chest pain while in the hospital, with EKG during chest pain showing no abnormalities. The pain lasted for seconds and went away without medication.

The patient is being discharged with the following medications: Lente and regular insulin — 45 units of Lente and 15 units of regular in the AM, and 15 units of Lente and 5 units of regular in the PM. Tylenol and codeine, one po q4h prn for low back pain.

DISCHARGE DIAGNOSIS

Diabetes, out of control, secondary to noncompliance
Epigastric pain
Low back pain
Chest pain

    N. J. Hopew, MD

Consultation Letter to Referring Physician

October 1, 19_____

W.F. Mayhan, MD
124 Medical Drive
San Francisco, CA 94119

Dear Doctor Mayhan:

Ms. Catherine Holmes was seen for neurological evaluation on September 28, 19_____.

She is a 21-year-old, white, right-handed, single, supermarket checker who complains of headaches.

The patient stated that on the evening of September 27, 19_____, she fell and struck the back of her head against an upholstered arm of a couch. She was not rendered unconscious but did have a headache afterwards. Nevertheless, the remainder of the evening passed uneventfully, and she did go to bed. The following morning she woke up and went to work. However, at approximately 10 o'clock she had the onset of a relatively severe headache with a feeling that her ears were popping and her eyes were glassy. In addition, she felt very fatigued. She complained of some nausea but did not progress to any vomiting. She took aspirin, which has given her some degree of relief.

At the time of her examination, the patient was continuing to complain of a mild headache, but one that was not severe. She did feel extremely tired and felt that she wished to rest at home. Approximately 1 year ago the patient did have a concussion; however, she was not hospitalized and suffered no long-term adverse effects. She denies any history of other neurological or general medical problems. She did have eye surgery a number of years ago for an extraocular muscle imbalance. She denied any history of surgery, fractures, or allergies. She smokes approximately a package of cigarettes per day and occasionally partakes of wine. Currently she is taking birth control medication, but no other agents.

Family history reveals her father to be suffering from hypertension. Her mother died approximately a year ago at the age of 46 from a cerebral hemorrhage, which, from her description, may have been a ruptured aneurysm. While speaking of her mother, the patient did become quite tearful.

EXAMINATION: The examination revealed a well-developed, well-nourished, white female. She was in no acute distress. She was alert, oriented, and cooperative.

Cranial nerve examination was normal. Deep tendon reflexes were active and symmetrical. Plantar responses were downgoing.

Motor testing showed no upper extremity drift. No other evidence of gross or focal motor weakness was noted.

Sensory testing was intact to pinprick as well as vibratory sensation. Romberg test was negative.

Cerebellar testing showed no incoordination or decomposition of movements.

The patient's gait was normal for all modalities including heel, toe, and tandem. No cranial or carotid bruits were heard. There was a full range of motion to her head and neck. Blood pressure was 100/60, right arm, sitting.

IMPRESSION: Status 1 day after head injury.

DISCUSSION: Currently, this patient's neurological examination is unremarkable. She does complain of a residual headache that is the result of the blow she received to her head the evening before this examination. Currently she is feeling better with very minimal symptomatic treatment, and it is quite possible that this will resolve without any further aggressive management. I have given her a prescription for Darvocet-N 50 mg in the event her headache recurs or becomes more severe. In addition, I have indicated to her that if further difficulties arise, she should again contact us.

Thank you for giving me the opportunity to meet this very nice patient.

With best personal regards,

E. Schroeder, MD

REVIEW QUESTIONS

1. Information gathered on a history and physical examination is used for varied purposes. List four of these purposes.
2. List and define the six parts of a patient's history.
3. The following information has been obtained from physician's notes. For each statement, indicate the correct component of the patient's record where this information would be recorded. Choose your answers from the following headings: chief complaint; history of present illness; past history; family history; social or occupational history; review of systems; physical examination; and impression.
   a. The patient is a 25-year-old white obese female who was in good health until approximately 10 PM last evening.
   b. There is no history of past operations.
   c. Neck: thyroid is not enlarged.
   d. Head: there is no history of headaches, sinus pain, or trauma.
   e. The arteries are full, soft, and readily compressible.
   f. "I have a lump in my left breast."
   g. Patient had measles and chickenpox when she was a child.
   h. R/O diabetes.
   i. There is decreased muscle tone in all four extremities.
   j. Patient's father has a history of hypertension for 5 years.
   k. GU system: There is no history of dysuria, hematuria, frequency, or nocturia.
   l. The patient denies the use of alcohol, tobacco, and drugs of any kind.

4. Define the following methods of examination, and state one body part or system that is examined in each method.
   a. Inspection
   b. Percussion
   c. Palpation
   d. Auscultation
   e. Mensuration
5. Describe the difference between the ROS and the PE.
6. List five forms of treatment that may be used for the care of a patient.
7. List three reasons why diagnostic studies are important for patient care.
8. State the purpose of the problem-oriented medical record.
9. List and explain the four parts of the problem-oriented medical record.

PERFORMANCE TEST

In a skills laboratory, a simulation of a job-like environment, the medical assistant student is to demonstrate knowledge and skill in obtaining identifying information and the medical history from a patient. The student may use a preprinted history form or make a list of questions that should be asked of the patient from the information presented in this unit. For these activities the student will need a person to play the role of the patient and the necessary supplies. Time limits for the performance of this procedure are to be assigned by the instructor.

Unit III

Preparing for and Assisting with Routine and Specialty Physical Examinations

COGNITIVE OBJECTIVES

On completion of Unit III, the medical assistant student should be able to apply the following cognitive objectives.

1. Define and pronounce the vocabulary terms listed.
2. State in summary form the medical assistant's responsibilities when assisting the physician during an examination of a patient.
3. List, identify, and state the function of each instrument commonly used during a complete physical examination, including rectal and vaginal examinations; a proctosigmoidoscopy; a neurological examination; an ear examination; an eye examination.
4. State two purposes for positioning a patient and three purposes for gowning and draping a patient for physical examinations.
5. State the purpose of and discuss the following special examinations: neurological; ear; eye; obstetrical; and breast self-examination.
6. Discuss the American Cancer Society's guidelines for examinations for the early detection of cancer in people without symptoms.

TERMINAL PERFORMANCE OBJECTIVES

On completion of Unit III, the medical assistant should be able to meet the following terminal performance objectives:

1. Prepare a patient for a physical examination by providing clear, simple instructions and explanations that are easy to understand.
2. Position and drape a patient in the positions outlined in this unit.
3. Select, identify, and prepare for use equipment and supplies required for:
   - Complete physical examination, which is to include a rectal examination and a pelvic examination with Papanicolaou smear
   - Proctosigmoidoscopy
4. Demonstrate correct assisting techniques during physical examinations.
5. Assist the patient before, during, and after the examination.
6. Record the procedures and results (when applicable) of physical examinations.
7. Measure the patient's distance visual acuity using the Snellen eye chart.

The student is to perform the above skills with 100% accuracy 90% of the time (9 out of 10 times).

Vocabulary

bimanual (bi-man'u-al)—With both hands, as bimanual palpation.

bronchoscopy (bron-kos'kō-pī)—Internal inspection of the tracheobronchial tree with the use of a bronchoscope; used for diagnostic or treatment purposes. For diagnosis, the physician will inspect the interior of the bronchi and may obtain a sample of secretions or a biopsy of tissue; for treatment, foreign bodies or mucus plugs that may be causing an obstruction to the air passages can be located and removed.

cystoscopy (sis-tos'kop-ī)—Internal examination of the bladder with a cystoscope. Samples of urine for diagnostic purposes can be obtained by passing a catheter through the cystoscope into the bladder or beyond, up into the ureters and kidneys. Also, radiopaque dyes may be injected through the cystoscope into the bladder or up into the ureters when taking x-ray films of the urinary tract.

digital (dij'it-al)—The use of a finger to insert into a body cavity, such as the rectum, for palpating the tissue.

endoscopy (en-dos'ko-pī)—Visual examination of internal cavities of the body with an endoscope, for example, a proctoscope, bronchoscope, cystoscope, gastroscope, and laryngoscope.

gastroscopy (gas'tros'ko-pĭ)—Internal inspection of the stomach with a gastroscope.

objective symptom—A symptom that is apparent to the observer; also called a sign, for example, rash, swelling.

oral examination—Examination pertaining to the mouth.

Papanicolaou smear or test (pap"ah-nik"o-la'oo) —A smear examined microscopically to detect cancer cells from body excretions (urine and feces), secretions (vaginal fluids, sputum, or prostatic fluid), or tissue scrapings (as obtained from the stomach or uterus); most commonly done on a cervical scraping to detect abnormal or cancerous cells in the mucus of the uterus and cervix. This test is often referred to as a Pap smear or test.

pelvic examination—Examination of the external and internal female reproductive organs.

physical signs—Objective manifestations of disease that are apparent on a physical examination; observable changes representing alterations resulting from a disease or dysfunction in the body (see also sign).

prodrome—An early symptom, indicating the onset of a disease, such as an achy feeling before having the flu.

roentgenological (rĕnt-gĕn-ŏl'ŏj-i-cal)—Pertaining to an examination with the use of x-ray film (radiographs).

sign—Any objective evidence (apparent to the observer) of disease or body dysfunction. Signs may be observed by others or revealed when a physician performs a physical examination; examples include swollen ankles, a distended rigid abdomen, elevated blood pressure, decreased sensation (see also physical sign).

symptom—Any subjective evidence of disease or body dysfunction; a change in the physical or mental state of the body that is perceptible or apparent only to the individual; examples include anorexia, nausea, headache, pain, itching.

syndrome—A combination of symptoms resulting from one cause or commonly occurring together to present a distinct clinical picture; an example is the dumping syndrome, which consists of nausea, weakness, varying degrees of syncope, sweating, palpitation, and sometimes diarrhea and a feeling of warmth. This may occur immediately after eating in patients who have had a partial gastrectomy.

subjective symptoms—Symptoms of internal origin that are apparent or perceptible only to the patient; examples include pain, dizziness (vertigo).

symmetry (sĭm'ĕt-rĭ)—Correspondence in form, size, and arrangement of parts on opposite sides of the body.

Instruments Used for Physical Examinations (Fig. 3-1)

anoscope (an'no-skōp)—A speculum or endoscope inserted into the anal canal for direct visual examination.

applicator—A slender rod of glass or wood with a pledget of cotton on one end used to apply medicine or to take a culture from the body.

biopsy (bi'op-se) **forceps**—Two-pronged instruments of varying sizes and shapes used to remove tissue from the body for examination.

bronchoscope (brong'ko-skōp)—An endoscope designed specifically for passage through the trachea to allow visual examination of the interior of the tracheobronchial tree.

cystoscope (sist'o-skōp)—A hollow metal tube instrument (endoscope) designed specifically for passing through the urethra into the urinary bladder to permit internal inspection. The bladder interior is illuminated by an electric bulb at the end of the cystoscope. Special lenses and mirrors allow the bladder mucosa to be examined for calculi (stones), inflammation, or tumors.

endoscope (en'do-skōp)—A specially designed instrument made of metal, rubber, or glass that is used for direct visual examination of hollow organs or body cavities. All endoscopes have similar working elements, even though the design will vary according to its specific use. The viewing part (scope) is a hollow tube fitted with a lens system that allows viewing in a variety of directions. Each endoscope has a light source, power cord, and power source; examples include bronchoscope, cystoscope, proctoscope, and sigmoidoscope.

insufflator (in'suf-fla-tor)—An instrument, device, or bag used for blowing air, powder, or gas into a cavity.

laryngeal (lar-in'je-al) **mirror**—An instrument used to view the pharynx and larynx, consisting of a small rounded mirror attached to the end of a slender (metal or chrome plate) handle.

laryngoscope (lar-in'go-skōp)—An endoscope used to examine the larynx. It is equipped with mirrors and a light for illumination of the larynx.

nasal speculum (na'zl spĕk'ū-lŭm)—A short, funnel-like instrument used to examine the nasal cavity.

ophthalmoscope (ŏf-thăl'mō-skōp)—An instrument used for examining the interior parts of the eye. It contains a perforated mirror and lens. When the ophthalmoscope is turned on and

(*Text continues on p. 66*)

Fig. 3-1. Instruments used for physical examinations. (Line drawings courtesy Miltex Instrument Co., Division of Miltenberg, Inc., Lake Success, NY)

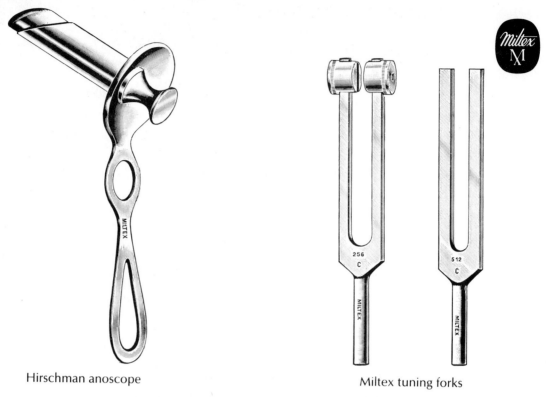

Hirschman anoscope

Miltex tuning forks

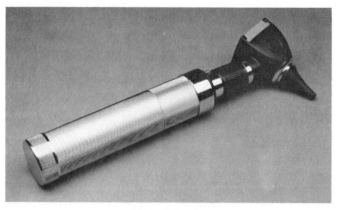

Otoscope

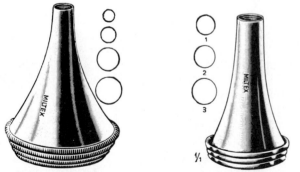

Boucheron and Toynbee ear specula to be used with an otoscope

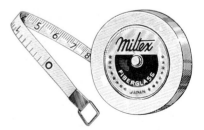

Miltex fiberglass tape measure

Fig. 3-1 *(continued)*

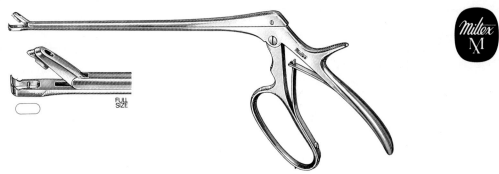

Tischler cervical biopsy punch forceps

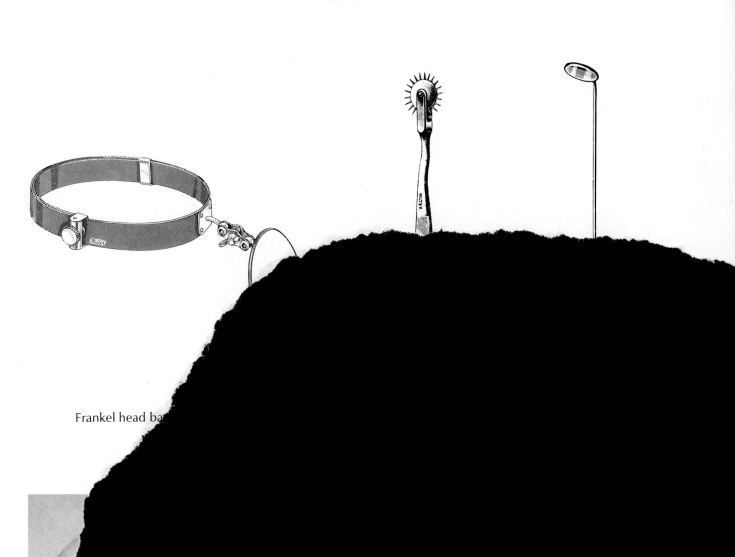

Frankel head ba

Fig. 3-1   *(continued)*

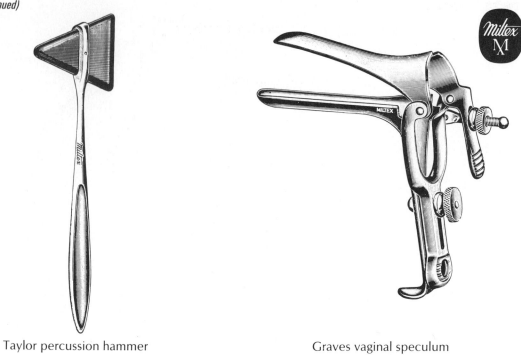

Taylor percussion hammer

Graves vaginal speculum

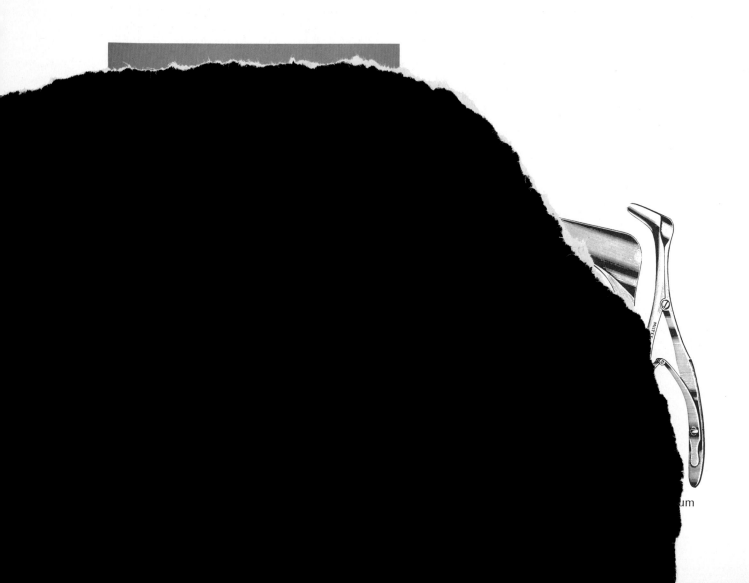

um

Fig. 3-1 *(continued)*

Schiotz tonometers

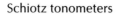

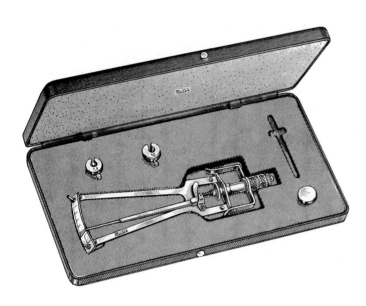

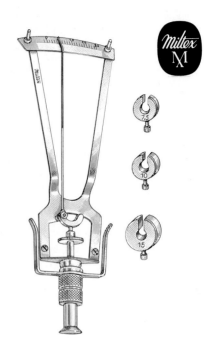

Original model with 3 weights (5.5, 7.5, and 10 g), plunger, footplate, and test block

Improved model with 4 weights (5.5, 7.5, 10, and 15 g), mirror insert on scale reduces error of parallax

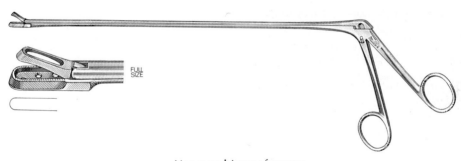

Yeoman biopsy forceps

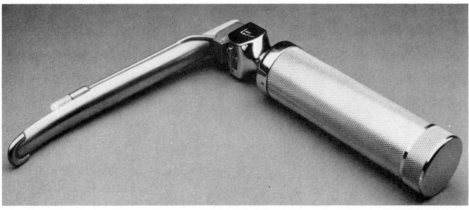

Laryngoscope

brought close to the eye, it sends a narrow, bright beam of light through the lens of the eye. By looking through the lens of the instrument, the physician is then able to examine the interior parts of the eye, including the lens, anterior chamber, retinal structures, and blood vessels, to detect any possible disorders. Many ophthalmoscopes come with an interchangeable otoscope, throat illuminator head, or nasal illuminator head.

otoscope (ō'tō-skōp)—An instrument used to examine the external ear canal and eardrum.

percussion (pur-kush'un) **hammer**—A small hammer with a triangular-shaped rubber head used for percussion.

proctoscope (prŏk'tō-skōp)—A specially designed tubular endoscope that is passed through the anus to permit internal inspection of the lower part of the large intestine.

sigmoidoscope (sĭg-moy'dō-skōp)—A tubular endoscope used to examine the interior of the sigmoid colon.

speculum (spĕk'ū-lŭm)—An instrument used for distending or opening a body cavity or orifice to allow visual inspection; a bivalve speculum is one having two parts or valves.

Sims vaginal speculum—A form of bivalve speculum used in the examination of the vagina and cervix.

stethoscope—An instrument used in auscultation to amplify the sounds produced by the lungs, heart, intestines, and other internal organs; also used when taking a blood pressure reading (see pp. **21**).

tongue blade—A flat, thin, smooth piece of wood or metal with rounded ends approximately 6 inches long; also called a tongue depressor. It is used for pressing tissue down to permit a better view when examining the mouth and throat. In addition, it may be used for application of ointments to the skin.

tonometer (to-nom'e-ter)—An instrument used to measure tension or pressure, especially intraocular pressure.

tuning fork—A steel, two-pronged, fork-like instrument used for testing hearing; the prongs give off a musical note when struck.

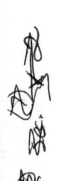

PREPARING FOR AND ASSISTING WITH PHYSICAL EXAMINATIONS

The physical examination is done in an examination or treatment room, whereas frequently the history is obtained from the patient in the physician's private office.

This unit covers gowning, positioning, and draping the patient for an examination, and preparing for and assisting with the common examinations performed by a physician—outlining *one* way in which examinations are conducted and listing *one* group of instruments and equipment for each. The physician(s) or agency for whom you work may utilize other methods and equipment; therefore, you must be able and willing to adapt to individual needs as required.

General instructions and responsibilities for medical assistants when assisting with examinations are given before the procedures. These instructions should be followed in every procedure that requires your assistance. Keep them in mind as you are preparing for all examinations, as they are not repeated in each individual procedure.

Frequently, during any of the examinations that are outlined in this unit, various types of specimens may be obtained. Detailed information for collecting and labeling specimens will be covered in Unit VI.

Cleansing and sterilization techniques to be utilized in the care of used, nondisposable equipment will be discussed in Unit IV. It is suggested that you refer to these units for more specific information.

GENERAL INSTRUCTIONS AND RESPONSIBILITIES FOR THE MEDICAL ASSISTANT

1. Always wash your hands thoroughly before setting up the required equipment for an examination and assisting the physician.
2. Prepare the patient, the examination room, and the equipment and instruments required by the physician for the examination according to office or agency policy.
3. Make certain that electrical and battery-operated equipment and all lights are in working condition.
4. Place the equipment for the examination so that it is conveniently located for the physician's use.
5. Check to make sure that the examination room is comfortably warm, well aired, and spotlessly clean.
6. Cover the examination table with a clean cover, either a cotton or muslin sheet, crepe paper, or a covered rubber sheet on the lower part of the table. A towel may be placed over a pillow at the end of the table.
7. Assist the patient as required. Have a sturdy step-stool for the patient to use when getting on and off the examining table. Offer support; guard against falling. Never leave a confused patient or a child alone on the examining table because of the danger of falling.
8. Assist the physician as required. You must learn the physician's methods and preferences for each examination.
9. Never expose the patient unnecessarily. Only

those parts of the body being examined are to be exposed.

10. A female assistant should remain in the room if the patient is female and the physician is male. Your presence may not only help the anxious patient to feel more relaxed, but it also protects the physician from unwarranted lawsuits. There can be no false allegations if you, as the witness, observe the entire examination.

11. Observe the patient for various types of reactions. A change in facial expression may indicate that the patient is apprehensive or experiencing pain. Note any unusual weakness, change in breathing pattern, change in skin color, or fainting. Your observations may provide the physician with important information that will help make a diagnosis and provide treatment for the patient.

12. Inform the patient of any special instructions. When the physician has completed the examination, inform the patient that he or she is free to leave after getting dressed, or if required, to check at the front desk to schedule a future appointment or a laboratory or x-ray examination. Often the physician requests that certain tests be run or specimens be gathered. Some offices and agencies have a printed sheet on which the physician can check each test that is to be performed on the patient. The medical assistant would make the proper arrangements, notify the technologist, or collect the specimens requested before the patient leaves.

13. Handle specimens obtained according to office or agency policy.

14. On completion of the examination, carry out your responsibilities for the disposal, cleansing, disinfecting, or sterilizing of the used equipment and the treatment room to prevent the spread of microorganisms.

15. Record findings from the examination accurately and completely. Use correct medical abbreviations, when applicable, in recording all information. Most physicians will record all the necessary information on the patient's chart, so frequently this will not be one of the medical assistant's responsibilities. The policy regarding this will vary and will be established by the physician or agency for whom you work. If it is your responsibility the following items are usually to be included:
    • Date, time, and type of examination and the findings/results, when applicable.
    • Name of the examiner.
    • If specimens were obtained, the type, how they were handled, the test(s) to be performed
    • Any pertinent observations that you have made that will help describe the patient's general condition. Be specific in the type of information you record; for example, patient com-

plained of slight nausea and a transient pain in the right lower abdominal quadrant.
    • Future directions given to the patient.
    • Your signature.

GOWNING, POSITIONING, AND DRAPING THE PATIENT FOR PHYSICAL EXAMINATIONS

A physical examination is facilitated by the use of an examining table and proper gowning, positioning, and draping of the patient. The purposes of positioning a patient are

• To allow for better visibility and accessibility for the physician during the examination of the patient
• To provide support for the patient when being examined

The purposes of gowning and draping the patient are

• To avoid unnecessary exposure of the patient's body during an examination, thereby protecting the patient's modesty
• To contribute to the patient's feeling of being cared for, which helps the patient relax
• To provide some comfort and warmth and to avoid chilling

The principle of gowning and draping is that only the part of the body that is being examined should be exposed, other than the head, arms and sometimes the legs, and only when the physician is about to begin the examination.

There are different positions used for various types of examinations. In all positions the patient must be well supported, as most positions are uncomfortable and difficult to maintain for any length of time. The position chosen will depend on the type of examination or procedure to be performed, and on the patient's age, sex, and physical and emotional condition. The various positions used most frequently in a general or special physical examination are presented along with the instructions for gowning, positioning, and draping the patient.

Equipment

Examination table
Patient gown, either cotton or disposable paper
Paper or sheet to cover the table
Small towel, cloth or paper
Small pillow
Drape sheet; two drape sheets are needed for the jackknife and Trendelenburg positions
Stirrups on the examining table for the lithotomy position
A binder to support the patient on the table when placed in the Trendelenburg position

Dorsal-Recumbent and Lithotomy Positions

In the lithotomy position the patient's feet are placed in stirrups that are raised approximately 12 inches from table level, although the stirrups on some examining tables cannot be elevated. These positions are used almost exclusively for pelvic, bladder, and rectal examinations (Figs. 3-2 and 3-3).

- The patient lies on the back with the legs separated and flexed.
- The feet are supported in stirrups, or the soles of the feet are flat on the table.
- The buttocks are brought to the edge of the examining table.
- The arms are placed either at the side or crossed over the chest or under the head.

Fig. 3-2. Dorsal-recumbent position.

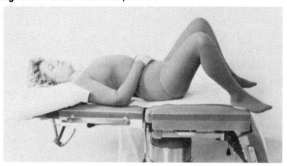

Fig. 3-3. Lithotomy position.

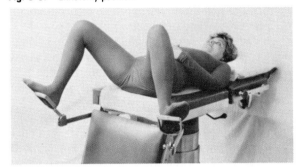

Procedure	Rationale
1. Place clean paper or sheet on the examination table.	
2. Identify the patient and explain the procedure.	The medical assistant must explain what is required and why it is necessary in order to gain full cooperation from the patient. Clear explanations also help reassure the patient.
3. Have the patient disrobe and put on the patient gown.	For a pelvic examination the patient should disrobe from the waist down. For a pelvic and breast examination, the patient should disrobe completely and put the gown on with the opening in the front.
4. Have the patient lie down on the table; place a small pillow under the head.	Help make the patient as comfortable as possible.
5. Cover the patient with a drape sheet, placing it in a rectangular arrangement.	One point of the sheet faces the patient's neck and covers the chest; the opposite corner is placed between the legs or feet. The other corners extend over the sides of the patient.
6. Have the patient move buttocks down to the extreme edge of the table with knees flexed and the feet firmly on the table, or at table level in stirrups.	
7. Place a small towel under the buttocks.	This will catch any discharge that may be excreted from the patient's body.
8. Have the patient cross arms under the head or over the chest, or place along the sides of the body.	
9. Take the lateral corners of the sheet and wrap them around the feet in a spiral fashion.	
10. When the examination begins, the corner of the sheet that covers the perineum is pulled back and upward toward the abdomen to expose the perineal area. Place this part of the sheet neatly over the patient's abdomen.	Avoid letting the sheet fall over the perineum, as it would obstruct the physician's examination.

Procedure	Rationale
11. If you are to position the patient in the lithotomy position, the same procedure is followed, *except* that the patient's legs are to be elevated in the stirrups.	In this position the lateral corners of the sheet are wrapped around the legs and feet that are supported in the stirrups. The stirrups will generally be raised at least 1 foot above table level and positioned to the sides of the table so that the knees are placed sufficiently apart to allow exposure of the perineum.

Jackknife or Proctological Position

The patient lies on the abdomen with both the head and legs lowered, so that the buttocks are elevated. Arms are placed along the side of the head.

This position is used for rectal examinations and occasionally for surgery. A special examining table that can be adjusted to facilitate this position is required (Fig. 3-4).

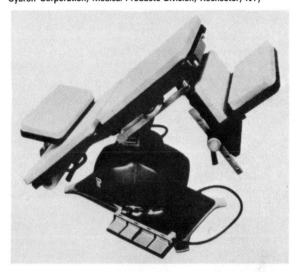

Fig. 3-4. The Ritter "75" Table raises, lowers, tilts, and rotates 315 degrees at the touch of your toe on the foot control. (Courtesy Sybron Corporation, Medical Products Division, Rochester, NY)

Procedure	Rationale
1. Place clean paper or sheet on table and a small towel over the area of the table where it will be split.	The small towel will help soak up any discharge that may be excreted from the patient during the examination, and can be removed or folded over before the patient gets up.
2. Identify the patient and explain the procedure.	This will help put the patient at ease somewhat and gain cooperation.
3. Have the patient disrobe completely and put on patient gown with the opening in the back.	If only a rectal exam is to be done, a female may leave her bra on.
4. Have the patient lie on the table and roll over onto the abdomen.	
5. The table is split so that the patient's head and legs are lowered, and the buttocks are elevated. Arms may be placed under the head or stretched out in front of the head.	The patient's legs are braced against the lowered part of the table. Good support is required, as this position is difficult to maintain.
6. Place a small pillow under the patient's head.	Make the patient as comfortable as possible.
7. Cover the patient's body with one sheet, and put another sheet over the legs.	Do not bind the legs together, as frequently it is necessary for them to be separated for proper examination.
8. When the examination begins, the lower part of the sheet covering the patient's body is drawn back, and folded over the lumbar region.	This exposes only the rectal region, which will be examined, and maintains the patient's modesty as well as can be expected.

Knee-Chest Position

The patient rests on the knees and chest, with the head turned to one side. Arms may be placed under the head to partially help support the patient. Buttocks extend up in the air, and the back is straight.

This position is used for the rectal examination and sometimes for vaginal and prostatic examinations (Fig. 3-5).

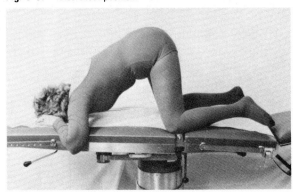

Fig. 3-5. Knee-chest position.

Procedure	Rationale
1. Place clean paper or sheet on the table.	
2. Identify the patient and explain the procedure.	This helps reassure the patient and helps the patient understand what to expect and the reason for assuming this position.
3. Have the patient disrobe and put on the patient gown.	The opening of the gown should be in the back.
4. Have the patient kneel on the table, keeping the buttocks elevated and back straight.	The patient will also be resting on the chest in this position. A small pillow may be placed under the chest for support and comfort.
5. Have the patient turn the head to one side.	
6. The arms should be flexed at the elbow and extended, placing them under or near the side of the head.	This helps support the patient.
7. Cover the patient's body with a drape sheet, and place a smaller drape sheet over the legs.	The patient should be fully draped.
8. When the examination begins, the drape sheet is pulled back and folded over the top of the buttocks.	This will expose only the rectal and vaginal areas, which are to be examined.

Sims or Left Lateral Position

The patient lies on the left side and chest, with the left leg slightly flexed and the right leg sharply flexed on the abdomen.

The left arm is drawn behind the body with the body inclining forward.

The right arm is positioned forward according to the patient's comfort.

The buttocks are brought up to the long edge of the table.

This position is used frequently for rectal examinations and when giving enemas. The vagina and abdomen can also be examined in this position, and it may be used for older women when the lithotomy position is too difficult to maintain (Fig. 3-6).

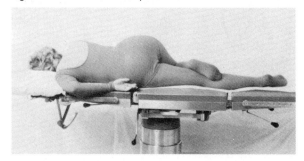

Fig. 3-6. Sims or left lateral position.

Procedure	Rationale
1. Place clean paper or sheet over table.	
2. Identify the patient, and explain the procedure.	This provides the patient with some understanding of why this position is to be assumed, thus enabling the patient to cooperate.
3. Have the patient disrobe completely and put on the patient gown.	The opening of the patient gown should be in the back.
4. Instruct the patient to lie down on the table, then to roll over onto the left side and chest, moving the buttocks up to the long edge of the table.	You may help the patient assume this position properly by placing your hand along the long side of the table, so that the patient's buttocks will touch your hand when they are over to the side far enough.
5. The left arm is drawn behind the body with the body inclining forward. The right arm is positioned in front of the body for support and where it is most comfortable for the patient.	
6. Place a small pillow under the patient's head. One may also be placed under or near the chest.	Provide comfort and support for the patient.
7. Instruct the patient to flex the right leg sharply over the abdomen, and to flex the left leg slightly.	This position provides good access to the anal canal, rectum, and sigmoid colon.
8. Place a small towel under the buttocks.	This will catch any discharge and can be removed before the patient gets up.
9. Cover the patient with the drape sheet.	
10. When the examination begins, fold back the drape sheet so that only the anal and vaginal areas are exposed.	

Trendelenburg Position

In the Trendelenburg (trĕn-dĕl'ĕn-burg) position, the patient lies on the back with the head lower than the rest of the body. The body is elevated at an angle of about 45 degrees, and the knees are flexed over the lower section of the examining table, which is lowered. The patient should be well supported to prevent slipping.

This position is not used routinely for an office examination, but often is used in the operating and x-ray rooms. It displaces the intestines into the upper abdomen.

An alternate form of the Trendelenburg position is one in which the patient's body is placed on an incline with the feet elevated at an angle of 45° and the head lowered. One may use this position to prevent shock or when the patient is in a state of shock or has low blood pressure. It is also used for some abdominal surgery. Some physicians will have the patient positioned in the Sims position along with this form of the Trendelenburg position for rectal examinations (Fig. 3-7).

Fig. 3-7. Trendelenburg positions.

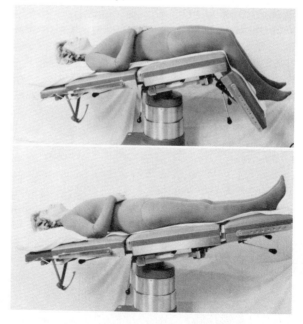

Trendelenburg Position (*continued*)

Procedure	Rationale
1. Place clean paper or sheet on the examining or x-ray table.	
2. Identify the patient and explain the procedure.	This enables the patient to understand the need for this position and what to expect. Your caring attitude will also help reassure the patient.
3. Have the patient disrobe and put on the patient gown.	Have the opening of the gown in the front.
4. Assist the patient onto the table and instruct the patient to assume a supine position. Place a small pillow under the head.	Make the patient as comfortable as possible.
5. Instruct the patient to cross arms over the chest region or place alongside the body.	
6. Cover the patient from the shoulders to the feet with a drape sheet.	
7. Support the patient with a binder to prevent slipping.	This will be placed over the abdominal region and secured to both sides of the table.
8. Adjust the examining table.	The body is on an inclined plane with the head slightly lowered. In the operating room the knees will be flexed over the lower end of the table. In the x-ray room, the table is raised so that the head is lowered and the feet are elevated. Feet and legs are straight.

Supine Position

The patient lies flat on the back, arms placed at the side, and head elevated slightly on a pillow. This position is used for examinations of the abdomen, breasts, some surgical and x-ray procedures, and on occasion for examination of the chest (Fig. 3-8).

Prone Position

The patient lies flat on the abdomen, arms flexed under the head, which is turned to one side. It may be used in examinations of the back in musculoskeletal and neurological examinations, and for some surgical procedures (Fig. 3-9).

Fowler's Position

The patient is sitting up. This position is used for examining the head, ears, eyes, nose and throat, neck, chest, and breasts (Fig. 3-10).

Semi-Fowler's Position

The patient is lying in a supine position, with the head of the table or bed raised 18 to 20 inches above the level of the feet. This may be used rather than the supine or Fowler positions when the comfort and physical condition of the patient require it, such as a patient with dyspnea (Fig. 3-11).

Fig. 3-8. Supine position.

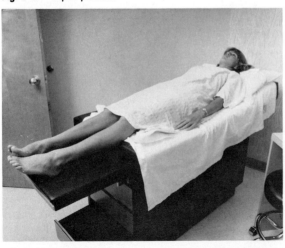

Fig. 3-9. Prone position.

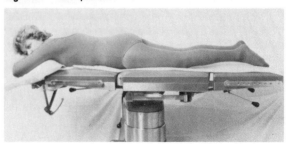

Fig. 3-10. Fowler's (sitting) position.

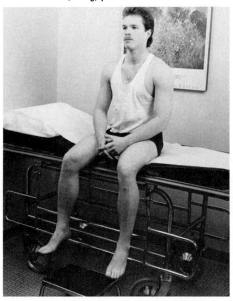

Fig. 3-12. Standing position.

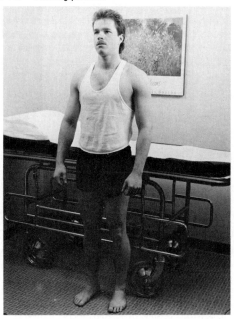

Erect or Standing Position

The patient stands erect with arms down at the sides, feet facing forward. This position is used for part of a neurological and musculoskeletal examination and also during some x-ray procedures (Fig. 3-12).

The following instructions apply to positioning and draping the patient in the supine, prone, Fowler's, and semi-Fowler's positions.

1. Provide the patient with a gown. Depending on the examination to be performed, the patient should be instructed to disrobe completely; at times the patient may leave underpants on. If the chest is to be examined, it is advisable to instruct the patient to put the gown on with the opening in the front, as this provides for comfort and easier accessibility to this region during the examination.

Fig. 3-11. Semi-Fowler's position.

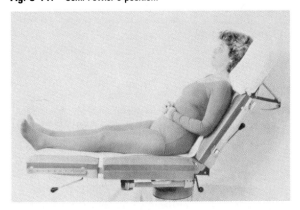

2. Instruct and assist the patient in assuming the correct position as required.
3. Place a drape sheet over the midtrunk and legs.
4. When the examination begins, the drape sheet may be folded back to expose the area on the body that will be examined.

PROCEDURE FOR A COMPLETE PHYSICAL EXAMINATION

Equipment

The exact amount and type of equipment to be assembled for a physical examination will depend on the following:

Purpose of the examination
Type and extent of the examination
Preferences of the physician
Condition of the patient

In some physician's offices and agencies, the equipment required for examinations will be kept on a special tray ready for use and in a central location. In others it may be necessary for you to assemble all the equipment that will be needed.

Although there are differences among physicians and agencies, the following list includes items that are commonly used, and should be available, ready for use (Fig. 3-13):

Examination table covered with a clean sheet
Patient gown, either cloth or paper

Fig. 3-13. Instruments and supplies commonly used for a physical examination. *Left to right:* nasal speculum, laryngeal mirror, otoscope *(top)* and ophthalmoscope *(bottom)* attachments with battery-operated handle, tuning fork, percussion hammer, vaginal speculum, anoscope, sponge stick (forceps) with sponge. *Top left corner:* tongue blade, cotton-tipped applicators.

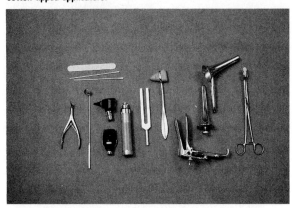

Draping material, drape sheet, small towel
Watch with a second hand
Stethoscope
Thermometer
Sphygmomanometer
Scale with height measure rod
Tape measure
Tuning fork
Percussion or reflex hammer
Tongue blades
Laryngeal mirror
Head mirror
Flashlight and/or gooseneck lamp
Otoscope
Ophthalmoscope
Nasal speculum
Safety pin
Tissues
Cotton balls

Alcohol or prepackaged alcohol swabs
Urine specimen bottle
Laboratory request form
X-ray request form
Emesis basin or waste container used for soiled equipment and/or waste

Additional equipment is required for a visual acuity test, vaginal, and rectal examinations. This will vary with the purpose of the examination, the condition of the patient, and the physician's preference.

Visual acuity test
 A Snellen eye chart is used most frequently to measure distance visual acuity.
Vaginal examination
 Vaginal speculum
 Sterile rubber gloves
 Lubricant, such as K-Y jelly
 Uterine sponge or uterine dressing forceps
 Sponges
 Two glass slides for smears; or one glass slide and one sterile culture tube with applicator
 Cotton-tipped applicators or wooden cervical spatulas
 Fixative spray or cytology jar with solution
 Plastic container for slides if using the fixative spray
 Laboratory request form
Rectal examination
 Rectal glove or sterile rubber gloves or rubber finger cot
 Lubricant, such as K-Y jelly
 Rectal speculum, proctoscope, or anoscope (depending on the extent of the examination)
 Tissues
 Sponge forceps
 Sponges
 Cotton-tipped applicators

Procedure	Rationale
1. Wash your hands.	
2. Assemble and prepare the necessary equipment for the physician.	Equipment is to be arranged on a table or tray covered with a clean towel.
3. Identify the patient, and explain the procedure.	An explanation allows the patient to understand what will be done, that is, what will occur, how it may feel, and how she or he can help in the examination. It also provides some reassurance for the patient.
4. Have the patient void in order to empty the bladder.	Instruct the patient how to collect a urine specimen if one is required (see pp. 196–198). When the bladder is full, it is difficult for the physician to palpate the abdomen adequately. It is also very uncomfortable for the patient to have a full bladder while being examined.
5. Take the following physical measurements and record accurately:	This will vary with your job requirements. At times the physician may wish to do these tests rather

Procedure	**Rationale**
TPR BP Height Weight	than have you do them. Height and weight should be taken after the patient removes shoes and heavy outer clothing.
6. Instruct the patient to disrobe completely and put on a patient gown with the opening in the front.	Gown donned with opening in the front permits access to the chest for examination while the shoulders and back are still covered.
7. Have the patient sit on the edge of the examining table with a towel under the buttocks. Place a drape sheet over the patient's lap.	
8. Call the doctor when the patient is ready and when you have all the necessary recordings completed and equipment assembled. The patient's chart should be given to the physician before the examination begins.	A female assistant should remain in the room if the patient is female and the physician is male, and/or if the physician requires your assistance when performing the examination (see p. 67, No. 10).
9. Assist the physician as required.	Depending on the physician's preference, you may have to be ready to hand up the instruments as needed. The physician will proceed with the examination from head to toe, examining the body systems and parts as described previously under the physical examination in Unit II.

Equipment
Tuning fork
Otoscope
Ophthalmoscope
Nasal speculum
Tongue blade
Flashlight
Head mirror
Laryngeal mirror
Stethoscope
Safety pin
Percussion hammer

Procedure	**Rationale**
10. While the patient is in a sitting position, the physician will examine the head, ears, eyes, nose, mouth, and throat; the neck and axillae; the chest, breasts, and heart; the neuromuscular reflexes and sensations, such as the pinprick; as well as a general observation of skin and body symmetry.	
11. When handing or accepting a tongue blade from the physician, hold it in the center. Break it at the center after use (without touching the end used) and then discard in the emesis basin or waste container.	By handling the tongue blade this way you avoid contamination to the patient and also to yourself.
12. Warm the laryngeal mirror by placing the mirrored end under warm running water or in a glass of warm water.	It must be warmed to prevent fogging. Be sure to dry it before it is used.
13. After step 10 is completed, the patient is to assume a supine position. Help the patient attain this position if necessary.	Give reassurance and support as needed. Often just placing your hand on the patient's shoulder or arm gives the patient a feeling of support and of being cared for.
14. Place the drape sheet to cover the patient from shoulders to feet. It can be moved down when the physician is ready to examine the breasts and abdomen. When the physician examines the breasts, fold the sheet down to the patient's waist, and open the patient's gown. When the abdomen is being examined, the patient's gown can be used to cover the breasts, and you are to fold the drape sheet down to the pubic hair line.	When the patient is in this position, the physician will palpate breasts, liver, spleen, and other abdominal organs. The groin will be checked for a possible hernia. The physician may use a stethoscope to listen to abdominal sounds as part of the examination of the abdomen.

Procedure for a Complete Physical Examination (*continued*)

Procedure	Rationale
15. For a vaginal and rectal examination, help the patient assume the correct position. Assist the physician as required.	Positions and procedures for these examinations are discussed next. Vaginal and rectal examinations are included in the complete physical examination of a female patient. For the male patient, the physician will examine the genitals, the rectum, and prostate gland.
16. Observe the patient for any unusual reactions, such as a feeling of weakness or pain, facial grimace, change in color.	
17. When the examination has been completed, the patient may sit up.	It may be advisable to allow the patient to remain in the supine position for a few minutes before getting up.
18. Check if patient has any questions to be answered.	Frequently a patient may have questions, but does not feel free to ask or may feel that there isn't time to do so.
19. Inform the patient of any special instructions (see No. 12, p. 67).	Frequently patients are left in the room after the examination not knowing if they are to talk further to the physician or are free to leave. Do not let this happen.
20. If necessary, help the patient dress; otherwise leave the room so that the patient may have some privacy.	
21. On returning to the examining room, assemble all used equipment and supplies to be disposed of properly.	Remove all linens and place in the soiled laundry. Place disposable equipment in a covered waste container. Take instruments to your cleanup area. Depending on the instrument and its requirements, you may rinse it with cool water, or wash or soak it in soap and water until you are ready to prepare it for sterilization or disinfection (see Unit IV). Others, such as the tuning fork, may be wiped off, then replaced in the usual storage area.
22. Resupply clean equipment as needed.	
23. Clean the examination table and put on a fresh cover.	
24. If smears or cultures were obtained, send them to the laboratory or place them in a refrigerator or a cool dark place until you can transfer them to the laboratory.	Make sure that specimens are properly labeled and that you have completely filled out the appropriate laboratory request form.
25. Wash your hands.	
26. Do any recording required of you completely and accurately (see No. 15, p. 67). Use accepted medical abbreviations when recording.	Charting example: Jan. 27, 19_____, 1 PM Complete physical examination done by Dr. Short. Patient referred to lab for a CBC (complete blood count) and UA (urinalysis) and to the x-ray department for a chest x-ray film. Patient to return in 1 week to discuss the results of these tests with the doctor. Ann O'Reilly, CMA

PELVIC EXAMINATION AND A PAPANICOLAOU SMEAR

Pelvic (vaginal) examinations and Papanicolaou (Pap) smears are essential for the adult female. Most general practitioners and internists as well as gynecologists and obstetricians will perform them routinely. These examinations, done for diagnostic purposes of the female reproductive system, include inspection of the vulva, vagina, and cervix for any abnormalities, and a bimanual palpation of the uterus, fallopian tubes, and ovaries. The physician notes the size, shape, position, and consistency of the uterus and whether any masses are present in the uterus, fallopian tubes, or ovaries. The purpose of the Pap smear is to detect precancerous conditions or any unusual cell growth and to detect cancer of the cervix or uterus. The value of the test is that it can detect potential problems early so that they can be treated.

You must instruct the patient not to put any creams or foams in the vagina, not to douche, and not to have sexual intercourse for 24 hours (some suggest 48 hours) before having a Pap smear taken. This is because any of these circumstances will interfere with the specimen obtained and make the test invalid. Also, a Pap smear must not be taken during the patient's menstrual period because the red blood cells will interfere with obtaining accurate findings.

The smear will be examined in the laboratory by a pathologist who will report the findings as one of five classifications that follow.

- Class I — Normal. Only normal cells are seen.
- Class II — Possibly abnormal. Some atypical cells are seen. These may be due to inflammation of the vagina or cervix.
- Class III — Abnormal. Mild dysplasia.
- Class IV — Abnormal. Severe dysplasia, suspicious cells.
- Class V — Abnormal. Carcinoma cells are seen.

When the Pap smear is abnormal it doesn't mean that the patient has cancer except if the findings were in Class V. Abnormal findings indicate the need for further diagnostic studies. Frequently a physician will first do a colposcopy. In this examination an instrument called a colposcope magnifies and focuses an intense light on the cervix. This allows the physician to observe the cervical anatomy in greater detail. If the colposcopy reveals an inflammatory process, a vaginal cream may be all that is needed for treatment. If the colposcopy reveals areas of abnormal tissues, the physician may use one or more diagnostic and therapeutic procedures which include a biopsy, cryosurgery, endocervical curettage, and possibly a cone biopsy or more extensive surgery. (Also see pp. 61 and 215.)

Equipment (Fig. 3-14)

Examination table (stirrups if available) covered with a clean sheet or paper
Patient gown
Drape sheet
Small towel
Small pillow
Gooseneck lamp
Vaginal speculum
Lubricant, such as K-Y jelly
Sterile rubber gloves
Uterine sponge or uterine dressing forceps
Sponges or cotton balls
Two glass slides for smears or one glass slide and one sterile culture tube with applicator
Two cotton-tipped applicators or wooden cervical spatulas
Fixative spray, such as Cyto-Fix, Spray-cyte; or cytology jar with solution; for example, 95% isopropyl alcohol solution is preferred, although formalin 10% may be used
Plastic container for slides when using the fixative spray
Tissues
Laboratory request form

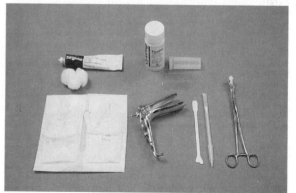

Fig. 3-14. Equipment for pelvic examination and Pap smear.

Procedure	Rationale
1. Wash your hands.	
2. Assemble and prepare the necessary instruments and equipment. Prepare the room.	Make sure the lamp is working and that there is a clean paper or sheet on the table.
3. Identify the patient. Explain the procedure, and reassure the patient.	An explanation gives the patient some understanding of the need for the examination and what to expect, that is, what will occur, how it may feel.
4. Have the patient empty her bladder.	Explain to the patient how to collect a specimen if a urinalysis is to be done.

Pelvic Examination and Papanicolaou Smear (*continued*)

Procedure	**Rationale**
5. You may be required to take the patient's pulse and blood pressure.	This is usually done if the woman is taking birth control pills; also frequently done routinely in many offices as a screening process for high BP.
6. Provide a patient gown, and have the patient remove all clothing from the waist down.	Shoes may be left on if the heels will fit into the stirrups.
7. Position the patient on the table in a dorsal-recumbent or lithotomy position and drape as explained previously. Remember to • Place the stirrups far enough out so the knees are apart; • Avoid exposing the patient unnecessarily; • Make sure that there is a small towel under the buttocks.	This will vary with the physician's preference and the patient's condition. The Sims position may also be used for a vaginal examination of an elderly woman.
8. Call the physician. NOTE: You may call the physician into the room and then have the patient assume the required position.	Remain in the room (refer to No. 10, p. 67).
9. Assist the physician as required. • Lower the foot of the examining table (if it is a table that splits), or push the foot piece in on newer model tables. • Pull back the drape sheet exposing *only* the perineal region.	If you do not have to assist the physician with the instruments and materials, give your attention to the patient. You may stand by the patient on one side and offer support and reassurance. Frequently support can be given just by having your hand placed gently on the patient's arm or shoulder.
10. Be prepared to hand the physician the various instruments and materials that may be needed. Some physicians will request that you put some K-Y jelly out on a gauze sponge; others will squeeze it out when they are ready to lubricate the rubber gloves and vaginal speculum. Direct the light on the area being examined.	The vaginal speculum may be warmed by running warm water over it. Alternatives used in some offices and agencies are to keep the instruments on a heating pad or in a warming pan. Other agencies use plastic disposable specula; warming these specula is not necessary.
11. If a smear is to be obtained, mark the patient's name on the slides and the cytology jar *or* on the container where they will be placed after using a fixative spray. Label the slides No. 1 and No. 2.	Paper clips should be attached to the ends of the slides to prevent them from sticking together if they are to be placed in a cytology jar with the isopropyl alcohol or formalin solution.
12. You may instruct the patient to breathe deeply through the mouth.	This helps relax muscles.
13. The *physician* will begin the examination. If a Pap smear is to be obtained, the *physician* will a. Insert a dry speculum into the vagina (Fig. 3-15). b. Open the speculum so that the cervix can be seen clearly. c. Insert a cotton-tipped applicator or wooden vaginal spatula and draw it across the cervix to obtain a specimen, which is then smeared evenly and moderately thinly across the No. 1 glass slide (Fig. 3-16). d. Insert another applicator or spatula and draw it across the posterior fornices or pools of the vaginal canal to obtain a second specimen, which is then smeared	NOTE: (a) If a smear is *not* to be obtained, the speculum would be lubricated for easier insertion into the vagina. Steps (c) through (e) would then be omitted. NOTE: Frequently an endocervical smear is more desirable than one obtained from the posterior vaginal pool. In this case, the physician would insert an applicator into the cervical os, rotating

Fig. 3-15. Procedure for vaginal examination. **A,** opening of the introitus. **B,** oblique insertion of the speculum. **C,** final insertion of the speculum. **D,** opening of the speculum blades. (From L. Malasanos, V. Barkauskas, M. Moss, and K. Stoltenberg-Allen, *Health Assessment,* St. Louis, 1977. The C.V. Mosby Co.)

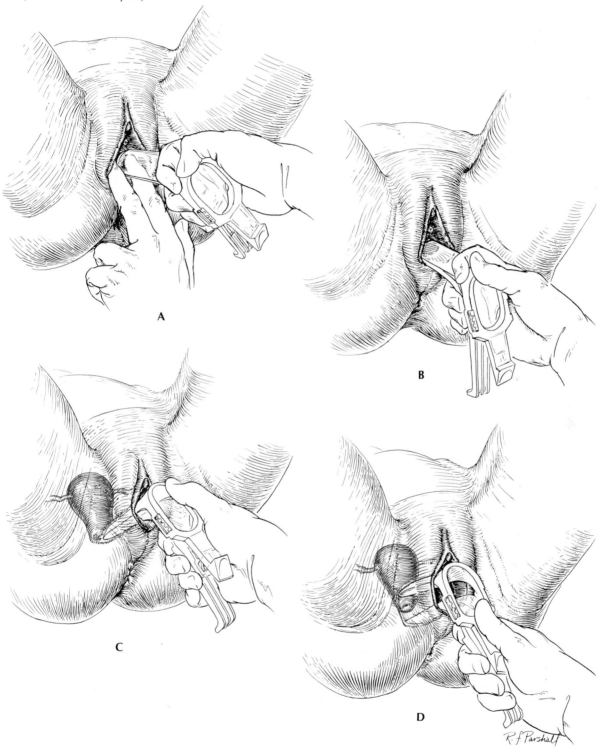

Pelvic Examination and Papanicolaou Smear (*continued*)

Procedure	Rationale
evenly and moderately across the No. 2 glass slide. If the material is spread too thickly, it will be difficult for the laboratory worker to visualize individual cells.	it completely around the os until the cotton is saturated. A smear is then prepared with this specimen (Fig. 3-17).

Procedure

evenly and moderately across the No. 2 glass slide. If the material is spread too thickly, it will be difficult for the laboratory worker to visualize individual cells.

e. Place these two slides immediately (within 4 seconds to prevent drying and death of cells) into the cytology jar with solution, or spray them thoroughly with the cytological fixative spray and place them in the designated container after the fixative has dried thoroughly (drying takes about 5 to 10 minutes).

f. Remove the speculum, and place in an area designated for used equipment.

g. Apply lubricant to the gloved index finger of the dominant hand.

h. Insert the gloved, lubricated finger into the vagina to palpate internaly for any abnormalities such as displacement or growths of the uterus, cervix, ovaries, and fallopian tubes. Place the other hand on the patient's abdomen and apply pressure so that the movable abdominal organs may be felt more easily during this bimanual examination (Fig. 3-20).

Rationale

it completely around the os until the cotton is saturated. A smear is then prepared with this specimen (Fig. 3-17).

NOTE: The *medical assistant* may be required to hold the slide while the physician smears the specimen on the slide and then spray the slide with the cytological fixative spray. When spraying the slides hold the nozzle of the can at least 5 to 6 inches away from the slide and spray lightly from left to right and then from right to left (Fig. 3-18). Allow the slides to dry thoroughly before placing them in the designated container for transport to an outside laboratory (Fig. 3-19).

NOTE: These slides will be sent with a properly labeled cytology laboratory request form to the laboratory for cytological examination. Enter the following on the request form:
- Date
- Physician's name and address
- Patient's name and age
- Source of specimen
- Test(s) requested

Also enter all of the following that apply:
- Date of last menstrual period (LMP)
- Hormone treatment (which includes birth control pills)
- Postmenopausal
- Postpartum
- Pregnant
- Previous surgery
- X-ray treatment
- Previous normal
- Previous abnormal and date

NOTE: Rather than making two smears, many agencies and physicians will obtain one endocervical smear for cytology studies and one culture for gonorrhea screening. This is done more frequently now, as often patients will have an infection present without any signs or symptoms. This has been found to be a very beneficial screening process that enables early treatment when an asymptomatic infection is present.

Fig. 3-16. Cervical smear. (From L. Malasanos, V. Barkauskas, M. Moss, and K. Stoltenberg-Allen, *Health Assessment,* St. Louis, 1977, The C. V. Mosby Co.)

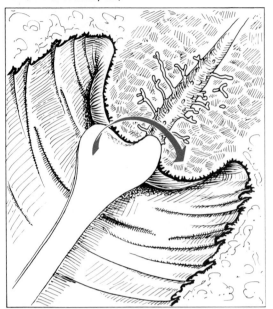

Fig. 3-17. Endocervical smear. (From L. Malasanos, V. Barkauskas, M. Moss, and K. Stoltenberg-Allen, *Health Assessment,* St. Louis, 1977, The C. V. Mosby Co.)

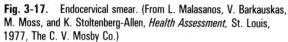

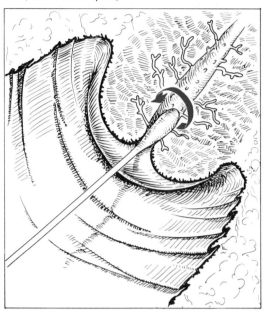

Fig. 3-18. Spraying smear with a cytological fixative spray.

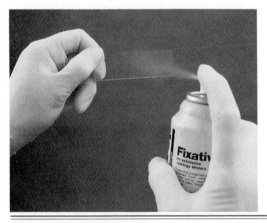

Fig. 3-19. Placing slides in container for transport to a laboratory.

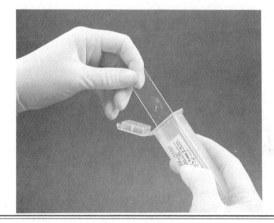

Fig. 3-20. **A,** bimanual palpation of the uterus. **B,** bimanual palpation of the adnexa. (From L. Malasanos, V. Barkauskas, M. Moss, and K. Stoltenberg-Allen, *Health Assessment,* St. Louis, 1977, The C. V. Mosby Co.)

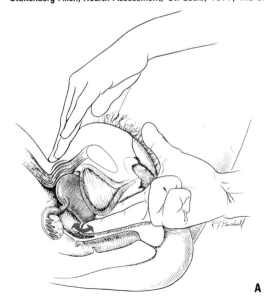

A

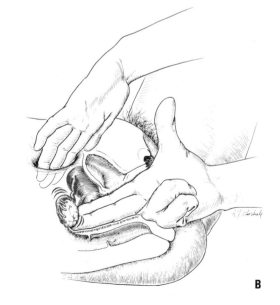

B

Pelvic Examination and Papanicolaou Smear (*continued*)

Procedure	Rationale
14. When the physician has completed the examination, wipe off the excess lubricant or discharge from the patient's perineal region.	You may use tissues or the small towel that was placed under the patient's buttocks.
15. Remove small towel from under the patient's buttocks.	
16. Raise or pull out the foot of the examining table.	This varies with the type of examining table used.
17. Help the patient remove her feet from the stirrups and place her legs down on the table.	If you are helping the patient lower her legs, lift and move both legs together to avoid any undue strain to the pelvic area.
18. The patient may now slide up toward the head of the table and then sit up.	Frequently it is desirable or advisable to allow the patient to rest for a few minutes before getting up.
19. Remove drape sheet.	
20. If necessary, help the patient get up and get dressed. Provide extra tissue and a sanitary pad and belt if required.	Always provide for the patient's safety, comfort, and well-being.
21. Inform the patient of any special instructions, if she is free to leave after she is dressed, or if the physician wishes to speak to her further. Ask the patient if she has any questions (see No. 12, p. 67).	Provide accurate and complete information, or refer the patient's questions to the physician if you cannot answer them. Part of patient care includes patient education and providing information and answers as necessary.
22. Leave the patient to dress in privacy if your assistance is not required.	
23. Return to the examining room to assemble all used equipment and supplies to be disposed of properly.	Remove any linens, and place in the soiled laundry. Place disposable equipment in a covered waste container.
	Take instruments to your cleanup area; rinse with cool water. These may be soaked in soap and water until you are ready to prepare them for sterilization (see Unit IV).
24. Resupply clean equipment as needed.	
25. Clean the examination table, and put on a fresh cover.	
26. If smears or cultures were taken, send them to the laboratory with request form, or place in a cool, dark place until you can transfer them to the laboratory.	It is important that all the required information appears on the cytology lab request, including notation of cervical and vaginal smears [see NOTE to No. 13(e), p. 80].
27. Wash your hands.	
28. Do any recording required of you completely and accurately (see No. 15, p. 67).	Charting example:
	January 27, 19_____, 2 PM
	Pelvic exam done by Dr. Short. Pap smear sent to laboratory for cytology studies. Patient had no specific complaints and left office in good spirits.
	Sandi Wilcox, CMA

RECTAL EXAMINATION

The rectal examination is used to detect polyps, early cancer, lesions, inflammatory conditions, and hemorrhoids. In addition, examination of the rectum can show how far the uterus is displaced, and if there are any masses in the rectum or pelvic region in a female; and the size, any enlargement, and texture of the prostate gland in a male. A more extensive examination of the interior surfaces of the rectum is done by a proctoscopy.

Equipment (Fig. 3-21)

Examination table
Sheet or paper to cover the table
Patient gown
Drape sheet
Small pillow
Small towel
Tissues
Rubber glove or finger cot
Lubricant (K-Y jelly)
Sponge forceps
Sponges
Rectal speculum and/or anoscope
Cotton-tipped applicators

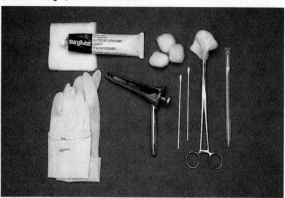

Fig. 3-21. Equipment for rectal examination including a Culturette (on the far right) to obtain a culture.

Procedure	Rationale
1. Wash your hands.	
2. Identify the patient and explain the procedure.	An explanation gives the patient some understanding of the need for the examination and provides some reassurance.
3. Have the patient empty the bladder.	Explain to the patient how to collect a specimen if a urinalysis is to be done (see Unit IV).
4. Provide a patient gown; have the patient remove all clothing from the waist down and put the gown on with the opening in the back.	
5. Assemble the necessary instruments and equipment.	This will vary somewhat depending on the extent of the examination to be done and the physician's preference. Frequently only the glove and lubricant will be necessary.
6. Position the patient on the examination table in a Sims, jackknife, or knee-chest position.	This will vary according to the physician's preference.
7. Drape the patient.	Refer to pp. 69–71 for positioning and draping techniques.
8. Call the physician.	NOTE: You may call the physician and then position the patient. By doing this, you prevent the patient from having to be in an uncomfortable position for an excessive period of time.
9. When the examination is ready to begin, pull the drape sheet back, exposing only the rectal area.	Avoid exposing the patient unnecessarily.
10. Assist the physician as required.	A female assistant should remain in the room if the patient is female and the physician is male even if she does not have to assist during the examination (see No. 10, p. 67).
11. Be prepared to hand the physician the various instruments and equipment. Some physicians will request that you put some K-Y jelly out on a piece of gauze; others will get it themselves in order to lubricate the gloved finger and anoscope if used. If a light is used, direct it on the part to be examined (the rectal region).	If you do not have to assist the physician, give your attention to the patient. Provide support and observe for any unusual reaction, such as a feeling of weakness, a change in skin color, or facial grimace, which may be an indication of pain.
12. The *physician* will begin the examination by inserting a gloved, lubricated finger into the rectum, then palpating the rectum internally to determine if there are any hemorrhoids,	

Rectal Examination (*continued*)

Procedure	Rationale
polyps or other obstructions, growths, or enlargements. This will be done gently, as it is often painful for the patient. If the anoscope is used, it will be lubricated, then the physician will insert it into the anal canal gently, and remove the obturator. If there is any bleeding or discharge, the physician may insert the sponge forceps and sponge through the anoscope to swab the area dry. This will allow better viewing of the internal surfaces. A good light will be needed so that the physician can view the internal lining of the anal canal. If a culture is to be taken, the physician will put a cotton-tipped applicator through the anoscope and swab the area. The cotton-tipped applicator will then be placed in a sterile culture tube, often one that has a special broth solution in it, so that the culture will not dry out.	
13. When the physician has completed the examination, wipe the patient's anal region for any excess lubricant or discharge.	You may use tissues, or the small towel under the patient's buttocks, which is then removed.
14. Help the patient, if required, assume a supine position.	Frequently it is desirable to allow the patient to remain lying down for a few minutes.
15. Remove the drape sheet.	
16. If required, assist the patient to a standing position and in getting dressed. Provide extra tissues to the patient, if required, for additional cleansing of the anal region.	Always provide for the comfort and welfare of the patient at the conclusion of an examination.
17. Tell the patient of any special instructions, if the patient is free to leave after getting dressed, or if the physician wishes to speak further to the patient in the office. Inquire if the patient has any questions (see No. 12, p. 67).	Always provide complete and accurate information. Refer the patient's questions to the physician if you cannot answer them completely and accurately. Never leave a patient in the examining room wondering if the office visit and examination are completed.
18. If your assistance is not required, leave the patient to dress in private.	
19. On returning to the examining room, assemble all used equipment and supplies to be disposed of properly.	Remove any linens and place in soiled laundry. Place disposable equipment in a covered waste container. Take instruments to your cleanup area; rinse with cool water. These may be soaked in soap and water until you are ready to prepare them for sterilization (see Unit IV).
20. Resupply clean equipment as needed.	
21. Clean the examination table and put on a fresh cover.	
22. If smears or cultures were obtained, send them to the laboratory or place them in a refrigerator or a cool, dark place until you can transfer them to the laboratory.	Make sure that specimens are properly labeled and that you have completely filled out the appropriate laboratory request form.
23. Wash your hands.	
24. Do any recording required of you completely and accurately (see No. 15, p. 67).	Charting example: Jan. 27, 19_____, 3 PM Rectal exam done by Dr. Short. No specimens were obtained. Patient complained of a sharp, continuous pain in the anal region when leaving the office and will call the doctor if it continues. Betty Fox, CMA

ENDOSCOPIC EXAMINATIONS: PROCTOSCOPY AND SIGMOIDOSCOPY

The purpose of a proctoscopy (prŏk-tŏs'kō-pĭ) and sigmoidoscopy (sig"moi-dos'ko-pĭ) is to examine the rectum and lower sigmoid colon for possible lesions, tumors, ulcers, polyps, inflammatory conditions, strictures, varicosities, and hemorrhages. Carcinoma will appear as a nodular, often cauliflower-like growth with superficial ulceration. Polyps are recognized easily by their pedicle. In doubtful cases, a biopsy of the growth will be done.

If found early and treated properly, 75% to 80% of all cases of cancer of the rectum and lower bowel can be cured. Most cases occur in individuals 55 to 75 years of age. Bowel cancers tend to grow slowly and are possible to detect at the most curable stage, before symptoms appear. Anyone with a personal or family history of rectal or colon cancer, or of polyps in the rectum or colon, or of ulcerative colitis should be examined carefully.

The American Cancer Society recommends that individuals have the following:

- An annual digital rectal examination after the age of 40
- An annual stool test for occult (hidden) blood after the age of 50 (see Unit VI)
- A proctosigmoidoscopy examination every 3 to 5 years after the age of 50 (*following* two initial negative annual examinations that were performed 1 year apart)

Many physicians also recommend that a sigmoidoscopy be included as part of the annual physical examination for men over age 40 because of the relatively high incidence of cancer of the rectum and sigmoid colon in this age group.

A proctosigmoidoscopy takes approximately 10 to 15 minutes and requires special preparation of the patient beforehand.

Check with your physician or agency for specific instructions. It is the medical assistant's responsibility to check that the patient is prepared before the examination begins. Generally the preparation includes

- A laxative the evening before (type and amount as prescribed by the physician)
- Only liquids for breakfast
- Tap water or saline enemas until the return is clear, usually 1 hour before the examination

NOTE: Enemas are usually avoided for patients who have colitis or bleeding from the rectum or who have Crohn's disease.

Equipment

Examination table covered with a clean sheet

Patient gown
Drape towel
Drape sheet
Small towel
Small pillow

Place and assemble the following equipment from the contents of the rectal diagnostic set on a clean drape towel (Fig. 3-22):

Sigmoidoscope with obturator (depending on the physician's request either a 30 to 65 cm flexible fiberoptic sigmoidoscope or a rigid 30 cm sigmoidoscope)
A rigid 15 cm proctoscope with obturator (depending on the physician's request)
Transilluminators (light source)
Rheostat
Extension cord
Insufflator with bulb attachment
Suction tip for suction machine
Biopsy forceps (sterile)
Metal sponge holder

When the above have been assembled add:

Rubber gloves
Doctor's gown
Rectal dressing forceps
Cotton-ball sponges
4 × 4 inch gauze
Tissues
Lubricant (K-Y jelly)
Specimen bottle with preservative if biopsy is to be taken
Laboratory request form
Kidney basin
Suction machine

Fig. 3-22. Equipment for sigmoidoscopy. *Top to bottom:* insufflator with bulb attachment, metal sponge holder, suction tip, light source, sigmoidoscope with obturator, disposable glove, sponges and lubricating jelly. Biopsy forceps may be added when required.

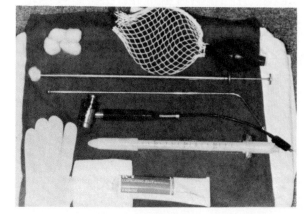

Procedure for Proctoscopy and Sigmoidoscopy

Procedure	**Rationale**
1. Wash your hands.	
2. Assemble and prepare the necessary equipment and supplies on a clean drape towel.	Disposable scopes may be used instead of the metal ones.
3. Test the suction apparatus and the light on the scopes to make sure that they are working properly.	
4. Identify the patient, and explain the procedure carefully.	This provides the patient with some understanding of the need for the examination and what to expect; that is, what will occur and how it may feel; it also enables the patient to cooperate more readily and to feel somewhat reassured.
5. Have the patient empty the bladder.	Explain to the patient how to collect a specimen if a urinalysis is to be done. (Refer to Unit VI for specimen collection procedure).
6. Have the patient remove all clothing from the waist down and put on the patient gown.	Patient gown should have the opening in the back.
7. Position the patient.	
a. Knee-chest position: Many examining rooms have a special proctoscopic table that is tilted in a way that supports the patient in the knee-chest position (see Figs. 3-4 and 3-5). Draping remains the same.	This is often preferred as it allows the abdominal contents to fall away from the pelvis, making it easier and less painful for the patient to be examined. NOTE: This is an uncomfortable position and usually cannot be tolerated for a long period.
b. Sims or left lateral position: Position of the patient may vary with the physician's preference.	This may be more comfortable for the patient, depending on age, weight, and condition.
8. Drape the patient completely.	Refer to draping procedures on pp. 70–71.
9. Call the physician into the room.	NOTE: You may call the physician into the room and then position the patient, as this would avoid the necessity of having the patient in an uncomfortable position for an excessive period of time.
10. When the physician is ready to begin the examination, pull the drape sheet back to expose only the anal area.	Avoid exposing the patient unnecessarily.
11. Assist the physician as required. Be prepared to hand the physician the various instruments and equipment.	A female assistant should always remain in the room if the patient is female and the physician is male (see No. 10, p. 67). If not assisting the physician, give your full attention to the patient. Provide support and reassurance. Observe the patient for any unusual reaction.
12. The physician will begin the examination.	*Method of examination:*
a. Put a generous amount of lubricant on 4 × 4 inch gauze square, and place on the towel with the equipment. Use this for lubricating the instruments and the physician's gloved finger when the exam begins.	The physician will first do a manual rectal examination. A liberal amount of lubricant is applied to the gloved index finger for easier insertion into the anal canal.
b. Warm the metal scopes by placing them in warm water or by rubbing them with your hand. Avoid additional discomfort for the patient that a cold instrument would cause.	This will vary with office or agency preference. Disposable scopes do not need to be warmed.
c. Hand the physician the scope. Attach the inflation bulb to the scope.	The physician or you then lubricates the distal end of the scope with the obturator in place.
d. To help the patient relax the anal sphincter for easier insertion of the scope, instruct the patient to bear down slightly, as though	If right-handed, the physician will separate the buttocks with the left hand, and then slowly and gently insert the scope about 3 cm to 4 cm.

Procedure	**Rationale**
having a bowel movement at the time when the physician inserts the scope. Also, instruct the patient to take deep breaths through the mouth, as this also helps relax the anus and rectum.	Force is *never* used when inserting the scope, as injury to the bowel must be avoided. The obturator is removed and can be placed in the kidney basin.
e. Attach the light source to the scope and adjust the light to the proper intensity. NOTE: You may turn off the lights in the room when the physician begins the visual examination through the scope. This allows for better inspection.	The physician will visually inspect the bowel as he or she advances the scope to its full length. Complete inspection and observation of the bowel will be performed.
f. Observe the patient throughout the procedure for fatigue, weakness, or fainting.	Next, the physician pumps the inflator bulb attachment slowly, in order to inject a small amount of air into the bowel. Although this is quite painful for the patient, it is necessary for proper inspection of the bowel.
	NOTE: This step is omitted in cases of ulcerative colitis or diverticulitis, because of fragility of the bowel.
g. Turn on the suction machine if it is to be used.	When there is bleeding or loose discharge in the bowel, the physician may place a long metal sponge holder with a sponge through the scope, to swab the area clean, or the suction tip may be used.
h. You may hand the biopsy forceps to the physician.	A biopsy forcep will be placed through the scope if a biopsy is required.
i. Have ready a labeled specimen jar.	When a specimen is obtained, it should be placed immediately into the labeled specimen jar.
j. Continue to offer reassurance and support to the patient. Frequently, just placing your hand on the patient's shoulder, arm, or hand gives the patient a feeling of being cared for as an individual.	On completing the examination, the physician will remove the scope slowly, which may then be placed in the kidney basin.
13. At the completion of the examination, take tissues and wipe the anal area for any lubricant and/or body discharge.	Provide for the patient's comfort.
14. Help the patient assume a supine position.	Frequently, it is desirable to allow the patient to rest for a few minutes before getting up, as he or she may feel faint.
15. Remove the drape sheet.	
16. When required, help the patient get up and get dressed. Provide the patient with extra tissues to cleanse the anal region more completely.	Always provide for the safety and comfort of the patient.
17. Inform the patient of any special instructions. Inquire if the patient has any questions (see No. 12, p. 67).	Provide complete and accurate information. Never leave a patient alone in a room after an examination without an understanding of what is to be done after getting dressed.
18. If your assistance is not required, leave the patient to dress in privacy.	
19. If specimens were obtained, send them to the laboratory.	Be sure that all specimens are properly labeled and sent to the laboratory with the correct requisition form.
20. Return to the examining room to assemble all used equipment and supplies.	Remove linens and place in soiled laundry. Disposable equipment should be removed and placed in a covered waste container. Take the instruments to your cleanup area. Rinse

Procedure for Proctoscopy and Sigmoidoscopy (*continued*)

Procedure	Rationale
	thoroughly with running water. You may then soak the instruments in soap and water until you are ready to prepare them for sterilization.
	NOTE: Do not soak the light attachment for the scope; cleanse it thoroughly with an alcohol sponge.
21. Wash the examination table with a disinfectant solution, and cover with a clean sheet or paper.	Prepare the examination room for the next patient.
22. Resupply clean equipment as needed.	
23. Wash your hands.	
24. Do any recording required of you completely and accurately (see No. 15, p. 67).	Charting example: Jan. 29, 19_____, 1:15 PM Sigmoidoscopy done by Dr. Short. Tissue biopsy sent with requisition to laboratory. Gary Greaves, CMA

OTHER SPECIAL EXAMINATIONS

Numerous other special or more specific examinations may be performed to gain pertinent information about a body part or system.

NEUROLOGICAL EXAMINATION

The neurological examination tests for adequate functioning of the cranial nerves, the motor or sensory systems, and the superficial and deep tendon reflexes.

Equipment and Supplies

Pins and cotton to test the senses of touch, sensation, and pain on the external surfaces of the body (Figs. 3-23, 3-24, 3-25)

Tuning fork to test hearing

Ophthalmoscope to examine the interior of the eye

Flashlight to test pupil reactions and equality

Tongue depressor to test the gag and corneal reflexes, and also pharyngeal sensation

Percussion hammer to test superficial and deep tendon reflexes (Fig. 3-26)

Test tubes with hot and cold water to test the skin for heat and cold sensation

Fig. 3-23. Evaluation for sensation and superficial pain using the sharp point of a safety pin.

Fig. 3-24. Alternate use of the dull end of the pin for evaluation of sensation and pain.

Fig. 3-25. Test of light touch sensation using cotton applied to stimulate the sensory nerve endings.

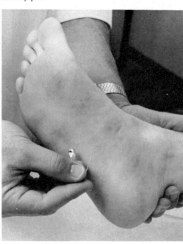

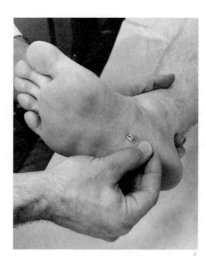

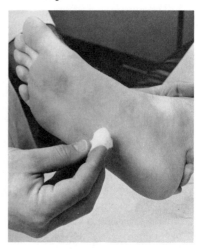

Fig. 3-26. Elicitation of the patellar reflex. A tap with the percussion hammer is applied directly inferior to the patella. **A,** with the patient sitting and legs hanging over the examination table. **B,** with the patient in a supine position. The normal response is the leg kicking out or extension of the leg.

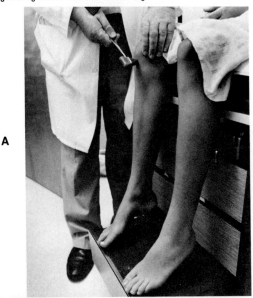

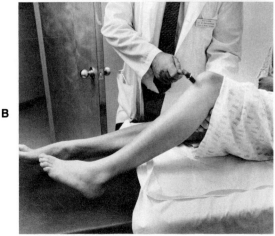

Equipment and Supplies (*continued*)

   Bottles of sweet, bitter, salty, and sour solutions to test the sense of taste

   Bottles of substances that have common familiar odors to test the sense of smell

   The physician also observes the patient's level of consciousness, behavior, and the higher functions of speech and writing. Coordination, balance, gait, muscle tone, and strength will be noted for adequate functioning of the motor system. The sense of touch, pain (deep and superficial), temperature, and discriminatory sensations are noted in the examination of the sensory system.

HEARING EXAMINATION

To detect impaired hearing, the physician will use an otoscope to inspect the external ear canal and eardrum (Fig. 3-27, *A* and *B*), and a tuning fork to test for hearing acuity.

   The tuning fork is used to determine the distance at which the patient can hear a certain sound (air conduction test) and for bone conduction tests. In the bone conduction test, the vibrating end of the tuning fork is placed on the patient's skull. This test is valuable in distinguishing between perceptive and transmission deafness (Fig. 3-28, *A* and *B*).

   A more accurate test to gauge and record the hearing sense is done with the use of an audiometer, a delicate instrument consisting of complex parts. For audiometry the patient is placed in a soundproof room and puts on earphones. Timing circuits, sound

Fig. 3-27. Examination of the ear with an otoscope. **A,** the patient's head is tipped toward the opposite shoulder. **B,** one way of holding the otoscope.

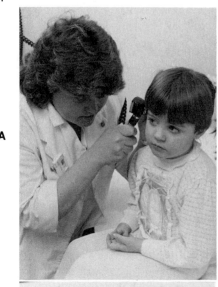

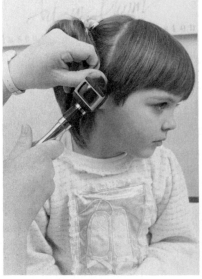

Fig. 3-28. Hearing examination. **A,** air conduction test. **B,** bone conduction test.

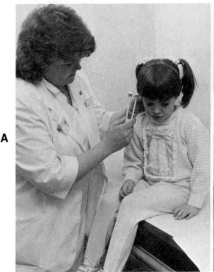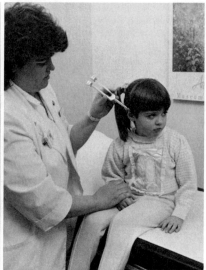

wave generators, and other complex pieces of equipment are utilized to measure the patient's acuity of hearing for the various frequencies of sound waves. Results are plotted on a graph called an audiogram. No special preparation of the patient is required for this test. Physicians, audiometric technicians, or other specially trained individuals will perform this test.

EYE EXAMINATION

External Eye Examinations

Distance Visual Acuity. Visual acuity means acuteness or clearness of vision. This may be measured on patients having complete physical examinations, but more specifically is measured on patients having a specific visual complaint and also on some patients because of employment requirements and for meeting the requirements as established by the Department of Motor Vehicles for obtaining specific types of drivers' licenses, such as a chauffeur's or truck driver's license. The visual acuity test is also performed in schools and on preschool-aged children as a means of vision screening. Imperfect refractive powers of the eye such as myopia (nearsightedness), hyperopia (farsightedness), and astigmatism (another refractive error of the eye resulting from irregularities in the curvature of the cornea and/or surfaces of the lens of the eye) can be detected by using the Snellen eye chart to measure distance visual acuity. The Snellen eye chart consists of varied-sized block letters arranged in rows in gradually decreasing sizes. Another chart used for preschoolers, individuals unable to speak English, slow learners, and those unable to read is the "E" chart, which consists of the letter "E" arranged in different directions in decreasing sizes.

Charts with pictures of common objects, such as a house and a truck, are available to use when testing preschoolers, although some children are unable to identify the objects because of lack of knowledge rather than a defect in visual acuity. On the Snellen chart there are two standardized numbers on the side of each row of letters; these numbers, shown one on top of the other, indicate the degree of visual acuity measured from a distance of 20 feet, the standard testing distance. The top number is 20, indicating the number of feet between the chart and the person taking the test; the bottom number indicates the distance in feet from which the normal eye can read the row of letters. The large letter on the top of the chart can be read by the normal eye at a distance of 200 feet. This is indicated as 20/200. In each of the succeeding rows, from top to bottom, the size of the letters decreases to where the normal eye can read the row of letters at distances of 100, 70, 50, 40, 30, 25, 20, 15, 13, and 10 feet. The row marked 20/20 indicates normal visual acuity and is expressed as 20/20 vision. A measurement of visual acuity of less than 20/20 vision is an indication of a refractive error or some other eye disorder. When the letters on the row marked 20/50 are read, the person is said to have 20/50 vision, and so on. This means that the person can read at only 20 feet what the normal eye can read at 50 feet. The larger the bottom number of the row read, the poorer the vision is. A reading of 20/15 indicates above average distance vision (Fig. 3-29, A and B). This test is to be given in a well-lit room with the person taking the test standing or sitting 20 feet away from the chart, with the chart placed at eye level to the person. Each eye is to be tested separately, with and without glasses or contact lenses. However, reading glasses should not be worn during the test, as they tend to blur distant vision. The results must be recorded indicating the reading for each eye without

Fig. 3-29. **A,** a Snellen eye chart consisting of varied-sized letters arranged in rows in gradually decreasing sizes. **B,** a Snellen Big E eye chart consisting of the letter "E" arranged in different directions in decreasing sizes.

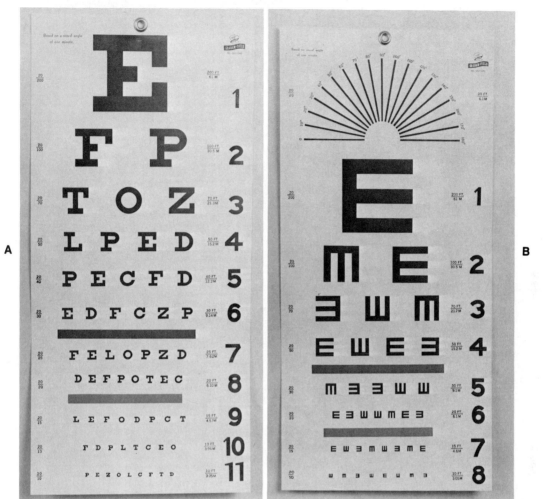

and with glasses or contact lenses. Both eyes are not usually tested together, as the stronger eye will usually compensate for the weaker eye. Patients who are unable to see even the largest numbers on the Snellen chart (top line 20/200) are given additional tests to determine if they can see enough to count fingers (this is recorded as C.F.), perceive hand movements (H.M.), perceive light (L.P.), or perceive light with projection (L.P.cP.). N.L.P. is used to record "no light projection." An ophthalmologist considers patients to be blind when they cannot even perceive light. Legal blindness is defined as vision of 20/200 or less in both eyes when wearing correction glasses.

There are also electric testing devices on the market, such as the Titmus II Vision Tester which is the product of advances in computer designed optics (Fig. 3-30). This one compact instrument, using eight test slides, can screen patients of all ages (preschool through adults) for *all* common vision problems—problems that the standard wall chart misses. The Titmus II Vision Tester measures acuity (both far and near), hyperopia, binocularity, muscle balance, color perception, depth perception, and, with the optional equipment, peripheral vision and intermediate vi-

sion, all within 5 minutes. The standard wall chart measures only distance vision. The fiber optics perimeter system determines if peripheral vision is adequate, a basic requirement for employees who operate machinery and mobile equipment. The intermediate distance feature tests the intermediate distance (20 to 40 inches) viewing capabilities important to machine workers and to the increasing number of video display terminal operators. Because of its extremely compact and lightweight design, the Titmus II Vision Tester can be used virtually anywhere. It is especially convenient when performing vision screening tests on large groups or in small areas where space is less than 20 feet. Only 5 square feet of space is required for using this instrument. Patients of all ages and statures can be easily screened because of the unit's balanced height adjustment. The unit's face mask, in addition to eliminating outside light, is designed to accommodate all sizes and types of eyeglasses. A training manual complete with an instructional cassette supplied as standard equipment provides correct testing techniques that are easy to learn. The Titmus II Vision Tester is a complete system for all vision screening in each individual office situation.

Fig. 3-30. Titmus II Vision Tester. (Courtesy Titmus Optical, Inc., Petersburg, VA)

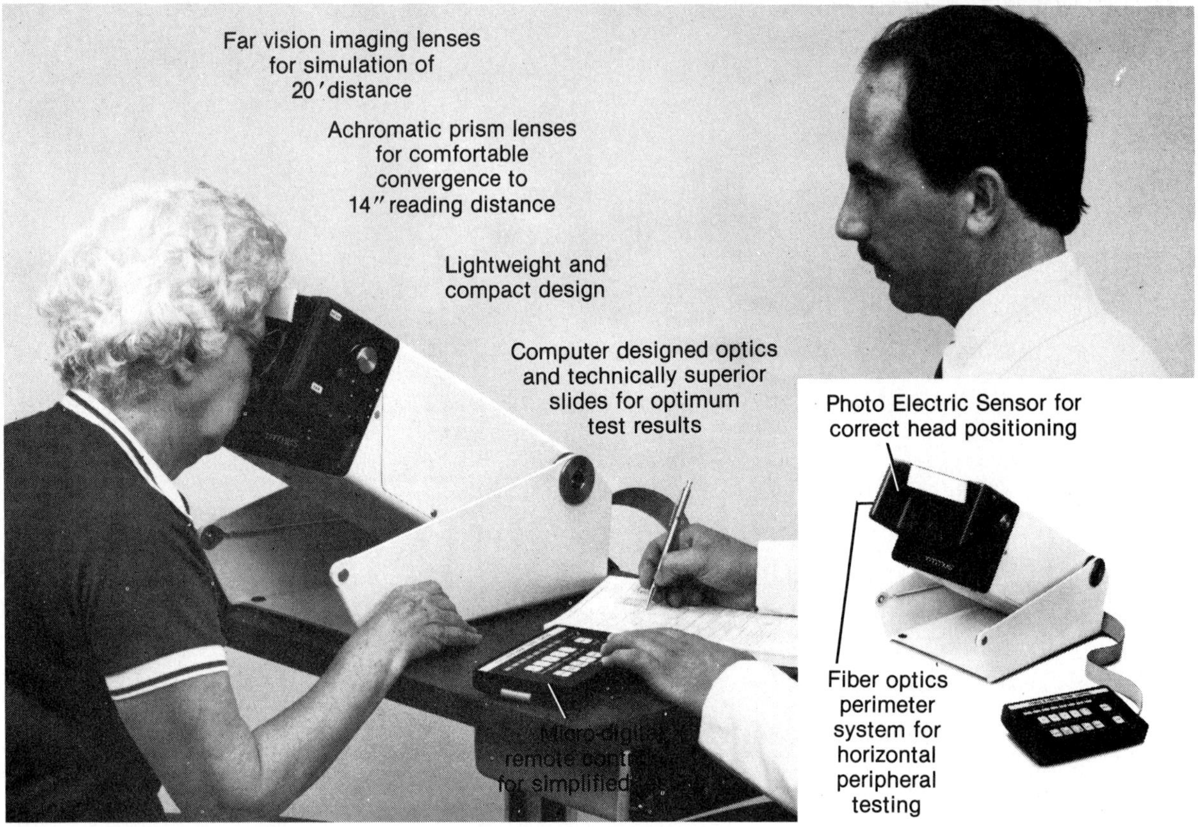

Far vision imaging lenses
for simulation of
20' distance

Achromatic prism lenses
for comfortable
convergence to
14" reading distance

Lightweight and
compact design

Computer designed optics
and technically superior
slides for optimum
test results

Photo Electric Sensor for
correct head positioning

Fiber optics
perimeter
system for
horizontal
peripheral
testing

Micro-digital
remote control
for simplified

Measuring Distance Visual Acuity Using the Snellen Chart

Equipment

Snellen eye chart (Fig. 3-29 *A*, and *B*)   Pen
Opaque card or eye cover   Paper

Procedure	Rationale
1. Wash your hands.	
2. Prepare the room; determine location of 20 feet from where the chart will be posted to where the patient will be positioned.	When this test is used frequently, this distance can be permanently marked to save time.
3. Assemble the supplies and equipment.	
4. Identify the patient and explain the procedure. Do not allow time for the patient to study and memorize the chart before the examination begins.	Explanations help the patient to feel comfortable and more relaxed, in addition to gaining the patient's confidence as you proceed with the examination.
5. Position the patient comfortably, either standing or sitting, 20 feet from the location of the chart.	Twenty feet is the standard testing distance.
6. Position the center of the Snellen eye chart at eye level to the patient.	To position the chart correctly, the patient must first be positioned.
7. Provide the patient with the opaque card or eye cover. Instruct the patient to cover the left eye with the card, and to keep the left eye open at all times.	The right eye (OD) is traditionally tested first. The hand or fingers are not to be used to cover the eye not being tested. The covered eye is to be kept open because closing one eye often causes the other to squint inadvertently.

Procedure	Rationale
8. Instruct the patient to use the right eye and to verbally identify the letters as you point to each row. Start at row 20/70 (or a row several rows above the 20/20 row) (Fig. 3-31).	The patient is to read as many letters as possible in the rows as you point to them. Starting with row 20/70, which has larger letters than those on row 20/20, allows the patient to gain confidence in identifying the letters.
9. As the patient identifies the letters in the first row that you point to, proceed down the chart until the patient has identified as many rows of letters as possible. If the patient is unable to identify row 20/70, proceed up the chart having the patient identify the rows of letters until the smallest row of letters is identified.	To obtain the correct visual acuity measurement, the patient is to identify the smallest letters possible.
10. Provide instructions to the patient during the test, such as what line to read and not to squint. Observe the patient for any unusual reactions, such as tearing in the eyes, blinking, squinting, or leaning forward to read the chart.	These reactions may indicate that the patient is experiencing difficulty with the test and must be recorded.
11. Continue testing until the smallest line of letters that the patient can read is reached, or until a letter is misread.	
12. Record the results of visual acuity of the right eye on a piece of paper.	It is important to write the results down when determined so that errors are avoided when charting the results on the patient's record.
13. Instruct the patient to cover the right eye with the opaque card or eye cover and keep the eye open (Fig. 3-31).	
14. Measure the visual acuity of the left eye (OS) using the method described in steps 8 through 12.	
15. Give further instructions to the patient as required.	
16. Replace equipment, and leave the room neat and clean.	

Fig. 3-31. Using the Snellen chart for distance visual acuity testing.

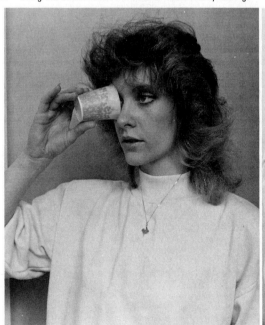 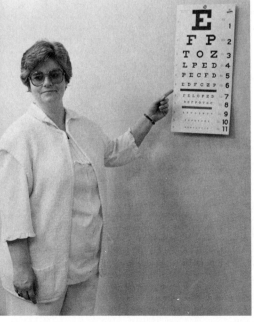

Procedure	Rationale
17. Record the results for each eye on the patient's chart using proper medical abbreviations. When one or two letters are missed or misread in a row, the results are recorded with a minus sign and the number of letters missed or misread next to the bottom number. That is, if the patient identified the rows of letters down to row 20/25 and could not read two letters in this row, you would record this result as 20/25-2. Record as sc (without correction) when the patient isn't wearing glasses or contact lenses, and cc (with correction) when the patient is wearing glasses or contact lenses.	Charting example: October 31, 19_____, 5 PM Snellen chart eye test given. Results without glasses: OD 20/20 sc OS 20/15-2 sc H. McMullen CMA

Visual Fields. The patient will be asked to look directly at a central point, then the extent of peripheral and side vision is spot checked with an instrument called a perimeter. A target screen method may also be used. The patient is asked to focus on a small target that is moved to different points on a screen. The patient has a visual field defect in the areas where the target cannot be seen.

Color Vision. The patient will be asked to identify colored figures and numbers on a color plate from a standardized distance, usually 75 cm.

Refraction. A physician will instill atropine drops (or any mydriatic, a drug used to dilate the eyes) into the eye. With the use of these drops, the lens of the eye is unable to accommodate, thus allowing the physician to determine eye function when the lens is at rest.

Internal Eye Examinations

Ophthalmoscopic Examination. With the use of the ophthalmoscope, the physician examines the anterior chamber, the lens, the vitreous body, and the retina of the eye. When using the ophthalmoscope, the physician may want the room darkened, as this causes the pupils to dilate and thus aids the examination. Visualization of the retina with the ophthalmoscope is known as a funduscopic examination (Fig. 3-32, A and B).

Tonometry. After the instillation of a local anesthetic into the eye, a tonometer is gently rested on the eyeball to measure the tension of the eyeball and intraocular pressure. This is an important test to determine the presence of an eye condition termed glaucoma, in which the pressure within the eyeball is increased.

Fig. 3-32. **A,** the physician using the ophthalmoscope to examine the lens and vitreous body of the eye from a distance of about 12 inches. **B,** the physician using the ophthalmoscope to examine the retina of the eye. The physician uses the right hand and right eye to examine the patient's right eye.

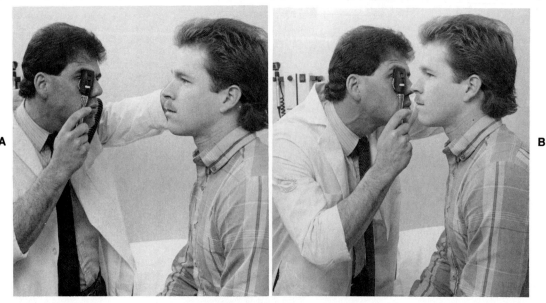

Glaucoma is the most frequent cause of blindness in adults. Normal tonometry reading is 11 to 22 mm Hg. A reading of 24 to 32 mm Hg suggests glaucoma.

OBSTETRICAL EXAMINATIONS AND RECORD

Obstetrics is the branch of medicine that deals with the care of the mother and fetus during pregnancy, labor and delivery, and the immediate postpartum period, which is called the puerperium. Pregnancy lasts approximately 280 days or 40 weeks from the day of fertilization. The puerperium lasts about 6 weeks after delivery. It is during that time that the mother's body, which has undergone many anatomical and physiological changes during pregnancy, returns to a normal pre-pregnancy state and the mother adjusts to the new responsibilities of motherhood. When a woman suspects that she may be pregnant after missing her regular menstrual period, she may call the physician's office or clinic for an appointment to be tested for pregnancy. To test for pregnancy most laboratories now do a blood test, called the HCG (human chorionic gonadotropin) beta subunit test, commonly referred to as the serum pregnancy test. This test can be done 10 to 14 days after the woman feels she may have conceived. Other laboratories prefer to do the blood test 6 weeks after the date of the first day of the woman's last menstrual period, or 1 – 2 weeks after the first missed menstrual period. The results of this test are reported as either + (positive) or − (negative). Results of 100 mIU/ml HCG or greater are positive. In special circumstances, a HCG quantitative serum pregnancy test may be ordered to rule out the possibility of an ectopic pregnancy or of a SAB (spontaneous abortion). The results of this test are reported as a number. Any number less than 5 mIU/ml HCG indicates a negative result (Fig. 3-33).

After pregnancy has been confirmed, monitoring both the physical well-being of mother and fetus and the progress of the pregnancy is highly recommended and considered vital by some. Prevention of health problems or the early detection, diagnosis, and treatment of health problems is accomplished by close supervision of the mother throughout the entire pregnancy. The mother should be seen by the physician at regular intervals. After the initial visit, the expectant mother should see the physician once a

Fig. 3-33. Laboratory request form to order a pregnancy test.

RIA — PLEASE PRINT — PRESS HARD

RIA GL 4063 | ST | BD

DRAWN BY | REMARKS

LAST NAME FIRST NAME

ADDRESS

ROUTINE REQUEST DRAWN AT: ______ TIME ______ DATE

BIRTHDATE AGE SEX CLASS

IF REQUEST IS OTHER THAN ROUTINE, PLACE STICKER WITH APPROPRIATE INSTRUCTIONS IN THIS SPACE

PHYSICIAN ROOM NO. HOSP. NO.

DATE | VERIFYING NURSE | DIAGNOSIS

DATE PHONE

CODE	TEST	NORMAL	RESULTS
3150	T_3 AND T_4 COMBINATION (includes free thyroxine index)		
3151	T_3 UPTAKE	30-40%	%
3153	T_4	4.5-11.5 ug%	ug%
	FREE THYROXINE INDEX	0.5-1.7	
3163	FERRITIN	25-125 ng/ml	ng/ml
3579	HB_SAG	NEG.	
3165	SERUM PREGNANCY		
6268	SERUM ESTRIOL		
3384	TSH	0.8-5.0 mIu/ml	
3167	HCG QUANT		

TIME IN TECHNOLOGIST TIME TELEPHONED OR TELETYPED TIME OUT

MEDICAL RECORD

month for the first 6 months, then every 2 weeks during the 7th and 8th months, and then once a week until the baby is born. For patients with medical problems such as diabetes, these prenatal visits will often be scheduled every week throughout the pregnancy.

About 6 weeks after the baby is born, the mother should return to the office or clinic for a postpartum physical examination to have her general physical condition evaluated.

Health Care During Pregnancy

In order to provide the best care and supervision of the expectant mother during her pregnancy, the physician must know the patient as an individual and as a member of her family. Based on her health status the physician can then determine what, how much, and when care will be required. The initial assessment will be made based on the mother's medical history and the results of a physical examination. The data gathered will initiate the prenatal or antepartum record (Fig. 3-34, *A, B,* and *C*). This record contains much of the same information as the health history and physical examination discussed in Unit II. The data collected are also essential to help in identifying high-risk patients. Follow-up visits and examinations will monitor the progress of the pregnancy.

Patient History.   This includes the patient's past medical history and also an obstetrical history if this is not the first pregnancy; the family history, which also includes information on the father's health and family history; the social and occupational history; the review of systems including the history of the patient's menstrual cycles—the age at onset, regularity, amount, duration, and the date of the last menstrual period (LMP) (see p. 49 and Fig. 3-34). Particular attention is given to habits, conditions, or diseases that could influence the health of the mother and fetus during the pregnancy. The physician will plan to watch and give more care during and after the pregnancy if the patient has a present or past history of one or more of the following:

- Age under 17 or over 35 years
- Problematic pregnancies, which may include repeated spontaneous abortions, premature deliveries, stillbirths, eclampsia, or toxemia
- Previous cesarean section(s)
- An infectious disease such as a sexually transmitted disease or a urinary tract infection
- Medical conditions such as kidney, cardiovascular, or respiratory diseases, hypertension, obesity, and nutritional deficiencies
- A metabolic disorder such as hyperthyroidism or diabetes
- A family history of genetic diseases
- Rh negative blood when the father has Rh positive blood

- Use of alcohol, tobacco, and/or drugs (which includes over-the-counter, prescription, or street drugs)

Personal History of the Present Pregnancy.   This includes the date of the first day of the last menstrual period (LMP), symptoms of pregnancy, warning signs, and the expected date of confinement (EDC).

The patient is asked to explain what, if any, early symptoms of pregnancy she has experienced. These symptoms may include fatigue, nausea and vomiting (morning sickness), frequent urination, and breast changes such as a tingling sensation in the breasts, tenderness, enlargement of the nipples, and darkening of the areolae.

The patient is also asked if she has experienced any warning signs. It must be explained to the patient what these are and to notify the physician if and when any of the following appear:

- Sudden increase in vaginal discharge
- Bleeding from the vagina
- Sudden continuous or intermittent abdominal pain or cramping
- Continuous or severe nausea and vomiting
- Blurred vision or seeing spots before her eyes
- Chills and/or fever

In addition, later in the pregnancy additional warning signs to watch for and report include the following:

- Pelvic pressure
- Sudden gush of water from the vagina with subsequent leakage
- Fainting spells or loss of consciousness
- Swelling or puffiness of the hands or face, and/or marked swelling of the ankles and feet
- Rapid weight gain in a short period of time
- Pain or a burning sensation on urination
- Painless contractions
- Low, dull backache
- Rashes or lesions

By using Nägele's rule and the date of the first day of the LMP you or the physician will determine the expected date of confinement (EDC). This is determined by adding 7 days to the date of the first day of the LMP, subtracting 3 months, and adding 1 year.

EXAMPLE:

EDC = date of first day of LMP
+ 7 days − 3 months + 1 year

EDC = April 4, 19_____ + 7 days
= April 11, 19_____

− (minus) 3 months
= January 11, 19_____

+ (plus) 1 year
= January 11 of the following year

Thus the baby will be delivered on approximately January 11 of the following year, or more commonly within 1 week before or 1 week after the EDC.

Fig. 3-34. Prenatal records.

OBSTETRICS AND GYNECOLOGY CLINIC

PROBLEM LIST	ONSET	COMMENTS	PLAN
1.			
2.			
3.			
4.			
5.			
6.			
7.			

DATING SHEET

LNMP _____ ⟶ EDC _____   LMP _____ ⟶ EDC _____

FIRST SYMPTOMS OF PREGNANCY (date) _____

(+)   PREGNANCY TEST   a.   URINE (date) _____ at _____ wks

b.   SERUM (date) _____ at _____ wks

FIRST EXAM (date) _____ SIZE _____ at _____ wks GA

QUICKENING (date) _____ at _____ wks GA

20 WK STETH FHT (date) _____ at _____ wks GA

Utx at umbilicus? _____

SIZE = DATES?

SONO #1 (date) _____ (findings) _____ ⟶ SONO EDC

SONO #2 (date) _____ (findings) _____ ⟶ SONO EDC

BEST ESTIMATE OF EDC

(*Fig. 3-34 continues*)

Fig. 3-34 *(continued)*

LAST NAME		FIRST NAME	
ADDRESS			
BIRTHDATE	AGE	SEX	CLASS
PHYSICIAN			
DATE		PHONE	

ANTEPARTUM RECORD

☐ IDENTIFIED HIGH RISK

PEDIATRICIAN

PATIENT (LAST NAME - FIRST NAME)	MAIDEN NAME	REFERRED BY

PATIENT'S ADDRESS (STREET, CITY, STATE, ZIP CODE)	HOME PHONE	BUSINESS PHONE

AGE	BIRTHDATE	BIRTHPLACE	RELIGION	HEIGHT	AVER. WT.	OCCUPATION	MAY WORK UNTIL (DATE)
				FT. IN.	LB.		

MARRIED YES ☐ NO ☐	FATHER'S NAME	AGE	HEIGHT	WEIGHT	BLOOD TYPE	OCCUPATION
				LB.		

FATHER'S HEALTH HISTORY

FATHER'S FAMILY HISTORY

HISTORY

CTA ONSET DATE	INTERVAL (DAYS)	DURATION (DAYS)	AMOUNT	DYSMENORRHEA	LMP	EDC	

PRESENT PREGNANCY HISTORY

	QUICKENING DATE	MOTHER TO NURSE? ☐ YES ☐ NO	ANESTHETIC

PREVIOUS PREGNANCIES – PARITY

YEAR	DURATION	LABOR	ANESTHESIA	SEX	WEIGHT	RHOGAM	* PREMATURITY	* FETAL LOSS

* RECORD REASON

FAMILY

DIABETES	HYPERTENSION	TWINS	CONGENITAL DEFECTS

PERSONAL

RH. FEV.	DIABETES	HEPATITIS	RUBELLA	ANEMIA	CARDIAC	THYROID	ALLERGIES

DRUGS	TRANSFUSIONS	URINARY TRACT	CONVULSIONS	PHLEBITIS	VARICOSITIES

SERIOUS ILLNESS, SURGERY, HOSPITALIZED:

INITIAL PHYSICAL EXAMINATION

BLOOD PRES.	PULSE	ENT	TEETH	HEART	LUNGS	EXTREMITIES

ABDOMEN	BREASTS

PELVIMETRY	PELVIC
D.C.	OUTLET
BIS	VAGINA
SPINES	CERVIX
S.S. LIG.	CORPUS
ARCH.	ADNEXA
SACRAL HOLLOW	RECTUM
FORE PELVIS	
DATE	SIGNATURE

INITIAL LABORATORY WORK

PCV.	HGB.	SEROLOGY	BLOOD TYPE	RH.	ALBUMIN	SUGAR	ATYPICAL ANTIBODIES	Rh TITRE	CYTOLOGY

COPY TO HOSPITAL IN APPROXIMATELY 30 WEEKS

PHYSICIAN

Fig. 3-34   *(continued)*

ANTEPARTUM RECORD

(CONTINUATION)

NAME

LAST NAME   FIRST NAME

ADDRESS

BIRTHDATE   AGE   SEX   CLASS

PHYSICIAN

DATE   PHONE

SUBSEQUENT VISITS

DATE	WEIGHT	BLOOD PRESSURE	HEIGHT OF FUNDUS	POSITION AND PRESENTATION	FETAL HEART	ALBUMIN	URINE SUGAR	HEMOGLOBIN	HEADACHE	DIZZINESS	EDEMA	NAUSEA & VOMITING	BLEEDING		INITIALS

(Columns under SYMPTOMS: HEADACHE, DIZZINESS, EDEMA, NAUSEA & VOMITING, BLEEDING)

DATE	PROGRESS NOTES	TEST	DATE	FINDINGS
		Rh TITRE		
		AMNIO-CENTESIS		
		ULTRA-SONOGRAM		
		X-RAY		
		OTHER		

QUICKENING DATE	MOTHER TO NURSE? ☐ YES ☐ NO	ANESTHETIC	PEDIATRICIAN

SEND COPY TO HOSPITAL AT APPROXIMATELY 38 WEEKS.

_____ M.D.
SIGNATURE

PHYSICIAN

Initial Prenatal Physical Examination and Diagnostic Tests. The initial prenatal examination includes a physical examination as described on pp. 50–52. Among other findings the patient's blood pressure and weight will be recorded at this visit and all subsequent visits. By keeping a continuous record of the blood pressure and weight, the physician can determine any excessive elevation of the BP or a sudden and rapid weight gain from one visit to the next. Such elevations may be early warning signs of a serious problem such as preeclampsia and will require further follow-up. Weight measurements are also helpful in determining the stages of fetal growth. The American College of Obstetrics and Gynecology recommends a weight gain of 22 to 26 pounds during pregnancy. Just as important as total weight gain is the rate of the gain. The mother's weight should increase only slightly in the first 3 months — about 1 pound per month. Then she should begin a steady rate of gain of ½ to 1 pound per week until the birth of the baby. It is critical that the added weight gain be from increased consumption of the necessary food groups, not simply overloading on calories.

Of particular importance during the physical examination are the breast, abdomen, and pelvic examinations. In addition to the routine examinations of these areas of the body, the breasts will be observed for any breast changes that accompany pregnancy as described previously. During the abdominal examination the initial measurement of the height of the fundus of the uterus will be recorded. This is the distance in centimeters between the superior aspect of the symphysis pubis and the top of the fundus of the uterus (Fig. 3-35). This provides a baseline for future measurements. During the pelvic examination a Pap smear and a culture for gonorrhea will usually be taken. By feeling the uterus, the physician can learn about its position, shape, and size, and how long the patient has been pregnant. An estimation of pelvic measurements will also be made to determine a diffi-cult delivery in cases of cephalopelvic disproportions. The vaginal examination will be done to check the birth canal for any abnormalities and obtain further pelvic measurements.

Samples of urine and blood will be collected for the following tests. (At times the patient may be sent to an outside laboratory to have these specimens collected.) On the first visit a complete urinalysis will be performed, then on subsequent visits the urine will be checked for albumin and sugar. The presence of albumin in the urine could be an early warning sign of toxemia. The presence of sugar in the urine could be a warning sign of a pre-diabetic state or diabetes. Both of these conditions will require careful medical supervision and treatment. Blood tests to be performed include a complete blood count to assess the general health status of the expectant mother. Of special importance are the hemoglobin and hematocrit results, which will determine if the mother is anemic. If anemia is present, special treatment will be given and further hemoglobin and hematocrit evaluations will be done. Other blood tests include the Rh factor and blood typing of the ABO blood groups, a VDRL (Venereal Disease Research Laboratory) or a RPR (rapid plasma reagin) test for syphilis, and a rubella titer to determine if the patient has immunity to rubella (German measles) (see also Units X and XI).

Also in California and a few other states, it is now a state mandate that the AFP (alpha fetoprotein) blood test be offered to the mother around the 16th week of pregnancy. The mother is at liberty to accept or deny this test. The AFP is a nondefinitive test and is used *only* as a screening test. It may be used to help rule out conditions such as neural tube defects, abdominal wall defects, chromosome problems, Down's syndrome, fetal demise, and also twins. If the results of this test are positive, *further testing is required.* First an ultrasound examination would be performed to check for the exact gestational time as AFP levels will vary at different times during pregnancy. This may be followed by a repeat serum test and/or an amniocentesis and possibly another ultrasound examination. Counseling and patient education are vital during all of this testing.

For other high-risk patients, a blood test that screens for hepatitis B may also be performed. This is a blood serum test that tests for the presence of the HBsAG (hepatitis B surface antigen). If the results are positive, a liver function test may then be performed.

Some physicians may order a Tine or Mantoux test to screen the patient for tuberculosis (see also Unit XIII). The physician will usually only order a chest x-ray to screen for tuberculosis if the patient has had a positive Tine or Mantoux test in the past, when the mother has been exposed to tuberculosis, or if other family members have tuberculosis.

After the examination has been completed, the physician will discuss with the patient general health care during pregnancy, care of the teeth, proper diet,

Fig. 3-35. Measuring the height of the uterine fundus.

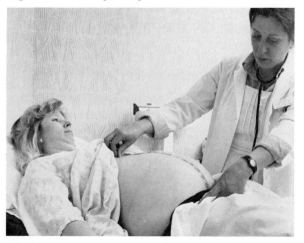

the need for rest and relaxation, types of exercise and work that can be continued, weight gain, the use of tobacco, alcohol and drugs, and the need for follow-up prenatal visits. Pamphlets containing similar information may be given to the patient to use as a reference. Many obstetric offices also have videotapes on pregnancy for the patient to watch and learn from.

Follow-up Prenatal Visits.   The antepartum record will also include essential data obtained during the follow-up prenatal visits (see Fig. 3-34C). Data measured and recorded include the patient's weight, blood pressure, height of the uterine fundus, position and presentation of the fetus, the fetal heart rate after the fourth month (Fig. 3-36), urine tests for albumin and sugar, blood tests for hemoglobin and a hematocrit or a complete blood count if deemed necessary, any symptoms or early warning signs experienced by the patient, and any concerns or questions that the patient may have. A vaginal examination is done only periodically and usually 2 to 3 weeks before the EDC. All this information aids the physician in determining and evaluating the progress of the pregnancy and in planning good patient care.

All visits should also include educating the mother in healthful living habits and various aspects of her pregnancy, as education is an integral part of antepartum care. The follow-up visits provide the perfect opportunity to reinforce healthful living habits to the mother and to provide explanations of the physical and emotional changes that she is experiencing and explanations on the growth pattern of the fetus. Information on the LaMaze method of childbirth may be given later in the pregnancy. You may be responsible for scheduling the LaMaze childbirth classes and possibly classes on the fundamentals of newborn care for the mother and father.

Other topics to be discussed and reviewed include exercise, rest, diet, sexual intercourse, partner support, labor (the signs of labor, how long it will last, anesthetics), delivery of the baby, postpartum care, and, possibly, family planning.

Medical Assistant's Responsibilities

In addition to the general instructions and responsibilities for the medical assistant listed on pages 66–67, and the procedures for assisting with a physical examination, a pelvic, and a rectal examination as outlined on pages 73–84, the medical assistant's responsibilities include the following:

- Acquire some of the information to be recorded on the antepartum record (see Fig. 3-34). The amount of information collected by the medical assistant will vary according to the physician's preference. Some physicians may obtain all of the history and have the medical assistant obtain only the vital signs and height and weight measurements.
- Assemble additional equipment that will be required for prenatal examinations. This would include:

    A flexible centimeter tape measure used to measure the height of the fundus of the uterus

    A pelvimeter used for taking pelvic measurements

    A fetoscope or Doppler fetal pulse detector and an ultrasound coupling agent used to listen to the fetal heart tones

- Develop a good rapport with the patient so that she will feel comfortable and confident enough to ask questions of you and the physician; help the patient to relax and gain confidence in your abilities and functions.
- Schedule the follow-up prenatal visits.
- Make certain that the patient understands all of the instructions that were given to her.

Fig. 3-36.   A, Doppler device used to detect fetal heart rate. **B,** listening to the fetal heart rate.

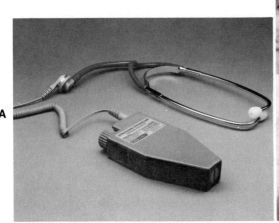

A

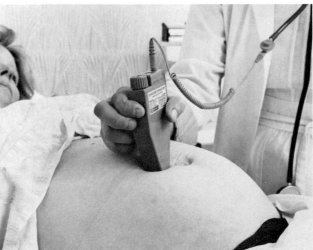

B

- Reinforce the need for healthful living habits.
- Take part in patient education as discussed previously.
- Remind the patient to call the physician immediately if she experiences any of the early warning signs of problems during the pregnancy.
- Remind the patient to call the office with any questions she may have about the pregnancy and her care.

BREAST SELF-EXAMINATION

Generally, the physician will examine the patient's breasts at each physical examination. During the time that individuals are unattended by a physician, they should examine their own breasts to detect any abnormality, which can be brought to the physician's attention immediately. The following information is supplied to the public for their general information by the American Cancer Society.

Why You Should Examine Your Breasts Monthly

Most breast cancers are first discovered by women themselves. Since breast cancers found early and treated promptly have excellent chances for cure, learning how to examine your breasts properly can help save your life. Use the sample six-step breast self-examination (BSE) procedure shown here (Fig. 3-37).

For the Best Time to Examine Your Breasts

Follow the same procedure once a month about a week after your period, when breasts are usually not tender or swollen. After menopause, check breasts

Fig. 3-37. How to examine your breast. (Courtesy American Cancer Society, New York, NY)

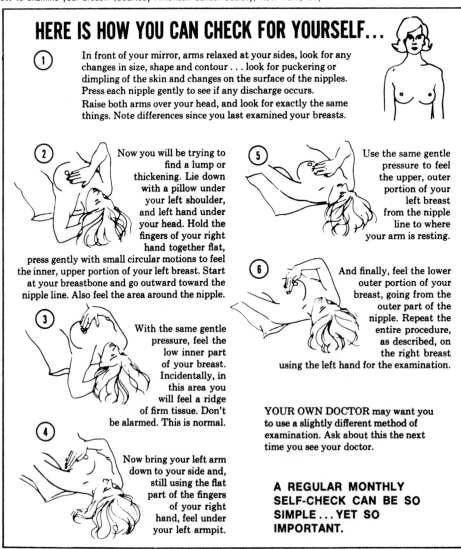

HERE IS HOW YOU CAN CHECK FOR YOURSELF...

① In front of your mirror, arms relaxed at your sides, look for any changes in size, shape and contour . . . look for puckering or dimpling of the skin and changes on the surface of the nipples. Press each nipple gently to see if any discharge occurs.
Raise both arms over your head, and look for exactly the same things. Note differences since you last examined your breasts.

② Now you will be trying to find a lump or thickening. Lie down with a pillow under your left shoulder, and left hand under your head. Hold the fingers of your right hand together flat, press gently with small circular motions to feel the inner, upper portion of your left breast. Start at your breastbone and go outward toward the nipple line. Also feel the area around the nipple.

③ With the same gentle pressure, feel the low inner part of your breast. Incidentally, in this area you will feel a ridge of firm tissue. Don't be alarmed. This is normal.

④ Now bring your left arm down to your side and, still using the flat part of the fingers of your right hand, feel under your left armpit.

⑤ Use the same gentle pressure to feel the upper, outer portion of your left breast from the nipple line to where your arm is resting.

⑥ And finally, feel the lower outer portion of your breast, going from the outer part of the nipple. Repeat the entire procedure, as described, on the right breast using the left hand for the examination.

YOUR OWN DOCTOR may want you to use a slightly different method of examination. Ask about this the next time you see your doctor.

A REGULAR MONTHLY SELF-CHECK CAN BE SO SIMPLE...YET SO IMPORTANT.

on the first day of each month. After hysterectomy, check with your doctor or clinic for an appropriate time of the month. Doing BSE will give you monthly peace of mind, and seeing your doctor once a year will reassure you there is nothing wrong.

What You Should Do If You Find a Lump or Thickening

If a lump or dimple or discharge is discovered during BSE, it is important to see your doctor as soon as possible. Don't be frightened. Most breast lumps or changes are not cancer, but only your doctor can make the diagnosis.

Know Cancer's Warning Signals!

C —Change in bowel or bladder habits
A —A sore that does not heal
U —Unusual bleeding or discharge
T —Thickening or lump in breast or elsewhere
I —Indigestion or difficulty in swallowing
O —Obvious change in wart or mole
N —Nagging cough or hoarseness

IF YOU HAVE A WARNING SIGNAL, SEE YOUR DOCTOR.

The medical assistant should see that the office or clinic has literature for women on this subject in addition to the information given in Figure 3-38. (See also "Mammography" in Unit XII.)

CONCLUSION

You have now completed the unit on Preparing for and Assisting with Routine and Specialty Physical Examinations. After you have practiced the procedures and are ready to demonstrate your skills and knowledge attained, arrange with your instructor to take the Performance Test. You will be expected to accurately demonstrate your ability in preparing for and assisting with procedures and examinations discussed in this unit and to measure a patient's distance visual acuity. In addition, you will be expected to identify by name the equipment and instruments used for each examination, if and when questioned by your instructor.

REVIEW OF VOCABULARY

The following are samples of a patient's admission note and a hospital discharge note as dictated by a physician. These are to help familiarize you with the format and contents of medical reports. Read these and be prepared to discuss the contents and define all

Fig. 3-38. Cancer related checkups. (Courtesy American Cancer Society, New York, NY)

The following guidelines for the early detection of cancer in people without symptoms are recommended by the American Cancer Society:

AGE 20-40	AGE 40 & OVER
Cancer-Related Checkup Every 3 Years	**Cancer-Related Checkup Every Year**

Cancer-Related Checkup Every 3 Years
Should include the procedures listed below plus health counseling (such as tips on quitting cigarettes) and examinations for cancers of the thyroid, testes, prostate, mouth, ovaries, skin and lymph nodes. Some people are at higher risk for certain cancers and may need to have tests more frequently.

Breast
- Exam by doctor every 3 years
- Self-exam every month
- One baseline breast X ray between ages 35-40
  Higher Risk for Breast Cancer: Personal or family history of breast cancer, never had children, first child after 30

Uterus
- Pelvic exam every 3 years

Cervix
- Pap test—after 2 initial negative tests 1 year apart—*at least* every 3 years, includes women under 20 if sexually active
  Higher Risk for Cervical Cancer: Early age at first intercourse, multiple sex partners

Remember, these guidelines are not rules and only apply to people without symptoms. Talk with your doctor. Ask how these guidelines relate to you.

Cancer-Related Checkup Every Year
Should include the procedures listed below plus health counseling (such as tips on quitting cigarettes) and examinations for cancers of the thyroid, testes, prostate, mouth, ovaries, skin and lymph nodes. Some people are at higher risk for certain cancers and may need to have tests more frequently.

Breast
- Exam by doctor every year
- Self-exam every month
- Breast X ray every year after 50. Between ages 40-50, breast X ray every 1-2 years.
  Higher Risk for Breast Cancer: Personal or family history of breast cancer, never had children, first child after 30

Uterus
- Pelvic exam every year

Cervix
- Pap test—after 2 initial negative tests 1 year apart—*at least* every 3 years
  Higher Risk for Cervical Cancer: Early age at first intercourse, multiple sex partners

Endometrium
- Endometrial tissue sample at menopause if at risk
  Higher Risk for Endometrial Cancer: Infertility, obesity, failure of ovulation, abnormal uterine bleeding, estrogen therapy

Colon & Rectum
- Digital rectal exam every year
- Stool blood test every year after 50
- Procto exam—after 2 initial negative tests 1 year apart—every 3 to 5 years after 50
  Higher Risk for Colorectal Cancer: Personal or family history of colon or rectal cancer, personal or family history of polyps in the colon or rectum, ulcerative colitis

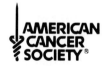
AMERICAN CANCER SOCIETY®

the medical terms that are used. You should recognize some of the terms; others are new, and you may have to refer to Appendix A or a medical dictionary for the definitions.

Medical Center
PHYSICIAN'S REPORT

PATIENT:
  McFerrin, Sandra
PHYSICIAN:
  Robert Scott, MD

☒ADMISSION NOTE
☐CONSULTATION

☐DISCHARGE SUMMARY
9/13/_____ Admitted
_____ Discharged

CHIEF COMPLAINT: Abdominal pain.
PRESENT ILLNESS:
  The patient is a 19-year-old woman who, for the

first 5 days, has had progressively severe abdominal pain. There has been no nausea until the day of admission, when she became nauseated driving over to the hospital. There has been no vomiting and there has been no chills or fever. The patient has not been bothered by constipation or diarrhea. She had a normal bowel movement the day prior to admission. The patient's menstrual period started the day before admission and the previous one approximately a month ago was normal.

The patient was seen in my office the day prior to admission and epigastric tenderness was noted. Donnatal and Maalox were prescribed, but this afforded little if any relief. The pain became more acute, more severe, and awoke the patient from sleep and prompted her present admission.

PAST HISTORY:

The patient's past health has been quite good except for an automobile accident approximately a year and a half ago in which her pelvis and bladder were fractured and lacerated respectively. No sequelae followed. Patient was treated prophylactically with INH for a year, approximately 7 to 8 years ago for exposure to tuberculosis.

FAMILY HISTORY:

There is no family history of diabetes, cancer, or premature cardiac disease. The patient's sister had pulmonary tuberculosis when the patient was young, and the patient received a year's course of prophylactic INH. The patient's skin test was positive.

REVIEW OF SYSTEMS:

There are no symptoms of respiratory, cardiac, or genitourinary disease.

PHYSICAL EXAMINATION:

Blood pressure 130/80, pulse 90, temperature 36.6 degrees centigrade.

General appearance: The patient is a young, well-developed woman who is lying in bed crying because of abdominal pain. Skin: no rash. Eyes: Sclera clear. The pupils are round, regular and equal. ENT: The tongue and mucous membrane are somewhat dry. Neck: Supple. Breasts: Clear. Heart: Normal sinus rhythm, no murmurs. Lungs: clear. Abdomen: Flat, the bowel sounds are hypoactive. There is marked epigastric and left upper quadrant tenderness. There is no guarding or rigidity. There is no rebound tenderness. There is no adnexal tenderness. Rectal examination negative. Extremities negative.

IMPRESSION:

Acute abdominal pain, etiology to be determined.

RS:vy
D:9/13/_____
T:9/13/_____

        _____

        Robert Scott, M.D.

DISCHARGE NOTE

PATIENT: Marion Dale

PHYSICIAN: Scott Douglas, MD
DATE: April 15, 19_____

The patient is a 45-year-old premenopausal white woman presenting a history of a recent dark vaginal discharge with a negative Papanicolaou test in April of last year, but a recent Papanicolaou test showed dyskeratotic cells and atypical class III cells. Biopsy the next month was positive for epidermoid carcinoma with lymphatic permeating present.

Pelvic examination revealed a lacerated eroded cervical canal, and, under anesthesia, pelvic examination showed uterine enlargement to approximately twice the normal size with a freely mobile uterus; however, no evidence of parametrial induration or other pelvic pathology was present.

Following endometrial curettage, a tandem and colpostat radium-containing applicator were inserted, with the applicator carrying a total of 90 milligrams homogenous distribution in a circular e.5 cm colpostat, 20 mg radium in the base and 20 mg in the tip of the tandem with ½ mm plantinum intrinsic filtration and 1.5 mm Monel extrinsic-filtration, representing total equivalent of 1 mm plantinum filtration.

The applicator was inserted to be removed after 72 hours for a total dosage of 6480 milligram hours. Following the course of radium, a complete pelvic cycle with external irradiation is recommended. Intravenous pyelogram showed no obstructive nephropathy or ureteral constriction or displacement. Portable AP and lateral views of the pelvis confirming the position of the applicator in situ are to be obtained. Three rolls of iodoform packing in the vaginal canal firmly secured the applicator in contact with the cervical lips, and a loose ligature affixed the colpostat to the anterior cervical lip during the surgical procedure.

        Scott Douglas, MD

REVIEW QUESTIONS

1. List and summarize the medical assistant's general responsibilities when assisting the physician with a complete physical examination.
2. Indicate what body part or system is examined with the following instruments:
   a. Otoscope
   b. Laryngeal mirror
   c. Ophthalmoscope
   d. Anoscope
   e. Tuning fork
   f. Bronchoscope
   g. Cystoscope
   h. Percussion hammer
   i. Stethoscope
3. In what position is the patient placed for
   • A vaginal or pelvic exam?
   • A rectal examination and proctosigmoidoscopy?
   • A chest examination?
   • An examination of the ears and eyes?
4. List the purpose(s) and the common instruments required for the following examinations:

- General physical examination
- Vaginal examination
- Pap smear or test
- Rectal examination
- Proctosigmoidoscopy

5. If a physician suspects a growth in the sigmoid colon that is considered doubtful as to being benign or malignant, what procedure will the physician usually perform?
6. You have a 50-year-old obese patient who cannot tolerate the jackknife position for a sigmoidoscopy. Name an alternate position that may be used for this examination.
7. Explain why it is important for a female assistant to remain in the room when a female patient is being examined by a male physician.
8. List some of the common unusual reactions for which you will observe a patient during an examination.
9. Explain why it is important that you check battery-operated and electrical equipment before an examination.
10. List the instruments and equipment that would be used for a neurological examination.
11. What is a Snellen chart, and how is it used?
12. When increased pressure is present in the eyeball, what common condition is suspected?
13. Albumin in the urine during a pregnancy is thought to be a serious sign of what condition?
14. List seven warning signals of cancer.
15. Explain how a woman can perform a breast self-examination.
16. Why should every woman examine her breasts monthly?
17. When is the best time of the month for a woman to examine her breasts for any unusual lump or thickening?

PERFORMANCE TEST

In a skills laboratory, a simulation of a joblike environment, the medical assistant student is to demonstrate knowledge and skill in performing the following procedures without reference to source materials. For these activities, the student will need a person to play the role of a patient, and all the necessary equipment and supplies. Time limits for the performance of each procedure are to be assigned by the instructor.

1. Given an ambulatory patient, the student is to position and drape the patient in the following positions, and state when each is used:
   a. Dorsal-recumbent
   b. Lithotomy
   c. Sims
   d. Knee-chest
   e. Supine
   f. Prone
   g. Trendelenburg

2. Given an ambulatory patient, the student is to prepare for and assist with
   a. A complete physical examination that is to include a vaginal and rectal examination
   b. A proctosigmoidoscopy, including a description of the patient preparation that is to be completed before the examination
3. Given an ambulatory patient, the student is to prepare for and measure distance visual acuity using the Snellen eye chart.

The student is expected to perform the above activities with 100% accuracy 90% of the time (9 out of 10 times).

PERFORMANCE CHECKLISTS

Preparing for and Assisting with a Complete Physical Examination, Including a Vaginal and Rectal Examination

1. Wash your hands.
2. Assemble and prepare the equipment and supplies needed, and be able to identify each instrument by name.
3. Identify the patient, and explain the procedure.
4. Take the following physical measurements of the patient, and record the results accurately on the patient's chart:
   - Temperature, pulse, and respiration rate
   - Blood pressure
   - Weight and height
5. Prepare the patient for the examination:
   - Have the patient void; save specimen if needed.
   - Have the patient disrobe completely and put on patient gown.
   - Position the patient on the examining table in a sitting or supine position.
   - Drape the patient.
6. Assist the physician as required during the examination (supply or hand supplies and equipment to the physician as needed).
7. Assist the patient during the examination, giving reassurance and support; observe the patient for any unusual reactions.
8. Assist the patient in changing positions to the Sims for the rectal examination, drape the patient, and have the required equipment ready for the physician.
9. Help the patient change positions to the lithotomy for the vaginal examination, drape the patient, and have the required equipment ready for the physician.
10. Provide for the patient's comfort at the conclusion of the examination by removing drapes, answering any questions the patient may have, informing the patient of special or future instructions, and helping the patient to get dressed.
11. Carry out the physician's orders for additional examinations or tests. If specimens were obtained, prepare them properly to be sent to the laboratory.

12. Collect, dispose of, clean, return, and replace all used equipment as needed.
13. Wash your hands.
14. Record on the patient's chart (neatly) complete and accurate information. Include: date, hour, procedure, and results (where applicable).
15. Complete the procedure in the time limit assigned by the instructor.

Preparing for and Assisting with a Proctosigmoidoscopy

1. Describe the preparation of the patient for the examination.
   • A laxative the evening before
   • Only liquids for breakfast
   • Tap water or saline enemas until clear, 1 hour before the examination
2. Wash your hands.
3. Assemble and prepare the supplies and equipment needed, and be able to identify all equipment by name. Test suction apparatus and the light on the scopes.
4. Identify patient and explain the procedure.
5. Prepare the patient for the examination.
   • Have the patient void; save a specimen if needed.
   • Have patient disrobe and put on patient gown.
   • Position patient in the knee-chest position or Sims position, as requested.
   • Drape the patient.
6. Assist the physician as required during the examination (supply or hand supplies and equipment to the physician as needed).
7. Assist the patient during the examination, giving reassurance and support; observe the patient for any unusual reaction.
8. Provide for the patient's comfort at the conclusion of the examination by assisting to a supine position, removing drapes, answering questions, providing any further instructions, and helping to dress.
9. Carry out the physician's orders for additional examinations or tests. If specimens were obtained, prepare them properly to be sent to the laboratory.
10. Collect, dispose of, clean, return, and replace all used equipment and supplies.
11. Wash your hands.

12. Record on the patient's chart complete and accurate information. Include: date, hour, procedure, source and disposal of specimens (when obtained), results (when applicable), condition of the patient (when pertinent).
13. Complete the procedure in the time limit assigned by the instructor.

Measuring Distance Visual Acuity with the Snellen Eye Chart

1. Wash your hands.
2. Prepare room; determine location of 20 feet from the chart where patient is to be positioned.
3. Assemble supplies and equipment.
4. Identify the patient and explain the procedure.
5. Position patient comfortably (sitting or standing) 20 feet from the eye chart.
6. Position the center of the Snellen eye chart at the patient's eye level.
7. Instruct the patient to cover the left eye with opaque card or eye cover, and to keep the left eye open.
8. Instruct the patient to use the right eye and to orally identify one row at a time on the chart as you point to each row, starting at row 20/70 (or several lines above row 20/20).
9. Proceed down the chart if the patient identifies the 20/70 row, or proceed up the chart if the patient is unable to identify the 20/70 row.
10. Continue testing until the smallest row of letters that the patient can read is reached.
11. Provide instructions to the patient during the test, and observe for any unusual reaction(s).
12. Record the results of visual acuity on a piece of paper.
13. Instruct the patient to cover the right eye and to keep it open.
14. Measure visual acuity of the left eye using steps 8 through 12.
15. Give further instructions to the patient as required.
16. Return equipment and leave room neat and clean.
17. Record the results on the patient's chart.
18. Complete the procedure in time limit assigned by the instructor, such as 10 minutes.

Unit IV

Infection Control: Practices of Medical Asepsis and Sterilization

COGNITIVE OBJECTIVES

On completion of Unit IV, the medical assistant student should be able to apply the following cognitive objectives.

1. Define and pronounce the terms presented in the vocabulary and throughout the unit.
2. List the five classifications of microorganisms that are capable of causing a disease process, giving examples of diseases caused by each.
3. List the six factors that are essential for the development of an infectious process, discussing briefly components in each.
4. Differentiate between the types of human reservoirs — overt cases, subclinical cases, and human carriers.
5. Compare direct transmission with indirect transmission of a disease process.
6. List and describe the body's natural defense mechanisms used to control or prevent disease and infection.
7. Discuss and compare the various types of immunity.
8. List the classical signs and symptoms of inflammation and briefly describe the inflammatory process.
9. List five diagnostic tests that may be used to diagnose an infectious process.
10. Differentiate between medical and surgical asepsis; list and describe procedures used to accomplish each and medical situations in which each is employed.
11. Differentiate between sanitization, disinfection, and sterilization; describe the procedures employed by these methods when working with contaminated instruments, syringes and needles, rubber goods, and other equipment, selecting the most effective method for controlling microscopic agents.
12. Explain the importance of sterilizing instruments and supplies before using them for medical procedures.
13. List and briefly describe five methods used for sterilizing equipment and two methods used for disinfecting equipment.
14. Describe how items are to be wrapped, positioned, and removed from a sterilizer for sterilization to be effective, and how items are to be positioned and removed from a boiler.
15. State the recommended exposure times for sterilizing and disinfecting the various types of equipment and supplies that are used in the physician's office.
16. Describe types of and state the reason for using sterilization indicators.
17. Discuss how, where, and the length of time sterile supplies should be stored.
18. Discuss infection precautions to use for AIDS (Acquired Immune Deficiency Syndrome) and other diseases that may be seen in AIDS patients.

TERMINAL PERFORMANCE OBJECTIVES

On completion of Unit IV, the medical assistant should be able to do the following terminal performance objectives.

1. Demonstrate how to wash hands, wrists, and forearms, explaining the reasons for the actions taken.
2. Given various items assumed to be contaminated, demonstrate how to sanitize, disinfect, and sterilize each, using the methods discussed in this unit.
3. Given packs that have been removed from an autoclave, determine if sterilization has been effective and then store each for use at a later date.
4. Given items to be sterilized, demonstrate how each should be wrapped before placing it in the sterilizer.

The student is to perform the above skills with 100% accuracy 90% of the time (9 out of 10 times).

Vocabulary

antiseptic (an'tĭ-sep'tik)—A substance capable of inhibiting the growth or action of microorganisms, without necessarily killing them; generally safe for use on body tissues.

asepsis (ā-sep'sis)—The absence of all microorganisms causing disease; absence of contaminated matter.

bactericide (bak-tēr'ĭ-sīd)—A substance capable of destroying bacteria but not spores.

bacteriostatic (bak-te"re-o-stat'ik)—A substance that inhibits the growth of bacteria.

contaminated, contamination (kon-tam"ĭ-na'shun)—The act of making unclean, soiling, or staining, especially the introduction of disease germs or infectious material into or on normally sterile objects.

disinfectant (dis"in-fek'tant)—A substance capable of destroying pathogens, but usually not spores; generally not intended for use on body tissue, because it is too strong.

fungicide (fun'jĭ-sīd)—A substance that destroys fungi.

germicide (jer'mĭ-sīd)—A substance that is capable of destroying pathogens.

immunization (im"u-nĭ-za'shun)—The process of rendering a person immune (protected from or not susceptible to a disease) or of becoming immune; frequently called vaccination or inoculation. A process by which a person is artificially prepared to resist infection by a specific pathogen.

incubation (in"ku-ba'shun) **period**—The interval of time between the invasion of a pathogen into the body and the appearance of the first symptoms of disease.

infection (in-fek'shun)—A condition caused by the multiplication of pathogenic microorganisms that have invaded the body of a susceptible host.

- *acute*—rapid onset, severe symptoms, and usually subsides within a relatively short period of time.
- *chronic*—develops slowly, milder symptoms, and lasts for a long period of time.
- *latent*—dormant or concealed; pathogen is ever-present in the host, but symptoms are present only intermittently, often in response to a stimulus. At other times the pathogen is dormant.
- *localized*—restricted to a certain area.
- *generalized*—systemic; involving the whole body.

medical microbiology—The study and identification of pathogens, and the development of effective methods for their control or elimination.

necrosis (ne-kro'-sis)—The death of a cell or a group of cells because of injury or disease.

normal flora—Microorganisms that normally reside in various body locations such as in the vagina, intestine, urethra, upper respiratory tract, and on the skin. These microorganisms are nonpathogenic and do not cause any harm (although they may become pathogenic and cause harm if they are introduced into a body area in which they do not normally reside).

pathogenic (păth"ō-jĕn'ĭk)—Productive of disease. *p. microorganism*—one that produces disease in the body.

reservoir (rez'er-vwar)—The source in which pathogenic microorganisms grow and from which they leave to spread and cause disease.

resistance (re-zis'tans)—The ability of the body to resist disease or infection because of its own defense mechanisms.

sepsis (sep'sis)—A morbid state or condition resulting from the presence of pathogenic microorganisms.

spore (spōr)—A reproductive cell, usually unicellular, produced by plants and some protozoa, and possessing thick walls to withstand unfavorable environmental conditions. Bacterial spores are resistant to heat and must undergo a prolonged exposure to extremely high temperatures to be destroyed.

sterile (ster'il)—Free from all microorganisms.

toxin (tok'sin)—A poisonous substance produced by pathogenic bacteria and some animals and plants. The toxins produced by bacteria include toxic enzymes, exotoxins, and endotoxins. Toxins in the body cause antitoxins to form, which provide a means for establishing immunity to certain diseases.

vaccination (vak"sĭ-na'shun)—The introduction of weakened or dead microorganisms (inoculation) into the body to stimulate the production of antibodies and immunity to a specific disease.

virulence (vir'u-lens)—The degree of ability of a pathogen to produce disease.

BASIC CONCEPTS AND GOALS

Since the early days of civilization, there has been concern with the control of disease and the spread of infection. The history of medicine documents the wealth of knowledge attained by numerous individuals on the anatomy and physiology of the human body, certain diseases, and many therapeutic agents. However, not until the last half of the nineteenth century was a connection between disease and pathogenic microorganisms established through the work of Louis Pasteur and Robert Koch. Among the findings documented, Pasteur discovered important properties of bacteria, and Koch was credited with establishing the germ theory of disease. Koch's theory states that to prove an organism is actually the specific pathogen causing the disease, one must es-

*UBIQUITOUS.
everywhere

tablish a causal relationship between the microbe and the disease.

*Microorganisms (microbes) are defined as minute living creatures that are too small to be seen by the naked eye. The classifications or divisions of microscopic life include viruses, rickettsiae, bacteria, fungi, and parasites. Microorganisms in each of these divisions that cause disease are termed *pathogens*. It is important to keep in mind that many members of these microscopic divisions are either beneficial or harmless to humans or animals. The term *medical microbiology* implies the study of pathogens, involving identification and development of effective methods of control or elimination.

Pathogenic microorganisms are everywhere around us. They are easily spread directly from person to person, or indirectly by animate and inanimate vehicles to humans. Disease or infection transpires when pathogens invade a susceptible host. Although we have antibiotics for use in the treatment of many infectious processes, the best method available for infection control is to prevent the spread of disease-producing microorganisms. It is our responsibility as health professionals to take an active, conscientious role in the process of infection control. Lack of knowledge as to how pathogens spread or how to control the process is frequently the cause of major outbreaks of infection or disease. The goals of infection control are to prevent the spread of pathogenic microorganisms, to attain a state of asepsis (absence of pathogens), and to educate the public in the ways that they too can help. Asepsis, or aseptic technique, is divided into two categories: medical asepsis and surgical asepsis. It is important to distinguish between these two methods.

The rest of this unit discusses disease-producing organisms, how they are spread, the body's own defense mechanisms, and medical and surgical asepsis with techniques and sterilization procedures used to prevent transmission of pathogens. Surgical asepsis (aseptic technique) is discussed in greater length in Unit V.

INFECTIOUS PROCESS AND CAUSATIVE AGENTS

Six factors are essential for the development of the infectious process. The mere presence of a pathogenic microorganism is not enough to promote infection. There must be a sequential connection between the following factors:

1. A cause or an etiological (e-tĭ-o-loj′ik-ăl) agent (pathogen)
2. A source or a reservoir of the etiological agent
3. A means of escape of the etiological agent from the reservoir (portals of exit)

4. A means of transmission of the etiological agent from the reservoir to the new host
5. A means of entry of the etiological agent into the new susceptible host (portals of entry)
6. A susceptible host

Cause or Etiological Agent

Infection begins with the invasion of the body by a pathogen that is the causative agent of the disease in question. The pathogenic organisms must be present in a sufficiently high concentration and be adequately capable of causing disease. The causative agent or pathogen may be one or more of the following.

Viruses.   Viruses (vī′rŭs) are the smallest pathogens and require susceptible host cells for multiplication and activity. To observe viruses, an electron microscope must be used. A phenomenon that characterizes viral infections as the most insidious is the fact that viruses, as intracellular parasites, can only multiply inside a living cell. Viruses attach themselves to a living cell, inject a compound of protein and a nucleic acid, either DNA (deoxyribonucleic acid) or RNA (ribonucleic acid), and take over the normal cellular metabolism. The cell proceeds to make new cells in addition to new viruses, then bursts, dies, and releases numerous viruses that can then invade other cells. Chemotherapy for viral diseases is extremely difficult, because the viruses surviving an initial dose of a drug have the ability to change their characteristics so that they rapidly become resistant to the drug.

Viruses are also more resistant to chemical disinfection than bacteria, but can be destroyed by heat, as is done when sterilizing equipment in an autoclave.

There is a greater variety of viruses than of any other category of microbial agents of disease. Viruses are the causative agents of flu, poliomyelitis, colds, mumps, measles, rabies, smallpox, chickenpox, as well as hepatitis A, hepatitis B, and herpes simplex I, and herpes simplex II.

Rickettsiae.   Rickettsiae (rĭk-ĕt′sĭ-ă) are also obligate intracellular parasites. They differ from viruses in that they are visible under a conventional microscope by special staining techniques and are also susceptible to antibiotic suppression of replication.

Rickettsiae are the causative organisms for the various "spotted fevers" such as Rocky Mountain spotted fever, and also typhus, Q fever, and trench fever. They are generally tick-borne, and therefore are not common in sanitary urban areas.

Bacteria.   Bacteria (bak-te′re-ah) can readily multiply outside of living cells. Bacteria are single-celled organisms that can be cultivated on artificial media and then with appropriate staining techniques are readily visible under a microscope. These characteristics make bacteria much simpler to identify than viruses and rickettsiae. There are many varieties, only some of which cause disease; most are nonpathogenic, and many are useful. Bacteria are classified in three groups according to their shape and appearance (morphology) (Fig. 4-1):

1. Cocci (kok'si) are spherical bacteria; among the cocci are the following three types:
   Staphylococci (stăf"ĭl-ō-kŏk'sĭ) — forming grape-like clusters of cells, these are the most common pus-producing organisms known to man. They are readily found in pimples, boils, suture abscesses, and osteomyelitis.
   Streptococci (strĕp"tō-kŏk'sĭ) — forming chains of cells, these are the cause of strep throat, rheumatic heart disease (RHD), scarlet fever, and septicemia (infection in the blood stream).
   Diplococci (dĭp-lō-kŏk'sĭ) — forming pairs of cells, different types of diplococci are the causative organisms for gonorrhea, pneumonia, and meningitis.
2. Bacilli (bah-sil'i) are rod-shaped bacteria; these organisms cause tuberculosis (TB), typhoid and paratyphoid fever, tetanus (lockjaw), gas gangrene, bacillary dysentery, and diphtheria.
3. Spirilla (spi-ril'ah) are spiral organisms; these organisms cause cholera, syphilis, and relapsing fever.

Fungi. Fungi (fun'ji) are the lowest form of infectious agents that bridge the gap between free-living and host-dependent parasites.

Fungi are unicellular or multicellular. They can be grown on artificial media and then identified under the microscope. Fungi appear in the form of molds and mushrooms, as well as in microscopic growth. Disease-producing fungi are seen as the causative agent in some infections of the skin, such as athlete's foot and ringworm.

The fungus *Candida albicans* (Monilia) is responsible for the disease known as thrush (an infection of the mouth and throat) and also some vaginal infections.

Parasites. Parasites (par'ah-sīt) are organisms that live in or on another organism from which they gain their nourishment. Parasites include single-celled and multicelled animals, fungi, and bacteria. Viruses are sometimes considered to be parasitic. Examples include the following:

1. Protozoa (pro"to-zo'ah) are single-celled microscopic organisms. Some can be cultivated, fixed, and stained for viewing under a microscope. The most well-known protozoa cause malaria, amoebic dysentery, and trichomonas infections of the vagina.
2. Metazoal (met"ah-zo'al) parasites are multicellular organisms, causing conditions such as pinworms, hookworms, tapeworms, and trichinosis in pork.
3. Ectoparasites (ek"to-par'ah-sīt) can superficially affect the host, like lice and scabies mite, or can invade the integument, such as the larvae of dipterous flies.

Source or Reservoir of Etiological Agent

Areas where organisms grow and reproduce are called reservoirs and are found mainly in human beings and animals. Organisms may also exist in soil, water, and equipment.

Human reservoirs include:

- Overt cases: people who are obviously ill with the disease
- Subclinical cases: abortive and ambulatory (walking) cases of the disease, e.g., "walking" pneumonia
- Human carriers: people unaware of their condition who circulate freely in their communities until detected and diagnosed, for example, the "Typhoid Marys," or people who are in the convalescent stage of an infection.

Animal reservoirs include mainly domestic animals and rodents. Zoonosis (zo"o-no'sis) is the term given to an animal disease that is transmissible to humans. In this case, the infection is usually derived from the animal and is not further transmitted from human to human. An example is rabies.

Means of Escape of Etiological Agent from Reservoir (Portals of Exit)

Pathogens commonly exit from their reservoir through one or more of the following:

- Respiratory tract in secretions from the nose, nasal sinuses, nasopharynx, larynx, trachea, bronchial tree, and lungs
- Intestinal tract through discharge with the feces
- Urinary tract through discharge or in the urine
- Skin or mucous membranes, or open lesions or discharges on the surface of the body

Fig. 4-1. Classification of bacteria according to their morphology.

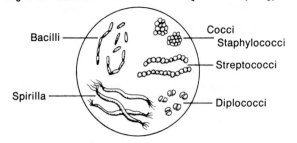

Bacilli

Cocci
Staphylococci

Streptococci

Spirilla

Diplococci

- Reproductive tract through discharges
- Blood
- Across the placenta

Means of Transmission of Etiological Agent from Reservoir to New Host

The means of transmission is the method by which the pathogen is transmitted from the portal of exit in the reservoir to the portal of entry in the new host. After an infecting organism has escaped from its reservoir, it can cause a new infection only if it finds its way to a new susceptible host. Transmission may occur by either of the following:

- *Direct transmission:* The organism passes from one person to another through inhalation or by actual physical contact, such as sexual contact, or by direct contact with an open lesion. The organism goes from one host to another without the aid of intermediate objects.
- *Indirect transmission:* The organism is capable of survival for a period of time outside the body and is transferred to the new host by a vehicle, which is either animate or inanimate. Animate vehicles are people who touch contaminated material, don't wash their hands, and then carry the microorganism on their hands to a susceptible host. Other animate vehicles are called vectors and include the various insects that spread infection. Inanimate vehicles are nonliving objects or substances and include water, milk, foods, soil, air, excreta, clothing, instruments, toiletries, or any contaminated article.

Means of Entry of Etiological Agent into New Susceptible Host

The infecting organism enters the new host through a part of the body, which is called the portal of entry. The main portals of entry follow:

- Respiratory tract—organisms may be inhaled
- Gastrointestinal tract—organisms may be ingested
- Skin or mucous membranes—organisms may be introduced via cuts, abrasions, or open wounds
- Urinary tract—organisms may be introduced through external body orifices
- Reproductive tract—organisms may be introduced through external body orifices
- Blood
- Across the placenta

Although avenues of escape or portals of exit correspond to the portals of entry, the pathogen can escape from one site in the reservoir and enter the new host in another site. An example of this is when the pathogen leaves from the respiratory tract in the reservoir (as through sputum or water droplets) and enters the new host through the skin (as through an open wound when a dressing is being changed).

Susceptible Host

For the infectious process to be completed, the pathogenic organism must enter a host whose resistance is so low that it cannot fight off the invading organism. Even though a pathogen gains entry to the body, disease or infection may not develop, since the body possesses certain defense mechanisms to protect itself. These mechanisms may also help destroy invading pathogens. Such defense mechanisms are called resistance, and if they are sufficiently great, they constitute immunity (ĭ-mū'nĭ-tē).

Table 4-1 outlines the six essential factors of the infectious process for two diseases. All infectious diseases can be outlined in this manner.

Stages of an Infectious Process

The stages of an infectious process generally include the following:

Table 4-1. Factors of infectious process

Disease	Cause/agent	Reservoir/ source	Means of escape from the reservoir	Means of transmission from reservoir to new host	Means of entry into new host	Susceptible host
German measles (rubella)	Virus	Humans	Mouth, nasopharynx	Water droplets	Mouth	Humans
Pneumonia	Bacteria	Humans	Mouth, nasopharynx	Droplets, sputum Fomites, such as a pencil (indirect transmission)	Mouth, respiratory mucosa	Humans

1. The invasion and multiplication of the pathogen in the body.
2. The incubation period, which may vary from a few days to months or years.
3. The prodromal period when the first mild signs and symptoms appear. The person is highly contagious during this period.
4. The acute period when signs and symptoms are at the most severe stage.
5. The recovery and convalescent period when signs and symptoms begin to subside and the body heals itself, returning to a state of health.

THE BODY'S DEFENSES AGAINST DISEASE AND INFECTION

The body's resistance level to undesirable microorganisms is influenced by the general health status of the individual and other related circumstances:

- Amount of rest, sufficient or insufficient
- Dietary intake of nutritional foods, adequate or inadequate
- How one copes with stress
- Age of the individual (the young and aged are most susceptible to infection because of the immaturity of the immune system in the young and the decline of this system in the aged)
- Presence of other disease processes in the body
- Condition of the external environment (such as poor living conditions)
- Influence of genetic traits (for example, people with diabetes mellitus and sickle cell anemia are more prone to some infections than are other individuals)

Physical and Chemical Barriers

The body has natural defense mechanisms, either physical or chemical, that act as barriers to the invasion of pathogenic organisms.

Skin. This tissue is the largest barrier against infection. As long as it remains intact, the skin serves as a physical barrier to a tremendous number of microorganisms. Chemical barriers of the skin include the acid pH of the skin (which inhibits bacterial infection), sweat, and lysozyme (which functions as an antibacterial enzyme in the skin).

Mucous Membrane. This tissue holds in check many microorganisms because of the repelling forces in the secretions that bathe these membranes. The cilia of some mucous membranes serve to keep their surfaces swept clean.

Respiratory Tract. The mucosal lining of this tract is very sensitive and thus readily stimulated by foreign matter. Certain reflexes, such as coughing or sneezing, help remove foreign matter, including microorganisms. The hairs lining the nostrils, along with the moist membranes, serve as a physical barrier. The cilia lining the bronchi beat upward to carry mucus and small, interfering foreign materials such as dust, bacteria, and soot to the throat. The tortuous passageway from the mouth to the lungs also serves as a barrier.

Gastrointestinal Tract. Hydrochloric acid in the stomach has an important bactericidal action, destroying many disease-producing agents. Bile, when in the small intestine, is thought to have a germicidal effect.

Blood and Lymphoid Tissue. These tissues contain and produce cells and antibodies that are able to exert a tremendous influence in protecting the body against disease. White blood cells (leukocytes) are particularly active when pathogenic microorganisms invade the body. In the inflammatory process, some leukocytes surround, engulf, and digest the pathogens. This process is known as phagocytosis (fag"o-si-tō'sis), which is basically the ingestion of the pathogen or "cell-eating." Lymphoid tissue produces antibodies, which are basically protein compounds that help combat infection.

Antigen-Antibody Reaction

Another internal defense mechanism that the body gradually develops against invasion by foreign substances (antigens) is the formation of antibodies. Antibodies are protein substances produced mainly in the lymph nodes, spleen, bone marrow, and lymphoid tissue in response to invasion by an antigen. Different types of antibodies are produced in response to different antigens, with each antibody being effective only against the specific antigen that stimulates its production. The antibodies can either neutralize the antigens, render them harmless, rupture their cell membrane, or prepare the antigen so that they are more susceptible to destruction by phagocytes (cells that ingest and destroy microorganisms, cells, and cell debris).

The antigen-antibody reaction is this reaction of the body to the invasion of antigens. When antibodies are produced in sufficient quantities, the body becomes immune. Since the body is capable of continuing to produce antibodies for weeks to several years, it is possible for immunity to last for months or years.

Immunity

Immunity, the resistance of the body to pathogenic microorganisms and their toxins, occurs as a result of the antigen-antibody reaction. Specific types of immunity follow:

- Active immunity develops when antigens are introduced into the body.
- Passive immunity develops when ready-made antibodies are introduced into the body.
- Natural immunity is an inborn resistance to a disease due to antibodies that are normally present in the blood.
- Acquired or induced immunity results from antibodies that are not normally present in the blood.

Both active and passive immunity are produced by natural and acquired means.

Natural Immunity. *Inherited (active) immunity* is acquired by being a member of a race or species. Some races are highly or less susceptible to certain diseases. The longer a race has been exposed to a certain disease, the less susceptible its members become. Humans do not contract many diseases common to lower species of animals, and lower species of animals do not contract most human diseases.

Congenital (passive) immunity is the immunity possessed at birth; antibodies are passed from the mother through the placenta to the fetus. The duration of this immunity may last from 5 to 6 months.

Acquired Immunity. *Natural active immunity* results from being a carrier, recovering from or having a disease, or having an atypical or subclinical case of the disease.

Artificial active immunity is acquired through vaccinations with inactivated (dead) or attenuated (weakened) organisms. Inactivated or dead vaccines include the typhoid, whooping cough, and influenza vaccines, and the Salk vaccine for polio. Attenuated vaccines include vaccines for polio (the Sabin vaccine), smallpox, measles (rubeola), mumps, and German measles (rubella). Toxoids are exotoxins that have been modified to reduce the toxicity. These include the diphtheria and tetanus toxoids.

Artificial passive immunity is obtained by injecting various products that are usually prepared commercially, to produce a high level of antibodies immediately. These products are used to modify, treat, or prevent disease and include gamma globulin and antitoxins.

Gamma globulin, obtained from the blood, is sometimes used for treatment, but is more frequently used for the prevention of viral hepatitis and measles. Antitoxins include the following:

- Diphtheria antitoxin, produced by vaccinating horses and then extracting the gamma globulin fraction of the blood, is used for the immediate prevention and treatment of diphtheria.
- Tetanus antitoxin, obtained by extracting the gamma globulin fraction from the blood of people recently vaccinated with the tetanus toxoid, is used for the immediate prevention and treatment of tetanus.
- Immune sera, either bacterial or viral in origin, are obtained from the gamma globulin fraction of blood from an artificially immunized animal. The rabies immune sera and the pertussis (whooping cough) immune sera are the most commonly used products.

For a guide to common vaccines and toxoids, see Tables 4-2 and 4-3.

Inflammatory Process

The inflammatory process is a nonspecific defense response of the body to an irritating, invasive, or injurious foreign substance. In other words, it is a process by which the body responds to injury. Acute inflammation is stimulated by necrosis and degeneration of tissue (injuries), invading microorganisms (infection), and antigen-antibody reactions (allergies). The inflammatory process includes dilation of the blood vessels because of increased blood flow, oozing of watery fluids and protein into tissue spaces (exudation) from the dilated blood vessels because of their increased permeability, and infiltration of neutrophils and monocytes (white blood cells) from the blood into the tissue of the injured area to phagocytize (ingest) necrotic tissue and bacteria, if present.

After phagocytosis is complete, the liquified remains diffuse back into the blood vessels or are carried away by the lymphatic vessels that drain into regional lymph nodes. Here the contents are filtered to prevent the spread of foreign substances or bacteria to other parts of the body. By now the process of repair has started at the original site of inflammation. Classical signs and symptoms of inflammation include both local signs and symptoms, which are a result of the changes seen in the blood vessels and the effect on the surrounding tissues, and systemic signs and symptoms.

Local

Redness
Heat or warmth
Swelling
Pain or tenderness
Limitation of function in the area

Systemic

Leukocytosis (increased number of white blood cells in the blood)
Fever
Increased pulse rate
Increased respiration rate

Table 4-2. Guide for use of selected vaccines and toxoids

This guide is intended to serve as a quick reference for commonly employed immunization procedures. It is based on recommendations made by the Public Health Service Advisory Committee on Immunization Practices (ACIP) and the Report of the Committee on Infectious Diseases 1982 (RED BOOK) of the American Academy of Pediatrics. Reference should be made to the complete published reports of these two committees for more detailed information on general considerations and specific applications of accepted immunization practices.

IMPORTANT: Avoid immunizing persons ill or febrile in preceding 24 hours. Carefully read the product description and directions supplied with each immunizing agent as potency (dosage) may vary with the manufacturer. In addition, agents may contain substances to which patients may be sensitive such as egg protein or antibiotics.

Disease	Immunizing Agent	Age Range	Administration (Intramuscular — IM) (Subcutaneous — sc)	Primary Immunization Interval(s)	Booster Doses	Comments
Diphtheria, tetanus, and pertussis	Toxoids of diphtheria and tetanus, alum precipitated or adsorbed, combined with pertussis antigen (DTP)	For infants and children ages 6 weeks through 6 years	Three doses: 0.5 ml each IM Fourth dose: 0.5 ml IM	4–8 weeks 6–12 months	At age 4–6 years, preferably at time of school entrance. Dose: 0.5 ml IM	Do not use after 7th birthday.
Tetanus and diphtheria (for adults)	Toxoids of tetanus and diphtheria, alum precipitated or adsorbed, combined (contains 1–2 Lf units diphtheria toxoid) (Td)	7 years through adult	Two doses: 0.5 ml each IM Third dose: 0.5 ml IM	4–8 weeks 6–12 months	Every 10 years for life	For severe wounds, it is unnecessary to use booster doses if the patient has completed a primary series and has had a booster dose within the preceding 5 years (within 10 years for clean minor wounds)
Influenza	Inactivated (killed) polyvalent, bivalent or monovalent influenza virus vaccine (grown in chick embryo tissue)	All ages, from 6 months. Seasonally for high risk groups such as the elderly and those with chronic illness	May change from year to year. See instructions on manufacturer's package insert	4 weeks or more, if 2 doses are needed	Seasonally for high risk groups	Does not protect after exposure. "Split", or "sub-unit" vaccine generally recommended for children
Poliomyelitis	Inactivated (killed) trivalent, poliovirus vaccine (IPV) Types 1,2,3 combined	All ages. Begin: 6 weeks	Three doses: 1.0 ml each IM Fourth dose: 1.0 ml IM	4–8 weeks 6–12 months	Booster dose every 5 years through age 17	To be used in persons with altered immune states and in their households

Vaccine	Description	Recommended age	Dose	Doses / schedule	Precautions
	Attenuated (live) trivalent oral poliovirus vaccine (TOPV). Types 1,2,3 combined	Begin: 6 weeks. Routine use in persons age 18 and over in the U.S. is not needed	Three oral doses	Between doses: 1 and 2: 6–8 weeks; 2 and 3: 6–12 months. Preschool age (4–6 years) and when traveling to endemic areas. Repeated "booster" doses are not needed	Can be given to pregnant women in outbreak situations. Avoid in persons with altered immune states
Measles (rubeola)*	Attenuated (live) measles virus vaccine	Age 15 months or older	One dose: 0.5 ml sc	One dose only. However, measles vaccine should be given again if there is a history of receiving a) killed measles vaccine only, or live vaccine within 2 years of receiving killed vaccine; b) vaccine before the first birthday; c) live *further* attenuated vaccine with immune serum globulin (ISG) or measles immune globulin (MIG).	Contraindications: Altered immune states such as leukemia, lymphoma, antimetabolite and radiation therapy, and generalized malignancy. As with any live virus vaccine, avoid during pregnancy
Mumps*	Attenuated (live) mumps virus vaccine	Age 12 months or older*	One dose: 0.5 ml sc	One dose only	As with any live virus vaccine, avoid during pregnancy and in persons with altered immune states.
Rubella*	Attenuated (live) rubella virus vaccine	Susceptibles age 12 months or older*	One dose: 0.5 ml sc	One dose only	SHOULD NOT BE GIVEN DURING PREGNANCY. Women of childbearing age may be considered for immunization if advised of necessity to avoid pregnancy for three months following vaccine administration. Avoid in persons with altered immune states

SMALLPOX: **As of 1980 there is no medical indication for smallpox vaccination in any part of the world except for persons handling variola/vaccinia-group viruses in research laboratories.**

*Combined live attenuated vaccines are available for these viruses (measles-mumps-rubella; measles-rubella; and mumps-rubella). If combined vaccine including measles vaccine is used, give at age 15 months or older.

(Courtesy State of California, Department of Health Services, Infectious Disease Section, revised April 1983.)

Table 4-3. Summary of pediatric immunization recommendations, effective November 1985. (Courtesy Infectious Disease Branch, California State Department of Health Services)

IMMUNIZATION SCHEDULES

Children Beginning Immunization in Early Infancy

Age	Vaccines
2 months (6-10 weeks)	DTP & OPV (polio)[1]
4 months	DTP & OPV (polio)
6 months	DTP[2]
15 months	MMR (measles, mumps & rubella)
15-18 months	DTP & OPV[3]
24 months	Hib[4]
4-6 years (before school entry)	DTP & OPV
14-16 years (and every 10 years thereafter)	Td

1. Can start at this age even for premature and/or low birthweight infants who are otherwise well.
2. An additional OPV dose at this time is optional in areas of high risk for polio exposure.
3. If child has not received MMR, can give MMR, DTP & OPV simultaneously, at separate sites.
4. May give to some high-risk children as early as age 18 months or as late as age 5 years.

Children Beginning Immunization After Early Infancy[1] But Before Age 7 Years

Date/Age	Vaccines
1st Visit	DTP, OPV, & MMR (if ≥ 15 mo. old)
6-8 weeks after 1st DTP & OPV	DTP & OPV
4-8 weeks after 2nd DTP & OPV	DTP[2]
6-12 mo. after 3rd DTP	DTP & OPV
24 months old	Hib[3]
4-6 years old (before school entry)	DTP & OPV[4]
14-16 years old (and every 10 years thereafter)	Td

1. If started in 1st year of life, give first three DTP doses and first two OPV doses as per this schedule and give MMR at 15 months
2. An additional OPV dose 6-8 weeks after the previous dose is optional in areas of high risk for polio exposure.
3. Hib may be given simultaneously at separate sites, with MMR, OPV and/or DTP
4. The USPHS considers these doses necessary unless the fourth DTP dose and the third OPV dose were given after the *4th* birthday. California's school entry law, which is a minimally acceptable standard rather than an optimum recommendation, does not require these doses unless the fourth DTP and third OPV doses, respectively, were given before the *2nd* birthday. Clinics should follow the USPHS recommendation.

Children Beginning Immunization at Ages 7-17 Years

Date	Vaccines
1st Visit	Td, OPV, & MMR
6-8 weeks after 1st Td & OPV	Td & OPV
6-12 mo. after 2nd Td & OPV	Td & OPV
10 years after 3rd Td (and every 10 years thereafter)	Td

Notes:

A If delay occurs between doses, regardless of the length, the series does not have to be restarted. Pick up the schedule where it left off

B TB skin testing is not a prerequisite to measles vaccine. If needed, a TB skin test can be given before or the same day as measles (or MMR) vaccine

C Record full dates of all vaccine doses given, as well as any continuing contraindications to immunizations on the yellow California Immunization Record Card (PM 298) and give to patient

D Different live vaccines (e.g. MMR, OPV) not given on the same day should be given no less than four weeks apart

VALID CONTRAINDICATIONS

Vaccine(s)		Condition
All	1.	Acutely ill; i.e., obvious fever and/or appears very sick.
MMR, MR Influenza	2.	*Anaphylactic* allergy to eggs (collapse, shock, tongue or mouth and throat swelling, hypotension, respiratory distress, hives)—Do *not* give measles and mumps-containing vaccines or influenza vaccine.
MMR, MR OPV	3.	*Anaphylactic* allergy to neomycin (cf. above for symptoms/signs)—Do not give measles, mumps or rubella-containing vaccines or OPV.
OPV	4.	*Anaphylactic* allergy to streptomycin (cf. above for symptoms/signs)—Do not give OPV.
Hib, DTP, DT, Td, Influenza	5.	Allergic hypersensitivity to thimerosal.
MMR, MR OPV	6.	Pregnancy (of vaccinee)—Do not give measles, mumps or rubella-containing vaccines. Give OPV only if at high risk of exposure.
MMR, MR	7.	Receipt of immune globulin or blood transfusion within past 3 months—Do not give measles, mumps or rubella-containing vaccines until 3 months have passed.
MMR, MR OPV	8.	Immunodeficiency or immunosuppression—Do not give measles, mumps, or rubella-containing vaccines or OPV. Also, do not give OPV if any other household member is immunodeficient or immunosuppressed.
DPT	9.	Serious reaction to prior DTP dose, i.e., a. Temp.≥105 F (≥40.5 C) within 48 hours. b. Convulsion(s) with or without fever within 3 days*. c. Persistent inconsolable crying for ≥3 hours, *or* unusual high-pitched crying or screaming (that does not have to last 3 hours), within 48 hours. d. Collapse or shock-like state (hypotonic-hyporesponsive episode) within 48 hours. e. Encephalopathy, incl. severe alteration in consciousness with generalized or focal neurologic signs, within 7 days. f. Allergic hypersensitivity (e.g. anaphylaxis). *If a convulsion occurs within 4-7 days, a full medical and neurologic evaluation should be made before deciding on continuing DTP.
DTP	10.	Evolving neurologic disorder, i.e., changing neurologic findings with or without a diagnosis—e.g., uncontrolled epilepsy, infantile spasms, progressive encephalopathy.
DTP	11.	Recently (<6 months) developed neurologic disorder or suspected underlying neurologic disease—e.g., recent convulsion(s). Defer DTP until neurologic status is evaluated and effect of treatment, if any, is assessed. If diagnosis is evolving disorder, give DT instead of DTP. If diagnosis is stable or resolved neurologic condition, can give DTP.

Schedule for DT for Infants and Children Who Cannot Take DTP

Infants under age 1 year—3 doses at 4-8 week intervals; a 4th dose 6-12 months after the 3rd, and a 5th dose at age 4-6 years, just before school entry. If 4th dose given after 4th birthday, the 5th dose is not necessary.

Children ages 1-6 years—2 doses 4-8 weeks apart, a 3rd dose 6-12 months after the 2nd, and a 4th dose at age 4-6 years, just before school entry. If 3rd dose given after 4th birthday, the 4th dose is not necessary.

VACCINE STORAGE AND HANDLING

1 DTP/DT/Td, Hib, Influenza—Store at 36°-46°F (refrigerate but do not freeze—check refrigerator periodically)
2 MMR, MR—Store at 35°-46°F (refrigerator) *Do not* allow to warm up or be exposed to light before use
3 OPV—Store in freezer. May be stored in refrigerator for up to 30 days if unopened, up to seven days if opened (multiple-dose vials). Do *not* allow to warm up to room temperature before use.

NON-CONTRAINDICATIONS

Immunizations generally *can* be given in these situations:

1. Mild acute illness (e.g., U.R.I.).
2. Allergy to ducks, chickens, or feathers.
3. Allergy to penicillin or other antibiotic (except anaphylactic allergy to neomycin or streptomycin).
4. "Allergies" in general, or relatives with allergies.
5. Currently taking antibiotics or other medicine (except immunosuppressive therapy).
6. Convalescent phase of illness—past febrile stage.
7. Mild, non-febrile diarrhea in otherwise well child.
8. Recent exposure to infectious illness.
9. Tuberculosis, or tuberculosis in family.
10. Convulsions in other family members.
11. Mother or other household contact is pregnant.
12. Lack of prior physical exam, even for infants.
13. Breastfeeding.
14. Concurrent or recent doses of other vaccines (Exception: Different live vaccines, if not given on the same day, should be given ≥ 1 month apart).
15. Prior history of immunization with or illness due to one or two of its three components is not a contraindication to MMR.
16. Childbearing age woman lacking negative pregnancy test, not in family planning program, not on contraception, or within 2 weeks of last menses. *Can* immunize with MMR or MR if she states she is not pregnant and does not plan pregnancy in next 3 months.

TETANUS PROPHYLAXIS IN WOUND MANAGEMENT

Prior Tetanus Doses	Clean, Minor Wounds		Other Wounds[1]	
	Td[2]	TIG[3]	Td[2]	TIG[3]
Uncertain, or<3	Yes	No	Yes	Yes
3 or more	No[4]	No	No[5]	No

1. E.g., Wound contaminated with dirt, feces, soil, etc.; puncture wound; avulsion, wound resulting from missile, crushing, burn, or frostbite; wound extends into muscle.
2. Substitute DTP for children under age 7 years.
3. TIG—Tetanus Immune Globulin.
4. Yes, if > 10 years since last dose.
5. Yes, if > 5 years since last dose.

MAKE SURE PARENTS KNOW THEIR CHILDREN WILL NOT BE FULLY PROTECTED UNTIL THE BASIC IMMUNIZATION SERIES HAS BEEN COMPLETED.

These guidelines, which have been derived principally from the published recommendations of the U.S. Public Health Service Immunization Practices Advisory Committee, should not be considered as unalterable rigid rules or regulations

SIGNS AND SYMPTOMS OF INFECTION

Common signs and symptoms of infection follow. The patient may have only a few of the signs and symptoms listed for each type of infection. At other times all of the listed signs and symptoms may be present.

Localized Infections

- Edema, redness of the area
- Exudate or drainage that is clear, cloudy, serous, purulent, or bloody
- Itching (in some infections)
- Pain

- Redness
- Swelling
- Tenderness
- Warmth

Generalized Infections

- Altered mental status
- Confusion
- Congestion
- Convulsions
- Decreased appetite
- Fatigue
- Fever
- Headache
- Hypotension
- Increased pulse rate
- Jaundice (in some infections)
- Joint pain
- Light-headedness
- Malaise
- Muscle aches
- Possible elevation of white blood cell count
- Shock

Gastrointestinal Infections

- Abnormal bowel sounds
- Abdominal cramps
- Anorexia
- Diarrhea
- Distention
- Elevated white blood cell count
- Fever
- Increased pulse rate
- Nausea
- Positive guaiac test
- Vomiting

Respiratory Infections

- Abnormal breath sounds
- Chest pain
- Congestion
- Cough
- Elevated white blood cell count
- Fever
- Increased pulse rate
- Positive sputum culture
- Positive throat culture
- Positive x-ray findings
- Productive cough (sputum)
- Rhinitis
- Shortness of breath
- Sore throat

Genitourinary Infections

- Dysuria
- Elevated white blood cell count
- Fever
- Flank or pelvic pain
- Frequency
- Hematuria
- Positive urine culture
- Purulent or foul discharge
- Urgency

DIAGNOSTIC DATA

None of the local or systemic signs and symptoms of the inflammatory process are diagnostic in themselves. Many of these signs and symptoms are seen in disease processes other than the infectious process. However, they do provide clues that aid in the diagnosis of a suspected infection. Diagnostic tests in conjunction with an evaluation of the patient's general health status are required to confirm a diagnosis and initiate therapeutic decisions. Examples of diagnostic tests used to obtain data follow. Each of these tests are discussed in detail in their respective units in this book.

- Microbiological tests—bacterial, viral, and fungal cultures and the Gram stain; cultures are commonly obtained from blood, sputum, urine, spinal fluid, aspirates of body fluids, and body discharges at any possible site of infection
- Blood counts
- Urinalysis
- Skin tests
- Radiological examinations
- Ultrasound examinations
- Gallium scans
- CT scans

It is essential that correct techniques for collecting and handling laboratory specimens occur to ensure accurate results. (See Unit VI for the methods to use for the proper handling and collection of specimens.) Inaccurate results will lead to a false diagnosis and an inappropriate form of therapy for the patient. Knowledge of the infectious disease process, of the signs and symptoms of an infectious process, and of prevention and control measures are vital to control and prevent all infectious disease processes.

INFECTION CONTROL

To control and prevent the infectious process, the sequential connection between the six factors involved must be broken at the weakest point. Various medical and surgical aseptic practices can break this cycle so that microorganisms cannot spread to and invade a susceptible host.

Medical Asepsis

keep your pens out of mouth

Medical asepsis refers to the destruction of organisms after they leave the body. Techniques employed to accomplish this include those practices that help reduce the number and transfer of pathogens. We observe many of these practices in everyday living, such as washing one's hands after using the bathroom or before handling food, covering one's nose and mouth when sneezing or coughing, and using one's own hair comb, toothbrush, and eating utensils.

Common medical aseptic practices to follow to break the cycle of the infectious process when working with patients include the following:

- Wash your hands before and after handling supplies and equipment, and before and after assisting with each patient. The handwashing procedure is discussed in detail in this unit.
- Handle all specimens as though they contain pathogens.
- Use disposable equipment when available, and dispose of properly according to office policy. All equipment is considered contaminated after patient use.
- Clean nondisposable equipment before and after patient use.
- Use gloves to protect yourself when handling highly contaminated articles
- Use clean or sterile equipment and supplies for each patient.
- Avoid contact of used supplies with your uniform to prevent the transfer of pathogens to yourself and to other patients.
- Place damp or wet dressings, bandages, and cottonballs in a waterproof bag when discarding these items to prevent the possible spread of infection to individuals who will handle the garbage.
- Cover any break in your skin as a protective measure against self-infection.
- Discard items that fall on the floor or clean before using, because all floors are contaminated.
- Use damp cloths for dusting or cleaning to avoid raising dust, which carries airborne microorganisms.
- If you are unsure whether supplies are clean or sterile, clean or sterilize them before use.

These practices are utilized during "clean" procedures, which involve parts of the body that are not normally sterile. Specific examples include aseptic procedures used when taking a temperature; obtaining urine, stool, or sputum specimens; obtaining smears or cultures from the throat or vagina; administering oral medications; removing and discarding used supplies; and cleaning a treatment room after use. See Appendix E, Universal Precautions.

Handwashing. To prevent the spread of microorganisms, handwashing is one of the first procedures that all health personnel must learn. *Correct handwashing is the foundation of aseptic technique.* Hands that are not properly cleansed are frequently the cause in spreading infection, as the hands are in constant use when working with or around patients. This procedure must become an automatic part of your work, as its importance *cannot* be overemphasized, and conscientiousness on your part *cannot* be overstressed. The time involved to wash the hands, wrists, and forearms well should be 1 to 2 minutes—2 to 4 minutes if they are highly contaminated. See Barrier Precautions and Handwashing in Appendix E.

Equipment

Clean paper towels
Sink with running water
Soap

Procedure	Rationale
1. Stand in front of the sink, making sure that your clothing does not touch the sink.	Sinks are always contaminated.
2. Turn water on; adjust it to a lukewarm temperature and a moderate flow to avoid splashing.	Warm water makes better suds than cold water; hot water may burn or dry the skin.
3. Wet hands and apply soap. When using bar soap, keep the bar in your hands throughout the whole procedure. *liquid soap*	Apply enough soap to develop a good lather. If you drop the bar of soap, you must repeat the procedure. Only the inside of a bar of soap is sterile when in use; all other objects are considered contaminated.
4. Wash hands (palm, sides, and back), fingers, knuckles, and between each finger, using a vigorous rubbing and circular motion (Fig. 4-2).	Friction caused by vigorous rubbing mechanically removes dirt and organisms. You must wash *all* areas on the hands.

Procedure	Rationale
5. During the procedure, keep the hands and forearms at elbow level or below (see Fig. 4-2).	This prevents water from running down to the elbows, which are areas of less contamination than the hands.
6. Rinse hands well under the running water. 7. Wash wrists and forearms as high as contamination is likely.	Washing the wrists and forearms after the hands prevents the spread of microorganisms from the hands to these areas.
8. Rinse ~~soap bar~~ off, and drop in the dish without touching the dish. *liquid soap*	Soap bars are excellent media for bacteria to grow on; therefore, they must be rinsed after use. The soap dish is considered contaminated and therefore must not be touched. *liquid soap*
9. Rinse hands, wrists, and forearms under running water.	Running water rinses away the dirt and organisms that have been loosened during the washing process.
10. Clean nails with an orangewood stick or nail brush at least once a day when starting work and each time when hands are highly contaminated; then rinse well under running water.	Microorganisms collect and can remain under the nails unless cleansed away.
11. Repeat steps 3 through 10 when the hands are highly contaminated.	A second washing is necessary when the hands are heavily contaminated to ensure that all the microorganisms have been removed.
12. Use a paper towel to turn water faucet off (Fig. 4-3).	The faucet is contaminated; using a paper towel allows the hands to remain clean.
13. Take another paper towel to thoroughly dry hands, wrists, and forearms.	Drying the skin completely prevents chapping.
14. Use hand lotion as necessary.	Lotion helps replace the skin's natural oils and prevents chapping. Chapped skin is more difficult to keep clean and more likely to crack. Once the skin is broken, microorganisms can easily enter and cause an infection.

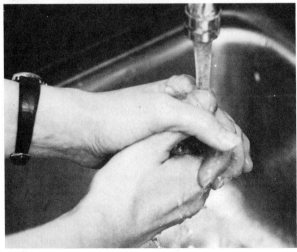

Fig. 4-2. Handwashing technique.

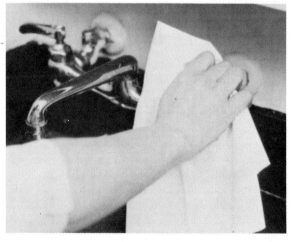

Fig. 4-3. Turn water faucet off using a paper towel after washing your hands.

Surgical Asepsis

Surgical asepsis refers to the destruction of all microorganisms, pathogenic as well as nonpathogenic, before they enter the body. The goal of surgical asepsis is to prevent infection or the introduction of microorganisms into the body.

Practices of surgical asepsis are usually referred to as sterile techniques. These techniques are used in all procedures in which entry into normally sterile body parts occurs, for example, when administering injections and during all surgical procedures. Surgical asepsis or sterile techniques are those practices followed when an area and supplies in that area are made sterile and kept sterile at all times. As an additional example, when changing dressings on a wound, a sterile field, sterile equipment, and sterile technique are maintained to prevent infection from developing.

Measures used to obtain and provide surgical asepsis include absolute sterilization of all instruments and supplies that will come in contact with normally sterile body parts and open wounds, thorough washing of the hands with a detergent or surgical soap, and wearing sterile gloves during sterile procedures, other than when administering injections. During surgical procedures, the physician and those directly involved with the procedure also wear a sterile gown, cap, and mask to help prevent contamination.

Methods of sterilization and disinfection are discussed in this unit. The use of other surgical aseptic or sterile techniques and practices is discussed in Unit V.

STERILIZATION

Sterilization is a precise scientific term with a single exact meaning when applied to medical supplies and instruments. We define sterilization as those processes/methods that completely destroy all microorganisms on objects.

Using specific procedures, sterilization is accomplished by subjecting the object(s) to chemical or physical agents that are capable of killing the microorganisms. It must be emphasized that there are no degrees of sterility — objects are either sterile or unsterile.

Sterilization plays a vital role in protecting the health and life of patients who seek treatment in both physicians' offices and hospitals. The use of presterilized disposable equipment has greatly helped reduce the spread of microorganisms and the need for sterilization procedures. Almost all equipment that may be used in a physician's office or clinic is now available in disposable materials. Nonetheless, there are certain items that are used repeatedly on many patients, such as a stethoscope, in addition to the nondisposable equipment still used by many. Therefore, the microorganisms that contaminate nondisposable supplies must be destroyed by appropriate measures.

The preceding information in this unit should aid your understanding of the need for and importance of correct sterilization methods.

METHODS TO CONTROL MICROSCOPIC AGENTS

Sanitization, disinfection, and sterilization are the three principal methods used for inhibiting the growth of and destroying microscopic life. Each represents a different level of decontamination, and though often used jointly, one must not be confused or substituted for the other.

Sanitization, the first step that must always be done before items can be reliably disinfected or sterilized, is a process of cleansing and scrubbing items with agents such as water and soap, detergents, or chemicals.

Disinfection involves methods that destroy "most" infectious microorganisms. However, some resistant and spore-forming bacteria and some viruses, such as the virus of hepatitis B, are not adequately destroyed by these methods. Agents employed to disinfect items include various types of chemical germicides and boiling water or flowing steam.

Sterilization is the complete destruction of all forms of microscopic life. Methods used to accomplish sterilization include:

- Dry heat
- Moderately heated chemical gas mixtures
- Chemical agents
- Steam under pressure (autoclaves)
- Unsaturated chemical vapor (Chemiclaves)

The first three methods are limited to certain applications and require longer exposure periods to sterilize items; therefore, they are not often employed. The autoclave, the most commonly used sterilizing method, and the Chemiclave are considered the most efficient, reliable, and practical answers to meet the sterilizing needs in the physician's office or clinic.

PREPARATION OF MATERIALS FOR STERILIZATION OR DISINFECTION

The initial step when sterilizing or disinfecting contaminated items is to remove them from the treatment room to the work area that is designated for dirty equipment. Care must be taken to avoid contamination to yourself or injury from any sharp instrument, and to prevent dulling any sharp blade or scissors while you are handling instruments. When handling heavily contaminated items or if you have any break in your skin, wear rubber gloves when sanitizing supplies. After cleaning all supplies, your hands are contaminated. Wash them as described previously.

Sanitizing Instruments

Procedure	Rationale
1. Bulk rinse the instruments in water containing a blood solvent or low-sudsing detergent or any approved germicide solution.	This first step is to clean all debris, oil, blood, and grease off the instruments.
2. Rinse the instruments in another sink or pan of fresh water.	
3. Scrub each instrument thoroughly with a brush and a warm nonionizing detergent solution (such as Tide or Joy) (Fig. 4-4).	Special attention must be given to serrated edges and other areas where blood, oil, or grease may collect.
4. Using hot water, thoroughly rinse all detergent off the instruments.	Soap solutions are not to be used, as they are alkaline and not compatible with germicides. Any soap residue on an instrument will prevent disinfection.
5. Remove the excess moisture from the instruments by rolling them in a towel.	
6. Check all instruments for working condition, and check to see that they are thoroughly cleaned. Never oil instruments, even if they are stiff when using them.	Oil on an instrument may protect a contaminated area from a sterilizing agent.
7. Wrap the instruments for sterilization.	
8. When instruments cannot be cleaned immediately after use, soak them in a solution of water and an effective blood solvent.	

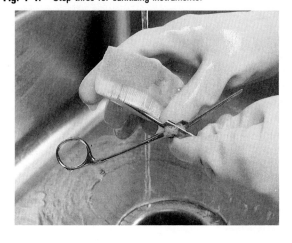

Fig. 4-4. Step three for sanitizing instruments.

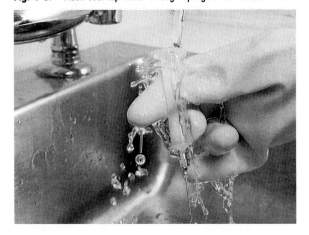

Fig. 4-5. Flush cool tap water through syringe and needle after use.

Sanitizing Syringes and Needles

Disposable syringes and needles have largely replaced the reusable units. However, if you are still using reusable units, special care must be taken before sterilizing the syringes and needles, because they are a common means of transmitting hepatitis B.

Procedure	Rationale
1. Rinse immediately by filling the syringe with cool tap water and flushing it through the needle (Fig. 4-5).	Rinsing immediately prevents coagulation of materials in the syringe and needle.

Sanitizing Syringes and Needles (*continued*)

Procedure	Rationale
2. Disassemble the unit.	
3. Place the needle in a separate tray; then put into the sterilizer for 30 minutes at 250°F.	Needles must first be decontaminated so they can be handled safely when cleaned.
4. Put syringe in water containing a low-sudsing, nonetching detergent, and thoroughly brush the interior of the syringe barrel.	All parts of the syringe must be cleaned to remove any foreign matter and contamination.
5. Clean the inside of the tip and the plunger.	
6. Flush the syringe twice with tap water and once with distilled water.	
7. The syringe is now ready to be wrapped and sterilized.	
8. Remove needles from sterilizer after the 30 minutes of exposure.	The needles are now decontaminated.
9. Clean the inside of the hub with a cotton-tipped applicator that is soaked with water and blood solvent or detergent solution (Fig. 4-6).	
10. Pass a stylet in and out of the interior (lumen) of the needle several times.	This removes any foreign matter or tissue left in the needle.
11. Check the point of the needle.	If it is damaged or dull, it must be resharpened and recleaned before sterilizing. Use a special whetstone or smooth oil stone (Arkansas stone) for sharpening. Directions for using these are provided by the manufacturer.
12. Thoroughly clean the exterior of the needle.	
13. Rinse the hub and exterior of the needle well under running tap water (Fig. 4-7).	
14. Using a syringe, flush tap water through the interior of the needle twice.	Both the exterior and the interior parts of the needle must be rinsed.
15. Rinse both the exterior and the interior with distilled water.	Rinsing is repeated with distilled water to ensure that all detergent is removed.
16. The needle is now ready to be wrapped and sterilized.	

Fig. 4-6. Cleaning inside hub of needle.

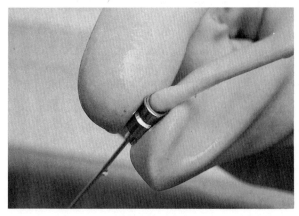

Fig. 4-7. Rinse hub and needle exterior well with water.

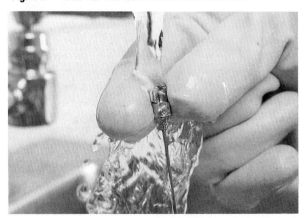

Sanitizing Rubber Goods

All rubber goods must also be cleaned and some must be sterilized. Such items as hot water bottles, ice caps, and rubber sheets should be covered with a towel or sheet before being used in patient care. Because they normally do not come in direct contact with the patient, these items are not usually sterilized, but must be thoroughly washed, rinsed, and dried after each usage. Other rubber goods, such as gloves, catheters, and tubing require special care and sterilization. Immediately after use they should be washed in cold water, then washed in warm water and a low-sudsing detergent, rinsed thoroughly, dried, and wrapped for sterilization.

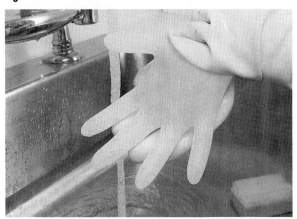

Fig. 4-8. Glove filled with water to check for holes or unremoved soil.

Procedure for Cleaning Rubber Gloves

Procedure	Rationale
1. Immediately after use, wash in cold water.	Cold water will remove blood and other soiling.
2. Wash thoroughly in warm water with a low-sudsing detergent, and rinse.	
3. Turn gloves inside out to wash and rinse again with fresh tap water.	Thorough rinsing is necessary to remove all detergent.
4. Fill gloves with water or air and inspect for punctures and unremoved soil (Fig. 4-8).	Water or air will leak out if any puncture hole is present.
5. Dry the gloves; pat with a towel to remove excess moisture, then allow to air dry. When exposed side is dry, turn to expose the inner surface for drying.	
6. The gloves are now ready to be wrapped for sterilization.	

Wrapping Instruments and Related Supplies for Sterilization. The next step before sterilizing items that are to be stored for future use is to wrap them in protective coverings, such as clean muslin or special disposable paper or bags. These materials are used because they can be permeated by steam or the chemical vapor from the sterilizer, but not by airborne or surface contaminants during handling and storage.

Items that will be used immediately or those that do not have to be sterile when used (for example, supplies used for "clean" procedures) can be sterilized by placing them in the sterilizer tray with muslin or other material designated by the manufacturer under and over them. When the sterilizing process has been completed, these items are to be removed with sterile transfer forceps and then either used or placed in the proper storage area.

However, those items that are to be kept sterile for future use must be wrapped. Materials and instru-

ments that will be used together may be wrapped together. Hinged instruments, such as hemostats, must be left open when being sterilized for immediate or future use. Also containers with lids are to be sterilized with the lid off; the lid is placed at the side or at the bottom of the container, with the inner surface facing outwards.

The method for wrapping instruments and other supplies, such as dressings, is the same. Figure 4-9 explains and illustrates the method to be used for wrapping these items. Study and practice this procedure of preparation.

Another aid to sterilization has been the introduction of disposable packaging materials. These include paper and pouches and tubing of paper and plastic. They are convenient for the sterilization and storage of syringes, tubing, and special purpose items.

ATI Steriline bags are made of a special surgical grade paper that allows rapid steam penetration during sterilization. They also act as a barrier against airborne bacteria during storage.

Each Steriline bag is printed with a temperature and steam-sensitive indicator consisting of an indicator line that changes color during sterilization to show that an item has been processed through the sterilizer (Fig. 4-10, A).

ATI pouches and tubing offer a clearly labeled package that can be used either for steam or ethylene oxide gas sterilization. They offer advantages similar to those of Steriline bags plus the benefits of content visibility and an easy, peel-open feature. Their use minimizes the risk of damaging expensive items by using the wrong sterilizing method. The steam indicator changes color from blue to grey/black during processing in either a gravity displacement or pre-vacuum, high temperature steam sterilizer. The gas indicator changes color from yellow to rust/red during processing in an ethylene oxide gas sterilizer (Fig. 4-10, B).

ATI Instrument Protectors are convenient, disposable holders for delicate surgical instruments. They protect instrument tips from being cracked or broken and help prevent the instrument from penetrating the pouch or package in which it is placed. Chemical indicators on each protector verify steam or ethylene oxide (EO) gas processing. To use these holders, first insert the instrument through the slots of the protector until the tip is completely covered by the plastic flap. Open hinged instruments, such as scissors, and fold the antilock flap forward between the handles. For added protection and holding ability, tuck the antilock flap into the topmost slot. Slide the loaded instrument protector into a sterilization pouch, with the instrument facing the film side. Seal the pouch in the normal manner and sterilize (Fig. 4-10, C).

Wrapping Reusable Syringes and Needles. Syringes are best wrapped in special disposable paper bags that are available for sterilization.

Fig. 4-9. Wrapping technique. (Courtesy of Wyeth Laboratories, Philadelphia, PA)

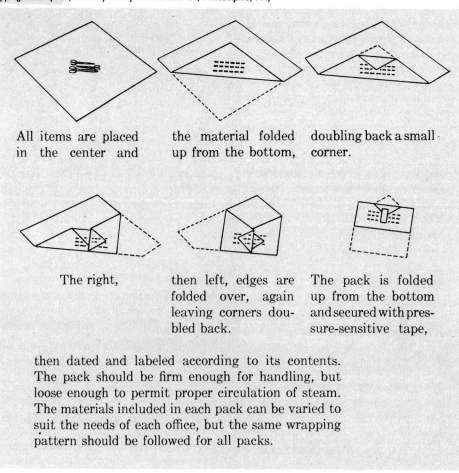

All items are placed in the center and

the material folded up from the bottom,

doubling back a small corner.

The right,

then left, edges are folded over, again leaving corners doubled back.

The pack is folded up from the bottom and secured with pressure-sensitive tape,

then dated and labeled according to its contents. The pack should be firm enough for handling, but loose enough to permit proper circulation of steam. The materials included in each pack can be varied to suit the needs of each office, but the same wrapping pattern should be followed for all packs.

Fig. 4-10. **A,** disposable bags used for sterilizing instruments, needles, and syringes. A line going across the bottom third of the bag is the sterilization indicator. If the line is green after autoclaving, it is your assurance that the contents have been subjected to sterilizing conditions. **B,** ATI Self-seal peel pouches and heat-sealable peel pouches. **C,** ATI instrument protector. (Courtesy Aseptic-Thermo Indicator, North Hollywood, CA)

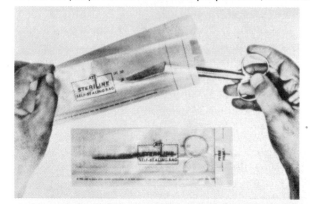

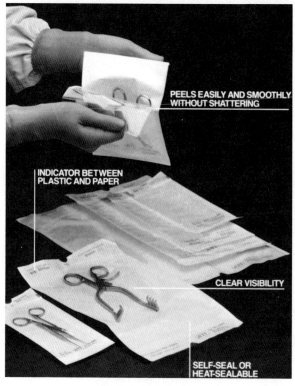

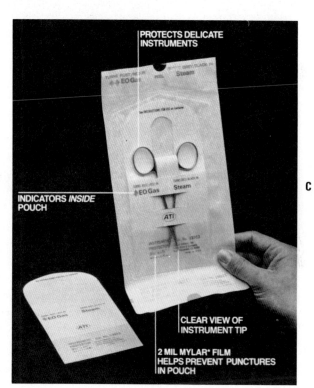

Procedure for Wrapping Reusable Syringes and Needles

Procedure	Rationale
1. Write the size of the syringe and the date on the outside of the bag.	Size must be indicated for identification. Date must be indicated, because if not used within 21 to 30 days (will vary with office or agency preference), it must be resterilized.
2. Place matching separated syringe and plunger inside the bag.	
3. Fold the top of the bag and seal securely.	

Wrapping Reusable Syringes and Needles (*continued*)

Procedure	Rationale
4. When the needle is to be sterilized with the syringe, place the needle in a disposable paper form (Fig. 4-11).	The paper form protects the point of the needle, provides a means for sterile handling when putting the needle on the syringe tip for use, and also prevents the needle from piercing the bag.
5. Label the bag with the size of syringe and needle and the date.	
6. Place the needle in the bag with the syringe and plunger; fold the top of the bag and seal.	
7. When the needle is to be sterilized individually, place it in a glass tube with constricted sides, and top the tube with a gauze, cotton or rubber stopper (Fig. 4-12).	The constriction in the tube prevents the sharp needle point from touching the bottom of the tube, thus preventing damage to the point.

Fig. 4-11. Reusable needle placed in paper form for sterilizing with a syringe in a disposable paper bag.

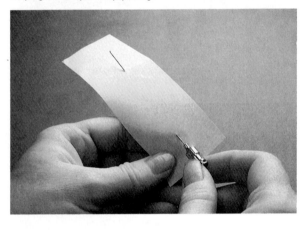

Fig. 4-12. Needle in glass tube with constricted neck ready for autoclaving.

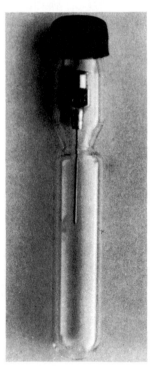

Wrapping Reusable Rubber Gloves.   Rubber gloves require special care. Study and practice the procedure outlined in Figure 4-13.

Autoclave – Steam Sterilization

Positioning Loads in Autoclave.   Proper positioning of all instruments and materials is extremely important be-cause of the pattern that steam follows as it circulates through the autoclave. *A direction booklet, which must be read carefully, is supplied with every sterilizer.* Usually, when the sterilizing cycle begins, steam will build up at the top of the inside chamber and will move downward from the point of admission. Dry, cool air will be forced downward and out an exhaust drain at the bottom front part of the chamber. All materials must be placed so that steam can flow be-

Fig. 4-13. Technique for wrapping reusable rubber gloves and placement in the autoclave. (Courtesy Wyeth Laboratories, Philadelphia, PA)

When dried rubber gloves are to be wrapped, they should first be powdered with a nonirritating starch preparation.

 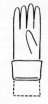 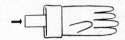

Then, using paper or gauze to separate the rubber surfaces from contact,

the cuffs of the powdered gloves are folded over.

The inside or palm is also held open by paper or gauze to allow free circulation of steam. The same procedure is repeated for both gloves.

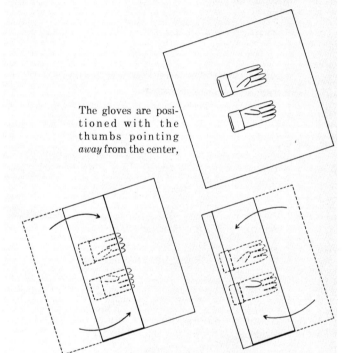

The gloves are positioned with the thumbs pointing *away* from the center,

and the wrapper folded neatly to protect the gloves from contamination. An alternate method is the use of glove envelopes which require an inner *and* an outer wrapper.

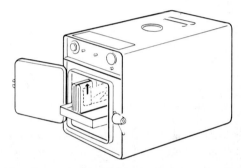

After the wrapper has been secured and labeled, the package can be placed in the sterilizer with the folded edges *up*. This will position the gloves so that steam can replace air in the thumbs for effective sterilization.

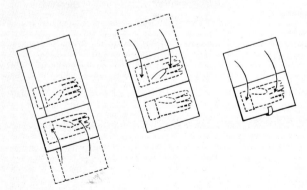

tween the packs and penetrate them. To avoid the formation of air pockets, you must place containers, tubes, cups, and similar items on their sides so that cool air can drain out in a downward direction and be replaced by steam. If they are placed upright, air will be trapped in the item, which in turn will prevent steam from contacting all surfaces, the result being incomplete sterilization.

Syringes wrapped in the disposable paper bags are to be placed horizontally (on their sides) in the sterilizer tray so steam will circulate inside the syringe barrel. Constriction tubes with needles are to be placed horizontally so that steam can circulate inside the tube. Packages with rubber gloves are to be placed on the sterilizer tray with the folded edges of the package facing upwards (see Fig. 4-13). This position will allow steam to replace air in the thumbs. Place linen and dressing packs in a vertical position.

When sterilizing linen packs and hard items in the same load, place the linen packs on top and the hard items on the bottom to prevent water condensation from dripping down on the linen packs. Items should not rest against plastic utensils so that the plastics will retain their shape even though exposed to very high temperatures.

Above all, *do not* overload the sterilizer chamber regardless of the items being sterilized. Place the articles as loosely as possible inside the chamber. Leave a space between all articles and the surrounding walls in the chamber. Correct positioning and spacing of all materials will allow effective sterilization to occur when the proper *temperature, pressure,* and *time* requirements are also met (Fig. 4-14).

Exposure Times. All loads placed in a sterilizer must be timed carefully after the sterilizer has attained the proper temperature. The length of sterilization time varies with the items and whether a wrapper, paper, or fabric is used. Suppliers of such materials will supply correct exposure data to ensure observance of adequate exposure periods.

The *high temperature* attained is the *sterilizing influence* that destroys the microorganisms. The amount of pressure used only makes it possible to develop the high temperature. An accurate thermometer should be used to provide a positive indication that sterilizing conditions have been met in the chamber. Thus, the three variables in the sterilizing cycle of an autoclave are *time, temperature,* and *pres-*

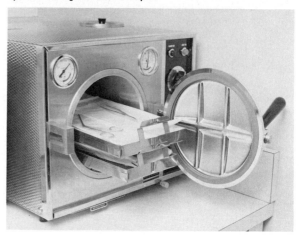

Fig. 4-14. Instruments in autoclave for sterilization must be well-spaced and hinged handles left open.

sure. Altering any one of these means that alterations are necessary for the others.

In the autoclave, when steam is in contact with all surfaces of the items, 15 minutes at 250°F is adequate time to kill all known microorganisms. However, in practice, longer periods are necessary to achieve this exposure. Recommended exposure times for items placed in an autoclave at 250°F (121°C) follow.

• Wrapped surgical instruments	30 minutes
• Wrapped syringes and needles	30 minutes
• Wrapped rubber goods (excessive exposure will cause heat damage to the rubber)	20 minutes
• Wrapped dressings	30 minutes
• Wrapped suture materials	30 minutes
• Wrapped treatment trays	30 minutes
• Unwrapped utensils, glassware and similar items, when inverted or placed on edge	15 minutes
• Unwrapped and unassembled syringes and needles	15 minutes
• Unwrapped instruments covered with muslin	20 minutes

Again, methods of wrapping, time of exposure, and the temperature must be scrupulously watched, since the purpose of autoclaving is to sterilize every article completely. Each manufacturer's direction booklet must be read and followed carefully to achieve adequate sterilization.

Removing Loads From the Sterilizer

Procedure	Rationale
1. Exhaust steam pressure from the chamber.	Read and follow precisely the manufacturer's directions for exhausting steam.

Procedure	Rationale
2. When the pressure has reached 0 and the temperature has decreased to 212°F, open the door of the autoclave slightly.	Stand back from the door to avoid steam burns to the face and hands.
3. Allow the contents to dry for approximately 15 minutes before removing them.	Some modern autoclaves automatically provide a sterilization cycle that includes drying, thus eliminating the need for these steps.
4. Regardless of the type of sterilizer you use, all dry, wrapped items and unwrapped items that do not have to remain sterile can then be removed with your clean and dry hands.	Do not remove unwrapped metal objects too soon with bare hands, because they retain heat, and you could get burned.
5. Remove unwrapped items that are to remain sterile for immediate use with sterile transfer forceps; place items to be used later in sterile storage containers.	

Sterilization Indicators.   Numerous commercial devices are used to indicate the effectiveness of the sterilization process. Used correctly, these devices, known as sterilization indicators, are adequate assurance of the sterility of items as long as the wrapper or container has not been torn or handled when moist, because that would contaminate the contents. These indicators work on the principle that specially prepared dyes will change color when exposed to the high temperature and saturated steam in the autoclave for a specific time. Individual disposable indicators for which color changes are to be observed after sterilization include the Sterilometer-Plus and Sterilometers (Fig. 4-15). Sterilometer-Plus represents the most precise, complete chemical indicator available. It consists of two indicator bars covered by a clear plastic overlay. The indicator bars contain a special reactive pigment that changes color from purple to green only in the presence of steam, not just heat (the water molecules in the steam actually are part of the color-change reaction, so that the reaction cannot take place without steam present). The clear plastic overlay prevents the indicator areas from coming into contact with items being sterilized.

When the indicator is exposed to steam in a sterilizer, the steam begins to work on the indicator inks.

Fig. 4-15.   **A,** Sterilometer-Plus sterilization indicators. The color changes from purple to green on the indicator bars point out when the conditions necessary for complete sterilization have been met. **B,** Sterilometer sterilization indicators. Sterilization is assured if the wide bar at one end has changed completely from white to black. (Courtesy Aseptic-Thermo Indicator, North Hollywood, CA)

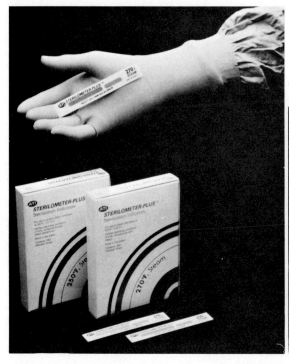

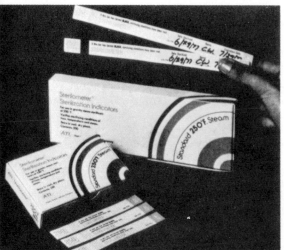

Fig. 4-16. Autoclave indicator tape used to seal and label packages before sterilization. Dark diagonal lines appear on the tape after the sterilization cycle to indicate that the pack has been exposed to steam and the autoclaving process. (Courtesy Aseptic-Thermo Indicator, North Hollywood, CA)

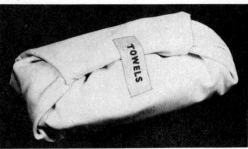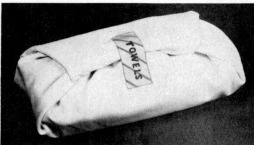

The heat energy and water content of the steam react with the purple pigment in the ink and cause it to turn green. The ink contains other chemicals that carefully control the amount of time necessary for the ink to completely change color, so that the indicator will change only when the conditions necessary for complete sterilization have been met.

The Sterilometer is a disposable tag that is placed in the center of a pack with the nonindicator end extended outside the wrapper. This enables the indicator to be removed without touching the contents of the pack. Sterilization is assured if the wide bar at the opposite end has changed completely from white to black. If these color change standards do not result, the pack must be resterilized.

Also, specific areas or markings on the outside of commercially prepared packages and on special disposable bags that are available for wrapping instruments, syringes, and needles will change color if sterilization standards have been met (see Fig. 4-10). These preceding indicators are superior to the frequently used autoclave tape indicators, because the dark diagonal lines that appear on the tape at the end of the sterilization cycle merely indicate that the pack has been exposed to steam and the autoclaving process (Fig. 4-16). There are many other indicators available for various types of sterilization processes (see Table 4-4). Figure 4-17 illustrates the dry heat sterilization indicator on a pressure-sensitive label, which changes from tan to black when exposed for 5 min-

Table 4-4. Sterilization monitors and indicators*

Steam Sterilization Monitors

Sterilometer-Plus®/270 — ⅝ × 4¼ inches (1.6 × 10.8 cm) strip with two purple ink bars that are sterilant specific and change color in sequence during exposure to 270°F (132°C) saturated steam. For use in pre-vacuum and "flash" sterilizers. A clear protective coating over the ink bars prevents the ink from touching items being sterilized. Packaged 200 indicators per box, 20 boxes per case.

Sterilometer-Plus®/270 — Long Form — ⅝ × 7⅜ inches (1.6 × 18.7 cm) strip with two purple ink bars that are sterilant specific and change color in sequence during exposure to 270°F (132°C) saturated steam. Packaged 200 indicators per box, 20 boxes per case.

Sterilometer-Plus®/250 — ⅝ × 4¼ inches (1.6 × 10.8 cm) strip with purple ink bars that are sterilant specific and change color in sequence during exposure to 250°F (121°C) saturated steam. A clear protective coating over the ink bars prevents the ink from touching items being sterilized. Packaged 200 indicators per box, 20 boxes per case.

Sterilometer®/270 — Short Form — ⅝ × 4¼ inches (1.6 × 10.8 cm). For use in pre-vacuum and "flash" sterilizers. Indicator changes color from white to black when exposed for 2–3 min. at 270°F (132°C) in saturated steam. Packaged 250 indicators per box, 20 boxes per case.

Sterilometer®/270 — Long Form — ⅝ × 8 ½ inches (1.6 × 21.6 cm). For pre-vacuum and "flash" sterilizers. Indicator changes color from white to black when exposed for 2–3 min. at 270°F (132°C) in saturated steam. Packaged 250 indicators per box, 20 boxes per case.

Sterilometer®/250 — Short Form — ⅝ × 4¼ inches (1.6 × 10.8 cm). For gravity sterilizers. Indicator changes color from white to black when exposed for 12–15 min. at 250°F (121°C) in saturated steam. Packaged 250 indicators per box, 20 boxes per case.

Sterilometer®/250 — Long Form — ⅝ × 8 inches (1.6 × 21.6 cm). For gravity sterilizers. Indicator changes color from white to black when exposed for 12–15 min. at 250°F (121°C) in saturated steam. Packaged 250 indicators per box, 20 boxes per case.

Steam Strip — ⅝ × 8½ inches (1.6 × 21.6 cm). For use in all 250°F (121°C), 270°F (132°C), and 285°F (143°C) sterilizers. Indicator changes color from white to black when exposed to steam sterilization conditions. Packaged 250 indicators per box, 20 boxes per case.

Steam Strip (Bulk Pack) — ⅝ × 8½ inches (1.6 × 21.6 cm). For use in all 250°F (121°C), 270°F (132°C), and 285°F (143°C) sterilizers. Indicator changes color from white to black when exposed to steam sterilization conditions. Packaged 1000 indicators per economical bulk box, 4 boxes per case.

Table 4-4 *(continued)*

Sterilometer-Plus® Wall Dispenser—wall mounted for Sterilometer-Plus® 250 and 270 short form indicators. 20 dispensers per case.

Daily-Autoclave-Chex® (Bowie-Dick Test)—For testing air leaks in pre-vacuum sterilizers, 270°F (132°C). Size 8½ × 11 inches (21.6 × 27.9 cm). Indicator stripes will uniformly change color from white to black when air has been eliminated and steam has penetrated the pack. Packaged 50 sheets per box, 5 boxes per case.

Disposable Bowie-Dick Type Test Pack—For testing air leaks in pre-vacuum sterilizers, 270°F (132°C). New, accurate, pre-packaged, disposable Bowie-Dick type test pack. Size 5 × 4⅜ inches (12.7 × 11.1 cm). Indicator stripes will uniformly change color from white to black when air has been eliminated and steam has penetrated the pack. Packaged 20 packs per box, 4 boxes per case.

EO Gas Sterilization Monitors

Sterilometer-Plus®/EO—⅝ × 4¼ inches (1.6 × 10.8 cm). A dual ink formulation breakthrough in indicator technology: Two indicator bars with different chemistries. Sterilant specific bar changes color from yellow to brown only in EO gas. Moisture specific bar changes color from yellow to blue/green if humidity level is above the required minimum. Packaged 200 indicators per box, 20 boxes per case.

EO Gas Sterilization Indicators—⅝ × 4¼ inches (1.6 × 10.8 cm) sterilization monitor for all EO gas sterilizers. Indicator changes color from yellow to blue when exposed for 30 to 45 min. in 600 mg/l of ethylene oxide at 54°C and at least 30% relative humidity. Packaged 200 indicators per box, 20 boxes per case.

EO Indicator (Bulk Pack)—⅝ × 4¼ inches (1.6 × 10.8 cm). Sterilization monitor for all EO gas sterilizers. Indicator changes color from yellow to blue when exposed for 30 to 45 min. in 600 mg/l of ethylene oxide at 54°C and at least 30% relative humidity. Packaged 800 indicators per economical bulk box, 4 boxes per case.

EO Monitor—Lightweight, pen-like stainless steel tube packed with ethylene oxide-sensitive material. Clips to lapel or pocket near breathing zone for passive monitoring of individual during a work shift. Monitor is mailed to ATI for analysis. Report is mailed to user (or telephoned if permissible exposure limits are exceeded). Size 3½ × ¼ inches. Packed 5 units per box, 1 box per case.

Sterilization Indicator Labels

Steam/EO Gas Label—Combination label for steam or EO gas sterilizers. Peel-off pressure-sensitive labels for hard surfaced items such as unwrapped glass or metal. Steam indicator bar changes color to black during steam sterilizing. EO gas indicator changes color to rust during EO gas sterilizing. Packaged 1 roll per box (1000 labels), 12 boxes per case.

Sterilabel®—For steam sterilizers. Peel-off pressure-sensitive labels for hard-surfaced items such as unwrapped glass or metal. Change color from purple to green during steam sterilization. Packaged 1 roll per box (1000 labels), 12 boxes per case.

Dry Heat Indicator Labels—Sterilization monitor for all dry heat sterilizers. Pressure-sensitive labels remain affixed during dry heat sterilization. Change color from tan to black after exposure in a dry heat sterilizer. Packaged 1 roll per box (1000 labels), 12 boxes per case.

Biological Sterilization Monitors

Disposable Biological Test Pack — Steam—Self-contained 3M Attest® Biological Indicator inside a precisely engineered pack. Designed to be equivalent to AAMI recommendations for steam biological test packs. Replaces tedious hand-made versions. 16 packs per box, 4 boxes per case.

Disposable Biological Test Pack-EO Gas—Self-contained 3M Attest® Biological Indicator inside a precisely engineered pack. Designed to be equivalent to AAMI recommendations for EO biological test packs. 16 packs per box, 4 boxes per case.

Dual-Temperature Incubator—Dry block incubator for steam and EO gas sterilization. Top tier operates at 54 ± 3°C (for steam), bottom tier operates at 37 ± 3°C (for EO gas).

Steam Incubator—Dry block incubator for steam sterilization. Operates at 56 ± 3°C.

EO Gas Incubator—Dry block incubator for EO gas sterilization. Operates at 37 ± 3°C.

Spore-O-Chex® (Bulk Pack)—500 indicators per box, in glassine envelopes. For EO gas sterilizers (Bacillus subtilis). 4 boxes per case.

Spore-O-Chex®—24 test sets (72 indicators) packed in a hinged-top plastic box, 10 boxes per case. For all steam sterilizers, EO gas sterilizers and dry heat sterilizers (Bacillus subtilis and Bacillus stearothermophilus).

Spore-O-Chex® Envelopes—For use with Spore-O-Chex® bulk pack indicators. Packaged 100 envelopes per box, 10 boxes per case.

Spore-O-Chex® (Bulk Pack)—500 indicators per box, in peel-back glassine envelopes. For all steam sterilizers, EO gas sterilizers and dry heat sterilizers. 4 boxes per case (Bacillus subtilis and Bacillus stearothermophilus).

Attest® is a registered trademark of 3M.

*Courtesy Aseptic-Thermo Indicator Co., North Hollywood, CA.

Fig. 4-17. Dry heat sterilization indicator labels. (Courtesy Aseptic-Thermo Indicator, North Hollywood, CA)

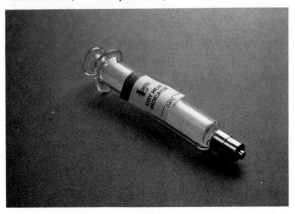

utes at 340°F. When any sterilization indicator is used, the manufacturer's directions for use must be followed. Sterilization indicators must be stored in a dry place and away from excessive heat.

Causes of Insufficient Sterilization

Failure of the indicators to change colors completely indicates a serious lack of steam penetration into the pack. This is a warning that there may be a sterilizer malfunction or an error in the sterilization technique. *Never neglect this warning.* Causes of sterilization failure are numerous, elusive, and often difficult to locate. The problem may require minute examination of every part of the sterilizer and/or a complete reexamination of your preparation, wrapping, and loading techniques. Some of the most common problems are as follows:

1. Faulty preparation of materials
2. Improper loading of the sterilizer
3. Faulty sterilizer
4. Air in the sterilizer
5. Wet steam

All materials must be sanitized completely beforehand, then wrapped and secured properly as described previously. You must position the load correctly in the sterilizer and not overload the chamber. Timing for adequate exposure times must begin *after* the sterilizer has attained the proper temperature. If all of these conditions have been met satisfactorily, it will be necessary to have the equipment checked for a defect and repaired as necessary.

Storing Sterile Supplies. Special storage places for each type of supply should be maintained away from areas where contaminated materials are handled. Storage places must be clean, dry, and dustproof. Sterile items wrapped in cloth or paper can safely be stored

for 21 to 30 days. Wrapped items that are placed in sterile plastic duster covers can be stored for 6 months, and items wrapped in plastic teel-packs (special envelopes with one side of transparent plastic and the other side of paper) for 3 months. After these time periods are exhausted, all packs should be reprocessed and resterilized before use. Instruments sterilized unwrapped are to be used immediately and are not to be stored if they are to be sterile when used.

In summary, the following points should be remembered when sterilizing items in an autoclave (steam sterilization). All items must be treated as follows:

- Sanitized (cleaned) properly before sterilization.
- Correctly wrapped, sealed, and labeled (for identification) or covered to prevent recontamination. When using cloth or paper wrapper, include a sterilization indicator in or on the pack.
- Positioned correctly in the sterilizer so steam will contact all surfaces.
- Able to fit easily into the chamber—*do not overload.*
- Exposed to saturated steam at 250°F (121°C) for 15 to 30 minutes (varies with the items).
- Allowed to dry before removal from the sterilizer.
- Stored in specific clean, dry, and dustproof places.
- Checked at intervals to determine if the period (date) of sterility has been exhausted.
- Reprocessed and resterilized when they are no longer sterile because of wrap damage or date expiration.

Unsaturated Chemical Vapor Sterilization

A practical, efficient, and reliable method of sterilization, the unsaturated chemical vapor sterilizer (now known as the MDT/Harvey Chemiclave, Fig. 4-18) depends on pressure, heat, and a specific solution, the Vapo-Sterile Solution, a formulation of proven effective liquid bactericidal chemicals and minimal water. When it is heated and pressurized to 270°F (132°C) and at least 20 pounds per square inch pressure, all living microorganisms are consistently killed within 20 minutes.

All items to be sterilized must first be cleaned. To avoid hand scrubbing of instruments and the possibility of transmitting pathogenic microorganisms among patients and medical personnel, an ultrasonic cleaning device, such as the Vibraclean 100 or 200, may be employed for this purpose (Fig. 4-19). Once cleansed, instruments must be thoroughly rinsed in cold running water to remove any residue or ultrasonic solution or soap, which would inhibit sterilization or damage the sterilizer, and then towel dried before being placed in the sterilizer. Small, hard-to-dry items should be dipped in a shallow tray of Vapo-

Fig. 4-18. A, early (evolving in 1936) to current models of the MDT/Harvey Chemiclave sterilization systems. Today's models represent the most sophisticated use of the basic principle of unsaturated chemical vapor sterilization. **B,** MDT/Harvey Chemiclave 5000. (Courtesy MDT Corporation, El Segundo, CA)

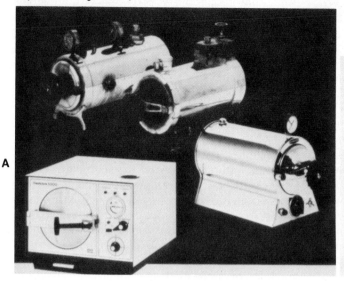
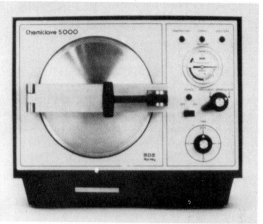

A

Steril solution in lieu of drying. The items are then to be placed in an instrument tray lined with a Harvey chemically pure hard surface tray liner. If storage of sterile instruments is desired, they are to be sterilized in Harvey Sterilization Indicator bags. These bags permit penetration by the chemical vapor but preclude contamination by air-borne bacteria.

The Chemiclave (the unsaturated chemical vapor sterilizer) uses mechanical principles substantially different from those of other systems. The sterilizer is preheated before the initial use and remains at 270°F (132°C) for immediate use. No further preheating is necessary. Unlike the steam autoclave, in which an unmeasured amount of water is recirculated over the heating element, the unsaturated vapor sterilizer valving system measures a precise amount of solution into the closed, preheated chamber. This solution

condenses on the cooler objects in the chamber to begin bactericidal activity. As the objects heat, vaporization of the solution occurs, and unsaturated chemical vapor acts to complete the sterilization cycle. Temperature monitoring is unnecessary, as this sterilizer provides both audible and visual signaling upon completion of the cycle. A thermostatically controlled heating unit maintains the chamber temperature, and a temperature indicator light registers that the heating element is functioning properly. Any failure in the system is immediately evident, as the pressure in the chamber will not be attained, and, unless all operating criteria are met, the pressure switch will not activate the cycle timer.

Cutting edges, even those of carbon steel, and surgical instruments, handpieces, forceps, and similar items vulnerable to dulling, corroding, rusting, or loss of temper in autoclaves or dry heat units are safely and effectively sterilized in a Chemiclave. Many "soft" items may also be safely sterilized in this unit; and since sterilization is achieved in a water-unsaturated environment, materials such as gauze and cotton are dry and ready for immediate use when the cycle is completed. Only low-grade plastic and rubber items, liquids, agars, and items damaged at 270°F (132°C) *should not* be placed in the Chemiclave. As with all sterilizers, the directions for operation from the manufacturer must be followed explicitly to obtain maximum results.

Dry Heat Sterilization

To sterilize items with dry heat, a special combined autoclave–dry heat sterilizer or an individual dry heat sterilizer is required. In essence they are like an oven.

Fig. 4-19. Harvey 100/Vibraclean, an ultrasonic cleaner. (Courtesy MDT Corporation, El Segundo, CA)

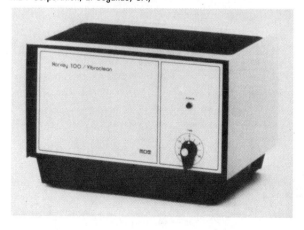

Before being sterilized, all items must be thoroughly cleaned. Instruments and glass items, such as syringes, should be placed on the tray or wrapped in aluminum foil. Sharp items should be placed on gauze in racks or wrapped in aluminum foil. Rubber goods and dressings must be well dispersed in a container or wrapped in aluminum foil. As for all methods of sterilization, both exposure time and temperature must be considered. Dry heat sterilizers require longer exposure periods and higher temperatures than do the autoclave (steam under pressure). The exposure time for dry heat is at least 1 hour at 320°F (160°C). If the items being sterilized cannot tolerate this temperature, reduce the temperature and extend the time proportionately. This method is suggested for instruments that corrode easily, sharp cutting instruments, and glass syringes, because moist heat will dull the cutting edges and the ground-glass portion of the syringe. Needles, powders, oils, ointments, lensed instruments, dressings, rubber goods, and polyethylene tubing can also be sterilized by this method.

Gas Sterilization

Gas sterilizers, using moderately heated mixtures of ethylene oxide gas, are useful for sterilizing heat and moisture-sensitive items, including rubber and plastic goods, delicate items such as lensed instruments, glass, ophthalmological surgical instruments, catheters, and anesthesia equipment. Items to be sterilized by this method should be cleaned, wrapped, and positioned in the gas chamber using the same steps that were discussed for autoclaving. The temperature in a gas sterilizer is lower (140°F or 50°C); thus the exposure time is extended to suit the temperature, moisture, and gas concentration being used. Time required is 2 to 6 hours plus additional time for aeration, which can be as long as 5 to 7 days for certain porous materials. Specific instructions for the times and temperatures required are supplied by the manufacturer with the sterilizer and must be followed explicitly.

Chemical Sterilization

Many studies have shown that chemical sterilization (cold sterilization) is difficult to accomplish. Therefore, this method is generally limited for items that are heat-sensitive, such as delicate cutting instruments and nonboilable sutures, or it is used when heat sterilization methods are not available. Chemical solutions are more commonly used for disinfection rather than for sterilization. Nonetheless, a variety of chemical solutions are on the market for sterilization and disinfection. They are classified as germicidal, bactericidal, disinfectants, antiseptics, and so on.

Three chemical solutions that have been recognized as reliable for both sterilization and disinfection procedures are Cidex, Ideal solution, and Formaldehyde Germicide. These solutions are capable of destroying bacteria (including spore-forming types) and viruses, and are safe to use on instruments, rubber, and plastic goods. Reliable manufacturers always indicate which microorganisms can be expected to be killed by the chemical solution, which items the solution can and cannot be used on, and specific directions for use.

Procedure for Chemical Sterilization

Procedure	Rationale
1. Sanitize items as discussed for autoclaving.	
2. Pour chemical solution into a designated container with an airtight cover (Fig. 4-20).	Follow the directions for each chemical accurately. Some may need to be diluted before use, but if diluted too much, the solution will lose its effectiveness.
3. Completely immerse the item into the solution, and close the cover.	
4. Leave for required time, which will vary with the chemical used. Exposure time may be from 20 minutes to 3 hours or more.	Correct exposure time is extremely important to ensure sterilization.
5. Before using, lift tray out of container, and rinse items in pan of sterile distilled water.	Often the solutions used are toxic; therefore, items must be thoroughly rinsed before being used on patients.
6. Using sterile transfer forceps, remove items from the tray for use.	
7. Change the solution in the container every 7 to 14 days or as recommended by the manufacturer.	

Fig. 4-20. Instrument container with airtight cover used for chemical disinfection and sterilization.

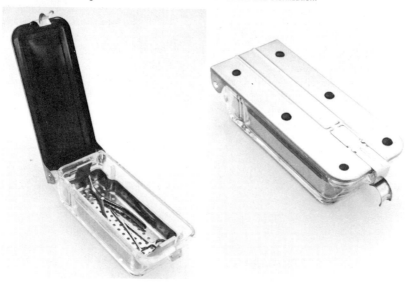

Disinfection Procedures

Chemical Disinfection

Many medical procedures are termed "clean" procedures; therefore, they do not require the use of strict aseptic (sterile) technique. Instruments and equipment used in clean procedures are in contact only with the patient's skin or shallow body orifices. Since they do not bypass the body's natural defenses, they can be used safely after being disinfected. Examples of such supplies are thermometers, percussion hammers, laryngeal mirrors, blunt instruments not used on open skin surfaces or on sterile materials, such as dressings that will touch an open wound, and stainless steel goods, such as kidney basins.

When disinfecting such items, thoroughly wash, rinse, and dry as for sterilization. Then apply a disinfectant or antiseptic solution to the surface of the item or immerse it completely in such a solution (refer to the procedure under chemical sterilization).

Certain items, such as sphygmomanometers, stethoscopes, and ophthalmoscopes may be ruined if washed and immersed in any solution. Disinfect these items only by wiping them off with gauze or cloth moistened with a disinfectant (Fig. 4-21). Chemical solutions suggested for use include Cidex, Ideal solution, Solucide, 70% to 90% isopropyl alcohol,

Deo-Fect, iodophor solutions, Zephiran chloride, Formaldehyde Germicide, and Chlorophenyl.

Boiling Water

The other method for disinfection involves the use of boiling water. Formerly considered safe for sterilization, investigations have now shown that many bacterial spores can withstand exposure to boiling water for several hours. Therefore, use boiling water only to disinfect items that do not penetrate body tissues.

Fig. 4-21. Disinfecting a stethoscope. Both earpieces and diaphragm should be disinfected after each use.

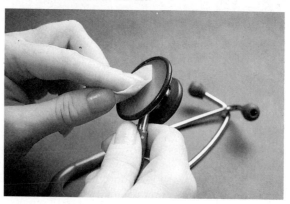

Procedure for Disinfection with Boiling Water

Procedure	Rationale
1. Fill boiler half full with cold water, preferably distilled water.	Distilled water does not leave sediment on the inside of the boiler as tap water would.

Procedure for Disinfection with Boiling Water (*continued*)

Procedure	Rationale
2. Clean items thoroughly.	All soil must be removed before the items are boiled.
3. Place items on the tray in the boiler. Hinges or clamps on instruments must be open; jars and similar containers must be placed on their side (Fig. 4-22).	The boiling water must come in contact with all surfaces to provide thorough disinfection of the item.
4. Lower the tray so items are completely immersed in the water.	
5. Close lid of boiler, and turn power switch on.	
6. Once the water is boiling (212°F or 100°C) vigorously, start timing the exposure period.	Recommended exposure time is 15 to 20 minutes. Do not boil for less than 15 minutes.
7. Once the cycle has been completed, stand back or to the side of the boiler, and open the lid to allow steam to escape.	Standing away from or to the side of the boiler prevents a steam burn.
8. Allow the items to cool, then remove and dry thoroughly.	Items can be removed with clean hands, or by using sterile transfer forceps.
9. Store the items in designated area, unless needed for immediate use.	

Fig. 4-22. Instruments correctly placed in a boiler for disinfecting process.

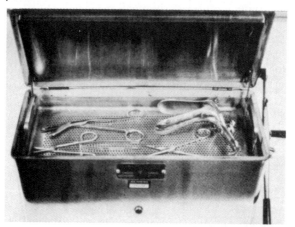

If you do not have access to an autoclave for sterilizing and must use the boiler, remove items from the boiler with sterile transfer forceps, dry with a sterile towel, and then transfer to a sterile field for use.

When the boiler is used frequently, it must be cleaned regularly to remove any sediment that has gathered on the sides. It may be necessary to scrub the interior surfaces with a stiff brush and cleanser. Follow the specific instructions provided by the manufacturer of the equipment that you use.

The limitations of disinfection procedures must be recognized; they must *not* be substituted for sterilization. These procedures can be effective in controlling many forms of microbial life on appropriate items, but may not destroy viruses. Also, spore-forming bacteria can withstand boiling water even after several hours exposure.

Summary

When instruments and other equipment are used, the spread of numerous pathogens can be prevented only by the proper sterilization of reusable items, or by the use of presterilized disposable items, in addition to meticulous aseptic technique.

Because few procedures more directly affect the continued health of the patient you attend, the physician, and yourself, conscientious attention must be given to sterilizing all items at all times. Periodic reexamination of the techniques employed should be done to check their adequacy.

The use of disposable equipment is highly recommended to help control infectious processes and has been found to be most economical in the long run.

AIDS (ACQUIRED IMMUNODEFICIENCY SYNDROME) INFECTION PRECAUTIONS

Purpose

The purpose of the following safeguards is the prevention of the possible transmission of the presumed AIDS infectious agent human T-Cell lymphotropic virus (HTLV-III,LAV, or ARV) to susceptible individuals, and to provide protection against other infectious agents that may infect patients with AIDS. The precautions described here are designed to protect individuals working with these patients, other patients, and employees. The infection precautions discussed here in general follow those recommended by the National Centers for Disease Control.

Introduction

The HTLV-III virus (also referred to as the HIV-human immunodeficiency virus; HIV is the internationally adopted name of the acquired immunodeficiency syndrome virus), which is related to AIDS, is transmitted by sexual contact or parenterally with blood or blood products. There is no evidence of transmission of HTLV-III or the AIDS-related retrovirus by respiratory means or casual contact with individuals infected by this virus. The transmission pattern of HTLV-III is similar to that of hepatitis B. The risk groups include males with homosexual contact, female sexual partners of bisexual males and drug abusers, persons with multiple sexual partners, children born to mothers who are infected with HTLV-III, intravenous drug abusers, and people who received frequent blood transfusions or blood products (e.g., Factor VIII given to hemophiliacs). Since the screening of donor blood for HTLV-III antibody and the heat treatment of blood products, transfusions of blood and blood products have a markedly diminished risk. Some AIDS patients may additionally have other infections that can be transmitted to healthy individuals (e.g., hepatitis B, CMV, EBV, tuberculosis, salmonellosis, and cryptosporidiosis).

Precautions beyond those recommended should be avoided because their use does not afford additional protection and may interfere with patient care. Health care workers should be well informed about the ways in which HTLV-III or ARV is transmitted and follow precautions appropriate for their protection. Use of excessive precautions by health care workers conveys misinformation to patients and other employees about the mode of transmission and appropriate precautions.

General Guidelines

In the health care setting, there is a risk of exposure to a number of infectious diseases upon exposure to blood or body fluids. The hepatitis viruses and the

AIDS-related virus, HTLV-III, may be carried in the blood of individuals who appear healthy and by individuals who are sick but do not have a complete diagnosis. All exposures to blood or body fluids from any individual should be considered potentially dangerous and appropriate precautions should be taken. The infection control precautions outlined here will help prevent the transmission of any blood- or body fluid-borne infection. In situations where considerable contact with blood or body fluids is expected, such as deliveries, operative procedures, and endoscopies, precautions should be used for all patients (i.e., gowns, gloves, goggles, and masks according to contact expected). All patients with blood-borne viruses may not be identified at the time of a procedure. Therefore, precautions as outlined are indicated for all anticipated blood exposure from any patient.

Diagnosis and Initiation of Infection Precautions

Identification of patients requiring isolation measures will be made by the physicians caring for the patients. Criteria for diagnoses that warrant AIDS precautions are as follows:

DOCUMENTED AIDS: This includes patients with Kaposi's sarcoma, *Pneumocystis carinii* pneumonia, and other opportunistic infections not associated with other underlying disease or therapy.

POSSIBLE AIDS: Unexplained fever, unexplained pulmonary symptoms and/or infiltrates, skin lesions highly suggestive of Kaposi's sarcoma, and systemic illnesses that are characterized by fever, weight loss, adenopathy, wasting, sweats, thrush, and diarrhea in persons from a high-risk group (gay males, hemophiliacs, and IV drug abusers). Patients being followed in an AIDS clinic for AIDS-related problems.

There is no indication for isolation of members of high-risk groups without symptoms suggestive of AIDS. Asymptomatic persons with antibody to HTLV-III who do not fit into the documented AIDS or possible AIDS categories as outlined above should not be placed in isolation. These individuals may have the virus in their blood, and the general precautions for handling blood and other body fluids for *ALL* patients should be followed (i.e., careful handwashing after any contact with body fluids, extreme care in avoidance of needlesticks, no recapping of needles, use of the puncture-resistant needle box for disposal of all sharps).

Precautions for AIDS

Procedure	Rationale
1. Patients requiring hospitalization will usually be given a private room. (If the medical assist-	To protect patients from infections to which he/she may be susceptible and to protect other im-

Precautions for AIDS (*continued*)

Procedure	Rationale
ant has to make arrangements for the patient to be admitted into a hospital, check with the physician and the hospital's policy if a private room should be requested).	munocompromised patients. A private room is indicated for patients who are too ill to use good hygiene, such as those with profuse diarrhea, fecal incontinence, or altered behavior secondary to central nervous system infection.

2. *Handwashing* before and after direct patient care.

3. *Needle disposal* in puncture resistant containers without breaking or recapping needle. Needle box should be in room or as close as possible to the area of use.

Guidelines for Preventing Needlesticks

a) Slow down and *think* when using or disposing of needles.

b) DO NOT *recap* needles unless absolutely necessary. If necessary, place cap on table top before inserting needle (insert needle into cap without holding cap).

c) Never put a needle down—dispose of it promptly in approved container.

d) Never put needles or other sharp instruments in trash cans.

e) Never leave needles or other sharp instruments on counter tops, examination tables, or disposable procedure trays.

f) Never push a needle into the red plastic needle disposal box with your hand. If the needle does not go into the opening easily, use a large syringe to push it in.

g) Never try to remove a needle or syringe from the red plastic needle box.

4. *Gloves* for contact with body secretions and blood.

5. *Gowns are not needed unless* gross contamination of your uniform is expected as in cases of expected direct contact between uniform and draining wounds, splatter during bronchoscopy, etc. If unexpected contamination of uniforms occurs, washing in a home washer with detergent is adequate for decontamination.

6. *Masks are not needed* for AIDS. However, a coughing patient with an undiagnosed pulmonary process should be on mask precautions until tuberculosis has been excluded as the cause of the pulmonary infiltrate. After 5 years experience with AIDS, there is no evidence that AIDS virus is spread by the respiratory route. However, since tuberculosis is a cause of pulmonary disease in a small percentage of cases, masks are a prudent precaution until tuberculosis is excluded. (See "Precautions for Other Diseases Which May Be Seen in AIDS Patients" for indications for masks.)

7. *Protective eyeware* (goggles, glasses, etc.)

Rationale (right column, continued):

To protect the immunocompromised patient and the health care worker.

To protect the physician, medical assistant, and janitorial staff. Needle recapping and disposal are frequent causes of needlesticks.

To protect health care workers from the transmissible agents of AIDS, hepatitis, herpes, CMV, and other infectious agents.

Procedure	Rationale

should be worn when spatter of blood is expected (operative procedures, endoscopies including bronchoscopies, deliveries, etc.)

8. *Hot water soluble laundry bags are not needed unless* the patient has draining wounds or is incontinent.

9. *Specimen handling:* All blood specimens from all patients whether known to be infected or not should be handled with caution. All specimens from AIDS patients must be labeled with "H/A (hepatitis/AIDS) Precautions" labels, placed in ZipLok bags and sealed for transport to prevent spills from broken tubes. A laboratory requisition should also be labeled and attached to the *outside* of the bag.

10. *Spills of blood and other body secretions:* Spills should be cleaned up promptly. Large spills should be cleaned up by a gloved employee, using paper towels, which should be placed in an infectious waste container. Then 5.25% sodium hypochlorite (household bleach) diluted 1:10 should be used to disinfect the area. Sodium hypochlorite should not be placed directly on large amounts of protein matter (urine, stool, blood, sputum, etc.), in order to protect the employee from noxious fumes. A 1:10 dilution of bleach may be ordered for the office or clinic from a hospital pharmacy.

11. *Laboratory procedures* should be adopted to prevent the formation of aerosols. Biological safety cabinets (Class I or II) and other primary containment devices (e.g., centrifuge safety cups) are advised whenever procedures are conducted that have a high potential for creating aerosols or infectious droplets. Other standard laboratory safety practices should be followed (MMWR, Nov. 5th 1982, Vol 31: 577).

12. *Decontamination of equipment:* Respiratory therapy ventilator tubing may be decontaminated by ethylene oxide or pasteurization. Any instrument that comes into contact with blood or other secretions must be thoroughly washed and sterilized or high-level disinfected before reuse. Lensed instruments must be thoroughly cleaned and then sterilized or high-level disinfected (that is, ethylene oxide sterilization or alkaline glutaraldehyde for 45 minutes).

   Other equipment such as EKG leads or EEG electrodes that contact intact skin only require washing with detergent and water prior to reuse.

   Decontamination of other equipment such as thermometers, tonometers, laryngoscopes, and spirometers should be done as for all patients.

Precautions for Other Diseases Which May Be Seen In AIDS Patients

Procedure	Rationale
Cytomegalovirus (CMV) 1. Pregnant women should not give direct care to excretors of CMV. Women trying to get pregnant should use very good personal hygiene (handwashing and gloves) with any body secretions from any patient.	Many AIDS patients excrete CMV. Because the CMV virus may cause birth defects, it is advisable for pregnant women not to have direct contact with known excretors. Although good hygiene has been shown to prevent acquisition of CMV, the standard community practice is for pregnant women to be excused from the care of any known CMV excretor. Pregnant women should be extremely cautious in the care of any patient, because not all CMV excretors are identified. Handwashing is extremely important after any patient or body fluid contact (see references 3 and 4).
Opportunistic and Other Infections 1. Masks (worn by others in the room or when the patient cannot wear a mask) when the patient has an undiagnosed pulmonary process, is coughing, and others have sustained close contact (until T.B. is excluded).	Until the patient's respiratory illness is diagnosed, others need to be protected from diseases spread by the respiratory route. Immunocompetent persons need protection from *Mycobacterium tuberculosis*. Immunocompromised persons need protection from *M. avium* and Pneumocystis. Although some AIDS patients have CMV in their lungs, it is not known if CMV can be transmitted by the respiratory route.
2. Other precautions should be as usual for the particular disease. See an Infection Control Manual for guidance.	

Employee Health Issues

Needlesticks, Mucous Membrane, or Conjunctival Exposure to Body Fluids from AIDS Patients. All needlesticks and other exposures to body fluids from AIDS patients must be reported to the physician, and to Employee Health if working at a hospital clinic. An accident report should be filled out. The employee will be evaluated as for hepatitis B exposure and treated accordingly. Gamma globulin is given as a part of this protocol. Employees with exposures must receive counseling by the physician or Employee Health Service and information regarding the availability of antibody testing for those who wish it.

Individuals with Immunosuppression. Individuals with immunosuppression as a result of disease or therapy should evaluate, with their personal physicians, their own risk of working in a hospital environment. Such individuals, if they feel they are at risk, should provide a letter from their physician to their supervisor indicating their ability to work and outlining any patient care areas where they should not work.

Employees with AIDS. Employees with AIDS should be handled on a case-by-case basis by an Employee Health physician in consultation with an AIDS Clinic physician. The final decision regarding work assignment will be made by the Infection Control Committee using advice from Employee Health and AIDS Clinic physicians on a case-by-case basis taking into account the safety of all employees and patients. Asymptomatic office, clinic, or hospital employees with AIDS, who have recovered from an intercurrent illness, may generally return to work. They should be instructed on health care precautions such as handwashing and wearing gloves for contact with mucous membranes or non-intact skin of patients. Any employee with exudative or weeping (*i.e.*, moist) skin lesions should be reassigned to nonpatient care areas. Evaluation of such employees will be by the physician or the Employee Health Service of the hospital.

In situations where it is not advisable for employees with AIDS to return to their clinical assignment, reassignment to another area should be coordinated with their supervisors.

Cardiopulmonary Resuscitation. Devices to protect employees from mucous membrane contact with blood and other secretions during any resuscitation should be made readily available. Ambu bags should be on all crash carts and are to be used in preference to mouth-to-mouth resuscitation on all patients.

CPR recertification standards should be maintained. Since the AIDS agent is in saliva and since blood may be present in saliva, employees with AIDS should not participate in manikin CPR training. For the protection of all CPR participants in two-person CPR, the second rescuer will simulate ventilation, and a solution of bleach will be used to decontaminate the manikin's face and mouth between all participants.

References

1. CDC: Acquired immune deficiency syndrome (AIDS): precautions for clinical and laboratory staffs. MMWR, **31** (43), 1982.
2. CDC: Recommendations for preventing transmission of infection with human T-lymphotropic virus type III/Lymphadenopathy-associated virus in the workplace. MMWR, **34**(45), 1985.
3. Voltra, E.M., et al.: Recommendations for pregnant employee interaction with patients having communicable diseases. Am. J. Inf. Control, **11**: 10, 1983.
4. Williams, W. W.: Guideline for infection control in hospital personnel. Infection Control, **4**: 326, 1983.
5. San Francisco General Hospital Infection Control Committee, 1987.

CONCLUSION

On completion of this unit, practice the procedures until you feel confident with the performance of your skills, then arrange with your instructor to take the performance test. You will be expected to demonstrate accurately your skill in preparing for and performing all of the procedures outlined in this unit. In addition, you should be prepared to discuss briefly the infectious process and the methods utilized for infection control.

REVIEW OF VOCABULARY

Read the following and define the italicized terms.

When *chemically disinfecting* supplies after use, you may use a variety of preparations that are on the market. These are designated as being a *bactericide* or *bacteriostatic*, a *germicide*, or a *disinfectant*. When making your choice for use, keep in mind that most of these solutions do not destroy *spores* and that the most effective method for decontaminating items is by using the process of *sterilization*. Remember also to keep *contaminated* supplies away from your clean working area.

Sterile or *aseptic technique* is a very important factor in *infection control* and is to be employed in numerous medical procedures. A basic and common example of a time when these techniques are used to prevent *infection* from developing is the administration of injections — the syringe and needle used must be *sterile*, and the patient's skin must be cleansed with an *antiseptic* before the injection is administered.

When a *pathogenic organism* leaves its *reservoir*, it may invade a new *susceptible host* and, depending on its *virulence* and the *resistance* of the new host, it may cause *infection*, *sepsis*, and even *necrosis* to the tissues involved.

Immunizations (vaccinations) are given to build up one's *resistance* to various infectious diseases, such as diphtheria, which has an *incubation period* of 2 to 5 days.

REVIEW QUESTIONS

1. State three goals of infection control, and explain how you and the general public can play an active role in this.
2. Differentiate between a local and generalized infection.
3. Differentiate between artificial passive and active immunity.
4. List five diagnostic tests that may be used to help diagnose an infection.
5. Describe the inflammatory process, listing five local and four systemic signs and symptoms of inflammation.
6. You are given three pieces of equipment: one is to be sanitized, one to be disinfected, and the other to be sterilized. Explain the differences among these three processes, and list methods used to accomplish each effectively.
7. At your place of employment you have an autoclave, a Chemiclave, a dry-heat sterilizer, a gas sterilizer, and chemical solutions. List at least three items that you would sterilize in each of these.
8. If you are busy and cannot clean soiled instruments immediately after use, what should you do?
9. When an instrument is to be boiled for 20 minutes, when do you start to time the exposure period?
10. Upon checking your storage area of sterile supplies, you find a pack that has been there for 1½ months. What should your next action be regarding this pack?
11. When removing a dry pack from the autoclave, you observe that the sterilization indicator has not changed color. What would you do?

PERFORMANCE TEST

In a skills laboratory, a simulation of a joblike environment, the medical assistant student will demonstrate skill in performing the following activities without reference to source materials. Time limits for the performance of each procedure are to be assigned by the instructor (see also pp. 32 and 35).

1. Given a bar of soap, perform a medical aseptic handwash.
2. Given reusable syringes and needles, rubber gloves, and instruments, sanitize these items and then wrap them for sterilization.
3. Given wrapped supplies for sterilization, position these correctly in the chamber of the sterilizer.
4. Given various types of sterilizers and the manufacturer's instructions, sterilize wrapped and unwrapped items, correctly remove them from the sterilizer on completion of the sterilizing cycle, and determine if sterilization has been effective.
5. Given thermometers, a percussion hammer, and a variety of blunt instruments, correctly disinfect these items using chemicals; disinfect blunt instruments using boiling water.

The student is to perform these activities with 100% accuracy 90% of the time (9 out of 10 times).

PERFORMANCE CHECKLISTS

Handwashing Technique

1. Stand in front of, but not touching, the sink.
2. Adjust the water flow and temperature.
3. Wet hands, and apply soap.
4. Wash hands well and rinse; keep hands and forearms at elbow level or below.
5. Wash wrists and forearms.
6. Rinse soap bar, and drop it into the dish without touching the dish.
7. Rinse hands, wrists, and forearms under running water.
8. Clean fingernails (at least once a day), and rinse well.
9. Repeat the wash if hands are highly contaminated.
10. Turn off water faucet using a paper towel.
11. Dry hand, wrists, and forearms well.

Sanitizing, Wrapping, and Positioning Instruments for Sterilization

1. Remove the instruments to work area, and bulk rinse in a solution of water and a blood solvent, low-sudsing detergent or germicide.
2. Rinse in fresh water.
3. Scrub each instrument thoroughly with a brush and warm detergent solution.
4. Rinse completely with hot water.
5. Dry the instruments, and check for working condition.

6. Place all instruments to be used together on a diagonal in the center of a square of muslin or disposable paper.
7. Fold the material up from the bottom, doubling back a small corner.
8. Fold the right then the left edges over, leaving the corners doubled back.
9. Fold the pack up from the bottom and secure with pressure-sensitive tape or special sterilizing masking tape.
10. Date and label the pack according to contents.
11. Place the pack in the sterilizer chamber correctly so that steam can flow between and penetrate the packs (place jars or similar containers on their side, hard packs on the bottom).

Sanitizing, Wrapping, and Positioning Gloves for Sterilization

1. Immediately after use, wash gloves in cold water.
2. Wash in warm water and detergent, then rinse.
3. Turn the gloves inside out, wash, and rinse well.
4. Fill the gloves with water or air to inspect for puncture holes.
5. Dry the gloves with towel, then allow to air dry. Both sides must be exposed to the air for drying.
6. When they are dry, powder the gloves with a nonirritating starch preparation.
7. Fold the cuffs over; use paper or gauze to separate the rubber surfaces.
8. Place paper or gauze inside the palm of the gloves.
9. Position the gloves in the center of disposable wrapping paper or muslin, with thumbs pointing away from the center.
10. Fold the bottom part of the paper or muslin up over the gloves.
11. Fold top part of paper or muslin down over the gloves already covered with the bottom fold of the material.
12. Fold the right side of the wrapper over the right glove and the left side of the wrapper over the left glove.
13. Fold the package in half (that is, left side over right side), and secure with sterilizing tape.
14. Label the package with the size of the gloves and the date.
15. Place the package in the chamber of the sterilizer with the folded edges up.

Sanitizing, Wrapping, and Positioning Syringes and Needles in the Sterilizer

1. Immediately after use, fill the syringe with cool water and flush it through the needle.
2. Disassemble the unit.
3. Place the needle in a tray and then into the sterilizer for 30 minutes at 250°F (121°C).
4. Soak the syringe in water and detergent, and thoroughly brush the interior of the barrel.
5. Clean the inside tip and the plunger.
6. Flush the syringe twice with tap water, once with distilled water.

7. After 30 minutes exposure time, remove the needles from the sterilizer.
8. Clean inside the needle hub.
9. Pass a stylet through the interior of the needle several times.
10. Check the needle point for sharpness and/or snags.
11. Clean the exterior of the needle.
12. Rinse the hub and the needle exterior well under running water.
13. With a syringe, flush tap water through the needle interior.
14. Rinse the exterior and interior of the needle with distilled water.
15. Label a disposable paper bag with the date and the size of the syringe.
16. Place matching separated plunger and syringe inside the bag.
17. Fold the top of the bag, and seal securely.
18. When the needle is to be sterilized with the syringe:
    - Place the needle in a disposable paper form.
    - Label the bag with the size of syringe, needle, and the date.
    - Place the needle in the bag with the syringe barrel and plunger.
    - Fold the top of the bag, and seal it securely.
19. When the needle is to be sterilized individually, place it in a glass tube with constricted sides, and top with a gauze, cotton, or rubber stopper.
20. Place a disposable bag with contents horizontally on the tray of the sterilizer; place a constriction tube with a needle horizontally on the sterilizer tray for the sterilization cycle.

Disinfecting/Sterilizing with Chemical Solutions

1. Sanitize items as for sterilization by autoclave.
2. Pour chemical solution into designated container with an airtight lid; dilute chemical if necessary, according to manufacturer's instructions.
3. Completely immerse item(s) in solution, and close the cover of container.
4. Leave for required time (time will vary from 20 minutes to 3 hours, depending on the solution used).
5. Remove the tray from the container, and rinse items in a pan of sterile distilled water before using.
6. Remove items for use from the tray using sterile transfer forceps.
7. Change the solution in the container every 7 to 14 days or as recommended by the manufacturer.
8. Items such as percussion hammers and stethoscopes can be disinfected by wiping these instruments off with a germicide or antiseptic solution.

Disinfection with Boiling Water

1. Fill the boiler half full with water.
2. Clean items thoroughly.
3. Position items on a tray in the boiler, hinges or clamps open, jars and so forth on their sides.
4. Lower the tray to completely immerse items in the water.
5. Close the lid, and turn the power switch on.
6. When the water is boiling, start timing the exposure period for 15 to 20 minutes.
7. When the cycle is completed, stand back or to the side, and open the lid of the boiler.
8. Allow the items to cool.
9. Remove and dry the items.
10. Store the items in a designated place, or use immediately.
11. When the boiler is used for sterilizing items because of the absence of an autoclave or other sterilizer, remove items from the boiler with a sterile transfer forcep, dry with a sterile towel, and transfer to a sterile field for immediate use.

Unit V

Surgical Asepsis and Minor Surgery

Vocabulary

anesthesia (an"es-the'ze-ah)—The loss of sensation or feeling.

asepsis (a-sep'sis)—The state of being free from infection or infectious matter.

144

biopsy (bi'op-se)—Removal of tissue from the body for examination.

    incisional biopsy—Incision into and removal of part of a lesion.

    excisional biopsy—Removal of an entire small lesion.

    aspiration/needle biopsy—Removal of material from an internal organ by means of a hollow needle inserted through the body wall and into the affected tissue.

cautery (kaw'ter-ē)—A hot instrument used to cut or destroy tissue, causing hemostasis at the time.

don—To put an article on, such as gloves or a gown.

ligate (li'gāt)—To apply a ligature.

ligature (lig'ah-tūr)—A suture; material used to tie off blood vessels to prevent bleeding, or to constrict tissues.

Mayo (mā'ō) **stand**—A stand with a flat metal tray used to hold sterile supplies during an aseptic procedure.

postoperative (post-op'er-ah-tiv)—Pertaining to the period of time following surgery.

preoperative (pre-op'er-ah-tiv)—Pertaining to the time preceding surgery.

sterile field—A work area prepared with sterile drapes (coverings) to hold sterile supplies during a sterile procedure.

sterile setup—Specific sterile supplies used in a specific sterile procedure.

suture (soo'cher)—Various types and sizes of absorbable and nonabsorbable materials used to close a wound with stitches.

transfer forceps—A type of instrument (forcep) that is kept in a chemical disinfectant or germicide and used for transferring or handling sterile supplies and equipment.

This unit discusses the common practices of, and some procedures requiring, surgical asepsis (sterile technique). In order to control the sources and spread of infection when one is performing and assisting with certain medical procedures, knowledge of and adherence to the correct performance of aseptic practices are essential.

A good preparation for studying this unit is to review Unit IV, which discussed concepts of infection control, medical and surgical asepsis, practices of medical asepsis, and the disinfection and sterilization of supplies.

BACKGROUND OF STERILE TECHNIQUE

Sterile techniques as we know them today have gradually evolved since the turn of the century. The history of medicine shows evidence of some understanding of asepsis as early as the time of Hippocrates, the father of medicine, in 460 BC. It was Hippocrates who started to use boiled water when irrigating wounds; then later, Galen (131–210 AD) boiled instruments before using them when caring for wounds. Throughout the centuries up to present times, numerous individuals, too many to mention here, played vital roles in describing diseases and their causes, theories for contagious diseases, the spread of infection by improperly washed hands, the role of bacteria in causing disease, the inhibition of the growth of microorganisms by heat, and the germ theory for the causes of disease.

It was Joseph Lister (1827–1912) who introduced the use of chemicals to destroy microorganisms in infected wounds (antisepsis) and later procedures to exclude bacteria from surgical fields (asepsis). Surgery as we know it today was essentially Lister's gift to humanity.

In the later years of the 19th century, the concepts of vaccinations against disease were introduced. Edward Jenner discovered the value of vaccination against smallpox. This was a discovery that led to further advances, such as Louis Pasteur's principle of inoculation by means of vaccines against viral and bacterial diseases.

Sterilization of items by boiling began around 1880, and the principles and practices of autoclaving (steam under pressure) began around 1886. Rubber gloves were first used to protect the hands from harsh antiseptics. Eventually they were accepted and used as a protective measure to prevent contamination to the patient. Thus, sterile technique or aseptic practices, as we know them, evolved.

PRINCIPLES AND PRACTICES OF SURGICAL ASEPSIS

Surgical asepsis, more commonly referred to as *sterile technique* or *aseptic technique*, is the practice used when an area and supplies in that area are to be made and kept sterile. These techniques are used in all procedures in which entry is made into normally sterile body parts, such as when administering an injection, when making a surgical incision, or when caring for any break in the skin, such as open wounds or skin ulcers. Strict sterile or aseptic technique is required at all times in such procedures, because body tissues can easily become infected. Breaks in technique may lead to infections that the body cannot combat. Even mild infections delay recovery and are costly—mentally, physically, and financially—to the patient. It is the responsibility of the medical assistant and the physician to adhere to the following principles and practices at all times when assisting with or performing a sterile procedure.

1. Sterilize all supplies used for sterile procedures either previously or at the time for immediate use.
2. When in doubt about the sterility of anything, consider it nonsterile.
3. When putting sterile gloves on, do not touch the outside of the gloves with bare hands.
4. People who are gloved must touch only sterile articles; people who are not gloved must touch only nonsterile articles, except when using sterile transfer forceps to move sterile items.
5. During a sterile procedure, if a glove is punctured by a needle or instrument, change the glove immediately, and remove the needle or instrument from the sterile field.
6. The outer wrappings and the edges of packs that contain sterile items are not sterile, and thus are handled and opened by the person who is not wearing sterile gloves.
7. Open sterile packages with the edges of the wrapper directed away from your body to avoid touching your uniform or reaching over a sterile field.
8. Touch only the outside of a sterile wrapper.
9. Once a sterile pack has been opened, use it; if it is not used, rewrap and resterilize it.
10. Avoid sneezing, coughing, or talking directly over a sterile field or object.
11. Do not reach across or above a sterile field or wound. Your clothes and skin are not sterile. If you touch the sterile field or drop debris onto it or into the wound, contamination results. Movements around the area should be kept to a minimum.
12. Avoid spilling solutions on a sterile setup. Any moisture that soaks through a sterile area to a nonsterile one produces a means of transporting bacteria to a sterile area. Thus, the wet areas are considered contaminated and must either be covered with sterile towels or drapes until the top surface is dry or be removed and redraped.
13. Hold sterile objects and gloved hands above waist level or level to the sterile field. Anything below this level is considered unsterile. Keeping objects or hands in sight helps avoid contamination.
14. Since skin cannot be sterilized, any object that touches it is considered contaminated.
15. Have a special receptacle or waxed paper or plastic bag to receive contaminated materials.
16. A sterile field should be away from drafts, fans, and windows. Microorganisms can be carried in air currents to the patient or the sterile field.
17. Store sterile packages in dry areas. If they become wet, they must be resterilized or discarded.
18. Hands are the greatest source of contamination; therefore, wash frequently using correct technique.
19. Be constantly aware of the need for very clean surroundings.

In summary, keep in mind these five basic rules:

- Know what is sterile.
- Know what is not sterile.
- Keep sterile items separate from nonsterile items.
- Prevent contamination.
- Remedy a contaminated situation immediately.

HANDLING STERILE SUPPLIES

Opening Sterile Packages

Many commercially prepared sterile packages have instructions for opening printed on them. Read these directions carefully before opening the package to avoid contamination of the contents. To open peel-down packages, such as those in which syringes and dressing materials are supplied, use the following procedure.

Opening Peel-Down Packages

Procedure	Rationale
1. Wash your hands.	
2. Using both hands, grasp both sides of the extended edges provided.	
3. Pull evenly along the sealed edges (Fig. 5-1, *A*).	Pull evenly in a downward motion to avoid tearing.
4. Do not touch the inside of the wrapper; place on a flat surface.	The inside of the wrapper is sterile and can be used as a sterile field until using the contents.
or	
Using sterile forceps, remove the contents from the wrapper and transfer to a sterile field, or use immediately in a sterile procedure, such as a dressing change (Fig. 5-1, *B*).	

Procedure	Rationale
or Holding the bottom of the package with the edges folded back, allow a person with sterile gloves on to take the contents (Fig. 5-1, *B*). *or* If the item is a syringe to be used by you, grasp the plunger end of the syringe with one hand while holding onto the package with your other hand.	Keep your fingers away from the contents to avoid contamination. The bottom part of the plunger does not have to remain sterile, because this is the way in which you take hold of the syringe to remove it from the sterile package.

Fig. 5-1. **A,** technique for opening peel-down package with sterile contents. **B,** technique for removing a sterile dressing from package.

A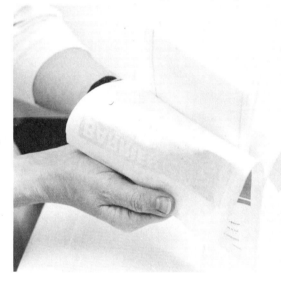

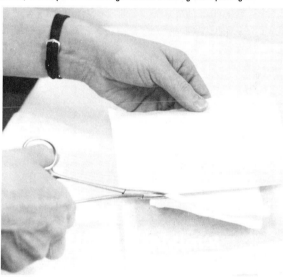 B

Opening an Envelope Wrap

Procedure	Rationale
1. Wash your hands. 2. Place package on a flat surface so that the folded edges are on top. 3. Remove tape or string fastener, and discard in waste container.	At this time you should also check the date and sterilization indicator to make sure that the contents are sterile.
4. Pull out the tucked under corner (if present), and unfold this top flap away from you (Fig. 5-2).	Unfolding away from you avoids the necessity of reaching over the sterile field later and causing contamination. Avoid touching the pack with your uniform or person.
5. Using both hands, grasp the second layer of folded corners, and open these flaps to the sides of the package (Fig. 5-3), or open first one side and then the other.	The contents of the package are still covered with the last layer of the wrapper.
6. Without reaching over any of the uncovered area, grasp the last fold or fourth corner, and open toward your body (Fig. 5-4).	Lift this corner up and toward you, dropping it on the surface holding the package. Do not touch the inside of the package or the contents with bare hands, as this would contaminate everything.

Fig. 5-2. Opening sterile pack. Unfold top flap away from you.

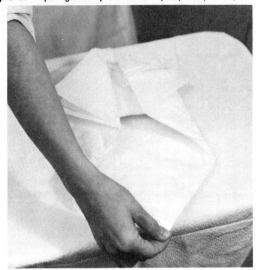

Fig. 5-3. Opening sterile pack, step 2. Open second layer of flaps to each side.

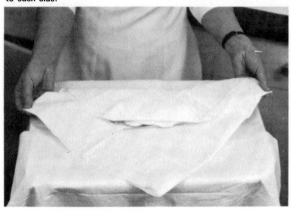

Fig. 5-4. Opening sterile pack, step 3. Open last flap toward your body.

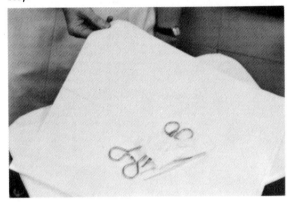

You now have a sterile field that can be used as a sterile work area. Additional sterile items that may be needed for the procedure may be added to this sterile field. To organize the items contained in the package you just opened, use sterile transfer forceps as discussed next (Fig. 5-5), or don sterile gloves.

Small packages can be held in the hand and unwrapped in the same fashion. Have someone who is wearing sterile gloves take the item from the opened wrap, or remove it with sterile transfer forceps, or carefully place the item on a sterile field, avoiding contamination to the item and field. Be sure that the wrapper corners do not touch the sterile field.

Handling Sterile Transfer Forceps

Sterile transfer forceps are used to transfer or handle sterile equipment to avoid contamination by the hands. The use of these forceps, which are kept in a container with a disinfectant or germicide solution, is being discouraged by many health care practitioners who feel that these forceps are highly vulnerable to contamination, and therefore, a cause of further con-

tamination. The more common and recommended practice is to use individually wrapped sterile forceps for each procedure when needed. Despite the fact that sterile transfer forceps are now not used as often, they remain standard equipment in many offices and clinics. The following describes how they are to be handled if and when you must use them.

Fig. 5-5. Using sterile forceps, arrange sterile supplies on sterile field for use.

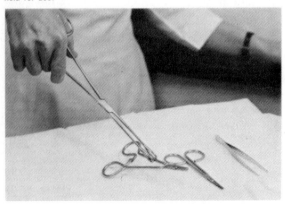

Procedure	Rationale
1. Keep only one forceps in the container of clean germicidal solution.	When more than one forceps is kept in the container, the chance of contaminating one against the other when removing one is too great.
2. Wash your hands.	
3. When removing from container, keep the prongs together and facing downward; grasp handles and lift vertically without touching any part of the container above the solution line (Fig. 5-6).	The container is not sterile above the solution line. Sterile parts are contaminated when touching unsterile parts.
4. You may tap the prongs together gently over the container to remove excess solution.	Excess solution falling on a sterile field would contaminate it. You must avoid this.
5. Keep forceps in a downward position when using to prevent any solution on prongs from flowing up to the handle.	The handle is not sterile. Solution that flows to the handle will flow back to the prongs when returned to a downward position, thus contaminating the forceps.
6. Use as required to handle, transfer, or assemble sterile supplies and equipment (see Fig. 5-5).	
7. Never touch the tip of the forceps to the sterile field when putting supplies on it after a procedure has begun.	After a procedure has begun, the forceps will be contaminated for any other procedure if you touch the present sterile field, and must be resterilized before being returned to the container.
8. After use, return the forceps to the container without touching any parts of the container.	Remember that the container is not sterile except inside below the solution level.
9. Sterilize the forceps and container, and refill container with fresh germicide solution weekly, or more frequently if indicated.	The more frequently these items are resterilized and the solution changed, the more likely this procedure will be safe to use.

Fig. 5-6. Removing sterile transfer forceps from container, keeping prongs together, facing downward.

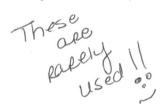

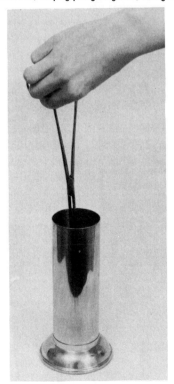

Pouring Sterile Solutions

When required to pour a sterile solution, you must use aseptic technique to avoid contamination to the solution.

Procedure	Rationale
1. Wash your hands. 2. Obtain the solution, and check the label.	Solutions are drugs. All drug labels must be checked three times before using or administering: • When removing from storage area • Before pouring • When replacing container in the storage area
3. Obtain sterile container to be used for the solution, and unwrap.	Follow procedure for unwrapping as described previously. NOTE: When using prepackaged sterile trays, a container for the solution may be included in the pack.
4. Remove bottle cap; place on a level surface with the top of the cap resting on the surface or hold it in your hand with the top facing downwards (Fig. 5-7).	The inner part of the cap is considered sterile. If you place the cap with top facing up, you have contaminated the inner surface, which then cannot be replaced on the container until it has been resterilized.
5. Hold the bottle with the label in the palm of your hand and about 6 inches above the container (or less, when pouring very small amounts of solution), and pour the solution (Fig. 5-7). 6. When pouring a solution on a sponge, pick up the sponge with forceps and pour the solution over the sponge. The excess solution will drip into the basin or discard container (Fig. 5-8).	Holding the bottle this way prevents damage to the label if the solution runs or spills; also undue splashing is avoided. Pour a small amount of solution into a waste container to cleanse the side of the bottle, and then pour from the same area.
7. Pick the cap up by the sides, and replace it on the bottle securely. 8. Check the label of the bottle, and replace it in the correct storage area.	Do not contaminate the inside of the cap, because it is considered sterile and must cover the sterile solution in the bottle.

Fig. 5-7. Pouring solution into container on sterile field. Hold top of container in your hand with top facing downwards.

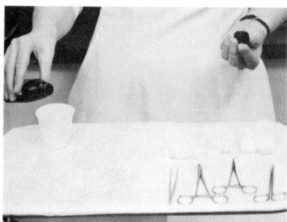

Fig. 5-8. Pouring solution onto sterile sponge.

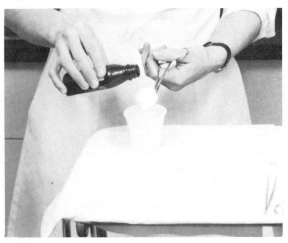

Donning Sterile Gloves

Sterile gloves are worn to protect the patient from infection caused by microorganisms that may be on your hands and to provide a means of safely handling sterile supplies and equipment without contaminating these items.

Procedure	Rationale
1. Wash your hands.	
2. Obtain wrapped gloves, and place on a clean, dry, flat surface with the cuff end toward you.	
3. Open the wrapper by handling only the outside.	The inside part of the wrapper is sterile.
4. Using your left hand, pick up the right-hand glove by grasping the folded edge of the cuff, and lift up and away from the wrapper (Fig. 5-9).	The folded edge of the cuff will be against your skin and is contaminated as soon as you touch it. *Do not* touch the outside of the glove with your ungloved hand.
5. Pulling on the edge of the cuff, pull the right glove on.	Keep your fingers away from the rest of the glove.
6. Place fingers of the right gloved hand under the cuff of the left-hand glove (Fig. 5-10).	Be sure that your gloved fingers do not touch your skin. The area inside the folded cuff is considered sterile.
7. Lift the glove up and away from the wrapper, and pull it onto your left hand.	Be sure that the left thumb does not stray up and touch the right glove. Keep the right gloved fingers under the cuff and straight; keep the right gloved thumb back to avoid touching skin.
8. Continue pulling the left glove up over your wrist.	
9. With the gloved left hand, place fingers under the cuff of the right glove and pull the cuff up over your right wrist (Fig. 5-11).	The area inside the folded cuff is considered sterile.
10. Adjust the fingers of the gloves as necessary.	If, when putting on either glove, the fingers get into the wrong space, you must proceed with the rest of the gloving procedure, and then adjust the gloves with gloved hands.
11. If either glove tears during the procedure, remove and discard, then begin the procedure again with a new pair of gloves.	

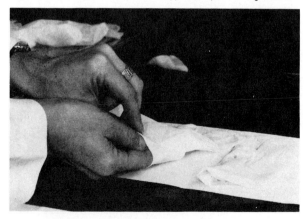

Fig. 5-9. Technique for donning first sterile glove. Grasp folded edge of cuff, lift up and away from wrapper, and pull onto right hand.

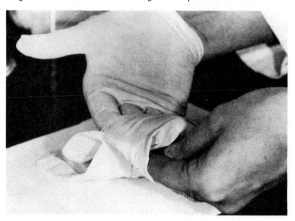

Fig. 5-10. Technique for donning second sterile glove. Place fingers of gloved hand under cuff of other glove and pull onto left hand.

Donning Sterile Gloves (*continued*)

Procedure	Rationale
12. *To remove gloves:* • Grasp the cuff of the right-hand glove with your left hand. • Pull the glove down over the hand. • Discard in appropriate place. • Repeat, using the right hand to remove left glove. Grasp the inside and top of the left-hand glove with your right hand, pull the glove down over the hand, and discard. Reusable gloves must be washed and resterilized; disposable gloves are discarded in the appropriate waste container.	The glove will turn inside out as it comes off. Do not touch the outside of the glove as it is considered contaminated after use.

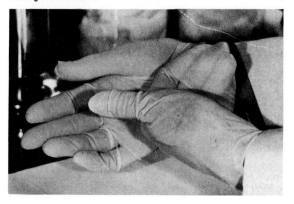

Fig. 5-11. Technique for donning sterile glove. Adjust cuffs on gloves, avoiding contamination.

MINOR SURGERY

Only "minor" surgery is performed in the physician's office, although frequently even these procedures are done in the emergency room or outpatient department of a hospital or in a clinic.

Minor surgical procedures include those that can be done with or without the use of a local anesthetic, such as the suturing of a laceration; the incision and drainage of an abscess or cyst; incision and removal of foreign bodies in subcutaneous tissues; removal of small growths such as warts, moles, and skin tags; various types of biopsies; cauterization of tissue (such as cauterization of the uterine cervix, or of a wart, mole, or skin tag); and insertion of an intrauterine device (IUD). After minor surgery performed in the office or at the hospital, the patient may come to the physician's office for dressing changes and for the removal of sutures as part of the postoperative care. Inspection of the wound is also done at that time to determine the amount of healing that has occurred and to ensure the absence of a developing infectious process.

As the physician's assistant, you may be called upon to assist with the surgical procedures or to change a dressing for a patient. Assisting in any surgical procedure is a highly responsible job, and strict aseptic technique must always be used. The nature of the surgery or postoperative care will govern the duties and responsibilities of the medical assistant.

Anesthesia

For minor surgery and extremely painful treatments, some type of local anesthesia is usually required. *Local anesthesia* refers to the absence of feeling or sensation and pain in a limited area of the body without the loss of consciousness. The extent and severity of the procedure will determine the type and amount of anesthetic used, which can be administered by injection or by topical application. Local anesthetics produce their effects in 5 to 15 minutes. These effects may last from 1 to 3 hours depending on the type and dose administered.

Types of Local Anesthesia

• Infiltration — The anesthetic solution is injected under the skin to anesthetize the nerve endings and nerve fibers at the site to be worked on. The sensory nerves become insensitive and remain so for several hours, depending on the amount of drug administered. (Rules for the administration of medications and injections as described in Unit VII apply here.) Examples of infiltration anesthetics include procaine (Novocaine) 1% to 2% and lidocaine (Xylocaine) 1% to 2%.

• Nerve block or block anesthesia — The anesthetic solution is injected into or adjacent to accessible main nerves, thus desensitizing all the adjacent tissue. Examples of nerve block anesthesia include procaine (Novocaine) 1% to 2% and lidocaine (Xylocaine) 1% to 2%.

- Topical or surface anesthesia — The anesthetic solution is painted or sprayed directly onto the skin or mucous membrane involved to deaden sensation and relieve pain. Examples of topical anesthetics include lidocaine 4% solution, for accessible mucous membranes of oral and nasal cavities, and ethyl chloride spray, for external topical use, because it is too harsh for use on mucous membranes. Before a topical anesthetic is applied, the patient's skin must be washed and dried well.

Allergic Reactions.   Before the administration of a local anesthetic, every patient must be asked if he or she is allergic to any drug, if he or she has any cardiac or respiratory problems, and if he or she has had any type of anesthetic before. This information is most important, as some local anesthetics can cause anaphylactic shock or violent allergic reactions in patients who are allergic to the drug. Frequently skin tests are made beforehand when deemed necessary. An emergency tray with sterile syringes and needles, sterile alcohol sponges, and ampules of a stimulant such as epinephrine (Adrenalin) must be kept in reach when an anesthetic is to be administered in case an emergency does arise.

Suture Materials and Needles

The purpose of sutures is to hold the edges of a wound together until healing occurs. When suture materials are needed for a procedure, they can be added to your sterile field. The most frequently used are the sterile prepackaged sutures with or without an attached suture needle (Fig. 5-12). The label on these packages indicates the type and size of the suture and needle enclosed. Sutures are prepared from materials that are either absorbable or nonabsorbable. *Absorbable sutures* do not have to be removed when used, as they are absorbed or digested by the body fluids and tissues during and after the healing process, for example, surgical gut (catgut). *Nonabsorbable sutures* used on outer skin surfaces are removed after the wound has healed, because body fluids and cells do not absorb or digest them, for example, cotton, silk, nylon, and wire. When used internally, they are not removed and remain as foreign bodies; usually they become encysted and cause no trouble. The size, or gauge, of most sutures is labeled in terms of 0s. That is, 0, which is the thickest, then 00, 000, and so on, each decreasing in size up to 10-0, which is the thinnest. Sizes 2-0 up to 6-0 are used most frequently; 10-0 silk, being extremely fine, is used for ophthalmological and vascular procedures. A few types of sutures are designated as 1, 2, 3, 4, and 5 (the thickest); others are designated simply as fine, medium, and coarse. The size of the suture used is determined by the area and the purpose for which it will be used. Thicker sutures are used when closing large wounds, medium ones are used on lacerations, and very fine sutures are used on more delicate tissues, such as the eye or facial tissues.

Suture needles are either straight or curved and have either a sharp, cutting point, or a round, noncutting point. They are supplied in individual packages or in packages with suture materials (Fig. 5-12). Some needles have an eye through which you thread the suture material. Other needles come attached to the suture material as one unit. These are called *swaged needles* (Fig. 5-13). Packages containing these will be labeled as to the type and size of the needle, and the type, size, and length of the suture material.

Sharp cutting needles are used on stable tissues, such as the skin, where the sharp point is useful in getting the needle through the tissue. Round, noncutting needles are used on less firm tissues, such as subcutaneous tissues and on the internal organs of body cavities. Curved needles are held in a needle holder (see Fig. 5-13, *D*) when used so as to be able to get in and out of the tissue, as when suturing small skin incisions. Straight needles are used by hand as they are pushed through adjoining tissues as when suturing large skin incisions. The size and type of suture needle used is determined by the area and the purpose for which it will be used.

An alternative to the use of sutures for holding the edges of tissue together is the use of adhesive skin closures. These are sterile nonallergic tapes that are supplied in a variety of lengths and widths. An example of a commercial adhesive skin closure is the Steri-Strip. The edges of the tissue are held together and the Steri-Strips are applied transversely across this area and left in place until the wound has healed.

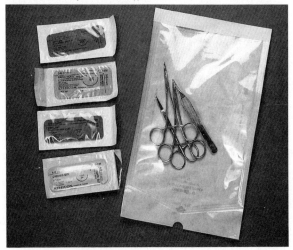

Fig. 5-12.   Prepackaged sterile suture materials. Cover of package indicates type and size of suture material, and the curved line under the suture label represents the type and size of needle included.

Fig. 5-13. Types of suture needles: **A,** straight; **B,** curved with sharp point; **C,** swaged; **D,** swaged needle positioned for use in needle holder. (**A, B,** and **C,** courtesy Miltex Instrument Company, Lake Success, NY)

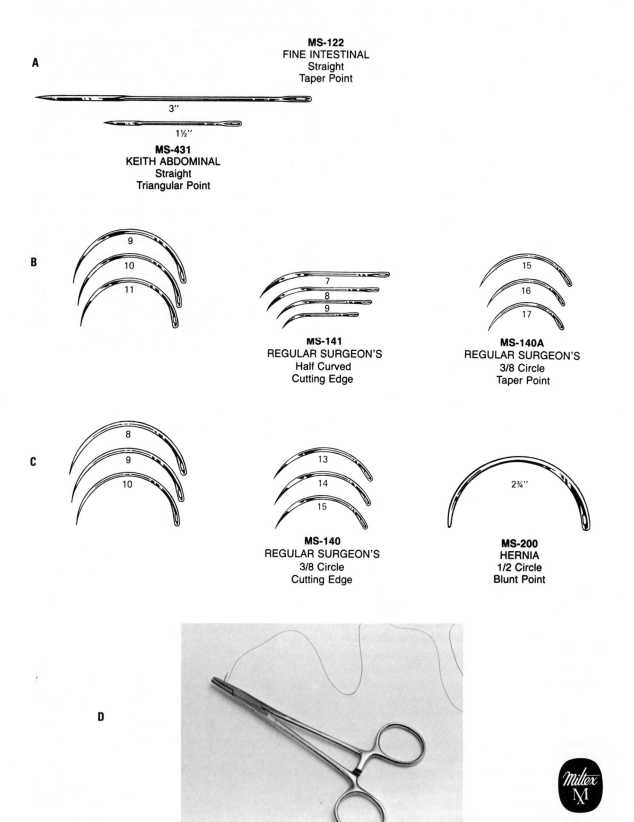

A

MS-122
FINE INTESTINAL
Straight
Taper Point

3″

1½″

MS-431
KEITH ABDOMINAL
Straight
Triangular Point

B

9
10
11

7
8
9

MS-141
REGULAR SURGEON'S
Half Curved
Cutting Edge

15
16
17

MS-140A
REGULAR SURGEON'S
3/8 Circle
Taper Point

C

8
9
10

13
14
15

MS-140
REGULAR SURGEON'S
3/8 Circle
Cutting Edge

2¾″

MS-200
HERNIA
1/2 Circle
Blunt Point

D

Instruments Used for Minor Surgery

Surgical instruments are tools or devices designed to perform a specific function, such as cutting, grasping, retracting, or suturing (Fig. 5-14). They are usually made of steel and are treated so that they are durable, rust-resistant, heat-resistant, and stain-proof. Proper care of all surgical instruments is essential. You must see that they are used correctly, handled carefully, inspected for any defects, and sterilized and stored correctly. As a medical assistant you should be able to identify a variety of surgical instruments, know how they are used, sterilized and stored, and be able to

select the correct instruments for a variety of minor surgical procedures that may be performed in the physician's office or clinic. Some of the more common surgical instruments will be discussed. Figure 5-14 illustrates many of these instruments. Additional figures in this unit illustrate tray set-ups for specific procedures with some of these instruments.

Scalpels (skal'pel). Scalpels are used to make incisions into tissues. They are small surgical knives that usually have a convex edge. Scalpel blades are supplied in various sizes and shapes that are designed for making different types of incisions in various tissues. Most scalpels are now disposable and some are sup-

(*Text continues on p. 159*)

Fig. 5-14. Instruments used for minor surgery. (Courtesy Miltex Instrument Co., Lake Success, NY)

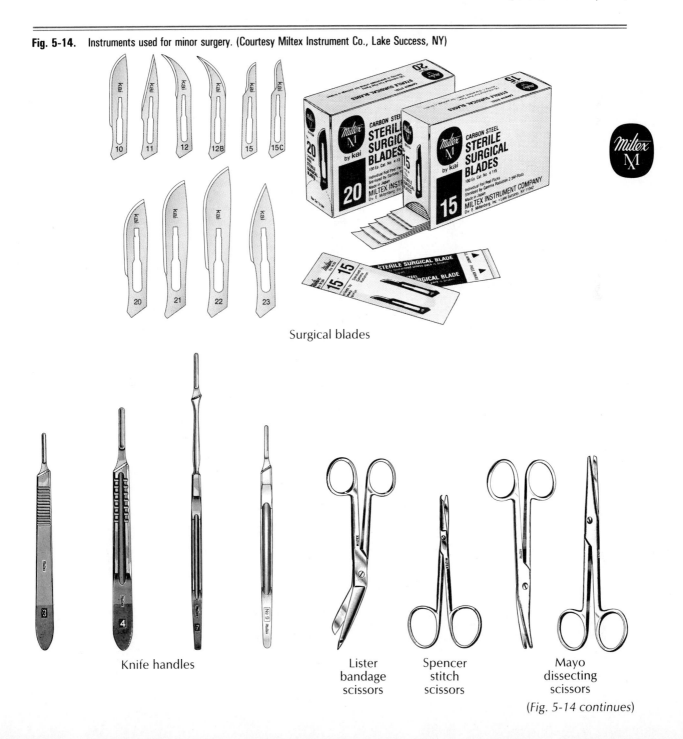

Surgical blades

Knife handles   Lister bandage scissors   Spencer stitch scissors   Mayo dissecting scissors

(*Fig. 5-14 continues*)

Fig. 5-14 *(continued)*

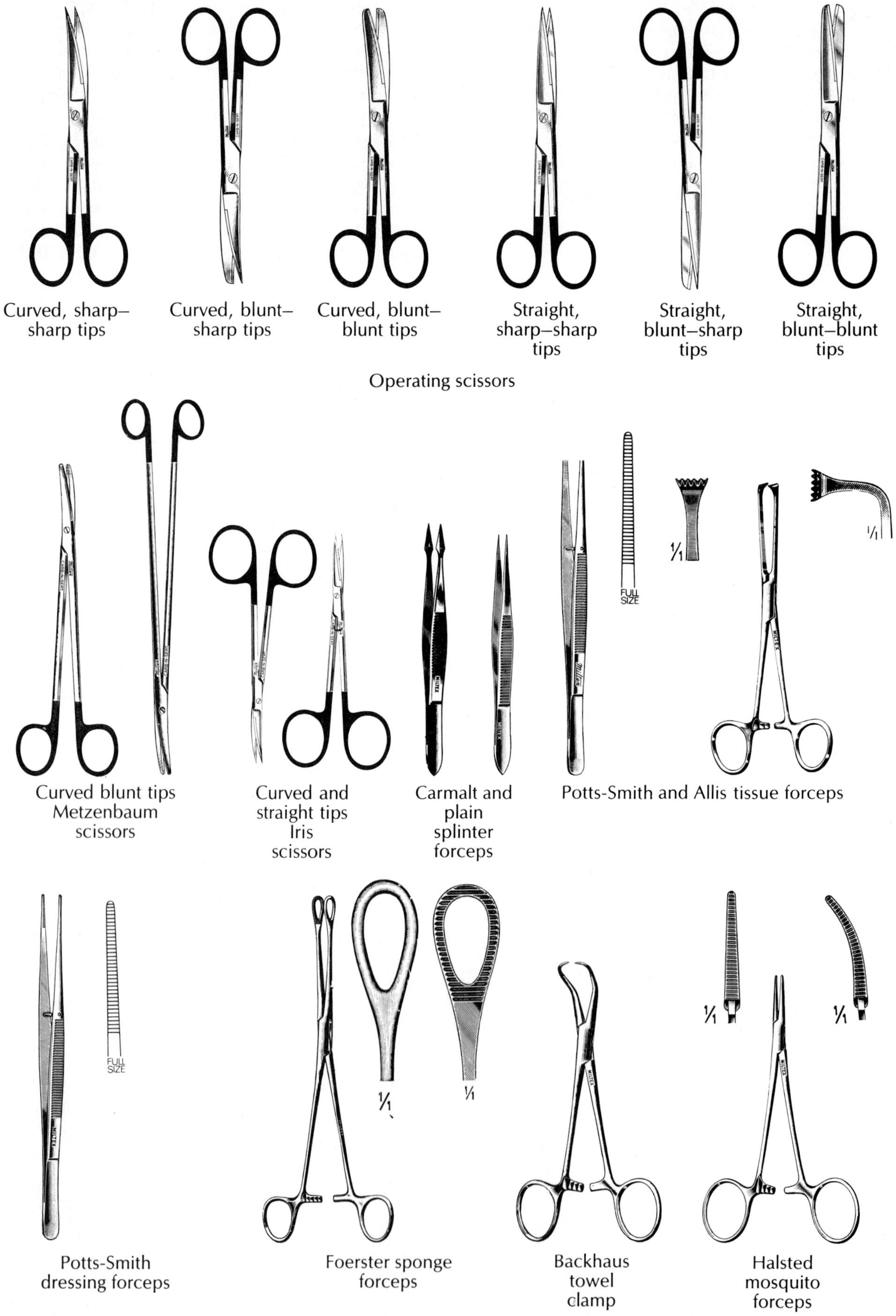

Curved, sharp–sharp tips
Curved, blunt–sharp tips
Curved, blunt–blunt tips
Straight, sharp–sharp tips
Straight, blunt–sharp tips
Straight, blunt–blunt tips
Operating scissors
1/1
FULL SIZE
1/1
Curved blunt tips Metzenbaum scissors
Curved and straight tips Iris scissors
Carmalt and plain splinter forceps
Potts-Smith and Allis tissue forceps
FULL SIZE
1/1
1/1
1/1
1/1
Potts-Smith dressing forceps
Foerster sponge forceps
Backhaus towel clamp
Halsted mosquito forceps

Fig. 5-14   *(continued)*

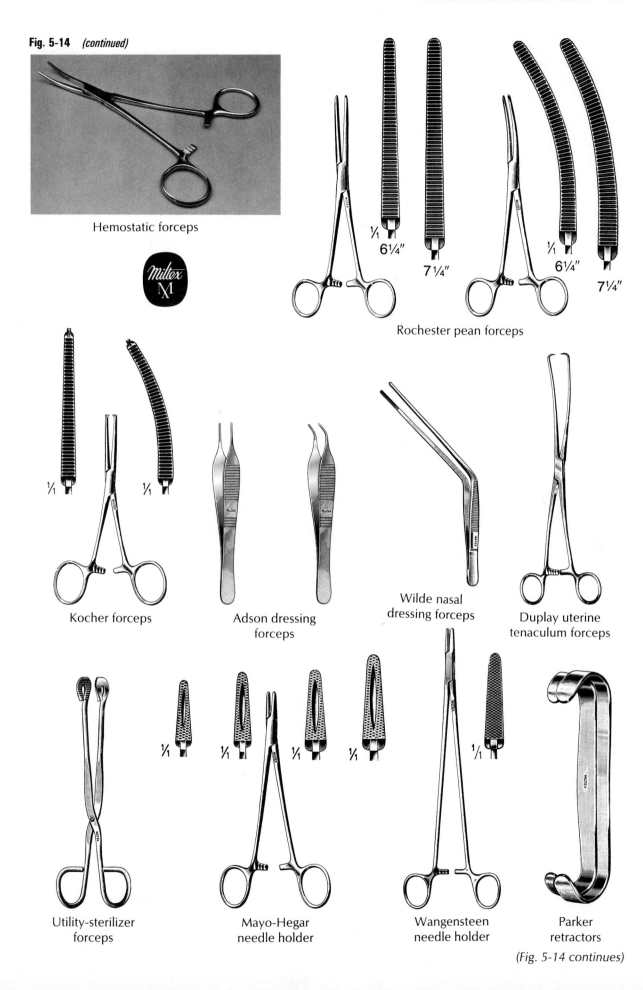

Hemostatic forceps

Rochester pean forceps

Kocher forceps

Adson dressing forceps

Wilde nasal dressing forceps

Duplay uterine tenaculum forceps

Utility-sterilizer forceps

Mayo-Hegar needle holder

Wangensteen needle holder

Parker retractors

(Fig. 5-14 continues)

Fig. 5-14 *(continued)*

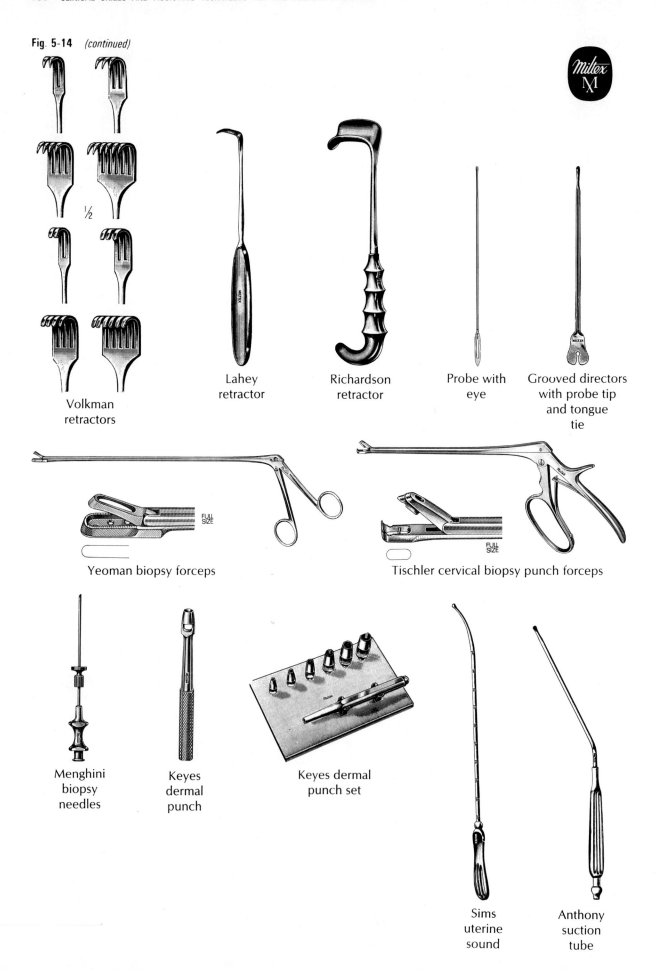

½

Volkman
retractors

Lahey
retractor

Richardson
retractor

Probe with
eye

Grooved directors
with probe tip
and tongue
tie

Yeoman biopsy forceps

Tischler cervical biopsy punch forceps

Menghini
biopsy
needles

Keyes
dermal
punch

Keyes dermal
punch set

Sims
uterine
sound

Anthony
suction
tube

plied with a disposable handle; others are reusable. The No. 3 and No. 7 handles are the most commonly used, the No. 7 handle being thinner.

Scissors. Surgical scissors are used to cut or dissect tissues and to cut sutures. Others are used to cut bandages when they are to be removed. These instruments consist of two opposing cutting blades, which may be straight or curved. The tips on the blades will vary. On some scissors both tips are sharp; on others both tips are blunt; others will have one sharp tip and one blunt tip. *Bandage scissors* have one blunt tip with the other tip having a flat blunt probe on it. These are used to remove bandages and dressings without puncturing the tissues. *Suture scissors,* used to remove sutures, have one blunt tip and a hook on the second tip. When removing sutures the hook goes under the suture. The blunt tip prevents one from puncturing the tissue. Common *dissecting scissors* are the straight or curved Mayo scissors; the short, curved Metzenbaum scissors, which is used on superficial, delicate tissue; and the long, blunt, curved Metzenbaum, which is used on deep, delicate tissue. The tips of dissecting scissors are blunt so that tissue will not be inadvertently punctured. *Operating scissors* have straight blades and may have any of the combination types of blades (sharp/sharp, blunt/blunt, or sharp/blunt). The type of scissor used in a procedure will vary depending on its intended function.

Forceps. Forceps are instruments of varied sizes and shapes used for grasping, compressing, or holding tissue or objects. They are two-pronged instruments with either a spring handle, or a ring handle with a ratchet closure. The ratchet is a toothed clasp that allows for different degrees of tightness to be applied to the tissue or object on which the instrument is used. The inner surfaces of some forceps have saw-like teeth that are called serrations (Fig.

5-15). Serrations prevent tissue from slipping out of the forceps jaw. The tips may be either plain-tipped or toothed-tipped. Plain-tipped forceps are used to pick up tissue, dressings, or other sterile objects. A toothed-tipped forcep is especially useful for grasping tissue. The teeth prevent the tissue from slipping out of the grasp of the instrument.

Examples of forceps with a *spring handle* are the thumb, tissue, splinter, and dressing forceps. Examples of forceps with a *ring handle* and ratchet closure are Allis tissue forceps, Foerster sponge forceps, Backhaus towel clamps, and straight or curved hemostatic forceps or hemostats. Hemostats include Halsted mosquito hemostatic forceps, Kelly hemostatic forceps, Rochester-Pean hemostatic forceps, and Ochsner-Kocher hemostatic forceps.

Forceps with a *toothed-tip* include standard tissue forceps, Allis tissue forceps, and Ochsner-Kocher hemostatic forceps. *Plain-tipped* forceps include standard thumb forceps, plain splinter forceps (these have sharp points), Adson dressing forceps, and the Halsted mosquito, Kelly, and Rochester-Pean hemostatic forceps.

Sponge forceps are used for holding sponges and have serrated ring-like tips. *Towel clamps,* having two sharp points, are used to hold the edges of sterile drapes or towels together. *Hemostats* are used to compress, hold, or grasp a blood vessel. They are also used by some people to apply or remove a dressing.

Needle holders. Needle holders have a ring handle, a ratchet closure, and serrated tips. Some needle holders have a groove in the middle of the serrations. (see Fig. 5-15). These instruments are designed to hold a curved needle used for suturing tissues.

Retractors. Retractors are instruments used to hold back the edges of tissues or organs to maintain exposure of the operative area. Examples include a double-ended Richardson retractor and a Volkmann rake retractor.

Probes. Probes are slender, long instruments used for exploring wounds or body cavities or passages. The end of a probe may be straight or curved. The body area being explored will determine the type of probe to be used.

Biopsy instruments. Biopsy instruments are used to obtain a small piece of tissue from the body for examination. There are various sizes and shapes of biopsy forceps. Three common ones that you may see in the office or clinic are the rectal biopsy punch, the cervical biopsy forceps, and a 6 mm biopsy punch used to obtain a small sample of skin.

Points to keep in mind for the care of instruments include the following:

1. Use the instrument *only* for the intended purpose and in the correct manner. "Handle with care."
2. Rinse or soak, then sanitize and sterilize instruments as described in Unit IV as soon as possible after use.

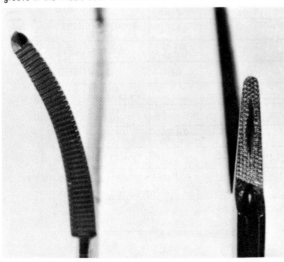

Fig. 5-15. *Left,* serrated tip on forceps. *Right,* serrated tip with groove in the middle seen on some needle holders.

3. Inspect each instrument for any defect and proper working condition.
4. Never toss instruments around or pile them on top of each other, as damage could result.
5. Keep sharp and lensed instruments separate from other instruments to prevent damage.
6. Keep ratchet handles open when not in use. This will prolong the usefulness of the instrument.

Preparing the Patient for Minor Surgery

When a patient is to have minor or major surgery, or other major forms of therapy, it is the duty of the physician to explain the nature of the procedure, the alternatives to the procedure, and the risks of the procedure. This allows the patient to give an *informed consent* for the procedure. Informed consent is a

Fig. 5-16. Sample consent form required for surgical procedures and other medical procedures.

CONSENT TO OPERATION, ADMINISTRATION OF ANESTHETICS, AND THE RENDERING OF OTHER MEDICAL SERVICES

Date _____

Time _____ ____M.

1. I authorize and direct _____ M.D. my surgeon and/or associates or assistants of his choice to perform the following operation upon me
_____ and/or to do any other therapeutic procedure that (his) (their) judgment may dictate to be advisable for my well-being.

2. The nature of the operation has been explained to me and no warranty or guarantee has been made as to the result or cure.

3. I hereby authorize and direct the above named surgeon and/or his associates or assistants to provide such additional services for me as he or they may deem reasonable and necessary, including, but not limited to, the administration and maintenance of the anesthesia, and the performance of services involving pathology and radiology, and I hereby consent thereto.

4. I hereby authorize the hospital pathologist to use his discretion in the disposal of any severed

tissue or member, except _____ .

(If patient is a minor or unable to sign, complete the following:)

Patient is a minor _____ , or is unable to sign, because _____

_____   _____
          Father   **Other Person and Relationship**

_____
          Mother

Patient's Signature _____

Witness _____

Witness _____

right . . . not merely a privilege. By law, the patient's consent is required for these types of treatment. A consent form (Fig. 5-16) must be signed by the patient before the procedure is started. This form gives the physician permission to perform the procedure. If this is not done, numerous legal complications may result. Although it is the physician's responsibility to give the patient an explanation, frequently the medical assistant will have to briefly explain the procedure once again on the day of surgery while preparing the patient and be ready to answer numerous questions that the patient may have. Remember, any surgical procedure is an invasion into body parts not normally interfered with; and although it may be a minor surgical procedure, it often does not appear minor to the patient. Many patients are somewhat anxious, nervous, or concerned about what is going to happen. The medical assistant can and must help the patient relax and allay any fears or apprehensions. Having everything ready when the patient arrives is the initial step. The room must be spotlessly clean, well lighted, and at a comfortable temperature. Supplies and equipment required for the procedure should be prepared in advance. Do not have instruments exposed for the patient's view, as these alone may make some patients more apprehensive.

On arrival of the patient in the office, greet and usher the patient into the treatment room. Have the consent form ready to sign. Provide a patient gown and give directions for the removal of clothing. Attend to the patient's needs for comfort and communi-

cation, and give emotional support and reassurance. Once again, a simple explanation of the procedure may be needed. Be willing to answer any questions that the patient may have. Always maintain a calm and confident manner as you are preparing the patient. This in itself can help to reassure and relax the patient.

The best of care can be enhanced by evaluating every patient and situation individually. In this way the most suitable environment can be provided for each individual. Also, when deemed necessary, have the patient arrange to have someone accompany her or him to the office or clinic and provide transportation home.

Assisting with Minor Surgery

Careful preparation and adherence to aseptic technique are required when preparing for office or clinic surgery. The responsibilities of the medical assistant during minor surgery include preparing the room and supplies; preparing the patient, both physically and mentally; and assisting the physician as needed. An efficient assistant can make the procedure easier for the patient and the physician by giving attention to both. Similar preparatory steps and equipment are utilized in most minor surgical procedures, although they may vary according to the physician's preferences.

Procedure	Rationale
1. Check that the room is spotlessly clean, well ventilated, and well lighted.	
2. Wash your hands.	
3. If electrical or battery-run equipment is to be used, check it for working order.	
4. Assemble and prepare supplies and equipment.	
• Open and place a sterile drape towel on a tray or Mayo stand.	This will be used as a sterile field.
• Place the required supplies and instruments on this sterile field.	Sterile supplies are to be handled with sterile transfer forceps or sterile gloved hands (refer to the section on handling sterile supplies).
When the required instruments come wrapped in the same package, or in a commercially prepared package, open the wrapper and use it for the sterile field. Then with sterile transfer forceps or gloved hands, organize the instruments for use (see Fig. 5-17, *A*).	Refer to the previous section on opening sterile packages.
5. Cover this sterile setup with a sterile towel until ready to use (Fig. 5-17, *B*).	Avoid contamination to the sterile setup.
6. Obtain any medications or solutions that will be required during the procedure.	
7. Open outer wrap of the sterile glove pack for the physician.	

Assisting with Minor Surgery (*continued*)

Procedure	Rationale
8. Prepare the patient. • Explain the procedure. Have the necessary consent forms ready for the patient to sign. • Provide a gown, and instruct what clothing must be removed. • Have the patient void if necessary. • Position the patient according to the type and location of surgery that is to be performed. • If required, wash the operative site with soap and water, and then shave the area. • Drape the patient. 9. Summon the physician.	Refer to the preceding discussion on preparing the patient for minor surgery. The patient must be made comfortable, whether sitting or in a prone or supine position, to avoid any undue tension or movement during the operation. The physician will drape the area with sterile drapes after painting the skin with an antiseptic solution.
10. When the physician has donned the sterile gloves, remove the sterile towel that is covering the tray of instruments.	Standing behind or to the side of the instrument tray, carefully grasp the two distal corners of the towel. Slowly lift the towel off by lifting it toward you. You must not touch anything but the two distal ends of the towel, otherwise you may contaminate the sterile setup.
11. Assist the physician as requested. If additional supplies are needed, you must use aseptic technique when handing them to the physician or placing them on the sterile field.	Refer to the previous section on Handling Sterile Supplies.
12. Offer physical and emotional support to the patient. It may be necessary for you to steady the patient's arm, hand, leg, head, or any body part so that moving or jerking is avoided while the physician is operating. Casually and calmly talk to the patient.	Casual and calm conversation may help to direct attention from any pain or discomfort being experienced and may help the patient relax.
13. Do not stand between the patient and the physician, or between the physician and the light source, or too near the sterile setup.	The operative area must not be obstructed. Sterile supplies must not be contaminated.
14. If you actually help the physician and handle the sterile supplies during the procedure, you must again scrub your hands thoroughly before the procedure is to begin, don sterile gloves, and, at times, also don a sterile gown.	When directly assisting the physician with the instruments, you must anticipate the physician's needs. That is, you must know when the physician will need each instrument or other supplies. You must hand an instrument over so that

Fig. 5-17. **A,** using sterile transfer forceps to organize instruments for minor surgery. **B,** cover sterile setup with a sterile towel until ready to use.

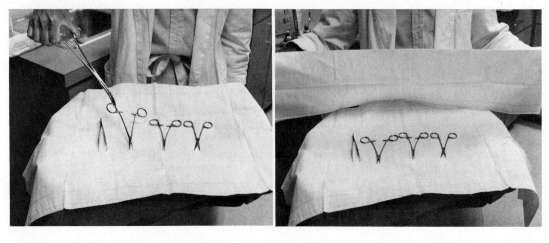

Procedure	Rationale
Then during the procedure, you will be expected to hand the instruments to the physician and to receive them after use.	when the physician grasps it, it is ready to use without need for adjustments.
15. Hold containers for collecting specimens or drainage or discharge near the work area when needed (Fig. 5-18).	
16. Place soiled instruments in a basin or container when they are no longer needed.	These should be placed out of the patient's view. Avoid contaminating the remaining sterile supplies.
17. Soiled sponges and dressings should be placed in a waxed paper or plastic bag.	Do not allow wet items to sit on a sterile field, because contamination will result.
18. When a biopsy is obtained, immediately place it into the designated jar containing a preservative solution (see Fig. 5-18).	

Fig. 5-18.   Hold container for receiving specimens or discards near the work area.

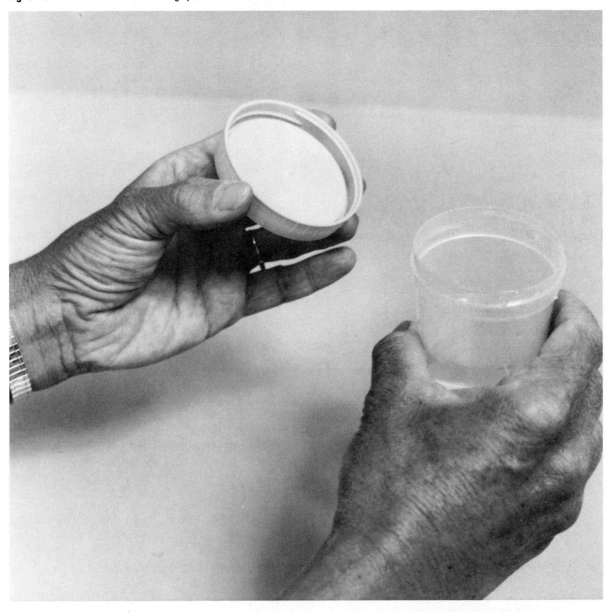

Assisting with Minor Surgery (*continued*)

Procedure	Rationale
19. After the surgery, it is often advisable to allow the patient to rest for a short while.	When sedation has been administered, *never leave the patient alone on the examining table* unless it has guard rails.
20. Help the patient prepare to leave the office. Do not allow the patient to leave the office without the physician's knowledge. Check with the physician regarding future treatments, medications, and appointments.	Frequently the physician will give the patient instructions regarding postoperative care to be performed at home by the patient.
21. Provide clear and concise postoperative instructions to the patient, when necessary.	When indicated, make sure that the patient knows and understands about • Compresses • Elevation of the affected part(s) • Presence of a drain • Changing dressing—how often, how it should be done, what to look for (drainage, healing, and so on), and how long to continue • The possibility of pain and the use of medications ordered for this
22. When the patient has left, attend to sanitization of the reusable instruments and supplies, discard disposables properly, and clean and prepare the room for the next patient. When time permits, clean all instruments for sterilization, sterilize, and return to the proper storage area.	
23. Wash your hands.	

Materials for Office Surgeries

The following are sample lists of equipment used for minor office surgeries that may vary with the individual physician's preferences and the case. Additional supplies and instruments can be added, or some deleted, to meet the requirements of the particular situation. Once you learn the physician's preferences, lists can be prepared for each procedure and used as a reference when preparing for minor surgery. In this way, the required instruments and supplies will not be omitted (Fig. 5-19). Figure 5-20 shows supplies and instruments used for procedures involving incisions *without* suture closure, and Figure 5-21 shows supplies and instruments used for procedures involving an excision of tissue and closure *with* sutures. Figure 5-22 shows a setup for major surgery.

Materials Basic to All Procedures

Sterile transfer forceps or individually wrapped sterile forceps
Sterile gloves for the physician
Sterile gloves for the assistant when directly assisting with the procedure
NOTE: When using instruments for the following setups that have been soaking in a chemical solution, rinse them in sterile water before using.

Materials for Preparing the Skin Area

Surgical detergent for washing the skin
Sterile sponges (cotton balls and gauze—2 × 2 inch and 4 × 4 inch)
Sterile forceps
Antiseptic solution such as Betadine (povidone-iodine) for disinfecting the skin
Razor and blade (if skin is to be shaved)
Draping materials

Materials to Administer Local Anesthesia

Sterile antiseptic in sterile container, such as Betadine solution
Applicators or cotton balls and a forceps to use when painting the skin. Prepackaged sterile Betadine applicators are available and may be used instead.
Sterile syringe (3 cc or 5 cc)
Sterile needles: 25 gauge, ½ inch, and 23- or 24 gauge, 1½ inch (size and gauge will vary with site to be infiltrated)
Local anesthetic: ampules or vials of lidocaine 1% or 2% or procaine hydrochloride 1% or 2%. For a topical spray anesthetic, ethyl chloride may be used

Fig. 5-19. Instruments used for medical-surgical purposes. **A,** types of scissors. *Left to right,* straight iris scissors, curved iris scissors, suture scissors, curved Metzenbaum blunt blade scissors, disposable suture scissors, bandage scissors with flat blunt tip to prevent puncturing skin when cutting away bandage. **B,** *Top (left to right),* punch biopsy forceps, #11 scalpel and handle. *Bottom (left to right),* Straight mosquito forceps, curved mosquito forceps, straight Kelly forceps, curved Kelly forceps, tissue forceps plain tip, tissue forceps toothed tip, Allis clamp, needle holder.

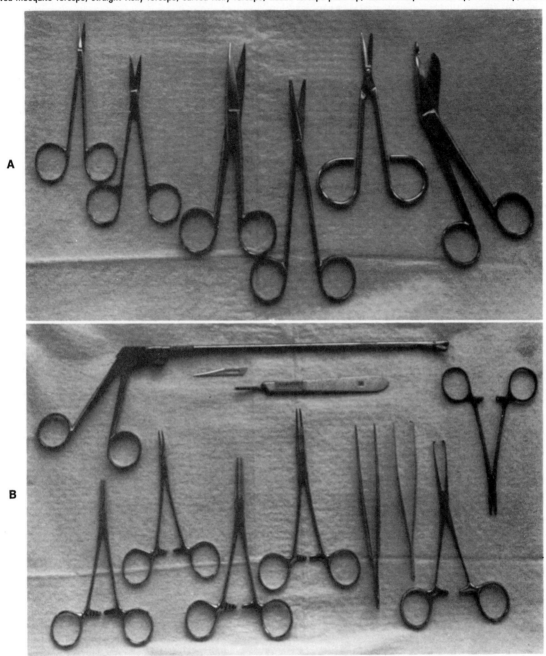

Sterile gloves (depending on physician's preference and procedure to be performed)
This setup may be prepared individually or added to the sterile setup used for the procedure.

Materials for Suturing Lacerations

Materials for preparing the skin
Local anesthetic setup
Sterile gloves

Toothed tissue forceps
Hemostat
Needle holder
Suture scissors
Suture material with suture needle
Sterile gauze 2 × 2 inch and 4 × 4 inch (for sponging and dressing wound; larger dressings are needed for lacerations larger than 3 inches)
Adhesive or, preferably, hypoallergenic tape and bandage scissors to cut it
Container for used instruments and sponges

Fig. 5-20.   Supplies and instruments used for minor surgery involving incision *without* suture closure. Materials for preparing the skin: container with sponges in surgical detergent and razor with blade. Materials for local anesthesia: vial of local anesthetic medication, 3 cc syringe with needle, alcohol sponge (other antiseptic solutions could be used rather than alcohol sponge). Other supplies and instruments: sterile gloves for the surgeon, 4 × 4 inch and 2 × 2 inch sponges, and instruments, *left to right*—No. 3 scalpel blade handle, scalpel blades (*top to bottom,* No. 11, No. 10, No. 15), curved iris scissors, straight mosquito forceps, tissue forceps (plain tip).

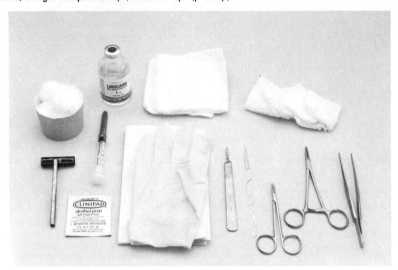

Fig. 5-21.   Supplies and instruments used for minor surgery when excising tissue and closing the skin *with* suture materials. Left side of picture and along the top includes materials for preparing the skin, administering local anesthesia, sponges, and sterile gloves for the surgeon. Additional supplies and instruments from left to right include: No. 3 scalpel blade handle, No. 10 *(top)* and No. 15 scalpel blades, toothed tissue forceps, curved iris scissors, curved and straight mosquito forceps, straight and curved Kelly forceps, suture scissors, needle holder with mounted curved atraumatic needle with suture material, and container for tissue specimen with preservative solution.

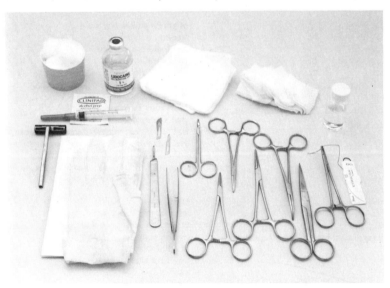

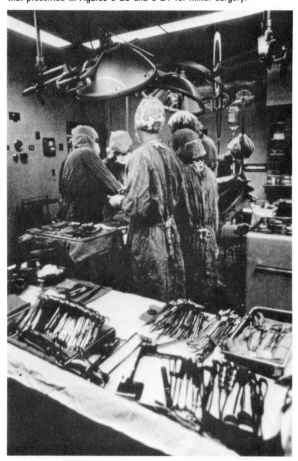

Fig. 5-22. Surgical team at work in major surgery. Note the difference in the instrument setup required for major surgery versus that presented in Figures 5-20 and 5-21 for minor surgery.

If the wound is infected or abscesses are to be incised, suture material is not needed because infected wounds are usually not sutured.

Materials for Incision and Drainage (I & D) of an Abscess or Cyst (Fig. 5-20)

Materials for preparing the skin
Local anesthetic setup
Sterile gloves
Scalpel handle and blade; usually a No. 11 blade — or a No. 15 blade for finer and smaller incisions
Iris (small) sharp scissors to dissect and cut with; sometimes larger blunt scissors will also be needed
Tissue forceps
Hemostat
Rubber drain to be inserted to provide for drainage during healing, when indicated. (Size will vary with the size of the incision and area drained. If this is sutured to the skin for support, suture material, suture needle, and needle holder are needed)
Sterile gauze for sponging and dressing the wound (2 × 2 inch and 4 × 4 inch)

Adhesive or, preferably, hypoallergenic tape and bandage scissors to cut it
Container for used instruments and gauze sponges

Materials for Removing Foreign Bodies in Subcutaneous Tissues, Small Growths, and Tissue Biopsy Specimens (Fig. 5-21)

Materials for preparing the skin
Local anesthetic setup
Sterile gloves
Mosquito forceps, straight and curved
Kelly forceps, straight and curved
Scalpel handle and blade (No. 10 or No. 15 blade) and the electrocautery unit, including a lubricated lead plate, which is placed under the patient for grounding purposes. This plate is not needed when the table is grounded. Some tables are supplied with an electrical system that is grounded to an electrical wall outlet
Iris scissors (small sharp scissors)
Toothed tissue forceps
Suture scissors
Suture material and needle
Needle holder
Sterile gauze for sponging and dressing the wound (2 × 2 inch and 4 × 4 inch)
Adhesive or, preferably, hypoallergenic tape and bandage scissors to cut it
Container for used instruments and sponges
Specimen bottle containing a preservative solution for a tissue biopsy specimen. Zenker's solution or formalin 10% are the preferred solutions used to preserve small tissues, warts, and moles
Biopsy forceps is also needed for obtaining a biopsy from certain body sites, such as the uterine cervix. In this case, dressing materials or tampons are needed to pack the area after the biopsy has been obtained, in addition to instruments used in pelvic examination (see p. 77)
Laboratory requisition

Materials for a Cervical Biopsy

• Materials for preparing the skin — skin antiseptic solution
• Sterile gloves
• Vaginal speculum
• Uterine dressing forceps
• Cervical biopsy punch
• Coagulant gel or foam
• Sponges
• Uterine tenaculum
• Vaginal packing or tampon
• Specimen bottle with preservative solution such as 10% Formalin
• Laboratory requisition

Materials for a 6 mm Skin Biopsy

• Materials for preparing the skin — skin antiseptic solution or an alcohol sponge

- Local anesthetic setup — sterile needle: 25 gauge, ⅝ inch *or* 30 gauge, ½ inch; 3 cc syringe; 1% lidocaine
- Sterile gloves
- Scalpel handle and a No. 15 blade
- 6 mm biopsy punch
- Suture set with straight sharp scissors (scissors used to remove the top two layers of skin)
- Suture material: 5-0 black silk and curved needle
- Needle holder
- Sterile gauze — 2 × 2 inch and 4 × 4 inch
- Specimen bottle with 10% formalin
- Band-Aid (used for the dressing over surgical site)
- Laboratory requisition

Materials for an Aspiration (Needle) Biopsy of the Breast

Syringe, a No. 18 needle, and a sterile culture tube to receive the specimen. Most laboratories prefer to receive the specimen in the culture tube, as each may use different procedures for fixing, staining, and examining the specimen. A Band-Aid is usually sufficient for the dressing.

Laboratory requisition when a specimen is sent for cytological or histological examination.

Materials for Removing Sutures (Fig. 5-23)

Suture removal kit that includes suture scissors, plain-tipped tissue forceps, sterile gauze 4 × 4 inch

Antiseptic solution in container (or disposable Betadine applicators)

Sterile applicators or gauze or cotton balls

Container for removed sutures, used instruments, and sponges

Materials for Electrocauterization (Fig. 5-24)

Materials for skin preparation

Local anesthetic setup (depending on extent and site of area to be cauterized; at times this may not be required)

Sterile gloves

Electrocautery unit

Extension electrode for the cautery and instruments used for a pelvic examination (see p. 77) for cauterization of the uterine cervix

Container for used instruments, sponges

Dressing materials: size and type determined by size and type of area cauterized. A Band-Aid may be applied to a small area to protect it from irritants; frequently dressings are not applied to small, superficial areas.

Fig. 5-24. Supplies and instruments for electrocauterization.

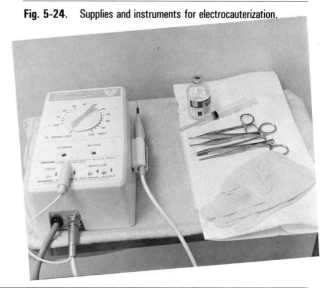

Fig. 5-23. Sterile disposable suture removal kits. (Courtesy Patient Care Division, Johnson and Johnson Products Inc., New Brunswick, NJ)

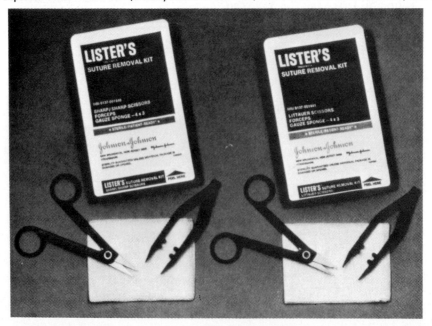

Insertion of an Intrauterine Device (IUD)

An intrauterine device is inserted into the uterus for the purpose of contraception. The Progestasert IUD is the only one now available. All others were taken off the market January 31, 1986. The physician will insert it usually on the third day of the patient's menstrual period, as at this time the cervix may be dilated some, and it is assumed that the patient is not pregnant. Before the insertion of an IUD, the patient should have had a Pap smear. On occasion, the physician may choose to insert an IUD 5 to 10 days after the patient's menstrual period. The patient is positioned and draped as for a pelvic examination (Fig. 5-25).

Equipment (Fig. 5-26)

Surgical soap and water
Alcohol or Betadine (povidone-iodine)
Sterile sponges
Vaginal speculum
Sterile gloves
Sterile single-toothed tenaculum
Sterile uterine sound
Sterile sponge stick
Sterile suture scissors
IUD and inserter

Fig. 5-25. Consent form for insertion of an IUD.

OB/GYN CLINIC
IUD CONSENT FORM

I have been informed by my physician of alternative methods of birth control and have chosen to use the IUD. I have received literature explaining the use of the IUD. I have read the literature and I understand it. I also understand the risks of insertion and use of an IUD. Some serious complications which may occur are an increased chance of infection, rarely leading to sterility, and possible uterine perforation. I understand that there is still a possibility of pregnancy with an increased risk of miscarriage or, rarely, a tubal pregnancy.

Signed_____
patient
Date_____

Date of insertion_____

Lot number of IUD_____

Name of IUD_____

Date to be changed_____

Fig. 5-26. Equipment for the insertion of an intrauterine device: IUD (not shown, to be added to tray), scissors, vaginal speculum *(on the left),* uterine sound, single tooth tenaculum.

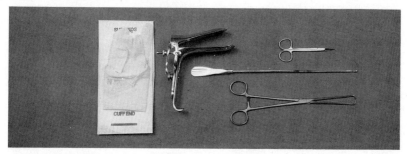

Procedure

The physician will

1. Introduce the vaginal speculum into the vagina.
2. Perform a pelvic examination.
3. Prepare the cervix with surgical soap and water, then with alcohol or Betadine.
4. Grasp the cervix with the single-toothed tenaculum.
5. Introduce the uterine sound into the uterus to check for depth.
6. Prepare and insert the IUD.
7. Withdraw the IUD inserter.
8. Cut the string attached to the IUD with suture scissors.
9. Perform a digital examination.

The medical assistant should now

10. Help the patient assume a supine position for 5 to 10 minutes to prevent the state of shock.

Procedure

11. Elevate the patient's head 45 degrees to 50 degrees for 5 minutes.
12. Have the patient sit up with legs over the side of the table and maintain this position for a few minutes to ensure that the patient's condition is stable.
13. Give the patient further instructions:
    - If bleeding, fever, or pain occurs, notify the physician.
    - Check for the presence of the IUD string in the vagina once a month after her menstrual period. (If she cannot find the string, she should make an appointment to see the physician.)
    - A yearly checkup with the physician is necessary.
    - The Progestasert IUD must be changed every year, as effectiveness decreases after that time span.
    - Once dressed, she is free to leave.
14. Ask the patient if she has any questions; answer them adequately, or refer the patient to the physician.

WOUNDS

A wound is a break in the continuity of external or internal soft body parts, caused by physical trauma to the tissues. An *open wound* is one in which the skin and mucous membranes are broken; in a *closed wound,* the skin is not broken, but there is a contusion (bruise) or a hematoma (hēm-a-to'ma), a tumor-like mass of blood.

Types of open wounds include the following (Fig. 5-27):

abrasion (ab-rā'zhun)—A scrape on the surface of the skin or on a mucous membrane; for example, a skinned knee.
avulsion (ā-vul'shun)—A piece of soft tissue torn loose or left hanging as a flap.
incision—A straight cut caused by a cutting instru-

Fig. 5-27. Types of wounds.

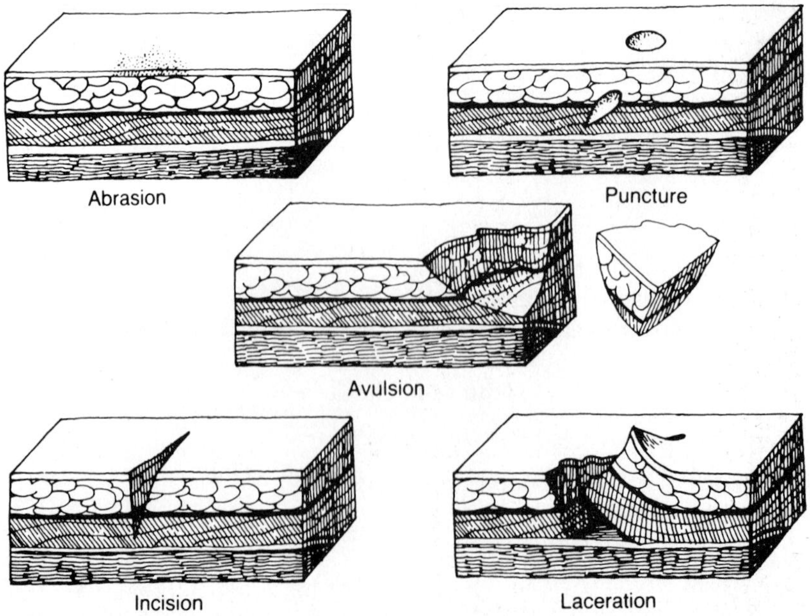

Abrasion

Puncture

Avulsion

Incision

Laceration

ment, such as a scalpel (surgical knife) for surgical purposes.

laceration (las"ĕ-rā'shun)—A tear or jagged-edged wound of body tissues.

puncture—A small external opening in the skin made by a sharp, pointed object, such as a needle or nail.

Microorganisms can invade both open and closed wounds, and an infection can result. Signs and symptoms that indicate the presence of an infection include redness, heat, pain, swelling, and at times, the presence of pus and a throbbing sensation at the wound site. Fever often accompanies infection. As the temperature rises, pulse and respiration rates also rise. An indication that an infection is spreading from a wound caused by needle pricks, splinters, or small cuts is the presence of a red streak running up the extremity from the wound site.

Wounds that are most susceptible to infection are those in which there is not a free flow of blood, wounds in which there is a crushing of the tissues, and those in which the break in the skin closes or falls back in place, thus preventing entrance of air, as seen in puncture wounds.

Common pathogenic organisms causing a wound infection include the following:

staphylococci (stăf-ĭl-ŏ-kŏk'sĭ)—Bacteria that occur in grapelike clusters; gram-positive cocci. Pathogenic species cause suppurative conditions

streptococci (strĕp"tō-kŏk'sĭ)—A type of bacteria occurring in chains; gram-positive cocci

colon bacillus (*Escherichia coli* or *E. coli*)—A type of bacteria; a normal inhabitant of the intestinal tract; gram-negative cocci. Pathogenic *E. coli* are responsible for many infections of the urinary tract and for many epidemic diarrheal diseases, especially in infants.

gas bacillus (*Clostridium perfringens*)—A type of bacteria; gram-positive cocci; anaerobic; the most common cause of gas gangrene. (Gas gangrene is a condition often resulting from dirty lacerated wounds in which the muscles and subcutaneous tissue become filled with gas and serosanguineous exudate. It is caused by the species of *Clostridium* that breaks down tissue by gas production and toxins. An exudate is material that has escaped from blood vessels and has been deposited in a body cavity, in tissues, or on the surface of tissues, usually as a result of inflammation).

tetanus bacillus (*Clostridium tetani*)—A type of bacteria; gram-positive cocci; anaerobic; spore-forming rods; the causative organism of tetanus or lockjaw. This organism enters the body through a break in the skin, especially through puncture wounds. In this case infec-

tion is often obvious. Tetanus and gas bacilli are common in puncture wounds because they are anaerobic, that is, they grow in the absence of oxygen.

One of the body's natural defense mechanisms against infection or trauma is the inflammatory process. It works to limit damage to the tissue, remove injured cells, and repair injured tissues (see also p. 113).

The Healing Process

Wounds heal by first intention or by second intention, depending on damage or loss of tissue. When the edges of wounds can be brought together, as in sutured surgical incisions, or when there is a minimal amount of tissue loss or damage, as in a relatively clean and small cut, they heal by first intention. There will be little inflammation and minimal scarring, if any.

Where the wound edges cannot be approximated because of extensive tissue loss or damage, healing by second intention occurs. This will be seen in open and infected trauma or surgical wounds, such as after the incision and drainage of abscesses, or in major lacerations. Since large amounts of granulation tissue form to fill the gap between the wound edges and to allow epithelial cells to migrate across the wound surfaces from the edges, this healing process is also known as healing by granulation or indirect healing. This is a slower process than healing by first intention; thus, it involves a greater risk of infection and usually produces greater scarring.

The healing process normally occurs in three stages.

1. Lag phase: Blood serum and cells form a fibrin network in the wound. A clot is formed that fills the wound and begins to knot the edges together with shreds of fibrin. Dried proteins then form a scab.
2. Fibroplasia: Granulation tissue (fragile, pinkish red tissue) forms as the fibrin network absorbs and epithelial cells start forming from the edges to form a scar.
3. Contraction phase: Small blood vessels are absorbed, fibroblasts (cells from which connective tissue develops) contract, and the scar begins to shrink and changes in color from red to white.

The body's ability to heal after any trauma is affected by the general health status of the individual. Good health helps the body deal successfully with injuries and infections.

Care of Wounds

The goals of wound care are to promote healing and prevent additional injury. There are two schools of thought regarding the care of a wound; that is, some prefer to leave the wound undressed, and others prefer to dress a wound.

Most closed wounds are left undressed, as well as some wounds that have sealed and can be protected from additional injury, irritation, and contamination. Exposure to the air helps keep the wound dry and can promote healing. Open wounds covered with a dressing provide a warm, dark, moist area that is suitable for the growth of microorganisms. Dressings applied incorrectly can interfere with adequate circulation to the area, which will interfere with the healing process; also, if a dressing does not stay in place, it can cause further irritation to the wound and possibly cross-contamination.

Regardless of the method used (dressed or undressed), a wound must be kept clean, have dead tissue removed, and then be allowed to drain freely.

When a dressing is changed, it and the wound must be inspected for the amount and character of drainage, if present. The amount is best described as scant, moderate, or large; the character refers to the color, odor, and consistency of the drainage.

Common terms to describe drainage

serous—Consisting of serum
sanguineous—Consisting of blood or blood in abundance
serosanguineous—Consisting of blood and serum
purulent—Consisting of or containing pus

The condition of the wound, the degree of healing, and the integrity of sutures and drains must also be observed during a dressing change.

DRESSINGS AND BANDAGES

Techniques of applying dressings and bandages vary according to the extent and location of wounds, injuries, or burns, the materials to be used, and the purpose for which they are applied.

Dressings

Dressings are materials of various types placed directly over wounds, open lesions, and burns as the immediate protective covering. When used correctly, dressings serve eight basic purposes.

1. To protect wounds from additional trauma
2. To help prevent contamination of the wound
3. To absorb drainage
4. To provide pressure for controlling hemorrhage, promoting drainage, and reducing edema
5. To immobilize and support the wound site
6. To ease pain
7. To provide a means for applying and keeping medications on the wound.
8. To provide psychological benefits for the patient by concealing, protecting, and giving support to the wound.

To prevent contamination and the possibility of an infection developing, sterile technique and sterile dressing materials must be used when applying or changing a dressing. The only exception is in emergency situations when the patient has serious bleeding. On those occasions it is more important to stop the bleeding than to worry about contaminating the wound with unsterile materials.

Dressing materials.   Various types and sizes of commercial sterile dressings are available (Fig. 5-28). Many are made of gauze, such as folded gauze sponges* available in sizes of 2 × 2 inch, 4 × 4 inch, 3 × 4 inch, and so on; and gauze fluffs, which are loosely folded large gauze squares used to absorb large amounts of drainage or to pack an opening. Some dressings are made from viscose rayon and cellulose materials, such as folded Topper* sponges supplied in 3 × 3 inch, 4 × 3 inch, and 4 × 4 inch sizes; still others are made from a unique, nonwoven binderless soft fabric called Sof-wik,* for example, Sof-wik dressing sponges, available in 4 × 4 inch and 2 × 2 inch sizes. Larger absorbent gauze and dressings made from similar materials are available for dressing large wounds, major burns or major surgical wounds, for example, Surgipad Combine Dressing* supplied in 5 × 9 inch, 8 × 7½ inch, and 8 × 10 inch sizes; and ABDs.

Other dressing materials have a special covering over the gauze to prevent them from sticking to an open or draining skin area. These are called nonadhering dressings. Examples of these include the Band-Aid Surgical Dressing,* which is a complete dressing in a single package, consisting of a nonadherent facing, enclosing an absorbent filler, and backed by Dermicel* tape, available with 4 × 6 inch tape and 4 × 3 inch pad; or 8 × 6 inch tape and 8 × 3 inch pad. Telfa** is a gauze dressing having a plastic-like covering on the side that is to be placed over the wound that is also available in various sizes. Steripak is another complete dressing, made of layers of absorbent cellulose and covered with a nonadhering perforated plastic material that is secured to a vented adhesive tape. Steripak is available in 4 × 8 inch, 4 × 4 inch, and 2 × 4½ inch sizes. The Adaptic* nonadhering single-layer dressing, made of a highly porous weave, is used as the immediate covering over a wound under an absorbent secondary dressing; it is available in a foil envelope in 3 × 3 inch, 3 × 8 inch, 3 × 16 inch sizes, and in a bottle in dimensions of ½ inch × 4 yards for a packing strip. Vaseline*** petrola-

---

*Johnson & Johnson, New Brunswick, NJ.

**Kendall Co., Greenwich, CT.

***Chesebrough Pond's Inc., Greenwich, CT.

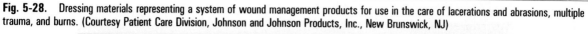

Fig. 5-28. Dressing materials representing a system of wound management products for use in the care of lacerations and abrasions, multiple trauma, and burns. (Courtesy Patient Care Division, Johnson and Johnson Products, Inc., New Brunswick, NJ)

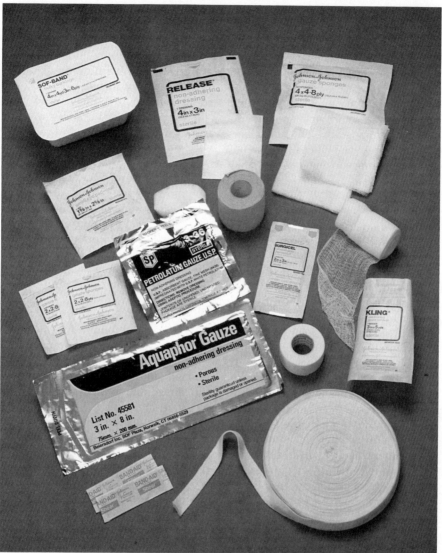

tum gauze, a fine mesh absorbent gauze impregnated with white petrolatum, is a nonadhering dressing that clings and conforms to the wound. This is used over open or draining wounds to prevent the top dressing from sticking to the wound or disrupting newly formed tissue.

A third type of dressing materials is kept moist in a package; some are premedicated. These are used for debriding tissue, for treating open or ulcerated wounds, and sometimes for dermatological conditions.

There are also spray-on dressing materials that, when sprayed over the wound, form a transparent protective film. These are nontoxic and somewhat bacteriostatic and allow for close observation of an incision or wound site. Fluff cotton or cotton balls are never to be used for dressings, because the fibers may get embedded in the wound and are difficult to remove if they do.

To hold dressings in place securely, various types and sizes of tape are available. The types of tape include hypoallergenic cloth tape, hypoallergenic paper tape, transparent tape, elastic cloth tape, and adhesive tape; sizes range from ½ inch to 3 inches.

When changing or applying an initial dressing, select the dressing materials according to the purposes to be accomplished; in other words, know why the wound is to be dressed. This will enable you to select the proper types and amounts of dressing materials. Any dressing must be large enough to cover the wound completely and extend at least an inch or more beyond.

In addition to patients who have had minor surgery in the office, patients who have had surgery in the hospital may come to the physician's office for a dressing change or wound culture when necessary. The medical assistant may assist the physician with these procedures or perform them alone.

Dressing Change with a Wound Culture

When infection is suspected, a wound culture is taken to determine the presence and type of microscopic organism that is causing the infection. Cultures can be obtained from wounds on any part of the body. Soiled dressings are removed and replaced by a clean sterile dressing.

Equipment (Fig. 5-29)

To obtain the culture
Sterile applicator(s) in a sterile culture tube(s) or a Culturette.* The type of culture tube will vary depending on the specific organism that is suspected. Check with your laboratory to ensure accuracy. Most laboratories request that an anaerobic Culturette* be used for wound cultures. Always check the expiration date on the outside wrapper before using to assure stability of the culture medium at the time of use. See Unit VI for additional information on cultures and materials used.

To change the dressing
Sterile dressing tray or a prepackaged sterile dressing set containing:

- Tissue forceps
- Hemostat
- Scissors
- Gauze sponges 2 × 2 inch, or cotton balls, or antiseptic swabs
- Dry dressings, for example, 4 × 4 inch gauze, Topper sponges, Sof-wik sponges
- Small container for antiseptic solution
- Antiseptic solution

Additional equipment

- Antiseptic solution, if not supplied in the prepackaged dressing set, such as Betadine (povidone-iodine), hydrogen peroxide, alcohol 70%, 1:750 aqueous benzalkonium chloride
- Tape, preferably hypoallergenic
- Waxed paper or plastic bag for soiled dressing and disposable equipment
- Sterile disposable gloves
- Draping materials, as needed
- Laboratory requisition

Optional equipment

- Acetone or benzine or commercial tape remover to moisten tape on old dressing for easier removal
- Sterile saline to moisten a dressing that has stuck to a wound, to allow for easier removal
- Sterile towels
- Additional dressing supplies appropriate to the condition of the wound site, for example, Telfa, adhesive bandages, Steripak, Surgipads, Adaptic dressing, roller gauze bandage, Kling elastic gauze bandage

Fig. 5-29. Supplies and instruments for dressing change with wound culture.

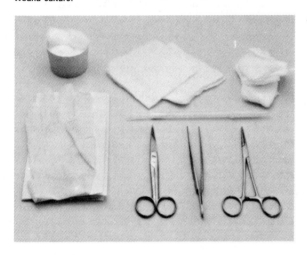

Procedure For Dressing Change With A Wound Culture

Procedure	Rationale
1. Wash your hands.	
2. Assemble your equipment.	Place the supplies on a flat, clean surface, convenient for use.
3. Identify the patient, and explain the procedure.	Provide reassurance, and gain the patient's cooperation. Explain that you will remove the soiled dressing, obtain a culture of the discharge from the wound, and apply a clean sterile dressing. The culture will then be sent to the laboratory for study. When the physician receives the laboratory report, the appropriate medication to

*Marion Scientific Corp.

Procedure	Rationale

eliminate the causative organism(s) of the infection may then be prescribed.

4. Have the patient put on a patient gown if necessary. Position the patient, providing for comfort and relaxation. Drape if and as needed, exposing the area where the wound is located. When the wound is on the arm or leg, place a towel under the area to be dressed. Remind the patient not to touch the open wound once the dressing has been removed, and not to talk over it, because microorganisms can spread into the wound.

Gowning, positioning, and draping will vary with the location of the wound. The important thing to remember is that the part of the body from which the culture is to be obtained and the dressing changed must be well supported and exposed. In addition, the patient's modesty must be protected.

5. a. Open the dressing set. Using sterile transfer forceps, arrange supplies in their order of use.

Use aseptic technique at all times. The wrapper on the dressing set is used for the sterile field.

   b. Open waxed paper or plastic bag.

Place the bag in a convenient place to receive the soiled dressing and used disposable supplies.

   c. Pour the antiseptic solution into the sterile container located on the sterile field.

NOTE: When the antiseptic solution is supplied in the dressing tray set, do not pour the solution until after you have donned sterile gloves.

   d. Cut pieces of tape that will be used to secure the clean sterile dressing when applied.

These may be tagged onto the side of your dressing tray.

6. Loosen tape on the present dressing (Fig. 5-30).

Loosen and pull tape gently, going toward the wound so you don't tear newly formed tissue. When the tape doesn't pull away easily, moisten it with a sponge soaked with acetone, benzine, baby oil, or a commercial tape remover.

7. Loosen and remove the soiled dressing with a sterile forcep (Fig. 5-31) or a gloved hand. Do not pull on the dressing. A dressing can also be removed by placing your hand inside a plastic bag. Then grasp and lift the dressing off, inspect for drainage, and invert bag over the dressing.

Handle all dressings as if they are contaminated. The forceps or glove is to be used for this step only, then set aside or, if disposable, discarded in the bag with the soiled dressing. If a dressing is difficult to remove, sterile saline may be applied to help loosen it.

8. Inspect the dressing, and then discard it in the waxed paper or plastic bag.

Observe the amount and type of drainage on the dressing.

Fig. 5-30. Technique for loosening tape on dressing.

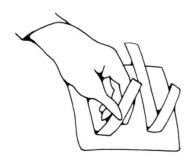

Fig. 5-31. Removing soiled dressing with forceps.

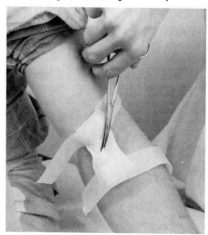

Procedure For Dressing Change with a Wound Culture (*continued*)

Procedure	Rationale
9. Observe the wound.	Note the location, type, and amount of drainage coming from the wound, and the presence of pus, necrosis, and/or a putrid odor. Note the degree of healing, and when sutures are present, if they are intact.
10. Remove the sterile applicator from the sterile culture tube or Culturette. Swab the drainage area of the wound once to obtain a specimen. If you need more of the drainage for culturing, you must use another applicator.	Swab only the draining area of the wound. Do not spread the infection to a clean area on the wound. Swab the wound only once in one direction. Never go back and forth over the area.
11. Place the applicator(s) in the culture tube(s), and set aside.	Secure the lid tightly to prevent air from getting into the tube. Air would cause the specimen to dry, thus destroying the microorganisms.
12. Don sterile gloves as described previously.	Gloves are donned to prevent any microorganisms that may be on your hands from entering the wound and also to keep your hands clean.
13. Pick up gauze sponge with forceps or hemostat (whichever is most comfortable for you to use).	
14. Dip the sponge into the antiseptic cleansing solution to wet through.	Do not oversaturate the sponge. Keep sponge and forceps facing downward.
15. Gently, but thoroughly, cleanse the wound using single strokes over and parallel to the incision, *one sponge per stroke*. Starting at the center of the wound, stroke toward the ends. Cleanse the side farthest from you, working outward from the incision, and then repeat on the side closest to you (Fig. 5-32).	Do not go back and forth over a cleansed area. Do not touch forceps to skin. Bacterial count is usually lowest at the center of the incision and greatest at the edges. Always work from the least contaminated areas to most contaminated areas to avoid contaminating uncontaminated sites.
16. Discard each sponge in the bag for waste after use.	Do not touch the bag with the forceps.
17. Repeat the process directly over the wound until it is cleansed to your satisfaction.	Use a clean sponge for each single stroke.
18. When cleansing a drain site or a very small wound, move the antiseptic sponge in a circle around the site (Fig. 5-33).	Cleanse around and away from the wound in an ever-widening circle. Do not go back over a clean area.
19. Discard the sponge, and repeat.	
20. Apply the sterile dressing. Center it over the wound area.	Forceps or gloved hands are used to apply the dressing. Additional layers of dressings are added as indicated by the type of wound and amount of drainage (when present).

Fig. 5-32. Cleansing wound starting at center going toward end. Use one sponge per stroke.

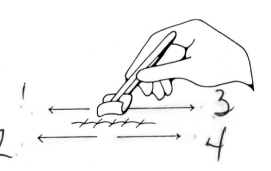

Fig. 5-33. Cleanse small wound or drain site using circular strokes, working from center to outside portion of wound site.

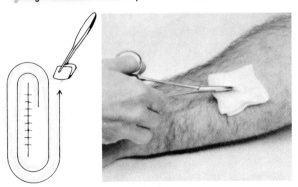

Procedure	**Rationale**
21. Discard disposable forceps and gloves in waste bag. Put reusable forceps and gloves to the side of the sterile field or in a container for used supplies.	Remove gloves by pulling on the cuff and turning inside out.
22. Secure the dressing with tape applied so that it conforms to body contours and movement. Ensure that it is adequately spaced; do not cover all the dressing with tape (Fig. 5-34). Place each strip of tape over the middle of the dressing and press down gently on both sides, working toward the ends.	Hypoallergenic tape is preferred. Have equal lengths of tape on both sides of the dressing— not too short or too long. Tape is not to cover the whole dressing, as it would interfere with air circulation. Distribute tension away from the incision. Do not tape too snugly, as this may constrict blood flow to the wound and interfere with the healing process.
23. Attend to the patient's comfort; you may reposition patient if necessary. Observe patient for any undue reaction. Provide further instructions as indicated or as ordered by physician.	Check if the patient has any questions. Inform the patient if he or she is free to leave. Help the patient dress when necessary.
24. Label culture tube(s) or Culturette(s) completely and accurately. Complete and attach the appropriate laboratory requisition.	The label should include • Patient's name • Physician's name • Date • Source of specimen • Test requested
25. Take or send the culture to the laboratory.	Avoid delay, to prevent drying of the specimen.
26. Remove used items from the treatment room; dispose of correctly.	Discard soiled items and disposable equipment in a covered container. Rinse reusable instruments under running water and then soak in detergent and water until you are ready to prepare them for sterilization.
27. Wash your hands.	
28. Replace supplies as needed. Leave the treatment room clean and neat.	

29. Record the procedure and observations on the patient's chart, using correct medical abbreviations.	Charting example:
	March 4, 19_____, 1 PM
	    Rt. forearm dressing changed.
	    Moderate amount of thick, yellow, purulent drainage on lower end of laceration.
	    Culture taken and sent to lab for C & S [culture and sensitivity].
	    Wound cleansed and dry dressing applied.
	    Ann Michaelson, CMA

Fig. 5-34. Correct method of securing a dressing to conform to body contour and movement.

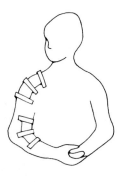
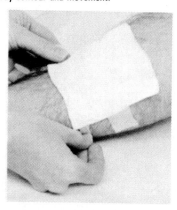

Bandages

Bandages are strips of soft, pliable materials used to wrap or cover a body part. When used correctly, bandages serve four basic purposes:

1. To hold dressings or splints in place
2. To immobilize or support body parts
3. To protect an injured body part
4. To apply pressure over an area

Bandaging materials should be clean, but not necessarily sterile, because they should never come into direct contact with an open wound, as do dressings.

Bandaging materials. There are several types of bandages prepared commercially.

Adhesive and elastic tape. Adhesive and elastic tape are supplied in rolls of various widths. When tape is used for a bandage, it is applied directly to the skin. Caution must be taken when wrapping a body part with tape so that circulation is not cut off by tape that has been wrapped too tightly. Elastoplast is an example of an elastic adhesive bandage.

Roller bandages. Roller bandages are available in various widths and materials. *Gauze*, a porous, lightweight, nonstretch material, has little absorbency, does not self-adhere, and does not conform readily to body contours. However, it is relatively inexpensive.

A preferred type of gauze bandage is the *elastic gauze bandage,* such as Kling. Kling conforms to all body contours, stretches, adheres to itself, and is absorbent; it will not slip with movement and therefore eliminates frequent rebandaging. It is nonocclusive, allowing for wound aeration; thus it will not interfere with wound healing.

Elastic bandages. Elastic bandages, made of woven cotton with elastic fibers, are particularly useful for bandaging areas that require firm support, immobilization, or the application of pressure. Frequently used are the Ace bandage or the Peg bandage, which is self-adhering. Once wrapped around a body part, nonadhering elastic bandages are secured with bandage clips. (See Fig. 5-37, which illustrates the application of a Peg bandage.)

Triangular bandages. Triangular bandages are large pieces of cloth, usually cotton, in the shape of a triangle. These bandages are usually used for slings on an injured arm, but can be adapted for use on almost any part of the body (Fig. 5-35). A cravat bandage can be made by folding the point of a triangular bandage to the midpoint of the base and continuing to fold it lengthwise until the desired width is obtained (Fig. 5-36). A cravat bandage can be used to hold a dressing in place, to help support an injured joint, to hold a splint in place, and if necessary, as a tourniquet.

Tubegauz. Tubegauz, a seamless, tubular-knitted, cotton bandage, is adaptable and conformable to all body areas. Because Tubegauz is tubular, it stays in place with little or no adhesive tape. A finger or cage-type appliance is used in the application of Tubegauz to provide a neat and strong bandage. Figure 5-39 has instructions for applying Tubegauz bandages.

Application of bandages. Important criteria for acceptable bandaging techniques are that the bandage perform its function and that it not cause additional problems or pain. The following measures promote safety and comfort when applying bandages.

• Observe the principles and practices of medical asepsis when applying a bandage.

Fig. 5-35. **A,** triangular bandage. **B,** triangular bandage used for arm sling.

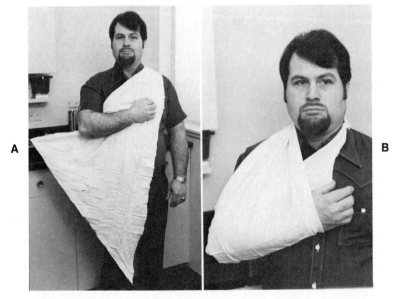

Fig. 5-36. Cravat bandage.

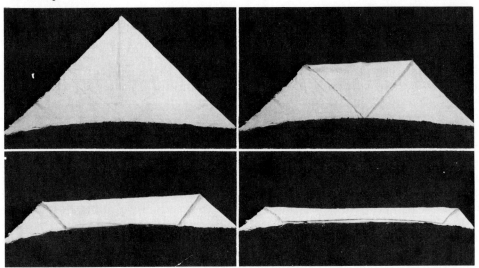

• Select a bandage of appropriate size for the area to be bandaged.

• Apply bandages to areas that are clean and dry. When an open wound is present, apply a bandage over a dressing.

• Do not have two skin surfaces touching each other under a bandage. Use absorbent material between touching skin surfaces under a bandage. For example, when bandaging two fingers together, place a padding between them to prevent the skin from rubbing together. Other areas that need similar techniques include the axillary areas (an individual's perspiration provides a moist environment that is conducive to the growth of microorganisms), the areas under the breasts, areas in the groin or folds of the abdomen, and areas between the toes.

• Pad bony prominences and joints over which a bandage must be placed to prevent skin irritation, to provide comfort, and to maintain equal pressure on body parts.

• Apply bandages on a body part while in its normal functioning position, and when placed in a resting position (1) so that deformities will not result and (2) to avoid muscle strain. Joints should be slightly flexed rather than extended or hyperextended.

• Apply bandages with sufficient pressure to attain the intended function, that is, pressure, support, or immobilization. However, do not apply the bandage too tightly, as this will interfere with circulation to the area. Ask the patient if the bandage feels comfortable.

• Wrap the bandage from the end of a limb toward the center of the body to avoid congestion and circulatory interferences in the distal part of the extremity.

• When possible, leave a small portion of an extremity, such as a finger or toe, exposed so that any change in circulation can be observed. Signs that indicate that the bandage is too tight include coldness and numbness to the part, pain, swelling, cyanosis, and pallor. If any of these signs occur, the bandage must be loosened immediately.

• Apply bandages so that they are secure and do not move about over the area causing irritation or the need for rebandaging frequently.

• Apply chest bandages so that they do not interfere with breathing.

• Avoid unnecessary layers of bandages; it will not be comfortable for the patient. Use only the amount of bandage material needed to accomplish its purpose.

• Place securing materials, such as clips, pins, or knots, well away from the wound or inflamed area to avoid undue pressure and irritation to the area.

• Check (or inform the patient to check) the bandage at regular intervals to note the circulation to the part and to see if the bandage needs to be reapplied, as when it has slipped out of place or loosened to the point where it would no longer be accomplishing its purpose. Also with injuries or burns involving swelling, it is very important to check bandages frequently to ensure that they are not becoming too tight.

• Replace clean bandages as required. Many bandages can be washed or autoclaved and then reused. Gauze should be discarded and replaced with clean gauze.

Basic wrapping techniques.   There are five basic turns used alone or in combination when applying a *roller bandage*. The type of turn used depends on the purpose and the area being bandaged.

When beginning a wrap with a roller bandage, you may anchor it by placing the outer portion on a bias next to the patient's skin; the bandage is circled around the body part, allowing the corner edge to protrude; the protruding edge is then folded down over the first turn and covered with the second encircling turn of the bandage.

The *circular turn* encircles the part with each layer of bandage overlapping the previous one. This turn is used most frequently for anchoring a bandage at the start and at the end, and on body parts that are even in size, such as the hand, fingers, toes and circumference of the head.

The *spiral turn* is applied by angling the turns of the bandage in a spiral fashion with each turn overlapping the previous one by one-third to one-half the width of the bandage. This turn is used on body parts that increase in size where circular turns are difficult to make, and on cylindrical parts, such as the forearm, fingers, legs, chest, and abdomen.

The *figure-eight turn* consists of diagonal turns that ascend and descend alternately around a part, making a figure eight. This turn is used over joint areas such as the wrist, ankle, elbow, or knee to support the joint, support a dressing, or to apply a pressure bandage.

Figure 5-37 illustrates the circular, spiral, and figure-eight turns, along with wrapping techniques for the Peg self-adhering, elastic bandage.

The *spiral-reverse turn* is a spiral turn in which reverses are made halfway through each turn; the bandage is directed downward and folded on itself, wrapped around the part so that when it circles around, it is parallel to the lower edge of the previous turn. Each turn overlaps the previous one by two-thirds the width of the bandage. Spiral-reverse turns allow for a neater fit because they take up the slack on the lower ends of the bandage applied to cone-shaped parts or parts that vary in width, such as the leg, thigh, or forearm.

The *recurrent turn* is a series of back-and-forth

Fig. 5-37. Bandage-wrapping techniques illustrating the circular, spiral, and figure-eight turns. The Peg self-adhering elastic bandage is used in these illustrations. (Courtesy Becton-Dickinson, Division Becton, Dickinson and Co., Rutherford, NJ)

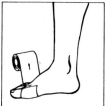 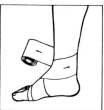 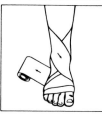 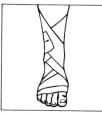

Foot and ankle Use 3-inch width. Hold foot at right angle to leg. Start bandage on ridge of foot just back of the toes.

Pass bandage around foot from inside to outside. After two or three complete turns around foot, ascending toward the ankle on each turn, make a figure eight turn by bringing bandage up over

the arch—to the inside of the ankle—around the ankle—down over the arch—and under the foot.

Repeat the figure eight wrapping two or three times. Fasten end by pressing the last 4 to 6 inches of <u>unstretched</u> bandage to the preceding layer.

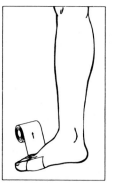 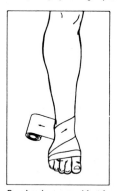 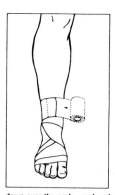 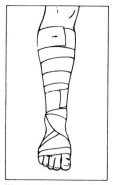

Lower leg Use 3- or 4-inch width depending on the size of the leg. A leg wrap requires two rolls of bandage. Hold foot at right angle to leg. Start bandage on ridge of foot just back of the toes.

Pass bandage around foot from inside to outside. After two complete turns around foot, make a figure eight turn by bringing bandage up over the arch—to the inside of the ankle—around the ankle—

down over the arch—and under the foot. Start circular bandaging, making the first turn around the ankle. To begin the second roll of bandage, simply overlap the <u>unstretched</u> ends by 4 to 6 inches, press firmly, and continue wrapping.

Wrap bandage in spiral turns to just below the kneecap. Fasten end by pressing the last 4 to 6 inches of <u>unstretched</u> bandage to the preceding layer.

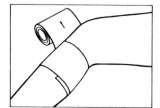 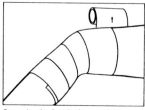 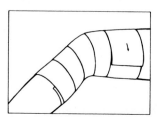

Knee Use 4-inch width. Bend knee slightly. Start with one complete circular turn around the leg just below the knee.

Start circular bandaging, applying only comfortable tension. Cover kneecap completely.

Continue wrapping to thigh just above the knee. Fasten end by pressing the last 4 to 6 inches of <u>unstretched</u> bandage to the preceding layer.

Fig. 5-37 *(continued)*

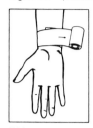 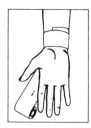 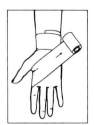 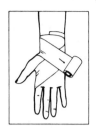 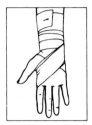

Wrist Use 2- or 3-inch width. Anchor bandage loosely at the wrist with one complete circular turn.

Carry the bandage across the back of the hand, through the web space between the thumb and index finger,

and across palm to the wrist. Make a circular turn around the

wrist and once more carry the bandage through the web space and back to the wrist.

Start circular bandaging, ascending the wrist. Fasten end by pressing the last 4 to 6 inches of underlined bandage to the preceding layer.

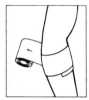 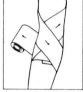 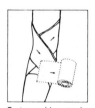 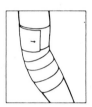

Elbow Use 3- or 4-inch width, depending on the size of the arm. Two rolls of bandage are required to complete the wrap. Start with a complete circular turn just below the elbow.

Wrap bandage in loose figure eights—

to form a protective bridge across the front of the elbow joint.

Fasten end by pressing 4 to 6 inches of underlined bandage to preceding layer. Start second bandage with a circular turn below the elbow—

over the first wrap. Continue spiral bandaging over the elbow, ascending to the lower portion of the upper arm. Fasten end with a circular turn.

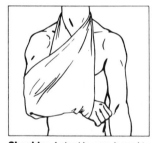 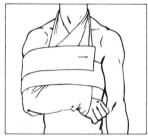 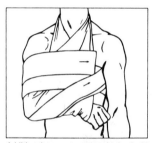

Shoulder A shoulder wrap is used to provide additional support for an arm in a sling. Use 4- or 6-inch width. One or two rolls of bandage may be used. Start under the free arm.

Carry the bandage across the back, over the arm in the sling, across the chest and back under the free arm in complete circular, overlapping turns. Fasten the end by pressing 4 to 6 inches of underlined bandage to underlying bandage.

Additional support can be obtained with a second bandage. Start at the back just behind the flexed elbow in the sling. Carry the bandage under the elbow, up over the forearm, around the chest and back, and repeat. Fasten end.

Fig. 5-38. Bandage wrapping technique: recurrent turn used for head bandage.

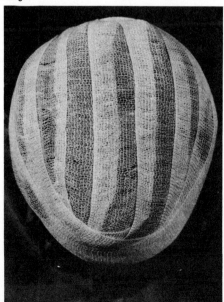

turns anchored by circular or spiral turns. After the bandage has been anchored, it is folded at right angles and passed across and back over the center of the part. Each subsequent fold is slightly angled and overlaps the previous fold by two-thirds the width of the bandage, first on one side and then on the other side of the center fold. To finish the bandage, a circular turn is made around the part and secured with tape, clips, pins, or a knot. The recurrent turn is used to bandage the head, fingers, toes, or the stump of an amputated limb (Fig. 5-38).

Application of Tubegauz bandages. When a *Tubegauz bandage* is applied, there is one basic method used for application to any body part being bandaged. Figure 5-39 illustrates areas where the Tubegauz may be applied, basic instructions for all Tubegauz applications, and a simple arm or leg bandage.

Fig. 5-39. Tubegauz bandage applications. (Courtesy Scholl, Inc., Hospital Products Division, Chicago, IL)

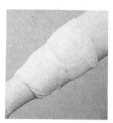

ARM or LEG

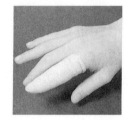

FINGER

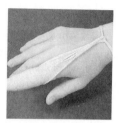

FINGER STALL

DOUBLE SEAL®
TUBEGAUZ®

Tubegauz is a seamless, tubular-knitted cotton bandage designed as an improved method of bandaging.

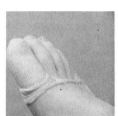

TOE

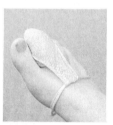

TOE SPLINT

TUBEGAUZ IS:

- QUICK AND EASY TO APPLY
- EFFICIENT AND NEATLY CONFORMABLE
- PRODUCED FROM QUALITY COTTON YARNS
- ADAPTABLE TO ALL BODY AREAS
- ECONOMICAL TO USE
- STRONG YET SOFT IN TEXTURE

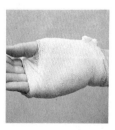

PALM of HAND

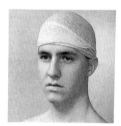

HEAD

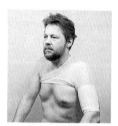

SHOULDER

Fig. 5-39 *(continued)*

BASIC INSTRUCTIONS FOR ALL TUBEGAUZ APPLICATIONS

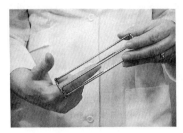

1   To apply any Tubegauz, first select a cage-type applicator that fits comfortably over the area to be bandaged.

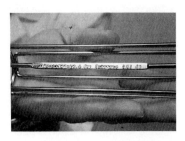

2   Next, select the size Tubegauz as printed on the cage-type applicator. For example, use Tubegauz size 01 for applicator No. 1.

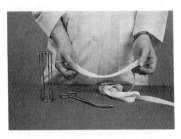

3   To load the Tubegauz onto the applicator, place the "channeled end" of the applicator on a flat surface and pull several feet of Tubegauz from the dispenser box.

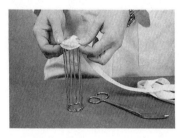

4   While spreading open the end of the tubular knit, slip the Tubegauz over the "smooth end" of the applicator.

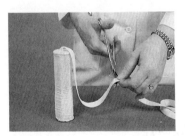

5   Complete loading by gathering sufficient Tubegauz to complete the bandage, onto the applicator and cut off near the dispenser box opening.

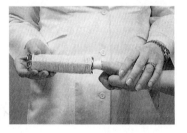

6   With the applicator loaded, pass the channeled end of the applicator over the limb to the middle of the dressing.

Fig. 5-39 *(continued)*

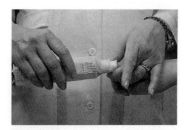

7 Pull the Tubegauz over the channeled end of the applicator, holding it lightly in place around the dressing.

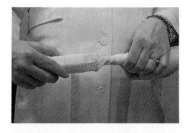

8 Continue to secure the dressing and Tubegauz end with one hand while slightly rotating clockwise to anchor as you withdraw the applicator over the limb.

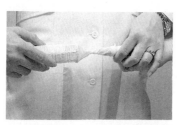

9 Withdraw the applicator several inches below the dressing or to the extremity, then rotate one full clockwise turn to anchor or close.

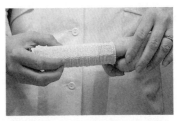

10 Move the applicator forward past the starting point and anchor with slight rotation several inches above the dressing.

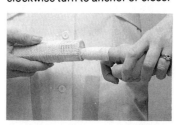

11 Continue this "back and forth" action until the desired layers of Tubegauz have been applied. Complete the last layer by stopping at the end of the bandage nearest the mesial plane.

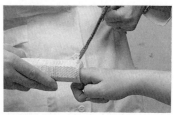

12 To finish, snip a small hole in the channeled rim, and continue cutting the Tubegauz from the applicator using the channeled rim as a cutting guide. If necessary, adhesive tape may be used to secure either end.

REMEMBER.....
Tubegauz is often applied over a sterile dressing which covers broken skin. Tubegauz is not sterile, but can be autoclaved on or off a metal applicator if desired.

Always load sufficient Tubegauz onto the applicator. It is difficult to complete a neat bandage when you have run out of Tubegauz in the middle of a procedure.

Fig. 5-39 *(continued)*

SIMPLE ARM OR LEG BANDAGE

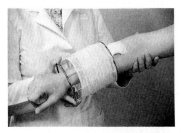

1 With applicator loaded as directed, bring the Tubegauz over the channeled end over sterile dressing.

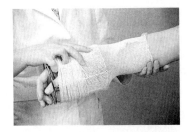

2 Hold the Tubegauz on the dressing with one hand and withdraw the applicator with the other hand letting the Tubegauz roll off the applicator to cover the desired area (usually just below the sterile dressing).

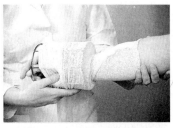

3 Rotate clockwise about ½ to ¾ turn to anchor slightly and proceed in opposite direction to above dressing.

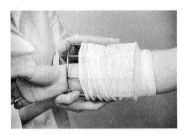

4 Rotate again in the same direction and return to base of bandage.

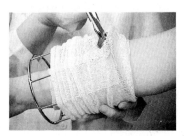

5 Cut Tubegauz off in channeled rim.

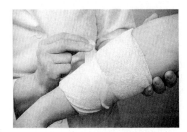

6 Secure with adhesive or slit and tie.

Adhesive tape may be applied at center of bandage by allowing a little more Tubegauz so that, after anchoring at base, the raw edge finishes in the center.

CONCLUSION

Strict aseptic technique is needed at all times when handling sterile supplies and assisting with sterile or surgical procedures. Never be reluctant to admit a possible break in technique.

Be honest, and admit contamination of sterile equipment, even if you are the only one who realizes that the equipment is not sterile. It is no disgrace to contaminate sterile equipment. The only disgrace is to use it after you know it is contaminated, because you would then subject the patient to the great danger of infection.

Learn the principles and practice the sterile techniques to be used when handling sterile supplies and equipment and when assisting with sterile procedures. Practice handing instruments so that the physician can grasp them in the way most convenient to use during a procedure. Be prepared to select and arrange the supplies and equipment required for the minor surgeries listed in this unit.

When ready to accurately demonstrate your skills, arrange with your instructor to take the performance test.

REVIEW OF VOCABULARY

The following is a sample of a minor surgery report using terms that have been defined for you. Read this, and be able to define or explain the terms that are italicized.

Operative Report

DIAGNOSIS: Lipomas in right buttock and posterior thigh (Rt); large mole, right posterior thigh.
POSTOPERATIVE DIAGNOSIS: Same.
OPERATION: Excision of lipomas; *cauterization* of mole.
ANESTHESIA: *Local infiltration — Lidocaine 1%.*
SURGEON: A. Joseph, MD
PROCEDURE
   Sterile field and setup prepared. *Sterile gloves donned.* With the patient in a prone position, the usual *skin preparation* was performed, and then *sterile drapes* were applied. The *local anesthetic* was administered. The tumors were excised without any difficulty, and two *biopsy* specimens were sent to the laboratory for cytology studies. The tissues were approximated with *000 black silk.*
   The *cautery* unit was then used to remove a questionable mole on the right posterior thigh.
   Dry dressings were applied to the surgical sites.
POSTOPERATIVE STATUS
   The patient left the office with minor complaints of discomfort in the surgical areas.
   Patient to return in 1 week for removal of *sutures* and for follow-up care.

Andrew Joseph, MD

Pathology Reports

The following minor surgery pathology reports were received in a physician's office. After reading these, you should be able to discuss the contents of these reports with your instructor. Reference sources may be used to obtain definitions of terms that you are not familiar with.

PATIENT NO. 1

CLINICAL DATA: 63-year-old black male, with sebaceous cyst of the left axilla and skin tag of the right arm.
CLINICAL DIAGNOSIS: Epidermoid inclusion cyst, left axilla, and right arm skin tag.
MATERIAL FROM: Excision of the above.
GROSS DESCRIPTION: The specimen is received in formalin in two parts:
   Part 1, labeled "left axilla," consists of a soft, round lesion with an opaque, glistening serosal surface, measuring 1.5 × 1.3 × 0.7 cm. Sectioning reveals a cystic character of the lesion, with brown, friable contents. Representative sections are submitted.
   Part 2, labeled "right upper arm," consists of a brown piece of tissue covered with skin and measuring 0.7 × 0.3 × 0.2 cm. Sectioning reveals a pale, pinkish tan, fibrous core. Representative sections are submitted.
MICROSCOPIC: Sections show features listed in the diagnosis.
DIAGNOSIS
   1. Epidermal inclusion cyst (excision biopsy, left axilla).
   2. Fibroepithelial skin tag with hyperkeratosis (excision biopsy, right upper arm).

J. D. Wynn, MD

PATIENT NO. 2

CLINICAL DATA: 29-year-old white female, with a recent onset of a right breast mass with nipple retraction.
CLINICAL DIAGNOSIS: Right breast mass.
MATERIAL FROM: Breast biopsy.
GROSS DESCRIPTION: Received fresh, labeled "breast mass," are two pieces of fibrofatty tissue measuring 1.8 × 1.3 × 1.3 cm and 1.7 × 1.7 × 0.6 cm, weighing 2.1 and 1.0 gm, respectively. Serial sections reveal homogeneous fibrofatty tissue. The specimen is submitted in its entirety.
MICROSCOPIC: Sections show features listed in the diagnosis.
DIAGNOSIS: Focally acute and chronically inflamed breast tissue with fat necrosis and fibrosis; see note (right breast biopsy).
NOTE: The peripheral nature of this inflammatory process suggests that it may represent the wall of an abscess.

J. D. Wynn, MD

PATIENT NO. 3

CLINICAL DATA: 34-year-old white female, with a lump in the upper outer left breast.
CLINICAL DIAGNOSIS: Same as above.
MATERIAL FROM: Left breast biopsy.
GROSS DESCRIPTION: Received in formalin are three pieces of pale tan, firm, fibrous tissue with attached yellow fat measuring $2.2 \times 1.4 \times 0.5$ cm, $1.1 \times 1.0 \times 0.3$ cm, and $0.4 \times 0.2 \times 0.1$ cm. Serial sectioning reveals similar homogenous, white, fibrous tissue. Representative sections are submitted.
MICROSCOPIC: Sections show features listed in the diagnosis.
DIAGNOSIS: Mammary dysplasia characterized by cyst, adenosis, and apocrine metaplasia (left breast biopsy).

J. D. Wynn, MD

REVIEW QUESTIONS

1. Having opened a sterile suture removal kit for use, the physician then decides not to remove the patient's sutures. What would you now do with these instruments?
2. When pouring a solution into a sterile container on a sterile field, you accidentally spill some of the solution on the sterile field. What would you do to remedy this contamination?
3. While directly assisting with a minor surgical procedure, you accidentally puncture your sterile glove with a needle. What should be your next actions?
4. Differentiate between a sterile field and a sterile setup.
5. When assisting with minor surgery, the physician asks for the thinnest black silk suture material. What size (number) would you provide?
6. Surgical asepsis is commonly referred to as sterile technique or aseptic technique. Explain what is meant by these terms.
7. List 15 of the principles and practices of aseptic (sterile) technique.
8. Why do you open envelope-wrapped sterile packages with the top flap going away from your body?
9. Before pouring a sterile solution for use, why do you first pour a small amount into a waste container?
10. List two reasons for wearing sterile gloves during a procedure.
11. Name and describe three methods used to administer a local anesthetic for a minor surgical procedure.
12. List the supplies and equipment that you would assemble and prepare when the physician is to
   - Incise and drain an abscess
   - Remove sutures
   - Repair a laceration by suturing
   - Obtain an aspiration (needle) biopsy of breast tissue

   - Remove a wart on the patient's left hand
   - Insert an IUD
13. Describe how to prepare a patient for minor surgery.
14. State the purpose of an IUD.
15. List and explain four terms that describe the character of drainage from a wound.
16. Describe the five types of open wounds, and explain the healing process.
17. List eight purposes of dressings and four purposes of bandages.
18. List and explain the five basic turns used to apply roller bandages, indicating when each may be most appropriately used.
19. List and briefly describe four types of dressing materials and four types of bandage materials.

PERFORMANCE TEST

In a skills laboratory, a simulation of a joblike environment, the medical assistant student will demonstrate skill and knowledge when performing the following activities without reference to source materials. Time limits for the performance of each procedure are to be assigned by the instructor.

1. Given a sterile syringe in a peel-down package and a sterile envelope-wrapped pack of instruments, open these packs and with a sterile transfer forceps arrange the contents for use, avoiding contamination.
2. Given a sterile solution and a sterile container, pour the solution into the container, avoiding contamination.
3. Given a pair of sterile gloves, don these, avoiding contamination, and then remove.
4. Given the choice of a variety of sterile instruments and prepackaged instrument sets, select, identify by name, and prepare for use those that will be used for
   - Preparing the patient's skin for minor surgery
   - Administering a local anesthetic
   - Suturing a laceration
   - Incision and drainage of an abscess or cyst
   - Removal of a foreign body in subcutaneous tissue, a wart and a mole, and a tissue biopsy from the skin surface
   - Cervical biopsy
   - Aspiration (needle) biopsy of breast tissue
   - Insertion of an IUD
   - Dressing change
5. Given a sterile hemostat while gloved, hand it to the physician in the way most convenient for immediate use.
6. Demonstrate the proper procedure for changing a dressing and obtaining a wound culture.
7. Demonstrate the application of a roller, triangular, and Tubegauz bandage.
8. At the completion of the preceding activities, be able to discuss with the instructor at least ten of the principles of aseptic technique, how to prepare a

patient physically and mentally for minor surgery, and how to assist the physician during a minor surgical procedure.

The student must be able to perform the above activities with 100% accuracy 90% of the time. If the student contaminates any item during the performance of these skills, the correct actions to remedy the contaminated site must be employed 100% of the time.

PERFORMANCE CHECKLISTS

Opening a sterile peel-down package

1. Wash your hands.
2. Obtain sterile package.
3. Using both hands, grasp the extended edges on the package, and pull evenly along the sealed edges.
4. Place opened package on a flat surface, ready for use; *or,* using sterile forceps, remove contents from wrapper and transfer to sterile field, avoiding contamination; *or,* holding bottom of the package with the edges folded back, allow someone with sterile gloves on to take the item; *or,* when the item is a syringe to be used by yourself, grasp the plunger end of the syringe, and remove from the package.

Opening an envelope-wrapped package

1. Wash your hands.
2. Obtain sterile package, and place on a flat surface.
3. Remove tape or string fastener, and discard.
4. Open top (distal) flap away from you.
5. Open the second layer of folded corners to the sides of the package.
6. Open fourth (last) flap toward you.
7. Do not at any time reach across the sterile field; do not touch the inside of the wrapper; handle only the outside of the wrapper.
8. Using sterile transfer forceps with prongs facing downward, or a gloved hand, arrange the items for use.
9. Use the same technique to open small packages to be opened while held in your hand; then carefully place the contents on a sterile field, avoiding contamination, or allow a person with sterile gloves to pick the item off the wrapper, or remove the item from the pack with sterile transfer forceps.

Handling sterile transfer forceps

1. Keep one forceps per container.
2. Wash your hands.
3. Grasp forceps by handle, lift vertically, prongs together and facing downward.
4. Do not touch the container above the solution line; prongs may be gently tapped together to remove excess solution.
5. Use to transfer or assemble sterile supplies,

avoiding contact of the prongs with the sterile field. Keep prongs facing downward at all times.
6. Replace the forceps in container, avoiding contamination.

Pouring sterile solutions

1. Wash your hands.
2. Obtain solution, and check label.
3. Obtain sterile container for solution, and unwrap correctly.
4. Remove bottle cap and place on a level surface, upside down.
5. Hold bottle with label facing the palm of your hand; pour small amount of solution into a waste container; and then, holding the bottle 6 inches above the sterile container, pour the solution for use. Do not splash.
6. To pour solution onto a sponge, hold the sponge in forceps, pour solution over sponge, and allow excess solution to drip into a waste basin.
7. Replace cap on the bottle without contaminating.
8. Check label, and return to storage area.

Donning sterile gloves

1. Wash your hands.
2. Place wrapped gloves on a clean, dry, flat surface, with cuff end toward you.
3. Open wrapper, handling outside only.
4. With left hand, grasp cuff of right-hand glove; lift up and away from wrapper.
5. Pull on glove.
6. Place gloved right fingers under cuff of left glove, and lift up and away from the wrapper.
7. Pull left glove over hand and wrist.
8. With left gloved hand, place fingers under right cuff and pull up over wrist.
9. Adjust fingers of both gloves as necessary.
10. To remove gloves, grasp cuff of one glove with opposite hand; pull glove down, turning inside out and discard.
11. Repeat to remove remaining glove.

Dressing change with a wound culture

1. Wash your hands.
2. Assemble equipment.
3. Identify the patient, and explain the procedure.
4. Prepare the patient; that is, gown, position, and drape as necessary.
5. Prepare supplies for use.
6. Loosen tape on the dressing.
7. Remove soiled dressing with a forceps or with a gloved hand, or grasp dressing with hand covered with a plastic bag.
8. Inspect dressing for type and amount of drainage; discard soiled dressing in the waxed or plastic bag.

9. Observe the wound for type and amount of drainage, degree of healing, presence of pus, necrosis, or a putrid odor. When sutures are present, note if they are intact.
10. Remove the sterile applicator from the tube, and swab the drainage area once to obtain a specimen.
11. Place applicator in the culture tube.
12. Don sterile gloves.
13. Cleanse the wound using aseptic technique.
14. Apply fresh sterile dressing, and secure correctly with tape.
15. Attend to the patient's comfort; give further instructions when indicated.
16. Label culture tube, complete laboratory requisition, and send together to the laboratory.
17. Assemble used supplies and dispose of according to office or agency policy.
18. Wash your hands.
19. Replace supplies as needed, leaving the room neat and tidy.
20. Record the procedure and observations on the patient's chart.

Unit VI

Collecting and Handling Specimens

On completion of Unit VI, the medical assistant student should be able to apply the following cognitive objectives:

1. Define and pronounce the vocabulary terms listed.
2. Discuss the proper care, handling, and storage of all specimens.
3. List the information that must be included on a laboratory requisition when sending a specimen for examination.
4. Explain how a specimen should be prepared for transportation through the mail to an outside laboratory.
5. List the purposes, the basic equipment and supplies required, and the medical assistant's usual assisting responsibilities for each procedure described in this unit.
6. State and define seven types of urine specimens, and discuss at least ten general facts relating to the collection of urine for examination.
7. Discuss the hemoccult slide test for stool specimens, stating why and how it is done; the special diagnostic diet that the patient may be on before and during the test; and medications that would interfere with the test.
8. Differentiate between upper and lower respiratory tract specimens.
9. Differentiate between a smear, a culture, and a culture medium.
10. Briefly discuss the Gram stain and the culture and sensitivity tests performed for bacteriological studies.
11. List seven types of smears that may be done to detect vaginal disorders and diseases.
12. Discuss patient care before and after a lumbar puncture.

TERMINAL PERFORMANCE OBJECTIVES

On completion of Unit VI, the medical assistant student should be able to do the following terminal performance objectives.

1. Demonstrate correct technique and proper communication to the patient for collecting the following specimens, preparing them to be sent to the laboratory, and completing the appropriate requisition form:
   • Urine specimen
   • Stool specimen
   • Sputum specimen
   • Throat culture
   • Nasopharyngeal culture
   • Wound culture
   • Vaginal smears and cultures
2. Demonstrate the correct technique for making a smear for cytology studies and a smear for bacteriology studies.
3. Demonstrate the correct procedure for performing a Gram stain.
4. Demonstrate the correct procedure for performing a hemoccult slide test on a stool specimen.
5. Demonstrate the correct technique for inoculating a culture medium with a specimen obtained on a cotton-tipped applicator.
6. Demonstrate the proper procedure for assisting with a lumbar puncture.
7. Demonstrate the correct method for recording information on a patient's chart after the specimen has been sent to the laboratory.
8. Demonstrate the correct method for completing various types of laboratory requisition forms that accompany a specimen that is sent to the laboratory.

The student is to perform the above activities with 100% accuracy 95% of the time.

Vocabulary

bacteriology (bak-te″-re-ol′o-je)—The study of bacteria.
bacteriolysis (bak-te″re-ol′ĭ-sis)—The destruction of bacteria.
biochemistry (bi-″-o-kem′is-tre)—The study of chemical changes occurring in living organisms.
culture (kul′tūr)—The reproduction or growth of microorganisms or of living tissue cells in special laboratory media (the material on which the

organisms grow) conducive to their growth. Various types of cultures include the following:

blood culture—Used in the diagnosis of specific infectious diseases. Blood is withdrawn from a vein and placed in or upon suitable culture media; then it is determined whether or not pathogens grow in the media. If organisms do grow, they are identified by bacteriological methods.

gelatin culture—A culture of bacteria on gelatin.

hanging drop culture—A culture in which the bacteria are inoculated into a drop of fluid on a coverglass, and then mounted into the depression on a concave slide.

negative culture—A culture made from suspected material that fails to reveal the suspected microorganism.

positive culture—A culture that reveals the suspected microorganism.

pure culture—A culture of a single microorganism.

smear culture—A culture prepared by smearing the specimen across the surface of the culture medium.

stab culture—A bacterial culture made by thrusting a needle inoculated with the microorganisms under examination deep into the culture medium.

streak culture—A bacterial culture in which the infectious material is implanted in streaks across the culture media.

tissue culture—The growing of tissue cells in artificial nutrient media.

type culture—A culture that is generally agreed to represent microorganisms of a particular species.

Culturette—A commercially prepared bacterial culture collection/transport system, consisting of a sterile plastic tube with applicator. Modified Stuart's transport medium is held in a glass ampule at the bottom end, to assure stability of medium at the time of use. Transport medium is released only after the sample is taken, by crushing the ampule. A moist environment (not immersion) is maintained up to 72 hours to preserve the specimen (see Fig. 6-7).

Culturette II culture collection system—This is identical to the Culturette, with the exception that the plastic tube contains two applicators and the ampule contains twice the medium (1ml) (see Fig. 6-7).

anaerobic Culturette culture collection system—This system offers the same basic properties of the Culturette, plus a standardized and dependable anaerobic environment for transport of anaerobic bacteria. The transport medium once released maintains an anaerobic environment for up to 48 hours. Many laboratories request that the anaerobic culture system be used when taking a wound culture.

culture medium—A commercial preparation used for the growth of microorganisms or other cells. (Types of culture media are described in this unit.)

cytology (sī-tol′ō-jē)—The study of the structure and function of cells.

dysplasia (dis-plā′ze-ah)—An abnormal development of tissue.

histology (hĭs-tol′ō-jē)—The study of the microscopic form and structure of tissue.

incubation (in-kū-bā′shun)—When pertaining to bacteriology, this term refers to the period of culture development.

inoculate (ĭ-nok″ū-lāt)—In microbiology, this refers to the introduction of infectious matter into a culture medium in an effort to produce growth of the causative organism.

macroscopic (mak-rō-skop′ĭk) **examination**—An examination in which the specimen is large enough to be seen by the naked eye.

medical microbiology—The study and identification of pathogens, and the development of effective methods for their control or elimination.

microorganism (mī-krō-or′gan-ism)—A minute, living body not perceptible to the naked eye, especially a bacterium or protozoon; these are viewed by use of a microscope.

microscopic (mī-krō-skọp′ik) **examination**—An examination in which the specimen is visible only with the aid of a microscope.

pathogen (păth′ō-jĕn)—A disease-producing substance or microorganism.

pathogenic (path′o-jĕn′ic)—Pertaining to a disease-producing microorganism or substance.

serological (sē-rō-lŏj′ik-al) **test**—A laboratory test involving the examination and study of blood serum.

smear (smēr)—Material spread thinly across a slide or culture medium with a swab, loop, or another slide in preparation for microscopic study.

fixation of a smear—Spraying with or immersing a slide into a special solution, or drying the slide over a flame, or air drying to harden and preserve the bacteria for future microscopic examination.

specimen (spec′ĭ-men)—A small part or sample taken to show kind and quality of the whole, as a specimen of urine, blood, or other body excretions, or a small piece of tissue for macroscopic and microscopic examinations.

sputum (spū′-tūm)—A mucus secretion from the trachea, bronchi, and lungs, ejected through the mouth, in contrast to saliva, which is the secretion of the salivary glands.

stool (stool)—Body waste material discharged from the large intestine; *synonym*: feces, bowel movement.

swab (swŏb)—A small piece of cotton or gauze wrapped around the end of a slender stick used for applying medications, cleansing cavities, or obtaining a piece of tissue or body secretion for bacteriological examination; *synonym* cotton-tipped applicator.

urine (ū'rine)—The fluid containing certain waste products and water that is secreted by the kidneys, stored in the bladder, and excreted through the urethra.

viable (vī'ah-bl)—Able to maintain an independent existence.

The science of laboratory technology is becoming increasingly sophisticated in methods used to process specimens obtained from a patient. Thus, it is rare, if not obsolete, that a medical assistant will be required to perform the actual tests on collected specimens in a physician's office or health agency, other than simple tests that may be performed several times a day, such as a routine urinalysis. Most physicians utilize the services of professional laboratories that perform tests under controlled conditions and use expensive equipment that is impractical for the physician's office. Frequently, the patient will be referred to a clinical laboratory where the specimen is obtained, processed, and the results prepared for report to the physician. At other times it will be necessary for the medical assistant to collect the specimen or to assist the physician when obtaining the specimen. Once the specimen has been properly obtained, the medical assistant's responsibility is to ensure that it is preserved and labeled correctly for submission to the laboratory for examination. It is therefore imperative that the medical assistant know how to collect various types of specimens and prepare a smear or culture from the specimen, so that specimens arrive at the laboratory in good condition for processing. When collecting specimens, the medical assistant must also be aware of any special preparation that is required by the patient, ensure that the patient is thoroughly informed (for example, collect the first morning specimen, or fast 12 hours before collection of the specimen), ascertain that this preparation has been followed, and be certain that the correct equipment is used for the specimen obtained. Most professional laboratories furnish manuals on request that outline the specific requirements for each study to be performed. In this unit you will learn techniques for obtaining and for helping the physician obtain different types of specimens, smears, and cultures, in addition to the care and handling of specimens.

Before beginning this unit you should be familiar with the infectious disease process, infection control, and medical and surgical aseptic techniques as presented in Units IV and V.

SPECIMENS

Samples of body fluids, secretions, excretions, or tissues can be removed from a patient's body for laboratory study. These materials, once removed, are called *specimens*. Serological, biochemical, and microscopic tests can be performed on all body specimens. These tests provide a means for evaluating the patient's health status and identifying pathogenic microorganisms and other abnormalities present. Once the suspected cause of a disease process is determined, appropriate methods of treatment can be provided.

It is important that a specimen be collected at the onset of a disease or condition, and when possible, before the administration of any antibiotics when an infectious process is suspected. Frequently the active participation of a patient is required to obtain a specimen; therefore, appropriate instructions must be given. Explain the procedure that is to be used in collecting the specimen (such as urine, sputum, or stool) completely and accurately.

Some tests require special preparation by the patient, and again the appropriate instructions must be given, along with an explanation of the necessity for following these instructions. Special preparation usually means a modification in diet or a period of fasting before the specimen collection. The time of day the specimen is to be collected may be specific; that is, the first morning urine is to be collected. For women, the use of vaginal medications, douches, or the time of the menstrual flow should be avoided when vaginal specimens are to be obtained.

Caring for, Handling, Transporting, and Storing Specimens

Essential considerations to remember with regard to each specimen follow. See Vocabulary for types of collection and transport systems used.

The specimen must be properly labeled and placed in the correct container. Each specimen is to be placed in the proper container or solution that is designed for the type of material collected with the lid fastened securely. The container with the specimen must be labeled with the patient's name, the date, the source of the specimen, and the attending physician's name.

The specimen must be protected when it is sent to outside laboratories or through the mail. Most outside laboratories will provide specific instructions for the transportation of specimens to them. Specimens that are sent to outside laboratories through the mail must be placed and secured in a proper transport container. This special container will protect and preserve the specimen for examination. Specimen containers sent by mail must be closed securely and wrapped in a protective covering such as corrugated cardboard or cotton, which will absorb shock or possible leakage. The wrapped specimen container should then be placed in a watertight metal container (Fig. 6-1), which is then placed with a laboratory requisition into a stiff cardboard mailing container that has shock-resistant insulating material (Fig. 6-2). The outside of this container must have a label that identifies it as a medical specimen.

The specimen must be uncontaminated. To prevent addition of microorganisms to the specimen obtained from the patient, sterile containers, sterile applicators, or other sterile devices, and clean or sterile techniques are to be used to collect the specimen.

- Cracked or broken containers and applicators must *not* be used.
- Only regulation tops or plugs are to be used on stopper bottles and test tubes. Cotton balls or gauze must *not* be used as a substitute. Many laboratories now use plastic-capped tubes, screw caps, and metal closure tubes; special vials or tubes with rubber stoppers are used for transporting suspected anaerobic organisms.
- Plugs or the inner surface of tops that come in contact with an unsterile surface are to be discarded.
- Containers should be filled only half-way. The top or plug must not be permitted to become wet, either from the specimen or other sources, in order to prevent contamination to the specimen and to personnel handling it.
- Specimen material must not be spilled on the outside of the container or on any surface. This is for the protection of everyone handling the specimen or near the area. If a specimen is accidentally spilled, call the laboratory to inquire how to destroy

Fig. 6-1. Wrap specimen container for mailing in corrugated cardboard or cotton and place in watertight metal container.

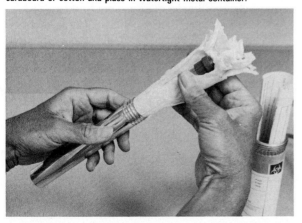

Fig. 6-2. Place watertight metal container containing specimen and laboratory requisition into a stiff cardboard mailing container.

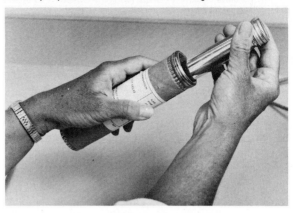

the pathogens that may be in the specimen and what to use. You must clean the work area immediately. A disinfectant such as phenol or cresol is frequently used to clean the area.

The specimen must contain living organisms collected from the proper source and reach the laboratory in a condition suitable for culturing, incubating, or examining. Specimens collected for a smear or culture may be taken from any body opening, whether natural, surgical, or accidental; for example, material may be collected from the ear, eye, nose, throat, urethra, vagina, rectum, or a wound. Body fluids such as urine, blood, and cerebrospinal fluid, and samples of tissue (biopsy) may also be obtained. To make sure that the pathogens remain viable (living), all specimens must be sent to the laboratory for processing without delay. If there is a delay, most specimens may be kept in a refrigerator for a few hours. Generally swabs from the throat, rectum, and wounds, and fecal (except when feces are to be examined for the presence of parasites) and sputum samples may be stored in a refrigerator for several hours. Spinal fluid may contain organisms that are sensitive to cold; therefore, this specimen should be placed in a bacteriological incubator.

Swabs of infectious matter must be prevented from drying before they are processed in the laboratory. Sometimes the sterile swab is moistened with a broth, or placed into tubes containing broth or a selected holding medium to prevent drying of the specimen. The broth is used to keep the air around the swab moist and is *not* a culture medium.

Special procedures for preservation and growth are used when an anaerobic organism (one able to live in the absence of oxygen) is believed to be the causative agent. Processing these specimens *immediately* is vital to maintaining the organism in a viable state. When there is a delay, inoculated culture plates may be placed in a candle jar (see Fig. 6-16) and then sent to the laboratory.

Urine specimens should be examined or sent to the laboratory immediately. If this is not possible, they must be refrigerated. (See No. 8 and 9 under "General Facts Relating to Urine Collection," which follows, and also Unit X, "Urinalysis.")

Most blood specimens must be examined within 8 hours or less from the time they were collected, and preferably, within 2 to 4 hours from the time they were collected. Blood for bacteriological studies must be collected in special containers and must not sit around. These specimens must be examined as soon as possible. Blood drawn for an electrolyte panel should be refrigerated if it is not tested immediately. Other blood samples may be left standing on the counter for 2 to 4 hours before testing, although some results may vary if the blood is left standing for 2 or more hours. (See Unit XI, "Hematology.")

When a specimen is to be examined in the physician's office or clinic, it should be tested, cultured, or examined microscopically immediately.

The specimen should be handled and transported in an upright position and should not be shaken. Remember that failure in successfully identifying pathogens may be caused by improper collection, care, and handling techniques.

Avoid and prevent contamination to yourself and other personnel who will be handling the specimen. All specimens obtained for microbiological study are presumed to contain potentially dangerous pathogens. Always keep in mind the possibility of spreading the infectious pathogen, know the necessary protective measures that must be adhered to (as listed), and utilize excellent aseptic technique when obtaining the specimen. In addition

- *Do not* eat, drink, or smoke while handling specimens because you could transmit pathogens to yourself by hand-to-mouth contact.
- *Do not* lick the label that will be placed on the specimen container.
- Cover any cut or scratch that you have with a Band-Aid.
- If you accidentally touch some of the specimen collected, immediately wash the contact area thoroughly with an antiseptic soap. If the contact area was on a cut or scratch, apply tincture of iodine or another antiseptic solution to the area.
- At the end of each work day, clean the work area with a disinfectant solution.

A laboratory requisition to accompany the specimen must always be filled out completely and accurately. The following information must be included.

- Date (time of day if relevant, for example, an early morning specimen)
- Name of the patient, address, age, and sex
- Name of the attending physician and address

- Source of the specimen
- Name of laboratory test(s) to be performed
- A notation if the patient is already taking antibiotics. [False-negative results could be obtained if the antibiotic has suppressed the growth of the microorganism(s).]

Additional information will depend on the type of specimen obtained and may include the following.

- Clinical history
- Previous normal or abnormal results
- Previous surgery
- X-ray treatment
- Clinical diagnosis

For vaginal and cervical specimens the following, if applicable, is also added:

- Hormone treatment
- Date of last menstrual period (LMP)
- Postpartum
- Postmenopausal
- Pregnant

All blood specimens from all patients whether known to be infected or not should be handled with caution.

All specimens from AIDS patients must be labeled with "H/A (hepatitis/AIDS) Precautions" labels, placed in ZipLok bags, and sealed for transport to prevent spills from broken tubes. A laboratory requisition should also be labeled and attached to the *outside* of the bag (see also Unit IV).

URINE SPECIMEN COLLECTION

A specimen of urine is collected to perform a urinalysis (u"rĭ-nal'ĭ-sis), which is an analysis of the physical, chemical, and microscopic properties of urine. The results of these examinations help determine the renal functions of the body, which in turn helps the physician diagnose and provide the appropriate treatment required for a disease process.

Many types of tests are used in analyzing the urine to determine whether it contains abnormal substances indicative of disease. (See Unit X for urinalysis procedures.) The most significant substances normally absent from urine and detected by a urinalysis are protein, glucose, acetone, blood, pus, casts, and bacteria.

Vocabulary

urination (u-"rĭ-na'shun), **voiding, micturition** (mik"tu-rish'un)—The act of passing urine from the body.

diuresis (di"u-re'sis)—An abnormal, increased secretion of urine as seen in diabetes mellitus, diabetes insipidus, or when large amounts of fluid have been drunk; this can be artificially produced by drugs with diuretic properties.

enuresis (en"u-re'sis)—The involuntary excretion of urine, especially at night during sleep; bedwetting; most frequently seen in children with either physical or emotional problems.

frequency—The need to urinate frequently.

incontinence (in-kon'tĭ-nens)—The inability to refrain from the urge to urinate. This may occur in times of stress, anxiety, anger, postoperatively, or from obstructions that prevent the normal emptying of the urinary bladder, spasms of the bladder, irritation due to injury or inflammation of the urinary tract, damage to the spinal cord or brain, or from the development of a fistula (an abnormal tubelike passage) between the bladder and the vagina or urethra.

urgency—The need to urinate immediately.

Types of Urine Specimens

Random or spot specimen. To collect a random or spot specimen, the patient voids at any time of the day or night, collecting a portion of the urine in a clean container.

Fasting specimen. To collect a fasting specimen, the patient voids 4 or more hours after ingestion of food and discards this urine. The next voided specimen is collected and regarded as the fasting specimen.

First morning specimen. To collect a first morning specimen, the patient voids and discards the specimen before going to bed. On arising the next morning, the patient collects the first morning specimen.

Postprandial specimen. To collect a postprandial specimen, the patient voids after eating and collects this specimen.

Midstream specimen. To collect a midstream specimen, the patient starts to void into the toilet or bedpan; then, without stopping the process of voiding, a portion of the urine is collected in a clean container. The last part of the urine flow is passed into the toilet or bedpan.

Clean-catch specimen. To collect a clean-catch specimen, the patient is instructed to wash the external genitalia using soap and water or some mild antiseptic solution. Then a midstream urine specimen is collected in a clean, dry container or in a sterile container if the specimen is being collected for bacterial examination. This yields a specimen with limited contamination by skin bacteria.

Multiple-glass specimens. The multiple-glass test is performed on men to evaluate a lower urinary tract infection. The man must have a full bladder, as 3 samples of urine will be collected. To collect a multiple-

DISEASE

glass specimen, the patient is instructed to wash the area around the urinary meatus with an antiseptic solution. Then he is to void about 100 ml (approximately 3½ ounces) into a clean, dry container. This specimen contains microorganisms and sediment "washed" from the urethra. Without interrupting the voiding process, another 100 ml of urine is then voided into a second clean, dry container. This specimen contains microorganisms and sediment representative of that in the bladder and kidney. Then the man is to stop voiding and the physician will gently massage the prostate gland. After this, the third urine specimen is collected in a clean, dry container. This last specimen contains secretions from the prostate gland.

Timed specimens (24 hour specimen). To collect a timed specimen, the patient discards the first morning specimen and then collects all urine for exactly 24 hours. (See No. 12, under "General Facts Relating To Urine Collection.")

A specific type of urine collection can provide optimum information when performing certain tests; for example, postprandial urine can be used for testing sugar content, and first morning specimens can be used for testing protein content.

General Facts Relating to Urine Collection

1. To minimize bacterial and chemical contamination, use only clean, dry, or sterile collection containers. Disposable containers are ideal.

2. The early morning urine specimen is the most concentrated; therefore, if at all possible, this is the specimen that should be obtained for simple routine testing. The concentration of urine will vary during a 24 hour period, partly due to the patient's food and water intake and level of activity.

3. A freshly voided specimen is adequate for *most* urinalysis when the first morning specimen cannot be obtained; although collection of a clean-catch midstream specimen is the method of choice.

4. To collect a freshly voided specimen in the office, give the patient a clean, wide-mouthed bottle, and instruct her or him to void directly into it. Inform the patient how much urine you want in the bottle — that is, up to what point in the bottle you want collected (usually 2 to 4 ounces is sufficient).

5. When urine is required for bacterial cultures, collect a clean-catch midstream specimen in a sterile container, and submit it to the bacteriology laboratory department as soon as possible for testing.

6. Ask patients if they are taking any medications, and the type, and if they are on a special diet, because certain medications and diets will affect

the findings of a urinalysis. NOTE: A note of medications and/or special diet should be recorded on the lab requisition and the patient's chart.

7. Inquire if a female patient is menstruating when a urine specimen is collected. The reason for knowing this is that if blood is found in the urine it may be from the vaginal canal, rather than from the urinary tract. A note of this must also be recorded, and another specimen may be required when the patient has finished menstruating.

8. Voided specimens should not be left standing at room temperature, because they become alkaline as a result of contamination by urea-splitting bacteria from the environment. Explain to the patient that refrigeration of the specimen is necessary if collected at home, until time to submit it for analysis. If examination is delayed in your office or the laboratory, the specimen should also be refrigerated.

9. Microscopic examination of urine should be performed within 1 hour after collection. Waiting for longer than 1 hour will cause dissolution of cellular elements and casts and bacterial overgrowth, unless the specimen was obtained under sterile conditions.

10. When more than one specimen is required, number each specimen according to its sequence.

11. If the patient is to collect the specimen at home, the procedure should have been explained previously. The patient should be told to use a thoroughly clean 3 to 4 ounce container in which to collect the specimen. Instruct the patient to boil the container that will be used for the collection for 20 minutes before using it. It is advisable to instruct the patient not to use a container that has held drugs or other solutions that may make the specimen unsuitable for examination.

12. When a 24 hour specimen is required, it is vital that the patient understand the procedure. *All urine must be collected within a 24 hour period.*
    a. The first early-morning specimen is discarded.
    b. All subsequent specimens are collected, including the first early-morning specimen the next day.
    c. The last specimen is collected 24 hours after collection was started.
    d. Urine is collected in a clean bottle into which a preservative has been added. (Preservative is prescribed by the laboratory.) This bottle must be refrigerated or kept cold by placing it in a bucket of ice.

Technique for Obtaining a Clean-Catch, Midstream, Voided Specimen

Equipment

Antiseptic solution (such as benzalkonium chloride) *or* soap and water
Washcloth
Sterile gauze sponges 4 × 4 inch
Sterile specimen container (with cover if sending out to a lab)
Tissues
Laboratory requisition

Procedure	Rationale
1. Wash your hands.	
2. Assemble supplies and equipment.	
3. Identify the patient, and explain the procedure.	Explanations help gain full cooperation from the patient, which is required to obtain a specimen successfully.
For a female patient:	
a. Ask patient to wash her perineal area using soap, water, and washcloth; separate labia and cleanse the area around the urinary meatus.	Careful cleansing is necessary to obtain a satisfactory specimen. The urethral orifice is colonized by bacteria. Urine readily becomes contaminated during voiding.
b. Repeat step (a) using water and 4 × 4 inch sponges. NOTE: Rather than using soap and water, the patient may wash herself with 4 × 4 inch sponges soaked with a mild antiseptic solution such as benzalkonium chloride.	It is important to remove all the soap, as a soap residue changes the results of the specimen analysis.
c. Instruct patient to start voiding into the toilet; then after she has voided for a few seconds, to move the specimen container into the urinary stream, in order to catch the midstream specimen in the sterile container.	This helps wash away urethral contaminants. You will need approximately 2 to 4 ounces of urine for analysis. Instruct the patient to fill the container no more than three-fourths full.

Procedure	Rationale
d. Instruct the patient to finish voiding into the toilet bowl.	Provide tissues for the patient to wipe herself and to wash the outside of the container if spillage should occur after collecting the specimen.
For a male patient:	
a. Instruct the patient to take the penis, retract the foreskin (if uncircumcised) to expose the urinary meatus, and cleanse thoroughly with soap and water using the washcloth.	Careful cleansing is necessary to obtain a satisfactory specimen. The urethral orifice is colonized by bacteria. Urine readily becomes contaminated during voiding.
b. Repeat step (a) using 4 × 4 inch sponges and water. NOTE: Rather than using soap and water, the patient may wash himself with 4 × 4 inch sponges soaked with a mild antiseptic solution such as benzalkonium chloride.	It is important to remove all soap, as a soap residue will change the result of the specimen analysis.
c. Instruct the patient to start voiding into the toilet and, after he has voided for a few seconds, to move the specimen container into the urinary stream in order to catch the midstream specimen.	This helps cleanse the urethral canal. Instruct the patient to fill the container no more than three-fourths full, as you will need only 2 to 4 ounces for the analysis.
d. Instruct the patient to then finish voiding into the toilet.	The patient is to avoid collecting the last few drops of urine, as prostatic secretions may be introduced into the urine at the end of the urinary stream.
4. Have the patient signal you when the specimen has been obtained, or instruct the patient where to place the specimen container.	
5. Send properly labeled specimen, with the correct laboratory requisition, to appropriate laboratory; or refrigerate it until it can either be tested or sent to the lab (Fig. 6-3).	Do not allow a urine specimen to stand at room temperature for any length of time, because it becomes worthless. It is best to put a cover on the container.

Fig. 6-3. Sample urinalysis laboratory requisition that is sent with urine specimen to the laboratory.

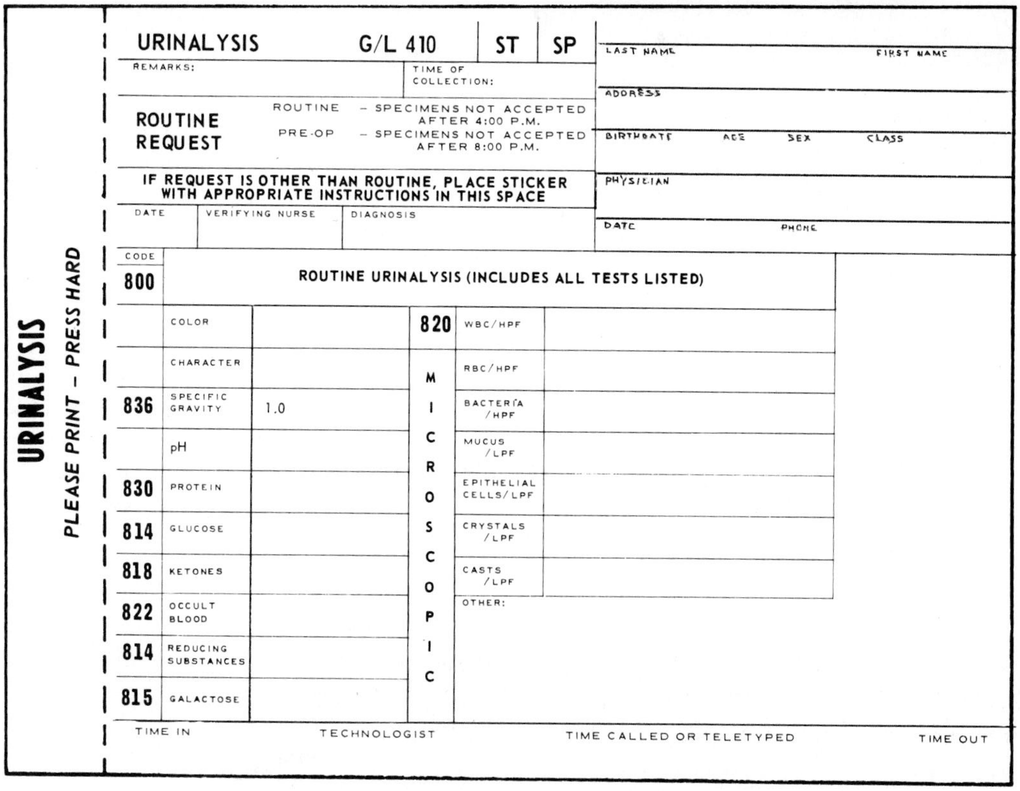
URINALYSIS G/L 410 ST SP

LAST NAME FIRST NAME

REMARKS: TIME OF COLLECTION:

ADDRESS

ROUTINE REQUEST — ROUTINE – SPECIMENS NOT ACCEPTED AFTER 4:00 P.M.; PRE-OP – SPECIMENS NOT ACCEPTED AFTER 8:00 P.M.

BIRTHDATE AGE SEX CLASS

IF REQUEST IS OTHER THAN ROUTINE, PLACE STICKER WITH APPROPRIATE INSTRUCTIONS IN THIS SPACE

PHYSICIAN

DATE | VERIFYING NURSE | DIAGNOSIS

DATE PHONE

CODE					
800	ROUTINE URINALYSIS (INCLUDES ALL TESTS LISTED)				
	COLOR		820	WBC/HPF	
	CHARACTER		M	RBC/HPF	
836	SPECIFIC GRAVITY	1.0	I	BACTERIA /HPF	
	pH		C	MUCUS /LPF	
830	PROTEIN		R O	EPITHELIAL CELLS/LPF	
814	GLUCOSE		S	CRYSTALS /LPF	
818	KETONES		C O	CASTS /LPF	
822	OCCULT BLOOD		P	OTHER:	
814	REDUCING SUBSTANCES		I C		
815	GALACTOSE				

TIME IN TECHNOLOGIST TIME CALLED OR TELETYPED TIME OUT

URINALYSIS

PLEASE PRINT – PRESS HARD

Technique for Obtaining a Clean-Catch, Midstream, Voided Specimen (*continued*)

Procedure	Rationale
6. Perform the urinalysis if this is required of you.	See Unit X for this procedure.
7. Wash your hands.	Avoid contamination.
8. Record on the chart the appropriate information. Always record on the chart if the urine appeared abnormal, that is, if blood appeared to be present, or if the urine was cloudy, and so on. Record the results if you have performed the analysis (as described in Unit X).	Charting example: February 25, 19_____, 4 PM Clean-catch urine specimen obtained and sent to the laboratory for routine UA [urinalysis]. Betty Bittinger, CMA

STOOL SPECIMEN COLLECTION

A stool specimen is collected for macroscopic, microscopic, and chemical examination to help diagnose the presence of parasites and ova, occult blood, fecal urobilinogen, pus or mucus, membranous shreds, worms, infectious diseases, foreign bodies, and to detect the amount of fat being eliminated and various disorders of metabolism.

The stool is examined macroscopically for its amount, consistency, color, and odor. Normal color varies from light to dark brown depending on urobilin content, a product formed from bilirubin. Various foods, medications, and conditions affect the color of the stool. For example, when a person has ingested the following, the color of the stool may be affected:

- Meat protein—the stool may be dark brown
- Spinach—the stool may be green
- Beets—the stool may be red
- Cocoa—the stool may be dark red or brown
- Bismuth, iron, or charcoal—the stool may be black
- Barium—the stool may be milky white

In conditions in which a patient is having upper gastrointestinal bleeding, the stool is tarry black; in lower gastrointestinal bleeding, it is bright red bloody; and in biliary obstruction, it is clay-colored. Other clinical conditions in which the stool has certain characteristics include the following:

- Steatorrhea (excess fat in the feces due to a malabsorption state caused by disease of the intestinal mucosa or pancreatic enzyme deficiency)—the stool will appear bulky, greasy, foamy, foul in odor, and gray or clay-colored with a silvery sheen.
- Chronic ulcerative colitis—mucus or pus may be visible in the stool.
- Constipation, obstipation, and fecal obstruction—the stool will appear as small, dry, rocky-hard masses.

As with most specimens, a fresh specimen is absolutely necessary and should be obtained before the administration of antibiotic therapy. Stool containing barium, mineral oils, or magnesia is usually unsuitable for diagnosis.

To best demonstrate parasitic infection, three fresh specimens collected on three different days are usually required. These must be sent to the laboratory immediately so that the parasites can be observed under the microscope while they are fresh, viable, and warm. Stool for occult blood testing should not be more than 1 hour old.

Some laboratories now prefer the new collection system that no longer requires that specimens be warm. The specimens are placed into two separate vials, each containing a special preservative and then are to be sent to the laboratory as soon as possible.

When forwarding the specimen to a hospital or large laboratory, send specimens to be tested for occult blood to the hematology laboratory, specimens for culture and acid-fast bacilli to the bacteriology laboratory, and specimens for parasites and ova to the parasitology laboratory. All specimens are to be accompanied by the appropriate clinical laboratory slips with accurate and completed information.

Vocabulary

bowel movement—The elimination/excretion of fecal material from the intestinal tract.

constipation (kŏn-stī-pā'shun)—A condition in which the waste material in the intestine is too hard to pass easily, or in which bowel movements are so infrequent that discomfort results.

diarrhea (di-ă-rē'ă)—Rapid movement of fecal material through the intestine, resulting in poor absorption, producing frequent, watery stools.

excrete—To eliminate useless matter, such as feces and urine.

excreta (ek-skre'tah)—Waste material excreted or eliminated from the body. Feces, urine, perspiration, and also mucus and carbon dioxide (CO_2) can be considered excreta.

excretion (ek-skrē'shun)—The elimination of waste materials from the body. Ordinarily, what is meant by excretion is the elimination of feces, but it can refer to the material eliminated from any part of the body.

feces (fē'sēz)—Body waste excreted from the intestine; also called stool, excreta, or excrement.

flatulence (flat'u-lens)—Excessive formation of gases in the stomach or intestine.

flatus (fla'tus)—Air or gas in the stomach or intestine.

guaiac (gwī'ak) **test**—The preferred chemical test to determine the presence of occult blood in feces.

melena (mē-lē-nah)—Darkening of stool by blood pigments.

obstipation (ob'stĭ-pa'shun)—Extreme constipation due to an obstruction.

occult blood—Obscure or hidden from view.

occult blood test—A microscopic or a chemical test performed on a specimen to determine the presence of blood not otherwise detectable. Stool is tested when intestinal bleeding is suspected but there is no visible evidence of blood in the stool.

parasite (par'ah-sīt)—An organism that lives on or in another organism, known as the host, from which it gains its nourishment, for example, fungi, bacteria, and single-celled and multi-celled animals.

stool—The fecal discharge from the bowels (see also feces).

   lienteric stool—Feces containing much undigested food.

urobilinogen—A colorless compound formed in the intestines by the reduction of bilirubin.

Technique for Obtaining a Stool Specimen

Equipment

Stool specimen container of waxed paper with a lid of glass or of plastic
Wooden tongue depressor or spatula
Clean bedpan with cover
Label for container
Small paper bag
Laboratory requisition

Procedure	Rationale
1. Wash your hands, and obtain a clean bedpan with a clean cover to give to the patient for use.	
2. Identify the patient. Explain to the patient that a stool specimen is needed and that a bedpan must be used.	Have the patient empty the bladder first if required, as urine should not be collected in the bedpan with the stool specimen. Explanations help gain the patient's full cooperation, which is essential for proper specimen collection.
3. Prepare the label for the specimen container. Fill out the laboratory requisition accurately and completely.	You can do this while the patient is collecting the specimen.
4. After the patient has used the bedpan, cover it and remove it to your work area.	Provide means for the patient to wash the hands.
5. Transfer a portion (1 to 2 teaspoons) of the stool into the specimen container by using the clean tongue depressor or spatula as a spoon. Place the lid on the container securely.	Be sure that there is no toilet tissue in the stool specimen. Do not smear the specimen on the edge or outside of the container. You may scrape the tongue depressor or spatula only on the inside of the container to rid it of feces.
6. Place the tongue depressor or spatula in the paper bag, and wrap it securely for proper disposal.	*Do not* throw it in the wastebasket, as it may be contaminated with infectious disease organisms. You should have a special container for used equipment such as this.
7. Empty and clean the bedpan. Avoid contaminating yourself or your work area.	*Before* emptying the bedpan, observe the feces for anything that appears abnormal to you; if so, report it at once.
8. Wash your hands thoroughly.	
9. Label the container, and attach the correct completed laboratory requisition to the container (Fig. 6–4).	The purpose of the examination must be stated on the requisition.
10. Send or take the labeled specimen to the laboratory immediately. If there is a delay, try to place the specimen for parasite examination in a warm place until it can be delivered to or	A stool specimen should be warm when it arrives in the laboratory for examination. This is especially important when looking for parasites so that they may be examined under the micro-

Technique for Obtaining a Stool Specimen (*continued*)

Procedure	Rationale
picked up by the laboratory. Refrigerate specimens for other examinations until delivered to the laboratory. NOTE: If more than one specimen is to be sent, indicate No. 1, No. 2, and so on.	scope while viable, fresh, and warm. Specimens for tests other than parasite detection can generally be refrigerated for a few hours when not sent immediately to the laboratory.
11. Wash your hands again.	Because of the chance of having disease organisms on your hands, wash them again to be safe.

12. Record on the patient's chart. If relevant, describe the appearance of the stool when charting.	Charting example:
	Feb. 27, 19_____, 10 AM
	    Stool specimen No. 1 sent to laboratory for ova and parasites, and fat content examinations.
	    Connie Hanks, CMA

Fig. 6-4. Sample laboratory requisition for fecal specimen.

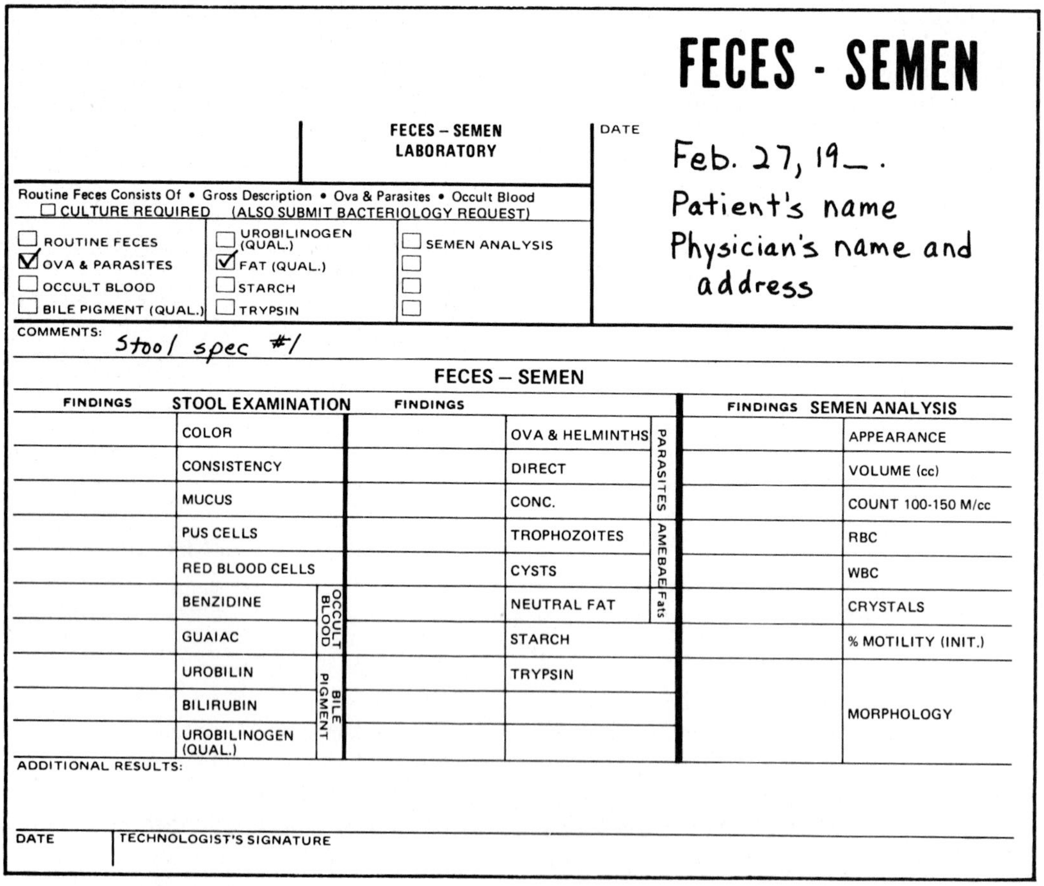

Hemoccult Slide Test On A Stool Specimen

The Hemoccult slide test is a rapid, convenient, and virtually odorless method for detecting the presence of fecal occult blood, as an aid to diagnosis of various gastrointestinal conditions:

• During routine physical examinations
• In newly admitted hospital patients
• In postoperative patients
• In newborn infants
• In screening programs for colorectal cancer

Because Hemoccult tests require only a small stool specimen, offensive odors are minimized and storage or transport of large stool specimens is unnecessary. See Figure 6–5 for more information, special instructions for the patient, and the equipment and proce-

(*Text continues on p. 204*)

Fig. 6-5. **A,** Hemoccult test and procedure. **B,** Hemoccult II slides. **C,** Hemoccult II Dispensapak with on-slide performance monitors. (**A, B,** and **C,** Courtesy SmithKline Diagnostics, Inc., Sunnyvale, CA) **D,** instructions to the patient for collecting fecal specimens for Hemoccult II slide test and Hemoccult II procedure. (Line art courtesy SmithKline Diagnostics, Inc., Sunnyvale, CA)

Hemoccult Single Slides are convenient for use when single stool specimens are to be tested.

Hemoccult II Slides, in cards of three tests, are designed so your patient can collect serial specimens at home over the course of three bowel movements. After the patient collects the specimens, the Hemoccult II test may be returned to a laboratory, a hospital, or a medical office for developing and evaluation. Serial fecal specimen analysis is recommended when screening asymptomatic patients (**B** and **D**).

Hemoccult Tape is designed to complement Hemoccult slides and is best suited for "on-the-spot" testing for occult blood during rectal or sigmoidoscopic examinations.

The Hemoccult test and other unmodified guaiac tests are *not recommended* for use with gastric specimens.

SUMMARY, EXPLANATION AND LIMITATIONS OF THE TEST
The Hemoccult test is a simplified, standardized variation of the guaiac test for occult blood. It contains specially prepared guaiac-impregnated paper and is ready for use without additional preparation.

When a small stool specimen containing occult blood is applied to Hemoccult test paper, the hemoglobin comes in contact with the guaiac. Application of Hemoccult Developer (a stabilized hydrogen peroxide solution) creates a guaiac/peroxidase-like re-action which turns the test paper blue within 60 seconds if occult blood is present.

The test reacts with hemoglobin released from lysed cells. When blood is present, hemolysis is promoted by substances in the stool, primarily water and salts. Typical positive reactions for occult blood are shown under READING AND INTERPRETATION OF THE HEMOCCULT TEST. As with any occult blood test, results with the Hemoccult test *cannot* be considered conclusive evidence of the presence or absence of gastrointestinal bleeding or pathology. Hemoccult tests are designed for *preliminary screening as a diagnostic aid* and are not intended to replace other diagnostic procedures such as proctosigmoidoscopic examination, barium enema, or other x-ray studies.

BIOLOGICAL PRINCIPLE
The discovery that gum guaiac was a useful indicator for occult blood is generally credited to Van Deen. The test depends on the oxidation of a phenolic compound, alpha guaiaconic acid, which yields a blue-covered, highly conjugated quinone structure. Hemoglobin exerts a peroxidase-like activity and facilitates the oxidation of this phenolic compound by hydrogen peroxide.

REAGENTS
Natural guaiac resin impregnated into standardized, high-quality filter paper.

A developing solution containing a stabilized dilute mixture of hydrogen peroxide (less than 6%) and 75% denatured ethyl alcohol in aqueous solution.

PERFORMANCE MONITORS
The function and stability of the slides and Developer can be tested using the on-slide Performance Monitor. Both a positive and negative Performance Monitor are located under the flap and below the specimen windows on the back of the Hemoccult II and Hemoccult single slides.

The positive Performance Monitor contains a hemoglobin-derived catalyst which, upon application of Developer, will turn blue within 10 seconds.

The negative Performance Monitor contains no such catalyst and should not turn blue upon application of Developer.

The Performance Monitors provide additional assurance that the guaiac-impregnated paper and Developer are functional. In the unlikely event that the Performance Monitors do not react as expected after application of Developer, the test results should be regarded as invalid. The manufacturer will provide further assistance should this occur.

PRECAUTIONS
For *in vitro* diagnostic use. Do not use after expiration date which appears on each slide or tape dispenser.

Prolonged exposure to some air pollutants and light may cause slides to turn blue. This does not affect the performance of the test and results can be read in the usual manner.

A

Hemoccult Developer should be protected from heat and the bottle kept tightly capped when not in use. It is flammable and subject to evaporation.

Hemoccult Developer is an irritant. Avoid contact with skin.

Do Not Use In Eyes. Should such contact occur, solution should be rinsed out promptly with water.

Do not use after expiration date on bottle.

STORAGE AND STABILITY
Do not refrigerate. Store at controlled room temperature 15°–30°C (59°–86°F) in original packaging. Protect from heat. Do not store with volatile chemicals (e.g., iodine, chlorine, bromine, or ammonia).

The Hemoccult test, stored as recommended, will maintain its sensitivity until the expiration date on the slide. The expiration date appears on each slide and tape dispenser.

Hemoccult Developer, stored as recommended, will remain stable until the expiration date on the bottle. The expiration date appears on each bottle.

SPECIMEN COLLECTION
Only a very small stool sample, about the size of a match-head, thinly applied, is necessary in preparing either slide or tape. When specimen is to be collected from toilet bowl, the patient should flush the toilet before defecating. The slides may be prepared and developed immediately or prepared and stored for up to 12 days.

Patients with bleeding from other conditions which may affect test results (e.g., hemorrhoids, menstrual bleeding, hematuria) are not appropriate test subjects while such bleeding is active.

Since bleeding from gastrointestinal lesions may be intermittent, it is recommended that stool smears for testing be collected from three consecutive bowel movements. To increase the probability of detecting occult blood, Greegor recommends that samples be taken from two different sections of each stool.

Patient Preparation
Whenever practicable, patients should be placed on the Special Diagnostic Diet (see below) starting two days before and continuing through the test period. Such a diet may increase the accuracy of the test and at the same time provide roughage to help uncover "silent" lesions which may bleed only intermittently.

An alternative procedure is to omit the special diet initially. Then if a patient has one or more positive tests in the initial three-slide series, he should be placed on the special diet and retested for three days.

Special Diagnostic Diet
(two days before and during the test period)

Foods to avoid
Rare red meat (beef, lamb, etc.)
Turnips
Horseradish
Melons

Drugs & Vitamins to avoid
Vitamin C in excess of 250 mg per day
Aspirin
Anti-inflammatory drugs

Foods to eat
Well-cooked meats, poultry and fish
Bran cereal daily
Cooked fruits and vegetables
Peanuts and popcorn

If any of the above are known from past experience to cause discomfort, patient is instructed to inform the physician.

Interfering Substances
Some oral medications (e.g., aspirin, indomethacin, phenylbuta-zone, corticosteroids, reserpine, etc.) can cause GI irritation and occult bleeding in some patients. These substances should be discontinued two days prior to and during testing.

Ascorbic acid (Vitamin C) in excess of 250 mg/day may cause false-negative results and should also be eliminated before testing.

Therapeutic dosages of iron can yield false-positive fecal occult blood test reactions. Use of iron preparations should be suspended before and during testing for fecal occult blood.

Fig. 6-5 *(continued)*

PROCEDURE: HEMOCCULT SLIDES

Identification	Preparation	Development of Test	Development of Performance Monitors

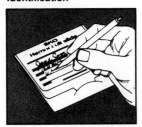

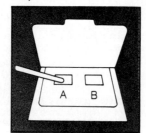

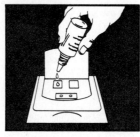

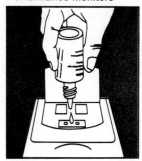

Identification

Write, or have patient write his or her name, age, address, phone number, and date specimen was collected in space provided on front of each slide.

Preparation

1. Collect small stool sample on one end of applicator.
2. Apply thin smear inside box A.
3. Reuse applicator to obtain second sample from different part of stool. Apply thin smear inside box B.
4. Close cover. Return slide to physician.

CAUTION: Protect from heat.

Development of Test

1. Open flap *in back* of slide and apply two drops of Hemoccult Developer to guaiac paper directly over each smear.
2. Read results within 60 seconds.

ANY TRACE OF BLUE ON OR AT THE EDGE OF THE SMEAR IS POSITIVE FOR OCCULT BLOOD.

Development of Performance Monitors

1. Apply ONE DROP ONLY of Hemoccult Developer between the positive and negative Performance Monitors.
2. Read results within 10 seconds.

A BLUE COLOR WILL APPEAR IN THE POSITIVE PERFORMANCE MONITOR, AND NO BLUE WILL APPEAR IN THE NEGATIVE PERFORMANCE MONITOR, IF THE SLIDES AND DEVELOPER ARE FUNCTIONAL.

IMPORTANT NOTE: Follow the procedure exactly as outlined above. Always develop the test, read the results, interpret them and make a decision as to whether the fecal specimen is positive or negative for occult blood BEFORE you develop the Performance Monitors. Do not apply Developer to Performance Monitors before interpreting test results. Any blue originating from the Performance Monitors should be ignored in the reading of the specimen test results.

READING AND INTERPRETATION OF THE HEMOCCULT TEST

Negative Smears*	Negative and Positive Smears*	Positive Smears*

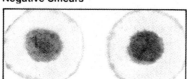

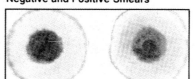

Specimen report: negative
No detectable blue on or at the edge of the smears indicates test is negative for occult blood.

Specimen report: Positive
Any trace of blue on or at the edge of one or more of the smears indicates test is positive for occult blood.

On-Slide Performance Monitors*

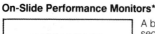

positive   negative

A blue color in the positive Performance Monitor will appear within 10 seconds if test system is functional.

No blue color will appear in the negative Performance Monitor if the test system is functional.

Neither the intensity nor the shade of the blue from the positive Performance Monitor should be regarded as an indication of what the blue from a positive fecal specimen should look like.

* The illustrations are an artist's rendition. Each specimen illustration is of two smears from a single stool specimen as displayed on a single Hemoccult test slide. A reaction on Hemoccult Tape may appear as any one of the illustrated smears.

HEMOCCULT TAPE

Preparation		Development

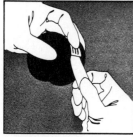

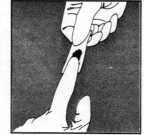

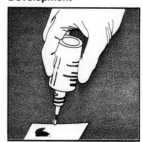

1. Tear strip of tape from dispenser.

2. Apply thin stool smear.

Development

1. Apply two drops of Hemoccult Developer to side opposite smear.
2. Read results on side opposite smear within 60 seconds.

ANY TRACE OF BLUE ON OR AT THE EDGE OF THE SMEAR IS POSITIVE FOR OCCULT BLOOD.

Fig. 6-5 *(continued)*

MATERIALS SUPPLIED (see panel **C**)
- Hemoccult guaiac paper slides (or tape in convenient dispenser)
- Specimen applicators (supplied with slides only)
- Patient envelopes with instructions for specimen collection and diet (supplied with Dispensapak™ units only)
- Hemoccult Developer (in plastic bottles)
- Hemoccult Identification Card

SATISFACTORY LIMITS OF PERFORMANCE; EXPECTED RESULTS
Results with the Hemoccult test are visually determined. The Hemoccult guaiac test paper should be observed for color change within 60 seconds after Developer has been applied.

This reading time is important because the color reaction may fade after two to four minutes.

If any trace of blue on or at the edge of the smear is seen, the test is positive for occult blood. For typical positive reaction, see READING AND INTERPRETATION OF THE HEMOCCULT TEST.

NOTE: Because this test is visually read and requires color differentiation, it should *not* be read by the visually impaired.

The function and stability of the Hemoccult slides and Developer can be tested using the on-slide Performance Monitors. The Hemoccult Tape may be tested by applying a drop of diluted whole blood (1 : 5,000 in distilled water) to an unused portion of the tape. Add Developer to opposite side. If any blue appears, the guaiac-impregnated paper and Developer are functional.

B

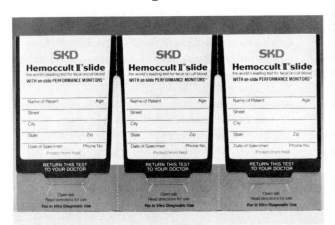

C

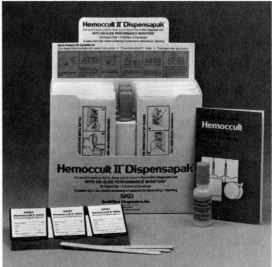

D

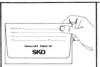 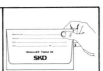

1. Fill in patient information on Hemoccult II* test. Give kit to patient.

2. Patient, at home, opens a cover flap and applies thin stool smear to Box A, a second smear from a different site to Box B. Patient performs procedure for three consecutive bowel movements.

3. Patient returns prepared slides to doctor's office or lab.

 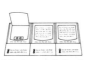

4.Doctor or medical assistant applies two drops of Developer on the back of the slide directly over each smear.

5. Doctor or medical assistant reads results within 60 seconds. Any trace of blue on or at the edge of the smear is positive for blood.

6. Doctor or medical assistant applies ONE DROP ONLY of Developer between the positive and negative Performance Monitors*. A blue color will appear within 10 seconds in the positive Performance Monitor, no blue in the negative Performance Monitor, if the slides and Developer are functional.

INSTRUCTIONS TO THE PATIENT FOR COLLECTING FECAL SPECIMENS FOR THE HEMOCCULT II SLIDE TEST

Hemoccult slides are used routinely to check the intestinal tract. Please follow these instructions carefully. Before you begin, put your name, address, age, and telephone number on the front of each of the three slide sets. Date each pair of specimens on the day that the two specimens are collected.

1. With wooden applicator stick, collect a small stool specimen from the toilet bowl.
2. Spread a very thin smear on box A of first slide. Repeat from a different portion of the stool for box B.
3. Repeat these instructions for the other two slides after your next two bowel movements.
4. Mail the 3 slides as soon as possible in the addressed envelope provided. You will need to add a 22¢ stamp.

IMPORTANT

1. Fecal specimens should not be collected during a menstrual period or while suffering from bleeding hemorrhoids.
2. Protect slides from heat, sunlight, and fluorescent light. Also, do not refrigerate the slides.
3. Follow the special diagnostic diet if your physician has instructed you to do so at least 48 hours before you collect the first stool specimen. Stay on this diet until all slides have been prepared.
4. Mail the 3 completed slides (or as many as you have completed) back to the laboratory *no later than 6 days from the time you collected the first stool specimen.*

dure for performing this test. The American Cancer Society recommends that a stool blood test be performed every year on patients aged 50 years and older.

RESPIRATORY TRACT SPECIMENS

Sputum Specimen Collection

Sputum specimens are examined to help determine the presence of infectious organisms or to identify tumor cells in the respiratory tract. The laboratory findings provide relevant information to the physician when making a diagnosis and initiating treatment.

Other specimens that may be obtained if a patient is unable to produce sputum include tracheal aspirates collected by aspiration with a suction catheter, and bronchial washings and transtracheal aspirates collected by the physician or a pulmonary technician. These specimens are of more value diagnostically than sputum, since they are not likely to become as contaminated with oropharyngeal flora. Nevertheless, because sputum is easy to collect and causes little discomfort to the patient, it is usually the first type of lower respiratory tract specimen to be obtained for examination and culture.

Procedures ordered on sputum specimens when sent to the laboratory include direct smears, routine culture and sensitivities, cultures for acid-fast bacilli (tuberculosis), fungus cultures, and sputum cytology (exfoliative cytology), which is performed to identify tumor cells.

Periodic sputum examinations may also be done on patients receiving antibiotics, steroids, and immunosuppressive agents for prolonged periods, as these agents give rise to opportunistic pulmonary infections.

When you collect sputum specimens, it is essential that you understand the physician's order. For example, if the order states "sputum cultures ×3," this means that you should collect three different specimens at different times or on three successive days. This order *does not* mean that you collect one specimen and divide it into three different containers. Even though these specimens would each be cultured, the findings will show that they were duplicates, thus the whole procedure would have to be repeated.

Vocabulary

exfoliative cytology—Microscopic examination of cells desquamated (shedding) from a body surface as a means of detecting malignant change.

expectorate—The ejection of sputum and other materials from the air passages.

hemoptysis (he-mop'-tĭ-sis)—Coughing up blood as a result of bleeding from any part of the respiratory tract. The appearance of the secretion in true hemoptysis is bright red and frothy with air bubbles.

immunosuppressive agents—Drugs that inhibit the formation of antibodies to antigens that may be present.

saliva (sah-li'vah)—The enzyme-containing secretion of the salivary glands in the mouth.

Technique For Obtaining A Sputum Specimen

Equipment

Sterile specimen container
Glass jar for acid-fast bacilli culture
Cardboard sputum container may be used for other studies
Label
Laboratory requisition
Paper bag and tape

Procedure	Rationale
1. Wash your hands, and assemble the supplies.	
2. Identify the patient, and explain the procedure. Give the sterile specimen container to the patient. Instruct the patient not to touch the inside of the container with the hands.	Obtain freshly expectorated sputum. If feasible, the specimen should be collected in the morning before eating or drinking. Usually a minimum of 5 ml of sputum is required by the laboratory for testing.
3. Instruct the patient to cough deeply and expectorate directly into the container, avoiding contamination to the outside of the container with the sputum.	Sputum (lung and bronchial specimen) is produced by a deep cough. You do not want a specimen of saliva from the mouth.
4. Label the container, and indicate test(s) required on the laboratory requisition (Fig. 6–6).	Accurate, complete information is always required: date, time, patient's name, type of specimen, test(s) to be performed, name of attending physician and, when available, the probable diagnosis.

Procedure	Rationale
5. Send the specimen to the laboratory. a. Secure the sputum container lid with tape. b. Place the container in a paper bag, and attach the laboratory requisition.	Specimens for culture and cytology should be sent to the laboratory within 30 minutes of collection, as any delay can cause organisms to multiply, which would result in misleading findings. Refrigerate the specimen to prevent bacteria overgrowth when it is not sent to the laboratory immediately.
NOTE: Specimens must be as fresh as possible except when accumulation over a specific length of time is ordered. Clearly mark on the label if the specimen is a 24 hour collection.	If a 24 hour specimen is to be obtained, instruct the patient to wrap a paper towel around the jar and secure it with a rubber band. Always keep the lid of the container closed except when in use.
6. Wash your hands.	Avoid contamination.
7. Record on chart. Note any abnormal quality that you may have observed, such as sputum which appears to be blood-tinged.	Charting example: February 25, 19____, 8 AM Sputum specimen obtained; sent to laboratory for C & S [culture and sensitivity]. Marjory Alving, CMA

Fig. 6-6. Sample laboratory requisition for sputum specimen for culture and sensitivity tests.

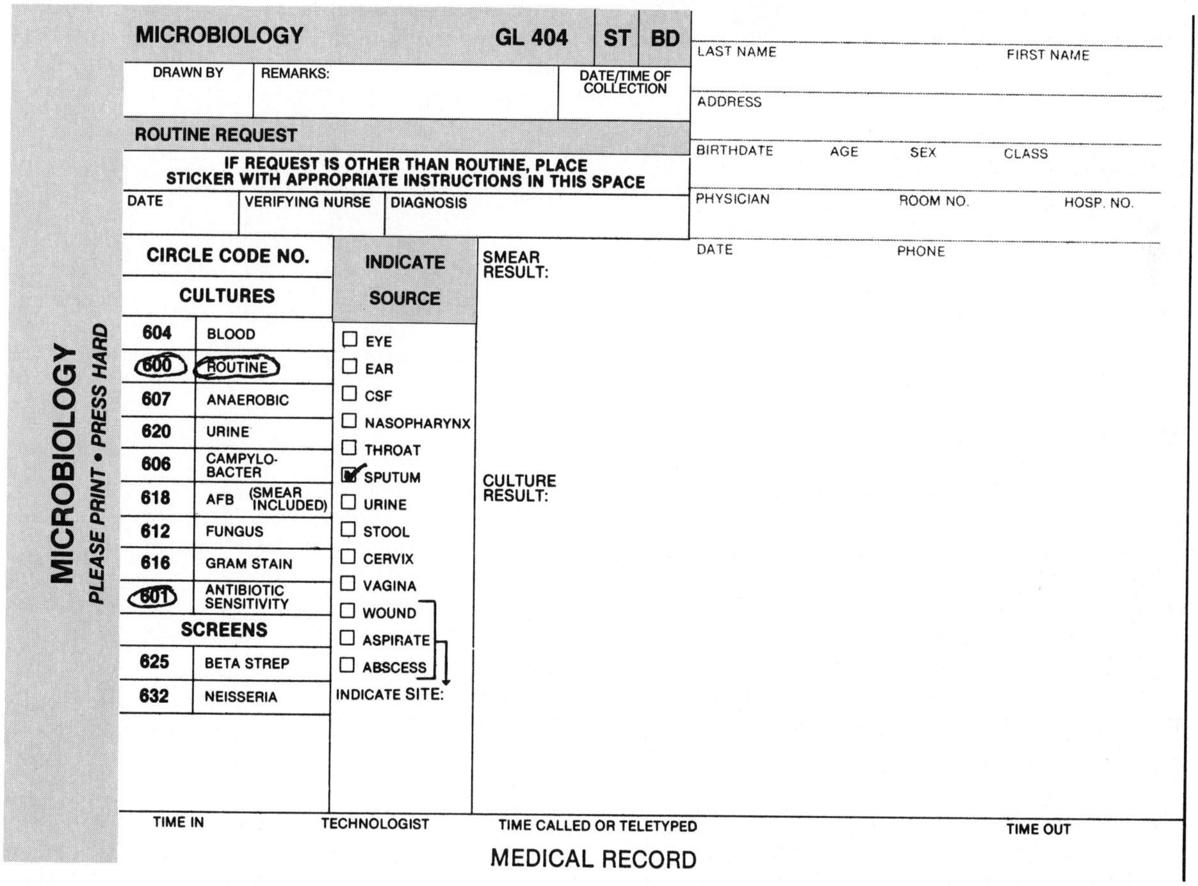
MICROBIOLOGY GL 404 ST BD

DRAWN BY | REMARKS: | DATE/TIME OF COLLECTION

ROUTINE REQUEST

IF REQUEST IS OTHER THAN ROUTINE, PLACE STICKER WITH APPROPRIATE INSTRUCTIONS IN THIS SPACE

DATE | VERIFYING NURSE | DIAGNOSIS

LAST NAME | FIRST NAME

ADDRESS

BIRTHDATE | AGE | SEX | CLASS

PHYSICIAN | ROOM NO. | HOSP. NO.

DATE | PHONE

MICROBIOLOGY
PLEASE PRINT • PRESS HARD

CIRCLE CODE NO. CULTURES		INDICATE SOURCE
604	BLOOD	☐ EYE
600	ROUTINE	☐ EAR
607	ANAEROBIC	☐ CSF
620	URINE	☐ NASOPHARYNX
606	CAMPYLOBACTER	☐ THROAT
618	AFB (SMEAR INCLUDED)	☑ SPUTUM
612	FUNGUS	☐ URINE
616	GRAM STAIN	☐ STOOL
601	ANTIBIOTIC SENSITIVITY	☐ CERVIX
SCREENS		☐ VAGINA
625	BETA STREP	☐ WOUND
632	NEISSERIA	☐ ASPIRATE
		☐ ABSCESS
		INDICATE SITE:

SMEAR RESULT:

CULTURE RESULT:

TIME IN | TECHNOLOGIST | TIME CALLED OR TELETYPED | TIME OUT

MEDICAL RECORD

Throat and Nasopharyngeal Cultures

Upper respiratory secretions most often obtained for examination are throat and nasopharyngeal cultures.

The throat is defined as the area of the body that includes the larynx and pharynx, passageways that link the nose and mouth with the respiratory and digestive systems. A sore throat is caused by inflammation, irritation, or infection of tissue in one or more of the areas in the pharynx or larynx. The common cause of throat infection is the invasion of the tissues by bacteria, such as streptococci, staphylococci, or pneumococci. Inflammation and discomfort in the throat are often caused by tonsillitis, as well as by just an overuse of the voice or excessive smoking.

Throat cultures are performed to determine the presence and the type of microscopic organism that is the cause of an infection. They are frequently ordered for patients suspected of having streptococcal pharyngitis and also for those with suspected cases of pertussis (whooping cough), diphtheria, and gonococcal pharyngitis. The nasopharynx (na"zo-far'ingks) is the part of the pharynx above the soft palate that is connected with the nasal cavities, and provides a passage for air during breathing.

Usually nasopharyngeal cultures are ordered on infants and children (when a sputum specimen cannot be obtained) who are suspected of having whooping cough, pneumonia, or croup. They may also be ordered for patients suspected of being carriers of pathogenic organisms that cause meningitis, diphtheria, scarlet fever, pneumonia, rheumatic fever, and other diseases.

Fig. 6-7. Culturette II and Culturette bacterial collection/transport systems. See the vocabulary for an explanation of these systems. (Courtesy Marion Scientific Corp., Kansas City, MO)

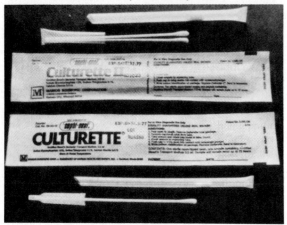

Throat Culture

Equipment

Sterile cotton-tipped applicator(s) in a sterile culture tube(s) or Culturette(s) (Fig. 6–7)
Clean tongue depressor
Laboratory requisition(s)

Procedure	Rationale
1. Wash your hands.	Avoid contamination.
2. Assemble the required equipment.	
3. Identify the patient, and explain the procedure.	Tell the patient that you are going to swab the back of the throat with the cotton-tipped applicator to obtain a specimen that will then be examined in the laboratory. This will help determine the cause of the patient's sore throat.
4. Have the patient assume an upright sitting position facing you.	The area where you are working should be well lighted. You may use an examination light that is positioned to give maximal illumination of the patient's throat.
5. Ask the patient to open the mouth as wide as possible, to extend the tongue, and to say "ah."	Saying "ah" will help relax the patient's throat muscle and minimize the gag reflex.
6. Remove the sterile cotton-tipped applicator(s) from the culture tube *or* from the Culturette tube.	There are commercially prepared culture tubes in which the applicator stick is secured in the lid of the tube.
7. Depress the patient's extended tongue with the tongue blade until the back of the throat is clearly visible (Fig. 6–8).	Place the tongue blade over two thirds of the tongue. This will help prevent the patient's tongue from touching the applicators as you are obtaining the throat specimen.
8. Using the cotton-tipped applicator, swab the area at the very back of the throat on both sides. Particular attention should be taken to swab any red, raw, or raised bumps along the side, and any areas coated with pus.	Care must be taken not to swab the tongue, but only the part of the throat from which the specimen should be obtained. Saliva must be avoided, as this will dilute the specimen, lead to overgrowth of nonpathogens, or inhibit the growth of the pharyngeal flora. Heavy mucus draining down the back of the throat from the nose is also undesirable culture material.

Procedure	**Rationale**

9. Remove the applicator quickly but gently, and place it into the culture tube, securing the lid. If a Culturette has been used, release the transport medium by crushing the ampule with your fingers. NOTE: On occasion, two cultures will be required — one from both the right and left tonsillar areas. Two culture tubes with applicators will be used when doing this, and each must be labeled specifically. Use a quick downward stroke, first on one side and then with *another* applicator, on the opposite side. Keep the tongue depressed while obtaining both specimens.

10. Remove the tongue blade, and discard into covered waste container.

11. Attend to the patient's comfort; you may reposition the patient if necessary.

12. Wash your hands.

13. Label the culture tube(s) completely and accurately.

Patient's name, doctor's name, date, and source of culture.

14. Complete and attach the appropriate laboratory requisition.

The above information is to be included, as well as the type of examination required.

15. Send the culture tube to the laboratory. Avoid delay, so that your specimen will not dry out before the laboratory can transfer it to a culture medium.

In the laboratory the culture will be transferred by the technician to a culture medium, which enables growth of the infectious organism for future examination.

16. Record on chart.

Charting example:

February 27, 19_____, 1PM

Throat culture obtained and sent to laboratory for C & S [culture and sensitivity].

Marcia Edwards, CMA

Nasopharyngeal Culture.   To obtain a better specimen with more organisms, you may induce the patient to cough by taking a throat culture first. Coughing can force organisms from the lower respiratory tract up to the nasopharyngeal area.

Fig. 6-8.   Obtaining a throat culture.

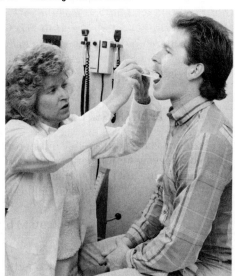

Procedure for Nasopharyngeal Culture

Procedure	Rationale
1. Obtain a throat culture first (if desired), then	
2. Insert a sterile cotton-tipped applicator through the nose into the nasopharyngeal area.	
3. Gently rotate the applicator to obtain the specimen.	
4. Remove the applicator, and place it into the sterile culture tube; secure the lid.	
5. Label and send the specimen to the laboratory with the correct laboratory requisition.	To prevent the drying of the specimen on the applicator, avoid delay.
6. Record the procedure on the patient's chart.	Charting example: February 27, 19_____, 1PM Throat and nasopharyngeal specimens obtained and sent to the laboratory for C & S [culture and sensitivity]. Abby Nelson, CMA

WOUND CULTURE

When it is suspected that a wound is infected, a wound culture is done to determine the presence and the type of microorganism that is causing the infection. Cultures can be obtained from wounds on any part of the body. The procedure for obtaining a wound culture is described on pp. 174–177 in Unit V.

SMEARS FOR CYTOLOGY STUDIES

Obtaining A Cytology Smear

Equipment

Sterile cotton-tipped applicators or Ayer spatulas (number depending on the number of smears to be obtained)

Frosted-end glass slide(s)

Fixative spray, such as Cyto-Fix (a water soluble antiseptic), Spray-Cyte, or bottle of fixative solution (solution of 95% isopropyl alcohol preferred; however, formalin 10% may also be used)

Cardboard or plastic slide holder, rubber band, and envelope provided by the laboratory if the slide is to be mailed

Laboratory requisition

Procedure	Rationale
1. Wash your hands.	
2. Write the patient's name and the date on the frosted end of the slide.	
3. When the physician has obtained the specimen on the applicator or spatula, be prepared to hold the slide while the physician makes the smear, or Take the applicator from the physician with your dominant hand, grasping the distal end of the stick.	
4. Hold the glass slide between your thumb and index finger of your nondominant hand.	
5. Starting near the unfrosted end of the slide,	

Procedure	Rationale

spread the specimen longitudinally along the slide by rotating the applicator in the opposite direction of spreading motion; that is, when spreading the specimen from right to left over the slide, rotate the cotton applicator clockwise (Fig. 6–9).

6. Spread the specimen onto the slide evenly and moderately thin so that individual cells will be able to be identified under a microscope.

7. *Do not touch* your thumb or fingers with the contaminated cotton-tipped applicator.

8. Discard the applicator in a covered waste container.

9. Fix the smear by immediately spraying it with the fixative spray or by immersing it in the bottle of fixative solution obtained from the laboratory. This should be done within 4 seconds to prevent drying and death of cells. Spray 5 to 6 inches away. With a continuous flow, make a stroke from left to right, then right to left. Allow to dry 4 to 6 minutes.

10. Wash your hands.

11. Send the smear in the designated container to the laboratory for cytological tests with the correct and completed requisition (Fig. 6–10).

   NOTE: If you are to mail the slide to a particular laboratory, place the slide inside the cardboard slide holder provided, once the fixative is dry. Close it with a rubber band.

   Fill out the requisition, giving the patient's name, age, LMP (last menstrual period), hormonal or other medication or treatment, pertinent clinical data, and history of any previous atypical Pap smears if this is a vaginal or cervical smear. Insert the slide and requisition into the envelope provided, seal, and mail (see Fig 3–19).

Rationale (for item 11):

In the laboratory, the smear will be incubated for a prescribed time (24 to 72 hours) at 37° C or room temperature, because excessive heating of the smear destroys the microorganisms. To identify specific organisms, the laboratory personnel will use various staining procedures and then examine the smear microscopically.

Fig. 6-9. Making a smear for cytology studies.

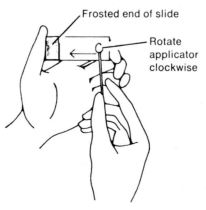

Frosted end of slide

Rotate applicator clockwise

Fig. 6-10. Sample laboratory requisition for cytology studies.

CYTOLOGY—SURGICAL PATHOLOGY REQUISITION. SEE BACK PAGE FOR INSTRUCTIONS

FOR LAB USE ONLY

CYTOLOGY - SLIDE NUMBER _____

PREVIOUS SMEARS: ☐ NO ☐ YES GRADE _____

PERTINENT HISTORY: (MUST BE COMPLETED)

PLEASE PRINT

MATERIAL SOURCE
☐ CERVIX
  ☐ GASTRIC
☐ VAGINA
  ☐ BREAST
☐ SPUTUM
  ☐ CSF
☐ URINE
☐ FLUID
OTHER _____

DATE & TIME OF COLLECT

LAST NAME   FIRST NAME

ADDRESS

BIRTHDATE   AGE   SEX   CLASS

PHYSICIAN   ROOM NO.   HOSP. NO.

DATE   PHONE

NAME OF INSURANCE CO.

NAME OF INSURED & I.D. NO.

ATTACH MEDI-CAL STICKER TO GREEN COPY

LMP / /   HORMONES   LAST PREG.   PREGNANT NOW? ☐ YES ☐ NO   IRRAD-IATION   SURGERY?   POST-MENOPAUSAL

MISCELLANEOUS FINDINGS					ESTROGEN EFFECT		HORMONAL PROFILE		
TEST	MANY	MOD-ERATE	FEW	NONE	HIGH		PB	I	S
RBC					MODERATE	MI			
WBC					LOW				
TRICHOMONAS					ATROPHY	☐ SPECIMEN UNSATISFACTORY			
CANDIDA									
BACTERIA					INVALID DUE TO INFLAMMATION	EXCESSIVE INFLAM.			
ENDOCERVICAL CELLS						SCANTY ☐ DRIED ☐ EXUDATE ☐			

CHARGE TO: ☐ PATIENT   ☐ PHYSICIAN

☐ NEGATIVE   ☐ ABNORMAL   SEE REPORT BELOW

TECHNOLOGIST/ PATHOLOGIST _____

TIME IN   TIME OUT

GENERAL INSTRUCTIONS:

1. Fill out history
2. Label all specimen containers and slides with patient's FULL name.
3. Deliver sputum, fluid and urine specimens within 1 hour of collection; REFRIGERATE until delivery

CERVICAL/VAGINAL PAP SMEAR
1. Prepare 1 or 2 smears of material from scraping of cervical canal and/or cervical os.
2. Place slides in fixative* immediately for a minimum of 10 minutes.

SPUTUM
1. Obtain first morning, deep-cough specimen.
2. Instruct patient to rinse mouth with water before stimulating cough.
3. Collect specimen in container with tightly fitted lid.
4. 50% Alcohol may be added as a preservative if specimen cannot be delivered to laboratory within 2 hours of collection.

BREAST (Nipple Secretion, Cyst Fluid)
1. Prepare 1 or 2 direct smears on a Dakin all-frosted slide.
2. Place slides in fixative* immediately.

BRONCHIAL WASH
PERICARDIAL FLUID
PERITONEAL FLUID
PLEURAL FLUID
} 1. Collect fluid in vacuum bottle or Vacu-Bag.

GASTRIC WASH   Contact Cytology 24 hours in advance for detailed instructions.

SPINAL FLUID
1. Collect 5 to 7 ml of fluid.

URINE
1. Collect 1st morning, clean catch specimen. A catherized specimen is suggested from female patients.

FLUIDS — DELIVER TO LAB IMMEDIATELY

* Fixative in bottle can be obtained in Cytology Lab.

SMEARS FOR BACTERIOLOGY STUDIES

Obtaining A Bacteriology Smear

The procedure for making a smear for bacteriology studies is the same as that for cytology smears (Steps 1 to 8), *except* to fix the smear.

Procedure	Rationale
9. Place the smear on a flat surface and allow to air dry for approximately a half hour.	Air drying allows the specimen cells to dry slowly.
10. Grasp the slide with slide forceps, and pass it quickly through the flame of a Bunsen burner three or four times to *heat fix* the slide. *Do not* overheat the slide, as this will distort the cells present.	Microorganisms are destroyed with the heat and attached to the slide so that they will not wash off when the slide is stained in preparation for examination.
11. Forward the slide to the laboratory in the container provided with the completed laboratory requisition.	

GRAM STAIN

Once a smear is sent to the laboratory it will be treated in various ways so that visualization of microorganisms under a microscope is possible. A method commonly used to identify bacterial organisms is the Gram stain. This staining method permits the classification of bacteria into four basic groups: gram-positive or gram-negative rods and gram-positive or gram-negative cocci. The technique involves the treatment of the smear with Gram crystal violet, Gram iodine solution, 95% ethyl alcohol-acetone decolorizer, and safranin counterstain, after which the forms and structure of the microorganisms can be visualized. Differentiation of bacteria is done on the basis of their color reaction to the above stains. Gram-positive organisms stain purple — for example, staphylococci, streptococci, and pneumococci. Gram-negative organisms are decolorized with the alcohol-acetone solution and will retain only the red color of the counterstain, safranin — for example, gonococci, meningococci, and *Escherichia coli* (*E. coli*). Such a classification has important clinical implications, as it immediately narrows down the differential diagnosis, thus guiding treatment until additional tests, such as culture and sensitivity, are completed. The type of groups in which bacteria are arranged, such as chains, pairs, and clusters, can also be seen on the Gram stain. This is another important guide for treatment.

The Gram stain is usually followed by a culture and sensitivity test to help determine definitive diagnosis and appropriate treatment of an infectious process.

Procedure For A Gram Stain (Fig. 6 – 11)

Equipment

Smear on a glass slide that has been *heat-fixed*
Slide forceps
Staining rack
Wash bottle containing distilled water
Gram crystal violet
Gram iodine solution
95% ethyl alcohol-acetone decolorizer
Safranin counterstain
Bibulous paper pad (absorbent paper pad)

Procedure
1. After making the smear and heat fixing it as described above, place the slide on the staining rack, smear side facing up.
2. Cover the slide with Gram crystal violet. Allow it to react for 1 minute (Fig. 6 – 11, *A*).

Procedure for a Gram Stain (*continued*)

Procedure

3. Grasp the slide with slide forceps and tilt it about 45 degrees to allow the Gram crystal violet to drain off (Fig. 6–11, *B*).

4. Rinse the slide thoroughly with distilled water for about 5 seconds (Fig. 6–11, *C*).

5. Replace the slide on the staining rack.

6. Cover the smear with Gram iodine solution allowing it to react for 1 to 2 minutes.

7. Grasp the slide with the slide forceps and tilt it to a 45 degree angle to allow the Gram iodine solution to drain off.

8. Rinse the slide in this position with distilled water from the wash bottle for 5 seconds.

9. With the slide still tilted at a 45 degree angle, slowly pour the alcohol-acetone solution over it. This will decolorize the smear. Gram-positive bacteria are resistant to decolorization and will retain the Gram crystal violet stain. These bacteria will remain purple. Gram-negative bacteria will now be clear or colorless as they are unable to retain the stain.

10. Rinse the slide with distilled water for 5 seconds.

11. Replace the slide on the staining rack, cover it with the safranin counterstain, and allow it to react for 30 to 60 seconds. The gram-negative bacteria must be counterstained to be seen under the microscope. The safranin counterstain will stain them pink or red.

12. Grasp the slide with the slide forceps and tilt it to a 45 degree angle to allow the safranin counterstain to drain off.

13. Rinse the slide thoroughly with distilled water for 5 seconds.

14. Blot the smear dry between the pages of the bibulous paper pad with the smear side facing down. *Do not rub the slide because you could rub the smear off the slide* (Fig. 6–11, *D*).

15. The slide is now ready to be examined microscopically. Position the slide on the microscope using the oil-immersion objective. Adjust the microscope for the examination of the smear, ensuring that the slide was prepared properly (Fig. 6–11, *E*). (Refer to Unit IX for instructions on using a microscope.)

16. Notify the physician that the smear is ready to be examined.

BACTERIAL CULTURE AND SENSITIVITY (C & S) TESTING

Identification of bacteria may be done by means of a culture. A specimen is put on a culture medium that is conducive to the growth of microorganisms (Fig. 6–12). The culture is then incubated for 24 to 48 hours to allow for the growth of the microorganisms. After this period the appropriate tests are performed to identify the microorganisms present. Most frequently the identification of a specific microorganism is accompanied by a sensitivity study. A sensitivity study determines the sensitivity of bacteria to antibiotics. The disc-plate method is most commonly used clinically (Fig. 6–13). This method measures the inhibition of growth of a microorganism, on the surface of an inoculated culture medium plate, by an antibiotic diffusing into the surrounding medium from an impregnated disc. The organism is reported as being either sensitive, intermediate, or resistant to the antibiotic. When the organism is sensitive to the antibiotic, there will be a clear zone around the impregnated disc. This indicates that the antibiotic was effective in destroying the organism. When there is growth around the impregnated disc, this indicates that the organism cannot be destroyed or inhibited by that antibiotic. The results obtained from a C & S provide the physician with information used to determine which antibiotic can be used to destroy pathogens causing a patient's infectious condition.

Fig. 6-11. Gram stain procedure. **A,** with smear side facing up on the staining rack, cover it with Gram crystal violet. **B,** grasp slide with slide forceps, and tilt it 45 degrees for Gram crystal violet to drain off. **C,** rinse slide with distilled water. **D,** blot the smear dry between pages of bibulous paper. **E,** position slide on microscope using the oil immersion objective for examination.

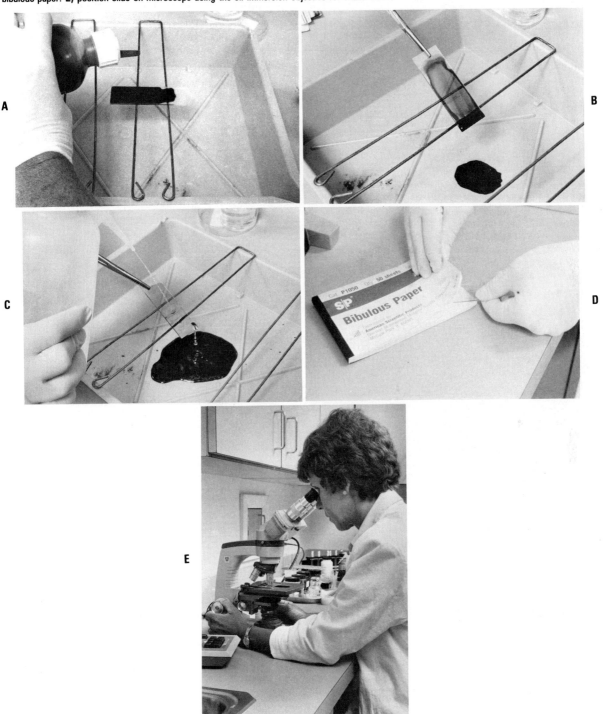

Fig. 6-12. Blood agar culture media contained in a Petri dish showing growth of bacterial colonies.

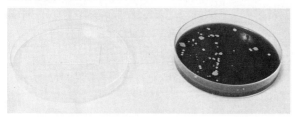

Fig. 6-13. Disc-plate method for sensitivity test. Microorganism being tested is inoculated on the agar medium. Paper discs containing antibiotics are placed on the medium. Clear zones represent inhibition of growth of the microorganism by the specific antibiotic. Zone size is significant. If zone size is smaller than prescribed for clinical effectiveness, the microorganism will be reported as *resistant* to the drug. When the microorganism is *sensitive* to the antibiotic, there will be a clear zone around the impregnated disc.

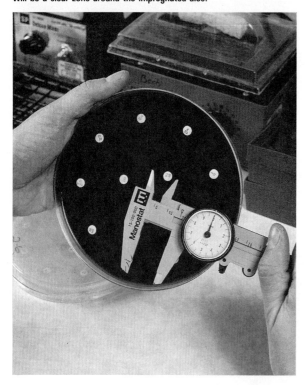

CULTURE MEDIA

A *culture medium* is a sterile commercial preparation used for the growth of microorganisms or other cells. The most commonly used media are broths (liquids), gelatin (solid), and agar (solid). The liquid media are usually prepared in test tubes; solid media are prepared in test tubes or in Petri dishes or plates (round, flat, covered dishes) (see Fig. 6–12).

Liquid media (broths) may be used for the growth of most organisms and for studying the production of gas, odor, and pH changes. Solid media (agar and gelatin base) are used for the growth of organisms, which then allows for the observation of colony size, shape, and color.

The classification of media according to their function and content follows:

- **Enrichment media.** These contain substances that inhibit the growth of various bacteria. They are used especially to isolate organisms that grow in the intestines and to prepare cultures from stool specimens. Examples include chocolate agar and blood agar.
- **Selective media.** These contain substances that suppress the growth of some organisms while enhancing the growth of others. They are used for the examination of stool and sputum specimens, for example, mannitol salt agar, and the modified Thayer Martin media, which are used mainly for suspected gonorrhea specimens and sometimes for detection of meningitis.
- **Differential media.** These contain substances that are used to distinguish between one microorganism and another. They are used to differentiate between forms of colony growth; for example, MacConkey agar is used for routine culturing of stool specimens, and eosin-methylene blue (EMB) agar is used for routine culturing of urine specimens.

Culture media are stored in a refrigerator and warmed to room temperature before being used. If the culture media are cold when used, the microorganisms placed on them will be destroyed. Petri plates are placed in the refrigerator with the media side facing up. Commercial plates come packaged in plastic bags that prevent the media from drying out. These plates will have an expiration date on them. If the expiration date has passed, these plates must not be used.

Inoculating a Culture Medium

Equipment

Sterile cotton-tipped applicators in a sterile tube, or Culturettes

Culture medium—this will vary with the type of specimen collected and the laboratory's preference; for example, Thayer Martin (TM) culture medium is used most frequently for vaginal, cervical, and rectal cultures

Bunsen burner and match

Sterile wire loop in container

Candle jar (see Fig. 6–16)

Procedure

1. Wash your hands.
2. When you or the physician has obtained the specimen, remove the top cover lid of the culture plate and place it upside down on a flat surface.
3. Inoculate the culture plate by rolling the applicator in a large **Z** pattern on the culture medium (Fig. 6–14).
4. Discard the applicator in a covered container for waste materials.
5. Replace the cover lid on the culture plate.
6. Obtain the wire loop and the Bunsen burner.
7. Light the burner, and place the wire loop over the flame until it is red hot.

8. Allow the loop to cool.

9. Remove the lid of the plate, placing it upside down on a flat surface.
10. Cross-streak the inoculated medium with the wire loop. With moderate pressure, crisscross the **Z** with the wire loop (Fig. 6–15).

11. Replace the lid on the culture plate.
12. Reflame the loop to destroy any organisms that were picked up during the streaking process.
13. Return the loop to the storage place. Store the loop with the wire extending out of the container so that the delicate wire will not be destroyed.
14. Label the cover plate with the patient's name, date, and source of specimen.
15. Place the culture plate in a candle jar, with the medium on the top side of the plate (Fig. 6–16).

Rationale

Prevent contamination.
Placing the lid in this manner avoids contamination to the inner surface of the lid, which will cover the culture.

This pattern provides adequate exposure of the organisms on the medium.

Heating the loop destroys unwanted organisms. If these organisms are not destroyed, a contaminated growth of organisms would be found in the culture medium.
If the loop is too hot, it will destroy the organisms that were inoculated on the medium.

Cross-streaking may be done in the laboratory. This spreads the organisms and isolates the colonies from the few contaminants that occasionally grow on selective media.

NOTE: A candle jar is a large gallon jar with a candle burning in it. The lid is tightly closed after the culture plate has been placed in it. When the

Fig. 6-14. Method for inoculating culture medium. (From "Criteria and Techniques for the Diagnosis of Gonorrhea," U.S. Department of HEW/Public Health Service, Centers for Disease Control, Atlanta, GA)

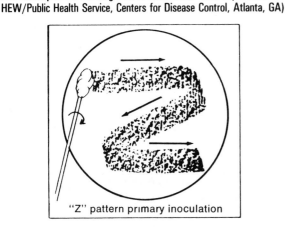

"Z" pattern primary inoculation

Fig. 6-15. Cross streaking inoculated medium with sterile wire loop. (From "Criteria and Techniques for the Diagnosis of Gonorrhea," U.S. Department of HEW/Public Health Service, Centers for Disease Control, Atlanta, GA)

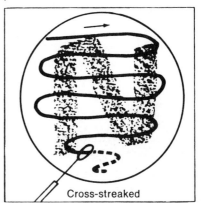

Cross-streaked

Inoculating a Culture Medium (*continued*)

Procedure	Rationale
	oxygen in the jar is depleted, the candle will go out. An appropriate carbon dioxide environment is thus established. The gonococcus bacteria grows best in an environment enriched with carbon dioxide. Each time you place a culture plate in this jar or remove a plate, the candle must be relit.
16. Wash your hands.	
17. Send the culture plate in the candle jar to the laboratory for incubation, along with the appropriate laboratory requisition completed correctly.	The jar will be kept at room temperature for 35° to 36° C. Incubation period is usually 20 to 24 hours. After this period the laboratory worker will examine the culture growth.
18. Record the procedure completely and accurately.	Charting example: February 20, 19_____, 5 PM Cervical and rectal specimens obtained by Dr. Edwards. Culture made and sent to the laboratory for C & S. Judy Dansie, CMA
19. NOTE: Following the determination of the type of organism that has grown on a culture plate, sensitivity tests are usually performed to determine the appropriate antibiotic to use for treatment. The organism grown is subjected to a special plate containing various samples of antibiotics. After a period of incubation, this plate is examined. When no growth is observed around a particular antibiotic sample, this indicates that the particular drug is effective in destroying or controlling the infectious organism causing the disease process in the patient (see Fig. 6-13).	

VAGINAL SMEARS AND CULTURE COLLECTION

To assist the physician in diagnosing various gynecological conditions (for example, cancer of the uterus or cervix, dysplasia, infections, sexually transmitted diseases, and estrogen levels), smears and cultures for cytological and bacteriological tests are obtained from the vagina, cervix, and sometimes the rectum. Some of the more common gynecological laboratory tests include the Pap smear, vaginal smears for trichomoniasis and candidiasis (moniliasis) (common vaginal infections), vaginal smears to determine estrogen levels, and smears and cultures for sexually transmitted diseases (STD); for example, gonorrhea, herpes simplex virus Type II, and chlamydia trachomatis.

General Instructions When Obtaining Vaginal Smears and Cultures For Cytological and Bacteriological Tests

1. Instruct the patient not to douche or use any vaginal medication or have sexual intercourse for 24

Fig. 6-16. Inoculated culture medium plate placed in a candle jar for incubation. The jar provides an environment where bacterial colonies will grow.

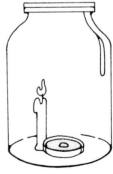

hours before having a specimen taken (some physicians request abstinence from these for 48 hours or up to 3 days before the specimen is obtained).
2. Do not collect vaginal or cervical smears when a woman is menstruating, because the microscopic

readings can be invalid because of the blood cells that are produced during that period.

3. Avoid doing a Pap smear for at least 6 weeks if the cervix has been cauterized and for a longer period if the woman has undergone radiation therapy, as these procedures cause distortion to the cervical cells.

4. Call the laboratory for specific instructions when in doubt on how to collect a particular specimen. Many laboratories will provide all the necessary equipment and instructions.

5. Always wash your hands extremely well before and after assisting with any of these procedures.

6. General preparatory and assisting techniques required are the same as those outlined for assisting with a pelvic examination (see pp. 76–82).

7. Proper and accurate procedures must always be adhered to in order to help the physician make a correct diagnosis and initiate the best treatment possible. It is the medical assistant's responsibility to see that specimens are handled and labeled correctly after the physician has collected them.

The Papanicolaou Smear or Test (Pap Smear). This is probably the most common vaginal and cervical smear done, since the specimen is easily obtained at the same time that a woman is having a pelvic examination. The Pap test is used to detect cervical or uterine cancer. The American Cancer Society recommends the following:

All asymptomatic women age 20 to 40, and those under 20 who are sexually active, have a Pap test annually for two negative examinations and then at least every 3 years.
All asymptomatic women age 40 and over have a Pap test annually for two negative examinations and then at least every 3 years.
Women who are at high risk of developing cervical cancer because of early age at first intercourse,

multiple sexual partners, or other risk factors may need to be tested more frequently.
A pelvic examination should be done as part of a general physical examination every 3 years from age 20 to 40 and annually thereafter.*

Refer to Unit III, Pelvic Examination with a Pap Smear, for more general information, the procedure, method, and assisting techniques used when obtaining this smear for examination.

Vaginal Secretions For Hormone Evaluation. Used to determine a woman's estrogen level, the specimen is obtained from the midlateral vaginal wall on a cotton-tipped applicator or spatula. A smear is then made and sent to the laboratory.

Smear For Trichomoniasis Vaginitis. *Trichomonas* is a genus of parasitic protozoa that occurs in vaginal secretions, causing a vaginal discharge, pruritus (itching), and sometimes a burning sensation when voiding. When trichomoniasis is diagnosed, specific medication such as Flagyl will be prescribed for treatment. This organism is generally passed from one person to another through sexual contact; therefore the patient's partner, who may be a carrier of the infection but is presenting no symptoms, should also be treated.

When obtaining a smear to diagnose this condition, follow the procedure for assembling equipment and preparing and assisting the patient as outlined for obtaining a Pap smear during a pelvic examination (Unit III, pp. 76–82), *except* that a vaginal aspirator may be used rather than an applicator to collect the vaginal discharge, depending on the physician's preference. Follow steps 1 through 13(b) as outlined for the pelvic examination in Unit III, pp. 77–78, then do the following:

*The American Cancer Society: Cancer-related checkups, 1986.

Procedure	Rationale
1. Place a small amount of normal saline on a slide.	The physician will obtain a vaginal specimen by saturating the cotton-tipped applicator with the vaginal discharge (or collect the fluid with the vaginal aspirator).
2. You or the physician then dip the saturated cotton-tipped applicator into the saline solution on the slide (or place the fluid in the aspirator into the saline).	
3. Discard the applicator in a covered container for waste disposal.	
4. Place a coverglass over the depressed section in the middle of the slide.	A *coverglass* is a small, thin piece of glass that will cover the saline and the specimen obtained on the glass slide so that any movement of the live cells can be viewed when the slide is examined under a microscope.

Obtaining a Smear for Trichomoniasis Vaginitis (*continued*)

Procedure	Rationale
5. Send the smear to the laboratory at once, because the organism, if present, will have to be identified immediately.	If the *Trichomonas* organism is present, the laboratory technician will observe a moving flagellated organism when the slide is viewed under the microscope.
6. Assist the patient as required. **7.** Assemble used equipment, and dispose of it according to office or agency policy. Resupply clean equipment as necessary. **8.** Wash your hands. **9.** Record on the patient's chart accurate and complete information.	Refer to steps 14 to 25 as outlined in the pelvic examination procedure in Unit III. Charting example: February 9, 19____, 1:15 PM Vaginal smear for *Trichomonas* obtained by Dr. Rouse. Specimen sent to the laboratory immediately. Patient sent home with a prescription to be filled pending positive test results from the lab. Mike King, CMA

Smear for Monilial Vaginitis. *Monilia,* now commonly referred to as *Candida,* is a yeastlike fungus. This is often referred to as simply a yeast infection by the general public. It is often in the female's vagina without causing any symptoms, and at other times it will produce an uncomfortable white, cheesy or curdlike vaginal discharge, itching, and irritation of the vulva.

Yeast infections are not commonly transmitted by sexual contact; the organisms are found everywhere. Frequently, infections tend to recur. The treatment generally includes the use of vaginal suppositories or creams that the physician will prescribe. The procedure for obtaining this smear is identical to the one just described for trichomoniasis, *except* the following three steps should be done first.

1. Place a small amount of saline on a slide.
2. Add (mix) 10% potassium hydroxide (KOH) to the saline.
3. Proceed as was described in steps 2 through 9.

NOTE: If the *Monilia* organism is present on the smear, the laboratory technician will observe the branching arms of the fungus when it is viewed under a microscope.

Smears and Cultures To Detect Gonorrhea. Gonorrhea is a highly contagious, sexually transmitted disease caused by the bacterial organism, *Neisseria gonorrhoeae,* or the gonococcus. Symptoms in a man usually occur within 1 week after exposure; a woman experiences no early symptoms. A man will have a burning sensation when voiding and a whitish fluid discharge or pus from the penis. Women may experience pain in the lower abdomen, with or without a whitish vaginal discharge or a burning sensation when voiding. Penicillin and other antibiotics or the sulfonamide drugs are all effective treatment. Cure for gonorrhea occurs relatively rapidly, although the patient is not considered cured until cultures taken of the discharge are negative for 3 to 4 weeks. Although gonorrhea is contracted through sexual contact, the gonococcus bacteria can infect the eyes (gonorrheal conjunctivitis) or a break in the skin or an open wound. Thus, the importance of preventing contamination to yourself and others with specimens obtained from patients suspected of having gonorrhea cannot be overemphasized. Avoid touching your eyes, and always wash your hands extremely well after assisting the physician when a specimen is obtained.

Procedure. For direct smears to be examined, urethral, endocervical, and vaginal specimens are collected and smeared evenly and moderately thinly on two glass slides, then fixed and dried for 4 to 6 minutes (as described previously). Some physicians may obtain a specimen from the anal canal, and also from the oropharynx, a common local source for disseminated gonococcal infection. The anal specimen is obtained by inserting a sterile cotton-tipped applicator approximately 1 inch into the anal canal. The applicator is moved from side to side; 10 to 30 seconds are allowed for absorption of the organisms on the applicator. A smear is then made and fixed. The oropharynx culture is obtained by swabbing the posterior pharynx and tonsillar crypts with a cotton-tipped applicator.

When a culture is desired, two sterile cotton-tipped applicators or Culturettes are used to collect the specimen. One is placed in a sterile culture tube or Culturette. The second applicator with the specimen is streaked across a special culture medium, such as the Thayer Martin medium. Both specimens are sent to the laboratory together.

CHLAMYDIA TRACHOMATIS: THE DIRECT SPECIMEN TEST*

The Chlamydiae are a large group of obligate intracellular parasites closely related to gram-negative bacteria. There are two species: *Chlamydia trachomatis*, primarily a human pathogen; and *Chlamydia psittaci*, primarily an animal pathogen.

The chlamydial infections of trachoma, inclusion conjunctivitis, and lymphogranuloma venereum have been recognized and studied for many years. However, the chlamydiae have only recently been identified as important etiological agents in sexually transmissible diseases. The prevalence of these chlamydia-related diseases and the population at risk are thought to exceed those of gonorrhea. *Chlamydia trachomatis*, the nation's most common sexually transmitted disease, is now known to cause urethritis, epididymitis, proctitis, cervicitis, pelvic inflammatory disease, infant pneumonia, and conjunctivitis. It has also been implicated in Reiter's syndrome and premature birth. In both sexes, the infection *may be asymptomatic.*

Females risk the most serious complication of chlamydial infection—acute salpingitis—and they can pass the infection to their newborn infants and sexual partners. Because of these risks, specific diagnosis of *C. trachomatis* in the large population of asymptomatic females is critical.

In addition to being undetected in large proportions of the female population, the organism is masked in another large population: men and women who have gonorrhea. Often chlamydia cannot be differentiated from gonorrhea on the basis of symptoms alone. The result—gonorrhea is treated, while the *C. trachomatis* goes undetected. Moreover, chlamydia and gonorrhea may require different antibiotic treatment.

The common thread running through all of these aspects, and the most significant element in terms of control, has been the difficulty of diagnosis. Clinically visible signs (e.g., macroscopic appearance of cervix, amount of vaginal discharge) are not specific for chlamydial infection, nor are cellular changes seen on Pap smears. Tissue culture, though extremely sensitive and specific, requires a considerable technical and financial commitment and, hence, is unavailable to most physicians. Also, results from tissue cultures are not available until 4 to 6 days later.

Current efforts to control chlamydial infections have been limited by this lack of adequate diagnosis. Asymptomatic and recurrent infections have gone undetected and coinfections have been treated inappropriately.

Practical Screening: The Direct Specimen Test*

Screening for chlamydial infections in asymptomatic women requires a diagnostic method that is less costly, less complex, and more available than tissue culture. *The MicroTrak™ Direct Specimen Test* meets these criteria while retaining the sensitivity and specificity of tissue culture.

Using monoclonal antibodies labeled with fluorescein, the direct specimen test can detect and identify the smallest forms of the organisms, elementary and reticulate bodies, in direct urethral or cervical smears. Diagnosis can be made within 30 minutes after specimen receipt in the laboratory. No cell culture is required.

As simple a procedure for a physician to perform as a Pap smear, the cervix (or, in the male, the urethra) is swabbed to remove a smear specimen. The specimen is rolled onto a glass slide, fixed with acetone and sent to the laboratory at room temperature. In the laboratory, the slide is stained with *MicroTrak's* antibody solution, causing chlamydia, if present, to appear as individual, bright apple-green pinpoints on a background of reddish cells when viewed through a fluorescence microscope, a typical item available in most large laboratories. MicroTrak Mounting Fluid contains photobleaching retardant to inhibit fading of fluorescence during examination of the specimen (Fig. 6-17).

This simple test design allows specific diagnosis of *Chlamydia trachomatis* in exactly the screening situations that must be tapped: prenatal clinics, family planning clinics, gynecologic offices, and abortion clinics. Further, any routine pelvic examination during which a Pap smear is taken can now be seen as an opportunity to screen for *C. trachomatis*. In populations of women under 25 years of age, where *C. trachomatis* is about forty times more prevalent than abnormal cytology, the rationale for such Pap/MicroTrak™ testing is apparent. With the rapid results afforded by the new test, physicians can prevent further spread to sexual partners or neonates by beginning specific treatment immediately, even while patients are still in the clinic. Follow-up testing to document cure also becomes more convenient.

These advances will undoubtedly contribute to a more targeted therapy and an eventual reduction in the number of chlamydial infections. Similar applications of monoclonal antibody technology are being developed for herpes simplex virus, gonorrhea, and other infectious diseases. The promise for improved diagnosis in these areas is equally great.

HERPES SIMPLEX VIRUSES; DISEASES, DIAGNOSIS, AND TYPING*

Herpes simplex viruses (HSV) are ubiquitous among humans. Once acquired, HSV can remain latent in the regional sensory ganglia and, when reactivated, move back along the sensory nerves to produce recurrent infections. HSV infections include genital le-

*Courtesy MicroTrak/Syva Company, Palo Alto, CA.

*Courtesy MicroTrak/Syva Company, Palo Alto, CA.

Fig. 6-17. Procedure for Chlamydia Trachomatis Direct Specimen Test. (Courtesy Micro Trak/Syva Company, Palo Alto, CA)

Procedure

Collection

The specimen is swabbed from the urethra, endocervical canal, rectum or neonatal conjunctiva and applied directly to the slide, where it is fixed and sent to the laboratory.
(Recommended: MicroTrak™ Specimen Collection Kit containing 2 swabs, slide with 8 mm well, acetone fixative, and transport pack.)

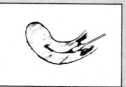

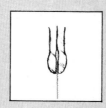

Staining

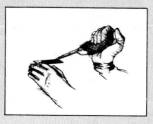

The fixed specimen is stained with MicroTrak™ Reagent and incubated at room temperature for 15 minutes.

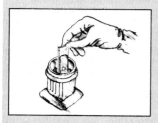

A rinse step removes unbound antibody. The slide is allowed to dry.

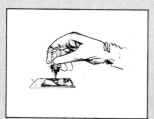

Mounting fluid (provided) is added and the coverslip is applied.

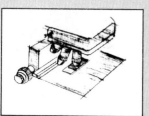

Viewed under the fluorescence microscope, positive specimens contain fluorescent apple-green chlamydial organisms.

See package insert for full instructions

sions, cold sores, pharyngitis, ocular keratitis, and encephalitis.

The viruses are classified as type 1 or 2 according to their genetic and antigenic composition. Although each type has been associated with a characteristic pattern of infection (oral HSV 1 and genital HSV 2), the site of infection is not an accurate predictor of the virus type. For example, HSV 1 is now suspected to cause a significant proportion of primary genital herpes.

Specific diagnosis of HSV infection is required in many situations, including infections of neonates, immunocompromised patients, or individuals suspected of having herpes encephalitis. In addition, specific diagnosis is useful in the counseling of sexually active individuals. Typing may have utility in (a) prognosis, since it has been reported that the recurrence rate of genital HSV 1 infection is less than that of genital HSV 2, (b) treatment, since it has been reported that the antiviral activity of chemotherapeutic agents can differ between the two HSV types, and (c) epidemiological research, where an association of HSV infection with other disease processes such as cervical carcinoma is being studied.

Virus isolation in tissue culture is routinely used for diagnosing HSV infections. Although tissue culture amplifies small numbers of infectious organisms for detection, it requires special facilities and 1 to 7 days before a result can be reported. Culture has stood as a generally recognized reference method, but recovery is recognized to be less than 100%.

Direct examination of viral antigen in cells obtained from lesions provides results more rapidly. A poorly prepared slide can be rapidly identified so that another specimen can be obtained promptly. It must be recognized, however, that viral antigen is identified by stained specimens, and no direct association with infectivity can be made.

Several laboratory methods of typing HSV have been reported, including plaque size, pock size on chorionic membrane, neutralization, ELISA, restriction endonuclease analysis, BVDU [E-5-(2-bromovinyl)-2'-deoxyuridine] sensitivity, and immunofluorescence.

The Syva MicroTrak HSV 1/HSV 2 Direct Specimen Identification/Typing Test and Culture Confirmation/Typing Test*

The Syva MicroTrak HSV 1/HSV 2 Direct Specimen Identification/Typing Test can provide typing results within 30 minutes of specimen receipt. The test can easily be used for the identification and typing of HSV in clinical specimens taken directly from external lesions (Fig. 6-18, *A* and *B*).

Cell culture must be initiated at the same time the direct specimen is taken. This allows recourse to the

*Courtesy MicroTrak/Syva Company.

Fig. 6-18.   A, Syva MicroTrak specimen Collection Kit. **B,** HSV 1/HSV 2 Direct Specimen Identification/Typing Test. (Courtesy MicroTrak/Syva Company)

A

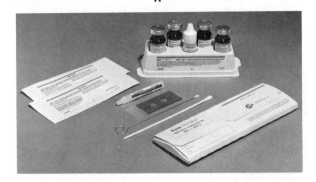

B

Procedure

Collection

The specimen is swabbed from the base of the lesion and applied directly to two slide wells, which are then fixed and sent to the laboratory. (Recommended: MicroTrak™ Specimen Collection Kit containing 2 swabs, slide with 8 mm wells, acetone fixative, and transport pack.)

Samples of poor quality may result in false negative determinations. A sample for isolation in cell culture must therefore be taken at the same time as the direct specimen. This allows recourse to the culture if a direct specimen is negative or inadequate for analysis.

Staining

culture result if a direct specimen is negative or inadequate for analysis.

Samples are taken by swabbing the base of the lesion with two Dacron-tipped swabs simultaneously. One swab is used to apply the specimen directly to a dual-well microscope slide, which is then air dried and fixed with acetone. The other swab is placed in a transport medium and both specimens are sent to the laboratory. Monoclonal antibodies that react specifically with HSV 1 or HSV 2 have been prepared and labeled with fluorescein isothiocyanate. At the laboratory, one well on the dual-well slide is stained with HSV 1 Reagent and the other well with HSV 2 Reagent.

The labeled antibodies bind specifically to their respective viral antigens, and rinse step removes unbound antibody. When slides are viewed under a fluorescence microscope, cells that are positive for the particular viral type show apple-green fluorescent staining that is characteristic of infection with HSV 1 and HSV 2, as demonstrated in the positive control wells; negative cells show only counterstaining, as demonstrated in the negative control wells. The absence of positive cells in the specimen wells should be interpreted cautiously.

In the culture procedure, the transport medium is inoculated into two tissue culture tubes. After the specimens have been cultured, cells are transferred to two slide wells, air dried, fixed with acetone, and tested with the Syva MicroTrak HSV 1/HSV 2 Culture Confirmation/Typing Reagents.

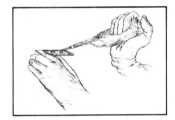

One fixed specimen is stained with HSV 1 Reagent and the other is stained with HSV 2 Reagent. The slide is incubated either at room temperature for 30 minutes or at 37 °C for 15 minutes.

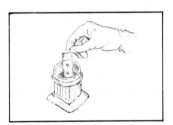

A rinse step removes unbound antibody. The slide is allowed to dry.

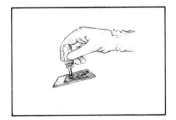

Mounting fluid (provided) is added and the coverslip is applied.

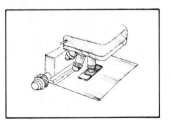

Viewed under the fluorescence microscope, positive cells display characteristic fluorescent apple-green staining. (Specimen quality is checked by evaluating the counterstained cells.)

LUMBAR PUNCTURE

A lumbar puncture (LP) is the insertion of a thin, hollow needle into the subarachnoid space of the spinal canal, usually between the third and fourth (L-3 and L-4) or between the fourth and fifth lumbar vertebrae (L-4 and L-5) to withdraw cerebrospinal fluid (CSF) or to inject air or a radiopaque contrast medium into this space. This procedure, also referred to as a spinal puncture or a spinal tap, is done under aseptic conditions for both diagnostic and therapeutic purposes.

For diagnostic purposes, a lumbar puncture is done to

- Obtain a specimen of CSF for laboratory examination, for example: microscopic examination to determine the presence of white blood cells, red blood cells, neoplastic cells, and microorganisms; chemical determinations for sugar and protein; serology tests to detect syphilis and certain viral infections
- Determine the presence of an obstruction to the flow of the CSF
- Measure the pressure within the cerebrospinal cavities
- Inject air into the subarachnoid space for certain x-ray examinations of the skull, such as a pneumoencephalogram
- Inject a radiopaque contrast medium into the subarachnoid space for an x-ray examination of the spinal canal and cord (myelogram)

For therapeutic purposes, a lumbar puncture may be performed to relieve cerebrospinal pressure, or to remove pus or blood from the subarachnoid space. It is also necessary for the injection of a spinal anesthetic.

Equipment for a Lumbar Puncture

A sterile prepackaged or disposable set containing the following:
   Lumbar puncture needles, 20 to 22 gauge, 3 to 5 inches long (size may be specified by the physician)
   Three way-stopcock
   Needles, 22 gauge, 1½ inch; and 25 gauge, ½ inch; and a 3 ml syringe for injecting a local anesthetic
   Spinal fluid manometer for measuring CSF pressure
   Local anesthetic—usually 1% lidocaine (Xylocaine) 10 mg/ml, or procaine
   Three sterile gauze sponges, 2 × 2 inch
   Sterile drape towel
   Sterile fenestrated drape (drape sheet with an open window or hole in it)
   Three swab sticks (stick with a small sponge on the end)
   Three sterile test tubes fitted with snap-top or screw-on caps, for the collection of the CSF
   Small sterile container for antiseptic solution, which will be used on the patient's skin
   Band-Aid or gauze and tape for dressing at site of puncture when the needle is withdrawn
Additional supplies needed:
   Sterile gloves
   Local anesthetic, if not on sterile tray
   Skin antiseptic, such as Betadine
   Soap and water
   Blood pressure cuff (may be used if a Queckenstedt test is to be performed)
   Laboratory requisition

This is a sterile procedure; excellent aseptic technique must be adhered to in order to avoid any possibility of introducing microorganisms into the spinal canal. It is more frequently done in a hospital or clinic where the patient may rest, lying flat for at least 6 hours after the procedure has been completed.

Procedure	Rationale
1. Wash your hands.	
2. Assemble the required supplies and equipment.	
3. Identify the patient, and explain the procedure. Explain what is to occur and how it may feel. This helps alleviate some fear of the unknown, thus allowing the patient to relax somewhat and cooperate during the procedure.	You may explain to the patient that there is no danger of injury to the spinal cord, as it does not extend past the second lumbar vertebra, and the physician will be inserting the needle at a location that is lower than that level.
4. Have the patient void; save a specimen if required.	A full bladder will only provide additional discomfort for the patient.
5. Provide a patient gown, and have the patient disrobe completely. The gown should be put on with the opening in the back.	
6. Summon the physician into the room.	
7. Using aseptic technique, open the sterile glove pack and the outer wraps of the LP tray for the physician.	The physician will don the sterile gloves, then prepare the supplies on the tray for use. The tray and all contents are sterile on all surfaces.

Procedure	Rationale

8. Position the patient on the side with a pillow under the head. The knees must be drawn up toward the chest and the head bent forward as close as possible to the knees.

9. Cleanse the skin with soap and water at and around the site to be entered; then prepare (swab) this area with the antiseptic solution by taking a sterile swab stick soaked in the desired antiseptic solution.

Because the patient's skin is the most likely source of contamination, it must be disinfected before the puncture is done. It is best to start at the area that will be punctured and cleanse and prepare in a circular outward fashion. The physician may choose to do the skin preparation after donning sterile gloves. In this case, the assistant pours the antiseptic solution into the small sterile container on the tray.

After the skin is prepared, the physician drapes the area with the fenestrated drape and the towel.

10. Assist the physician as required. When using a stock supply of local anesthetic solution, hold the vial, check the label, and repeat the name and dosage of the drug aloud so that the physician hears what you are saying. Then hold the vial so that the physician can also read the label before withdrawing the solution into the needle and syringe.

This step is omitted if the drug ampule is supplied on the tray, because the physician alone would check the label and withdraw the drug.

11. Help the patient maintain the correct position. Explain to the patient the importance of remaining very still. You may stand on the side facing the patient's front and hold onto the back of the knees and shoulder. Tell the patient to breathe slowly and deeply through the mouth.

Using the 3 ml syringe with the 25 gauge needle, the physician administers the local anesthetic. For deep infiltration, the 22 gauge, 1½ inch needle is used. The usual dose of lidocaine is 1 to 2 ml. Supporting the patient helps prevent sudden moves that (1) make it more difficult for the physician to insert the spinal needle or (2) cause the needle to break or (3) cause trauma to the surrounding tissues.

12. Once the spinal needle is in place, instruct and help the patient to slowly straighten the legs (this prevents a false increase in intraspinal pressure), and to breathe normally, that is, not to hold the breath or strain.

The spinal puncture needle is introduced into L3-4 or L4-5 interspace, which is below the level of the spinal cord. To take a pressure reading, the physician will attach the stopcock to the spinal needle and the manometer into the stopcock. At this time you may be asked to record the pressure reading.

13. Be ready to receive the specimens of CSF once the physician has obtained them. Check that the caps are secured tightly; stand tubes upright for sending to the laboratory. Some disposable trays have depressions in which the physician places the tubes upright, after securing the caps on tightly.

Approximately 2 ml of fluid is collected in each of the three test tubes for observation, comparison, and analysis. Normal CSF is clear, colorless, and sterile.

If asked to assist with a Queckenstedt test, which is done when a spinal tumor is suspected, follow this procedure.

14. Place a blood pressure cuff around the patient's neck and inflate it to a pressure of 22 mm Hg (the physician will attach the manometer),
    or
    you may be asked to compress the jugular veins for 10 seconds, then release either the cuff or your own pressure on the jugular veins.

Normally, there is a rapid rise in pressure of the CSF when the veins are compressed and a rapid return to normal when compression is released. When the pressure rises and falls slowly, this indicates a blockage due to a lesion or tumor that is compressing the spinal subarachnoid pathways.

Lumbar Puncture (*continued*)

Procedure	Rationale
These pressure readings are done at 10 second intervals and measured each time the veins are compressed.	
15. Note any unusual reaction in the patient, for example, a change in the patient's color, respiratory rate, or pulse rate. If you do note any of these changes, inform the physician in a manner that will not alarm the patient.	
16. After the needle is withdrawn, you may place a Band-Aid or gauze dressing over the puncture site.	
17. Assist the patient as required. It is highly advisable to keep the patient lying flat for 6 to 12 hours (up to 24 hours is recommended) to help avoid headaches. If this procedure was done in the office or clinic, keep the patient lying flat for as long as is possible before sending him or her home. Encourage the patient to take a liberal amount of fluids. Inform the patient of any special instructions.	Frequently glucose or saline is administered intravenously to a patient with a severe headache. An ice cap and aspirin may also be given to alleviate a headache.
18. Label and send specimens obtained to the laboratory with the completed requisition.	Spinal fluid is to be stored in an incubator, *not* a refrigerator, as it may contain organisms that are sensitive to cold.
19. Return to the examining room to assemble all used supplies and equipment, dispose of them properly, and replace clean equipment as necessary.	
20. Wash your hands.	

21. Do any recording required of you accurately and completely. NOTE: Physicians may wish to vary the procedural details according to their technique and judgment.	Charting example:
	    Feb. 11, 19_____, 2 PM
	        Lumbar puncture done by Dr. Cox. Three CSF specimens sent to lab for examination. Opening pressure reading was 250 mm H_2O. Spinal fluid appeared slightly blood-tinged.
	        Patient had no complaints at this time and is resting quietly in the office bed.
	        Susan Oliver, CMA

CONCLUSION

You have now completed the unit, Collecting and Handling Specimens. When you have practiced the procedures sufficiently, arrange with your instructor to take the Performance Test. You will be expected to demonstrate accurately your ability to prepare for and to assist with all the procedures outlined in this unit and to perform some of them. In addition you will be expected to identify accurately the supplies and equipment by the proper name when questioned by your instructor.

REVIEW OF VOCABULARY

The following are samples of information seen on various patient charts. In each of these samples, words that have been defined for you are used. Read these, and define the italicized terms.

1. Chief complaint: *Diuresis* and *frequency* for the past two months. Laboratory data: urine specimen obtained for *C & S*, and a routine urinalysis. Results: C & S showed no growth and no cells; *routine urinalysis*—sugar 4+; acetone, moderate.
2. History: This 35-year-old white female accountant has approximately nine *bowel movements* a day

times 4 months, increased by activity and eating either fatty or sugary foods. The *stools* are loose and have no form. There is some mucus in the stools and some *melena*. She had problems with *constipation* up until 4 months ago. Stools are extremely foul smelling. *Tarry stools* were followed with *guaiac tests; occult blood stools* were noted. Question of *GI bleeding*.

3. History: This 54-year-old gentleman stated that he first coughed up some bright red blood in his *sputum* about 3 weeks ago. The *hemoptysis* occurred again 1 week ago. He has a chronic cough and has smoked two packs of cigarettes daily for the past 15 years.
   Sputum exfoliative cytology: There was a single group of highly atypical cells present, with nuclear feature strongly suggestive of malignancy, although the nuclei are partially obscured by the blood and show some degenerative changes.

4. This patient was first seen 1 week ago, at which time she complained of lower abdominal pain and *dysuria*. The patient also indicated that she had noted progressive *vaginal discharge* during the past week. The patient had previously been followed in the *GYN* clinic at City Hospital because of repeated *Pap smears* that showed *dysplasia* consistent with malignancy. A cervical biopsy was done, but the pathology specimen showed no malignancy.
   Vaginal and endocervical smears were obtained and sent to the lab for *Trichomonas* and *Monilia examinations*. Treatment pending positive laboratory results.

5. This patient complained of severe, persistent pain in the lower back radiating down the right leg. After a complete examination was done, this patient was referred to the x-ray department for a *myelogram*.

6. *Rectal, cervical, and throat cultures* showed no *gonorrhea*.

7. *Vaginitis*, secondary to the steroid treatment. The patient has had well-documented *Candida* growth in her vaginal mucosa and has been treated with Mycostatin suppositories.

Pathology Report

The following is a pathology report received in the physician's office after the patient had surgery because of an abnormal Pap smear and postmenopausal bleeding. After reading this you should be able to discuss the contents with your instructor. A dictionary or other reference book may be used to define terms that are not familiar to you.

PATIENT: Pat Lewis
DATE OF BIRTH: 7-09-27
DATE RECEIVED: 12-12-87
PREOPERATIVE DIAGNOSIS: Abnormal Pap smear, postmenopausal bleeding.
POSTOPERATIVE DIAGNOSIS: Same.
SOURCE OF TISSUE: (A) D & C currettings (B) Cold cone biopsy
OPERATION: Biopsy

GROSS DESCRIPTION

A. Specimen consists of bits of glistening mucoid pink to reddish material, totaling about 1 cm in aggregate. Totally embedded in one cassette.
B. Specimen consists of a somewhat cone-shaped piece of pink rubbery tissue, 1.8 cm in maximum diameter and varying from 1 to 1.7 cm in height. A widely patulous, round external os, 1 cm in diameter, occupies the cervical aspect.

MICROSCOPIC DESCRIPTION

A. Sections show one intact fragment of endometrial tissue with a single nonsecretory gland and compact stroma along with fragments of glandular tissues lined usually by low columnar inactive cells. A rare gland shows slightly taller lining and some perinuclear vacuoles within the cytoplasm.
B. Sections show a moderately severe chronic and subacute cervicitis and endocervicitis with many of the endocervical glands located in the exocervical tissues and opening almost up to the surface. Some of these glands are lined by atypical reactive cells. The overlying squamous epithelium shows thickening and areas of parakeratosis and rather marked hyperkeratosis. Occasional granular cell layer is present, and the epithelium is infiltrated with occasional inflammatory cells. The endocervical mucosa is denuded, covered with fibrin and fresh blood. Stroma shows infiltrated chronic inflammatory cells along with an occasional lymphoid follicle. No evidence of malignancy.

DIAGNOSIS

A. Fragments of nonsecretory endometrial glands.
B. Severe chronic and subacute cervicitis and endocervicitis, conization.

M. L. McArthur, MD

REVIEW QUESTIONS

1. List four types of material that can be obtained from a patient's body for laboratory examination.
2. What is meant by "special preparation" of the patient before collecting a specimen?
3. List three types of specimens for which active participation of the patient is required.
4. After obtaining a throat culture, you accidentally drop the lid of the culture tube on the floor. What action would you take before sending the specimen to the laboratory?
5. What specimens should be kept refrigerated if you cannot send them to the laboratory immediately, and why do you refrigerate them?
6. Itemize all the information that should be written on a laboratory requisition when submitting a specimen to the laboratory for examination.

7. You have obtained a wound culture and have sent it to the laboratory for a C & S. Explain what types of testing will be performed on the culture and the purpose of these tests.
8. Why is it important for you to wash your hands before and after obtaining any type of specimen from a patient?
9. List information that you should provide to patients when they are collecting a urine specimen at home.
10. Explain the procedure for fixing a smear; state the value and use of smears.
11. Explain the procedure for inoculating culture media.
12. In what position would you place a patient who is to have a vaginal smear taken? Why?
13. When a physician is doing a lumbar puncture on the patient, where would the spinal needle be inserted and why at this location?
14. List and compare the three classifications of culture media as described in this unit.
15. What is the purpose of performing an occult blood test on a stool specimen?
16. List three substances that may affect the color of a stool specimen.
17. What is the purpose(s) of obtaining a sputum specimen from a patient? Describe the explanation that you would give to a patient who is to collect a sputum specimen.
18. Name two common vaginal infections that are diagnosed by means of vaginal smears.

PERFORMANCE TEST

In a skills laboratory, a simulation of a joblike environment, the medical assistant student is to demonstrate skill and knowledge in performing the following procedures without reference to source materials. For these activities the student will need a person to play the role of the patient. Time limits for the performance of each procedure are to be assigned by the instructor (see also pp. 32 and 35).

1. Given an ambulatory patient and the appropriate supplies, prepare for, give explanations to the patient for, and obtain the following: (a) urine specimen, (b) stool specimen, (c) sputum specimen, (d) throat culture, (e) nasopharyngeal culture, (f) wound culture.
2. Given an ambulatory patient and the required equipment, prepare for, give explanations to the patient for, and assist with the following procedures:
   (a) Vaginal smears and cultures
   (b) Preparing a smear from the specimen obtained by the physician
   (c) Lumbar puncture
3. Having obtained the above specimens, smears, and cultures, complete the appropriate laboratory requisition form, forward all to the laboratory for examination and record the procedure on the patient's chart.
4. Given the required supplies, demonstrate the correct procedure for staining a smear using the Gram stain.
5. Given the required supplies, demonstrate the proper procedure for performing a hemoccult slide test on a stool specimen.
6. Given the required supplies, demonstrate how to inoculate a culture medium.

The student is expected to perform the above with 100% accuracy 95% of the time.

PERFORMANCE CHECKLISTS

Clean-catch Urine Specimen

1. Wash your hands.
2. Assemble required equipment and supplies.
3. Identify the patient, and explain the procedure. Supply the patient with the appropriate supplies required to wash the genital area and collect the urine specimen.
4. Receive the specimen from the patient.
5. Label the specimen, and complete the laboratory requisition.
6. Send the specimen with the requisition to the laboratory.
7. Wash your hands.
8. Record the procedure on the patient's chart.

Stool Specimen

1. Wash your hands.
2. Assemble the required equipment and supplies.
3. Identify the patient, and explain the procedure.
4. Prepare the label for the specimen container, and complete the laboratory requisition.
5. Receive the bedpan with specimen from the patient, cover it, and take to your work area.
6. Transfer a portion of the specimen into the container, using a clean tongue blade as a spoon; place the lid securely on the container.
7. Discard the used tongue blade in a bag, close securely, and dispose of in a container for waste materials.
8. Clean and empty bedpan.
9. Wash your hands.
10. Send the specimen with a completed laboratory requisition to the laboratory.
11. Wash your hands.
12. Record the procedure on the patient's chart.

Sputum Specimen

1. Wash your hands.
2. Assemble the required equipment.
3. Identify the patient, and explain the procedure.
4. Receive the specimen from the patient; secure the container with paper tape.

5. Label the container, complete the laboratory requisition, and send together to the laboratory in a paper bag.
6. Wash your hands.
7. Record the procedure on the patient's chart.

Throat Culture

1. Wash your hands.
2. Assemble the equipment.
3. Identify the patient, and explain the procedure.
4. Have the patient sitting, facing you.
5. Have patient open mouth, extend tongue, and say "ah."
6. Remove the sterile cotton-tipped applicator from the sterile tube.
7. Depress the patient's tongue with the tongue blade.
8. Swab the back areas of the throat on both sides.
9. Place the applicator in a sterile tube, and secure the lid.
10. Obtain two specimens, one from both the right and left tonsillar areas if this is required.
11. Discard the tongue blade in the container for waste supplies.
12. Reposition the patient if necessary.
13. Wash your hands.
14. Label the culture tube(s), complete the laboratory requisition, and send together to the laboratory.
15. Record on the patient's chart.

Nasopharyngeal Culture After Throat Culture

1. Insert a sterile cotton-tipped applicator through the patient's nose into the nasopharyngeal area.
2. Rotate the applicator gently, and obtain the specimen.
3. Remove the applicator, place in the sterile culture tube, and secure the lid.
4. Label the tube, complete the laboratory requisition, and send together to the laboratory.
5. Record the procedure on the patient's chart.

Making a Smear

1. Wash your hands.
2. Assemble the required equipment and supplies.
3. Write the patient's name on the frosted end of the slide(s).
4. Receive the applicator from the physician with your dominant hand, grasping the distal end of the stick.
5. Hold the glass slide between your thumb and index finger of your nondominant hand.
6. Spread the specimen across the slide, starting at the unfrosted end, using the correct method.
7. Discard the applicator.
8. Fix the smear by spraying it from a distance of 5 to 6 inches, using a continuous flow going right to left, then left to right; or you may place the smear in a container of alcohol solution.
9. Allow the fixed smear to dry for 4 to 6 minutes.
10. Wash your hands.

11. Prepare the smear to be sent to the laboratory immediately with a completed requisition. If the smear is to be mailed, place it in the cardboard slide holder, secure it with a rubber band, and place this with a completed requisition in the mailing envelope provided by the laboratory. Seal and mail.
12. Record the procedure accurately and completely on the patient's chart.

Inoculating a Culture Medium

1. Wash your hands.
2. Assemble and prepare equipment for the examination to be done and for inoculating the culture media.
3. Identify and prepare the patient. Explain the procedure. Have the patient disrobe and put the patient gown on. Have the patient void. Position the patient for the examination.
4. Assist the physician and patient as required.
5. Receive the applicator with the specimen from the physician.
6. Remove top cover lid of culture plate, and place it upside down on a flat surface.
7. Inoculate the Thayer Martin culture plate; roll the applicator in a large **Z** pattern across the culture medium.
8. Discard the applicator.
9. Replace the cover lid on the culture plate.
10. Obtain the wire loop and Bunsen burner; light the burner, and heat the wire loop over the flame until it is red.
11. Allow time for loop to cool.
12. Remove cover lid of culture plate, placing it upside down on a flat surface.
13. Cross-streak the inoculated culture in a criss-cross fashion over the **Z** with the wire loop.
14. Replace the cover lid over the culture media.
15. Reflame the wire loop, and replace it in the appropriate container in the correct position.
16. Label the cover plate correctly and completely.
17. Place the culture plate in a candle jar with the medium on the top side of the plate.
18. Wash your hands.
19. Send the culture plate in the candle jar to the laboratory with the correct completed laboratory requisition.
20. Record the procedure promptly and accurately on the patient's chart.

Vaginal Smear for Trichomoniasis Vaginitis and Monilial Vaginitis

1. Wash your hands.
2. Assemble and prepare the required equipment and supplies.
3. Identify and prepare the patient. Explain the procedure. Have the patient void. Have the patient disrobe and put on a patient gown. Assist the patient in assuming a lithotomy or dorsal-

recumbent position for the vaginal exam. Drape the patient.

4. Assist the physician as needed.
5. Place a small amount of saline on the glass slide. Add KOH (potassium hydroxide) if testing for monilial vaginitis.
6. Receive the applicator with the specimen from the physician.
7. Dip the applicator into the solution on the slide.
8. Discard the applicator.
9. Place a coverglass over the depressed area in the middle of the slide.
10. Send the specimen to the laboratory with a completed requisition.
11. Assist the patient as required.
12. Assemble and dispose of used supplies according to office or agency policy.
13. Wash your hands.
14. Replace equipment and supplies as required.
15. Record the procedure on the patient's chart.

Procedure for a Gram Stain

1. Wash your hands.
2. Assemble and prepare the required equipment and supplies.
3. Make the smear and *heat fix* it.
4. Place the slide on the staining rack, smear side up.
5. Cover the slide with Gram crystal violet and allow it to react for 1 minute.
6. Grasp the slide with slide forceps and tilt it about 45 degrees to allow the Gram crystal violet to drain off.
7. Rinse the slide thoroughly with distilled water for 5 seconds.
8. Replace the slide on the staining rack.
9. Cover the smear with Gram iodine solution allowing it to react for 1 to 2 minutes.
10. Grasp the slide with the slide forceps and tilt it to a 45 degree angle to drain off the iodine solution.
11. Rinse the slide with distilled water in this position for 5 seconds.
12. With the slide remaining tilted, slowly pour the alcohol-acetone solution over it.
13. Rinse the slide with distilled water for 5 seconds.
14. Replace the slide on the staining rack, cover it with safranin counterstain, and allow it to react for 30 to 60 seconds.
15. Using a slide forceps, tilt the slide and allow the counterstain to drain off.
16. Rinse the slide thoroughly with distilled water for 5 seconds.
17. Blot the smear dry between the pages of the bibulous paper.
18. Position the slide on the microscope to be examined.
19. Notify the physician that the smear is ready to be examined.
20. Replace equipment and supplies as required.
21. Record the procedure on the patient's chart (if this is one of your responsibilities).

Assisting with a Lumbar Puncture

1. Wash your hands.
2. Assemble the required equipment and supplies.
3. Identify and prepare the patient. Explain the procedure. Furnish a patient robe; have the patient disrobe and put the gown on with the opening in the back. Have the patient void, and save the specimen if required.
4. Summon the physician into the room.
5. Using aseptic technique, open the sterile glove pack and the outer wrapping of the LP tray.
6. Position the patient correctly.
7. Cleanse the skin with soap and water.
8. Prepare the skin with an antiseptic solution. (Steps 7 and 8 may be done by the physician.)
9. When using a stock supply of local anesthetic, check the label, read aloud, and hold the vial for the physician to identify and withdraw the solution with the needle and syringe.
10. Help the patient maintain the proper position.
11. Give appropriate instructions to the patient to remain still and to breathe slowly and deeply through the mouth when the needle is being inserted; once the needle is in place, instruct and help the patient to straighten the legs and breathe normally.
12. Receive the test tubes with the specimens from the physician.
13. Check the caps for secure closure.
14. Place the tubes in an upright position.
15. Assist with the Queckenstedt test if it is performed.
16. Observe the patient for any unusual reaction.
17. Once the spinal needle is withdrawn, secure a Band-Aid or gauze dressing over the puncture site.
18. Assist the patient as required.
19. Send the specimen(s) to the laboratory with a completed requisition.
20. Assemble and dispose of used equipment according to office or clinic policy.
21. Wash your hands.
22. Replace equipment as necessary.
23. Chart the procedure (if this is one of your responsibilities).

Wound Culture and Dressing Change

1. Wash your hands.
2. Assemble equipment.
3. Identify the patient, and explain the procedure.
4. Prepare the patient. Position as required, and drape the wound site if necessary.
5. Prepare supplies for use.
6. Loosen the tape on the dressing.
7. Remove the soiled dressing either with forceps, or wear a sterile disposable vinyl or rubber glove, or grasp the dressing with your hand in a plastic bag.
8. Inspect the dressing for type and amount of drainage; then discard it in the waxed or plastic bag.
9. Observe the wound for the type and amount of drainage, the degree of healing, and presence of

pus, necrosis, or a putrid odor. If sutures are present, note if they are intact.

10. Remove the sterile applicator from the tube, and swab the drainage area once to obtain a specimen.
11. Place applicator in the culture tube.
12. Don sterile gloves.
13. Cleanse the wound using aseptic technique.
14. Apply fresh sterile dressing, and secure correctly with tape.
15. Attend to the patient's comfort; you may reposition the patient if necessary.
16. Label the culture tube, and complete the laboratory requisition; send both together to the laboratory.
17. Assemble and dispose of used supplies according to office or agency policy.
18. Wash your hands.
19. Replace supplies as needed, leaving the room neat and tidy.
20. Record the procedure on the patient's chart.

Unit VII

Principles of Pharmacology and Drug Administration

COGNITIVE OBJECTIVES

On completion of Unit VII, the medical assistant should be able to apply the following cognitive objectives.

1. Define and pronounce the terms listed in the vocabulary.
2. List and briefly describe the uses, sources, names, classification, and types of drugs.
3. Select and name official and other reference books on drugs.
4. Differentiate between a controlled substance, a prescription drug, and a nonprescription drug.
5. Define "prescription"; list and explain the seven parts of a prescription.
6. Differentiate between administering, dispensing, and prescribing medications.
7. Interpret abbreviations and symbols commonly used when administering medications.
8. State and discuss drug standards and the laws governing drug usage.
9. State and describe the various types of pharmaceutical preparations.
10. Explain how drugs should be stored, handled, and labeled.
11. List examples of drugs that may be kept on an emergency tray.
12. State and discuss the legal requirements for controlled substances inventory and the prescriber's record.
13. List ten routes by which medication may be administered, briefly describing each.
14. List at least 15 rules for administering medications and eight specific rules for administering injections.
15. Calculate the correct dosage of a medication to be administered.
16. List the five rights for preparing and administering medications.
17. State the correct size needle and syringe for intramuscular and subcutaneous injections; list factors that influence these choices.
18. List at least eight factors that will influence drug dosage and action.
19. Discuss aspects of patient education when on drug therapy.
20. State six reasons why medication is administered by an injection.
21. List six to eight dangers involved when giving injections and the sites that are to be avoided.
22. List anatomical sites for administering an intramuscular injection, a subcutaneous injection, and an intradermal injection.
23. Describe how drugs are placed into a syringe from a vial, from an ampule, and from a prefilled sterile cartridge-needle unit.
24. Explain how the skin is prepared before an injection is administered.
25. Explain what to do with a syringe and needle after use.
26. List three reasons for the administration of solutions by an intradermal injection.

TERMINAL PERFORMANCE OBJECTIVES

On completion of Unit VII, the medical assistant student should be able to do the following terminal performance objectives.

1. Given medication orders, interpret these, and calculate the dosage of drug to be administered.
2. Given a medication order, prepare and administer safely and efficiently a subcutaneous and an intramuscular injection using (a) a sterile disposable syringe and needle of the correct sizes, and (b) a metal reusable syringe with a prefilled sterile cartridge-needle unit.
3. Given a medication order, prepare and administer safely and efficiently an intramuscular injection using the Z-Track technique.
4. Demonstrate how to identify the correct sites for administering a subcutaneous and an intramuscular injection by palpating definite anatomical landmarks.
5. Demonstrate how to fill a syringe with a medication from a vial; from an ampule.

6. Given the PDR or other reference pharmacology book, obtain information on a variety of drugs.

The student must perform the above activities with 100% accuracy before passing this unit.

Vocabulary

addiction (ah-dik′shun)—An acquired physiologic and/or psychologic dependence on a drug with tendencies to increase its use.

AMA—American Medical Association.

anaphylactic (an″ah-fi-lak′tik) **shock**—An intense state of shock brought on by hypersensitivity to a drug, foreign toxin, or protein. Early symptoms resemble an allergic reaction, then increase in severity rapidly to dyspnea, cyanosis, and shock. This can be fatal if emergency measures are not taken immediately (see also Unit XVI, First Aid for Allergic Reactions to Drugs).

BNDD—Bureau of Narcotics and Dangerous Drugs (a federal government agency of the DEA).

chemotherapy (kē″mo-ther′ah-pē)—The use of drugs (chemicals) to treat disease; a type of therapy used for cancer patients in which powerful drugs are used to interfere with the reproduction of the fast-multiplying cancer cells.

contraindication (kon″tra-in″dĭ-kā′shun)—Condition in which the use of certain drugs or treatments should be withheld or limited.

crude drug—An unrefined drug.

cumulative action of a drug—A drug accumulates in the body; it is eliminated more slowly than it is absorbed.

DEA—Drug Enforcement Administration. This is the federal law enforcement agency charged with the responsibility of combating drug diversion.

dilute—To weaken the strength of a substance by adding something else.

drug idiosyncrasy (id″ē-ō-sing′krah-sē)—An unusual or abnormal response or susceptibility to a drug that is peculiar to the individual.

drug tolerance—The decreased susceptibility to the effects of a drug after continued use. In this case an increased dosage would be required to produce the desired effects, as the initial dose would be ineffective.

cross-tolerance—Cross-tolerance can develop when tolerance to one drug increases the body's tolerance to drugs in the same category. For example, a tolerance to one depressant drug leads to a tolerance of other depressant drugs.

FDA—Food and Drug Administration (a federal government agency).

habituation—Emotional dependence on a drug due to repeated use, but without tendencies to increase the amount of the drug.

HHS—Health and Human Services (a federal government agency).

PDR—Physician's Desk Reference, a book on drugs.

placebo (plah-sē′bō)—An inactive substance resembling and given in place of a medication for its psychological effects to satisfy the patient's need for the drug; it hopefully will produce the same effect as the real medication through psychological means. A placebo may be used experimentally.

prophylaxis (prō″fĭ-lak′sis)—Prevention of disease.

pure drug—A refined drug; one that has been processed to remove all impurities.

side effect—A response in addition to that for which the drug was used, especially an undesirable result.

untoward effect—An undesirable side effect.

stock supply—A large supply of medications kept in the physician's office or pharmacy.

toxicity (tok-sis′ĭ-te)—The nature of exerting harmful effects on a tissue or organism. The level at which a drug becomes toxic to the body. Minor or major damage may result.

unit-dose—A system that supplies prepackaged, premeasured, prelabeled, individual portions of a medication for patient use.

USP–NF—*United States Pharmacopeia–National Formulary*, a drug book listing all official drugs authorized for use in the United States.

Among the many duties of a medical assistant, the administration of medications holds high responsibility. As a member of a professional team involved with the medical care of the public, it is important that the medical assistant seek all possible knowledge of drugs—their use or abuse, correct dosages, methods and routes of administration, symptoms of overdose, and abnormal reactions that may occur when they are administered. Although it is beyond the scope of this book to include a detailed presentation of pharmacology, general concepts, basic information on drugs, and procedures for the correct methods of administration will be discussed. Reference sources for more detailed information on drugs will be cited. It is the responsibility of the medical assistant to obtain adequate knowledge of a drug before administering it to a patient.

PHARMACOLOGY AND DRUGS

Pharmacon is Greek for drugs. Pharmacology is the science that deals with the study of drugs—their origin, properties, uses, and actions. Drugs are any medicinal substances or mixtures of substances that are used for therapeutic, prophylactic, or diagnostic purposes. Drugs are either medicinal, therefore therapeutic, or poisonous, depending upon dosage and use. The therapeutic use of drugs includes the application of these substances to treat or cure a disease or condition, to relieve undesirable symptoms such as pain, and to provide substances that the body is not producing or not producing in sufficient amounts, for example, insulin, used for diabetes mellitus, and thyroid extract, used for hypothyroidism. Prophylactically, drugs are used to prevent diseases, such as vaccinations given to prevent communicable diseases. Drugs can also help a physician diagnose an illness, as seen when a contrast medium is given to a patient in a diagnostic x-ray procedure, or when antigens are used to detect skin allergies in a patient.

Pharmacology has undergone tremendous changes during the past few decades and continues to be dynamic. Through constant study and research, new drugs arrive on the market, and some old ones are withdrawn, either because newer ones are more effective, or because complications arising from the use of the older drugs prove to be too hazardous to the patient's health.

Drugs are derived from four main sources.

1. Plant sources — obtained from plant parts or products. Seeds, stem, roots, leaves, resin, and other parts yield these drugs; examples include digitalis and opium.
2. Animal sources — glandular products from animals are used, such as insulin and thyroid.
3. Mineral sources — some drugs are prepared from minerals, for example, potassium chloride and lithium carbonate (an antipsychotic).
4. Synthetic sources — laboratories duplicate natural processes. Frequently this can eliminate side effects and increase potency of the drug; examples include barbiturates, sulfonamides, and aspirin.

Drug Names: Brand (Trade), Generic, and Chemical

A typical drug may be known by as many as three names, as follows:

1. A brand or trade (proprietary) name
2. The generic name
3. The chemical name

When a drug is developed and marketed, it is assigned a specific name that is patented by the pharmaceutical company that has manufactured it. This is called the *trade or brand name* of the drug and is the exclusive property of the manufacturer. After a patent has expired (drug patents run 17 years), other companies may manufacture and sell the drug either under different brand names or under the drug's generic name. These exact copies of the original drug are often called generic drugs. Each drug has an official or nonproprietary name, which is also called the *generic name*. This name is often descriptive of the chemical composition or class of the drug and is assigned to the drug in the early stages of its development for general recognition purposes. Thus, every drug has a generic name. Generic names are established by the U.S. Adopted Name Council (USAN). Except in the case of older drugs, the generic (USAN) name is identical to the USP (United States Pharmacopeia) or NF (National Formulary) name. A generic drug may be manufactured by any number of companies and placed on the market under a different brand or trade name. Examples follow. Brand names are prominently used in advertising a drug to the medical profession, although the generic name must appear in advertising and labeling in letters at least half as big as that of the brand name.

Generic name	Brand or trade name	Pharmaceutical company
tetracycline	Tetracyn	Pfizer
meprobamate	Equanil	Wyeth
	Meprotabs	Wallace
	Miltown	Wallace
penicillin G	Bicillin	Wyeth
procaine penicillin	Crysticillin	Squibb

When prescribing a drug, the physician may use either the generic or the trade name. Currently the trend is to write more prescriptions using the generic name of the drug, if one is marketed (many trade names are still under patent protection and are not available from other manufacturers by the generic name), because it is generally less expensive for the patient to purchase. However, if the physician orders a specific trade name, most states now have laws that state that even though the prescription may be written under the trade name, the patient is entitled to ask the pharmacist for the medication under its generic name unless the physician has specifically directed otherwise, either orally or in handwriting. Also, the pharmacist filling the prescription order for a drug product prescribed by its trade or brand name may select another drug product of the same generic drug type (that is, the generic or chemical name of the drug that is considered to be therapeutically equivalent or "bioequivalent") unless the physician has specifically directed otherwise either orally or in handwriting, and only when the drug product selected costs the patient less than the prescribed drug product. Since both trade and generic named drugs represent the same chemical formula and must meet the same FDA standards, they can be used interchangeably according to most state laws. This provides one way to keep the cost of medical care down. When the substitution is made, the use of the cost-saving drug product dispensed must be communicated to the patient, and the name of the dispensed drug product must be indicated on the prescription label, except where the prescriber orders otherwise.

The third name a drug may be assigned is the chemical name. This represents the drug's exact formula, that is, the chemical makeup or molecular structure. Generally this name is used only by the manufacturer and on occasion by the pharmacy when compounding a drug, because, for most drugs, the chemical name is long and complex.

References and Official Books on Drugs

Established standards and up-to-date information on drugs are published in various books; some of the more common ones follow.

United States Pharmacopeia (USP)–National Formulary (NF). Once two individual books, the USP and NF are now published as a single volume. The National Formulary was acquired by the U.S. Pharmacopeial Convention, Inc., in 1975 and now publishes the USP–NF approximately every 5 years. This is an authoritative book establishing the standards for drugs. Only "official" drugs are listed in this book. All drugs sold under the name listed in the USP–NF must legally conform to the standards set forth. Detailed information on the description of drugs, standards for purity, strength and composition, storage, use, and dosage are given. Drugs that meet the standards set by the *Pharmacopeia* will bear the initials USP on their labels. Some drugs listed in the USP section of the book will be cross-referenced to the NF chapter. The NF chapter of the book deals primarily with the pharmaceutical ingredients of the drugs.

AMA Drug Evaluations. This book is published annually by the American Medical Association (AMA). New drugs that are not yet listed in the USP, but that have been evaluated by the Council on Drugs of the AMA, are presented.

Physician's Desk Reference (PDR). Although not official, the *PDR* is a common reference book used by most medical personnel. It is published annually by Medical Economics, Inc., and is automatically distributed free of charge to medical offices, agencies, and hospitals. The *PDR* has seven sections, which list the following:

1. Names, addresses, emergency telephone numbers, and a partial list of products available from the manufacturers who have provided information for the *PDR*.
2. Products by brand name in alphabetical order.

3. Products according to an appropriate drug category or classification.
4. Products under generic or chemical name headings.
5. Products shown in color and actual size under company headings, and a directory of Poison Control Centers and emergency telephone numbers for the 50 states, as well as Guam, Puerto Rico, and the Virgin Islands.
6. An alphabetical arrangement by manufacturer of over 2500 products. Each is described as to composition, uses and action, administration and dosage, precautions, contraindications, side effects, form in which each is supplied, and the common names and generic compositions or chemical names.
7. An alphabetical arrangement by manufacturer of diagnostic products with descriptions for use.

Inside the back cover is a Guide to Management of Drug Overdose. Supplements that provide new or revised product information developed after the *PDR* was published for the current year are published and distributed as necessary.

American Hospital Formulary Service (AHFS). This book is published by the American Hospital Formulary Service. Subscribed to by all hospital pharmacists, it contains extensive, unbiased drug information kept current by periodic supplements. The *AHFS* arranges drugs into therapeutic or pharmacological classes according to official (generic) names.

Medical assistants should be familiar with these publications and always keep one or more up-to-date copies in the physician's office as a reference source, for both the physician and themselves.

Drug Standards and Laws Governing Use

When physicians or other qualified medical practitioners prescribe, administer, or dispense drugs, including narcotics, they must comply with federal and state laws that regulate such transactions. Comprehensive laws have been passed by the United States Congress and individual state legislatures to regulate the manufacture, sale, possession, administration, dispensing, and prescribing of a range of drugs.

To assist physicians in complying with the legal obligations required of them, medical assistants should know and understand the laws regulating drugs and narcotics in the state in which they are employed, because individual states may supplement federal legislation with their own laws.

All drugs available for legal use are controlled by the Federal Food, Drug and Cosmetic Act of 1938. This act contains detailed regulations to assure the purity, strength, and composition of food, drugs, and cosmetics. The general purpose of this act, based on interstate commerce, is to control movement of impure and adulterated food and drugs. Amended periodically, the Federal Food, Drug and Cosmetic Act is enforced by the Food and Drug Administration (FDA), a department within the Department of Health and Human Services (HHS), formerly the Department of Health, Education, and Welfare (HEW). There are also other federal and differing state laws that regulate the development, sale, and use of drugs.

Legal Classification of Drugs

Controlled Substances.   Drugs having the potential for addiction and abuse, including narcotics, stimulants, and depressants, are termed controlled substances. Control of these drugs at all levels of manufacturing, distribution, and use is mandatory. Federal legislation that outlines these controls is the Controlled Substances Act of 1970 (the Comprehensive Drug Abuse Prevention and Control Act), which supersedes the Harrison Narcotic Act of 1917 and became effective May 1, 1971. This act is enforced by the Drug Enforcement Administration (DEA) in the U.S. Department of Justice. The law is designed to improve the administration and regulation of manufacturing, distribution, and the dispensing of controlled substances by providing a "closed" system for legitimate handlers of these drugs. Such a closed system should help reduce the widespread diversion of these substances out of legitimate channels into the illicit market. Under this act, drugs that are under federal control are classified into one of five schedules. Each schedule reflects decreasing levels of addiction and abuse potential, from Schedule I through Schedule V. Complete listings of the drugs in each schedule are available from district DEA offices. Only a few examples are included here. All controlled substances listed in the *Physician's Desk Reference (PDR)* are indicated by the symbol C with the Roman numeral II, III, IV, or V printed inside the C to designate the schedule in which the substance is classified.

Schedule I.   These drugs, having the highest potential for addiction and abuse, have not been accepted for medical use in the United States. Their use is limited to research purposes only after the research facility has obtained government approval and agreement to research protocol to test drugs for medical indications. Examples are heroin, marijuana, LSD, and mescaline.

(PCP)

Schedule II.   These drugs have a high potential for abuse and addiction, but have an acceptable medical use for treatment in the United States. Examples are amobarbital, amphetamine, cocaine, codeine, meperidine, methadone, methamphetamine, morphine, opium, and secobarbital.

(Valium)

Schedule III.   These drugs have less potential for abuse than the drugs in Schedules I or II and have a moderate or low addiction liability. They do have an acceptable medical use in treatment in the United States. Examples are APC with codeine, butabarbital, methyprylon, nalorphine, and paregoric.

Schedule IV.   These drugs have a lower potential for abuse and a more limited addiction liability than those in Schedule III. They do have an acceptable medical use in treatment in the United States. Examples are chloral hydrate, diazepam, meprobamate, paraldehyde, and phenobarbital.

Schedule V.   These drugs have a low potential for abuse and a limited addiction liability relative to drugs in Schedule IV. They do have an acceptable medical use in treatment in the United States. Examples are drugs of primarily low-strength codeine (less than those compounds included in Schedule III) combined with other medicinal ingredients. Other drugs in Schedule V are preparations containing limited quantities of certain narcotic drugs generally used for antitussive and antidiarrheal purposes.

For a complete listing of all the controlled substances contact any office of the DEA.

Under federal law, every practitioner who administers, dispenses, or prescribes a controlled substance (with the exception of interns, residents, law enforcement officials, and civil defense personnel who meet special conditions outlined in the Federal Code of Regulations) must be registered with the Drug Enforcement Administration. Medical practitioners must also have a valid license to practice medicine in their chosen state. The practitioner's office location from which controlled substances are handled must be registered, and the certificate of registration is to be kept at this location and available for official inspection. Applications for this registration can be obtained from any DEA regional office or from the DEA Section, PO Box 28083, Central Station, Washington, DC 20005. Registration must be renewed every 3 years.

Only DEA-registered practitioners can order and purchase controlled substances. Schedule II substances must be ordered with the Federal Triplicate Order Form (DEA-222). For example, the physician must fill out a Triplicate Order Form in order to obtain Demerol from the normal source of supply. Orders for Schedules III, IV, and V substances require only the practitioner's DEA registration number. In some states, when ordering Schedule II substances from out-of-state companies, a copy of the purchase agreement (*not* the Federal Triplicate Order Form) must be sent within 24 hours of placing the order to the office of the state attorney general.

Physicians who discontinue practice must return their Registration Certificate and any unused order forms to the nearest DEA office. It is suggested that the word "VOID" be written across the face of the order form before it is sent to the DEA. Physicians having controlled substances in their possession when they discontinue their practice should obtain information from the nearest field office of the DEA and from the responsible state agency on how to dispose of these drugs.

Some important duties of the medical assistant are to ensure that the physician is *currently* registered with the DEA, to obtain the correct federal forms for ordering and purchasing controlled substances, and to keep appropriate records of all transactions. Failure of the physician to comply with the laws regulating the use of controlled substances and other drugs could lead to considerable civil and criminal liability, in addition to the loss of the right to dispense or prescribe medications.

Prescription Drugs. These are drugs that may be obtained only when prescribed, administered, or dispensed by practitioners licensed by state law to prescribe drugs. The Federal Food, Drug and Cosmetic Act requires that these drugs bear on the label the legend *"Caution: Federal Law prohibits dispensing without prescription."* Examples include digoxin and penicillin.

Nonprescription Drugs. Drugs easily accessible to the general public fall into this category. They are frequently referred to as "over-the-counter" (OTC) drugs, as they can be obtained without a prescription, for example, vitamin tablets and aspirin.

Classification of Drugs

Drugs are classified in various ways. These classifications include the following:

- Drugs that have a principal action on the body, for example, analgesics, antidiarrheals
- Drugs used to treat or prevent specific diseases or conditions, for example, hormones, vaccines
- Drugs that act on specific organs or body systems, for example, cardiovascular drugs, gastrointestinal drugs
- Forms of drug preparations, for example, solids or liquids

You should be aware that frequently one drug may be used to treat varied conditions, because most drugs have multiple effects aside from the primary effects that they are assigned; or, the same drug can affect different body systems by exerting its primary effect. For example, a broad-spectrum antibiotic can be used to treat various types of infectious processes, or a diuretic may be used to exert an effect on the cardiovascular system or on the urinary system.

Table 7-1 is a classification of drugs based on their primary actions or effects on the body.

PRESCRIPTIONS

A prescription is an order written by a licensed physician giving instructions to a pharmacist to supply a certain patient with a particular drug of specific quantity, prepared according to the physician's directions. It is a *legal document*. A prescription consists of the following seven parts (Fig. 7-1):

1. Date, patient's name, and address (for children, age should be given)
2. Superscription, consisting of the symbol ℞, from the Latin *recipe*, meaning "take thou"
3. Inscription, specifying the ingredients and the quantities
4. Subscription, directing the pharmacist how to compound the drug(s)
5. Signa (Sig), from Latin, meaning "mark," which gives instructions to the patient indicating when and how to take the drug, and in what quantities
6. Physician's signature and address, registry number (this is the physician's license number), and when prescribing controlled substances, the BNDD number (this is the same as the DEA number)
7. Number of times, if any, that the prescription may be refilled; instructions to the pharmacist that the physician wants the drug identified on the label of the container

Current prescription writing has been greatly simplified, as pharmaceutical companies now prepare most drugs ready for administration. These preparations have largely eliminated the need for the pharmacist to compound or mix drugs and solutions.

When the physician writes a prescription, it is given to the patient to take to a pharmacist, who will dispense the required medication. Once the prescription has been filled, the pharmacist must keep a record of that sale for 2 years (3 years in four states).

Fig. 7-1. Sample of a prescription.

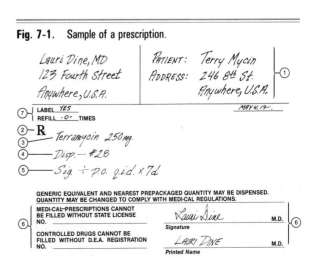

Table 7-1. Classification of drugs based on actions or effects on body

Drug	Action	Examples
Amphetamine	Acts as stimulant on central nervous system: has temporary effect of increasing energy and mental alertness; sometimes used to depress the appetite	Amphetamine (Benzedrine), dextroamphetamine (Dexedrine)
Analgesic	Relieves pain	Aspirin, Empirin Compound with codeine, codeine, acetaminophen (Tylenol), phenacetin
Anesthetic	Produces generalized or local loss of feeling	Thiopental sodium (Pentothal Sodium), tetracaine hydrochloride (Pontocaine Hydrochloride), lidocaine hydrochloride (Xylocaine Hydrochloride)
Angiotensin converting enzyme inhibitors	Used for hypertension	Capoten, Vasotec
Antacid	Counteracts acidity in stomach	Sodium bicarbonate, Maalox, Mylanta
Anthelminthics	Destructive to worms	Piperazine, mebendazole, Povan, Vermox
Antibiotic	Inhibits growth and reproduction of or eliminates pathogenic microorganisms	Penicillin, ampicillin, tetracycline
Antidiarrheal	Counteracts diarrhea	Lomotil, Kaopectate, codeine, paregoric
Anticoagulant	Inhibits blood clotting mechanism	Heparin sodium, dicumarol
Anticonvulsant	Inhibits convulsions, as in epilepsy. Prevents or reduces the frequency or severity of seizures related to idiopathic epilepsy, as well as seizures secondary to drug reactions, hypoglycemia, eclampsia, alcohol withdrawal, or traumatic brain injury	Phenytoin (Dilantin), bromides, ethotoin, phenobarbital, primidone, trimethadione
Antidepressant	Relieves depression; often called mood elevator or modifier	*Tricyclic antidepressants:* Imipramine (Tofranil), Amitriptyline (Elavil), Sinequan, Norpramin *Monoamine Oxidase Inhibitors (MAO):* Nardil, Parnate *Antimanic agents:* Lithium (Eskalith)
Antidote	Counteracts poison	Ipecac syrup
Antiemetic	Counteracts nausea and vomiting	Dimenhydrinate (Dramamine), prochlorperazine (Compazine), triethobenzamide (Tigan)
Antifungal	Destroys or checks the growth of fungi; controls Candida (Monilia) infections in vagina	Mycostatin, Nystatin
Antihistamine	Counteracts effect of histamine in the body; given to relieve symptoms of allergic reactions, such as hay fever, and also to relieve symptoms of common cold	Diphenhydramine (Benadryl), guaifenisen (Actifed), promethazine (Phenergan), chlorpheniramine (Chlor-Trimeton)
Antihypertensive (also referred to as hypotensive)	Reduces high blood pressure	Reserpine (Serpasil), guanethidine (Ismelin), hydrochlorothiazide (Esidrix)

Drug	Action	Examples
Antiinflammatory agent	Reduces or relieves inflammation	Indomethacin (Indocin), triamcinolone (Kenacort), triamcinolone acetonide (Kenalog), piroxicam (Feldene)
Antiarthritic preparation	Acts against arthritic symptoms	Indomethacin (Indocin), phenylbutazone (Butazolidin), prednisone, Feldene, Naprosyn
Antiseptic	Inhibits growth of microorganisms	
Skin antiseptic		70% alcohol
Urinary antiseptic to be taken internally		Nitrofurantoin (Furadantin), nalidixic acid (NegGram)
Antineoplastic	Inhibits growth and spread of malignant cells	Chlorambucil (Leukeran), busulfan (Myleran), melphalan (Alkeran)
Astringent	Constricts tissue and arrests discharges or bleeding	Silver nitrate, alum, zinc oxide
Beta-adrenergic blockers	Used to treat angina, hypertension, cardiac arrhythmias, myocardial infarctions. Act as a shield against excessive stimulation to the sympathetic nerve endings in the heart tissue. Slow down the heartbeat besides making the heart less responsive to stimulations. Thus the heart performs more work with less oxygen demand and pain can be prevented	Inderal, Corgard, Lopressor, Tenormin, Visken
Bronchodilator	Causes dilation of bronchi, eases breathing	Aminophylline, Bronkotabs, isoproterenol (Isuprel), epinephrine (Adrenalin)
Calcium channel blockers	Used for hypertension and angina	Cardizem, Ipoptin
Cardiogenic (heart stimulator)	Strengthens heart muscle action	Digitoxin, digitalis, digoxin (Lanoxin)
Cathartic	Relieves constipation and promotes defecation; often classified according to the increased intensity of their action as laxatives, purgatives, and drastic purgatives	Cascara, mineral oil, castor oil, bisacodyl (Dulcolax)
Contraceptive	Prevents or diminishes likelihood of conception	Enovid, Ortho-Novum
Cytotoxins	Toxic to certain cells. Used for treatment of cancer	Cytoxan, 6-mercaptopurine
Decongestant	Relieves swelling and congestion in upper respiratory tract	Ornade Spansule, Actifed, pseudoephedrine (Sudafed), phenylephrine (Neo-Synephrine)
Diuretic	Increases urinary output	Chlorothiazide (Diuril), furosemide (Lasix)
Emetic	Stimulates vomiting	Ipecac syrup
Expectorant	Liquifies mucus in bronchi and aids in the expectoration of sputum, mucus, or phlegm	Benylin expectorant, terpin hydrate, potassium iodide
Hemostatic	Arrests flow of blood by helping coagulation	Vitamin K
Hormone	Endocrine system produces hormones and secretes them directly into bloodstream. Commercial preparations are available for patients whose own glands are malfunctioning	Cortisone, insulin, thyroxin

(Table 7-1 continues)

Table 7-1 (*continued*)

Drug	Action	Examples
Hypnotic	Produces sleep	Glutethimide (Doriden), chloral hydrate
Laxative	Promotes movement of bowels	Mineral oil, docusate (Colace), senna (Senokot)
Miotic	Contracts pupils of eye	Pilocar ophthalmic solutions
Muscle relaxant	Relaxes muscles	Diazepam (Valium), carisoprodol (Soma) compound
Mydriatic	Dilates pupils of eye	Phenylephrine (Neo-Synephrine) solution, atropine sulfate ointment
Narcotic	Produces sound sleep, stupor, and relief of pain	Drugs derived from opium; morphine, codeine, meperidine (Demerol)
Psychedelic	Produces feelings of relaxation, freedom from anxiety, highly creative thought patterns, and perceptual changes; causes hallucinations, alters mental functions. Highly controversial, potentially very dangerous, and used only under controlled supervision for experimental purposes	LSD, mescaline
Sedative	Quiets and relaxes patient without producing sleep	Phenobarbital
Stimulant	Increases activity of an organ or body system	Caffeine, amphetamine (Benzedrine)
Styptic	Checks bleeding by means of astringent quality	Styptic pencil
Sulfa preparations	Antibacterial	Sulfisoxazole (Gantrisin)

Tranquilizers (also called ataractics)	Calms or quiets patients who are anxious or disturbed without causing drowsiness that a sedative would produce or the stimulation that antidepressants produce	*Antianxiety (anxiolytic)—minor tranquilizers*
		  Benzodiazepines
		    Librium, diazepam (Valium), Ativan, Serax, Halcion, Xanax, Dalmane
		  Nonbenzodiazepines
		    meprobamate (Equanil and Miltown)
		Antipsychotic (neuroleptic)—major tranquilizers:
		  Phenothiazines
		    chlorpromazine (Thorazine), Mellaril, prochlorperazine (Compazine), Haldol, Navane, Stelazine, Trilafon

Vaccine	Prevents infectious diseases	Salk polio vaccine, tetanus and typhoid vaccines, measles, mumps, and hepatitis B vaccines
Vasoconstrictor	Constricts blood vessels to increase force of heartbeat, relieve nasal congestion, raise blood pressure, or stop superficial hemorrhage	Epinephrine (Adrenalin), norepinephrine (Levophed), ephedrine sulfate
Vasodilator	Dilates blood vessels and reduces blood pressure	Nitroglycerin reserpine (Serpasil), amyl nitrite
Vitamins	Organic substances found in foods that are necessary for body to grow and maintain health; commercial preparations of all these vitamins are available	Fat-soluble vitamins; A, D, E, K Water-soluble vitamins: B, C

These records are subject to inspection and copying at any time by authorized employees of state and federal law enforcement and regulatory agencies. When a prescription is written for a Schedule II controlled substance (narcotic), a few states require the physician to use an official triplicate prescription blank. Where this is the case, one copy is kept for the physician's office files, and the original and other copy are given to the patient to take to the pharmacist. After filling the prescription, the pharmacist retains the original and endorses the copy, which is forwarded to the Department of Justice at the end of the month in which the prescription was filled.

All prescriptions written for controlled substances in Schedule II must be wholly written in ink or indelible pencil or typewritten, and must be signed by hand by the physician. A separate prescription blank is to be used for each controlled substance ordered. These prescriptions must contain the following information:

- Name and address of the patient
- Date of prescription
- Name and quantity of controlled substance prescribed
- Directions for use
- Physician's DEA registration number (the BNDD number)
- Signature and address of physician

Prescriptions for controlled substances in Schedule II cannot be refilled, and some states require that they be filled within 7 days from the date written.

In the case of a bonafide emergency, the physician may telephone a prescription order to a pharmacist for a Schedule II controlled substance. In these cases, the prescribed drug must be limited to the amount required to treat the patient during the emergency period. Within 72 hours the physician must furnish a written, signed prescription order to the pharmacy for the controlled substance prescribed. Pharmacies are required by law to notify the DEA if they have not received the written prescription order within the 72 hours. ("Emergency" means that the drug must be administered immediately for treatment, that there is no alternative treatment available, and that it is not possible for the physician to provide a written prescription form for the drug at that time.)

Prescriptions for controlled substances in Schedules III, IV, and V are written on the physician's standard prescription blank and need only to be signed by the prescriber. These prescriptions are limited to five refills within a 6 month period with proper authorization. A prescription for any controlled substance must be issued for a legitimate medical purpose by physicians acting in good faith in the course of their professional practice. Keep in mind that regulations for prescribing and dispensing controlled substances differ for each of the five schedules and may

also be subject to stricter controls passed by many states. It is therefore vital for medical assistants to learn what laws apply for their specific state.

Prescription pads should be kept in a safe place where they cannot be picked up easily by patients. Minimize the number of pads in use at one time. They are to be used only for writing prescriptions; *do not* use them for notes or memos. A drug abuser could easily erase the note and use the blank to forge a prescription. The Drug Enforcement Administration and local police department are to be contacted if your office experiences any theft or loss of controlled substances or official order forms. Contact a local police department if you are aware of forged prescriptions.

Although medical assistants do not write prescriptions, a knowledge of prescription abbreviations and terms used is valuable and may be required to carry out the physician's orders, transcribe medical notes, take telephone messages, answer questions for a patient regarding a prescription, verify information for a pharmacist, and understand instructions for the administration of medications. Table 7-2 is a list of the more common abbreviations and symbols used.

ADMINISTER, DISPENSE, PRESCRIBE

In the physician's office, medications may be handled in one of three ways: they may be administered, dispensed, or prescribed. A medication is administered when it is actually given to the patient to take by mouth, or when it is injected, inserted, or given by any other method used for administering medications. It is dispensed when it is given to a patient by the physician or pharmacist at the pharmacy to be taken at a later time; and it is prescribed when the physician gives the patient a written order, the prescription, to have filled by the pharmacist. Only the physician is licensed to prescribe medications. Depending on state law, varied medical personnel may administer medications, and the physician and pharmacist will dispense them. On occasion under the physician's order and supervision, the medical assistant may also dispense stock medications to a patient in the physician's office or health agency.

PHARMACEUTICAL PREPARATIONS

Because of the various properties and uses of different drugs, there are different ways in which they are prepared for patient use. Drugs are supplied in either a solid or liquid state.

Solid State (Fig. 7-2)

pills—Small, hard, molded objects of medication, either oval or round.

Table 7-2. Common prescription abbreviations and symbols*

Abbreviation or Symbol	Meaning	Abbreviation or Symbol	Meaning	Abbreviation or Symbol	Meaning
ā	before	kg	kilogram	qam	every morning
āā	of each	L	liter	qd	every day
ac	before meals	liq	liquid	qh	every hour
ad lib	as desired	m or min	minim	q2h or q2°	every 2 hours
amt	amount	mcg	microgram	(q3h or q3° and	every 3 hours
aq	aqueous	mEq	milliequivalent	so on)	
bid	twice a day	mEq/L	milliequivalents per	qhs	every night
c̄	with		liter	qid	four times a day
cap(s)	capsule(s)	mg	milligram	qod	every other day
cc	cubic centimeter	ml	milliliter	qs	quantity sufficient
dil	dilute	mm	millimeter	℞	take thou
Dx or Diag	diagnosis	npo (NPO)	nothing by mouth	s̄	without
D/C or d/c	discontinue	NS	normal saline	sc or subq or	subcutaneous
D/W	dextrose in water	noc(t)	night	SubQ	
dr	dram	od	daily or once a day	Sig	directions
℥	dram	OD	right eye	sol	solution
℥ᵢ	one dram	oint	ointment	ss or s̄s̄	one half
d	day	OS	left eye	subling	sublingual (under the
Dr	doctor	OU	both eyes		tongue)
fl or fld	fluid	oz	ounce	stat	immediately
gal	gallon	℥	ounce	S/W	saline in water
gm	gram	p̄	after, past	tid	three times a day
gr	grain	per	by or with	tinc or tr or	tincture
gt or gtt	drop(s)	pc	after meals	tinct	
H or hr	hour	po (or per os)	by mouth	tab	tablet
hs	hour of sleep or	prn	whenever	tsp	teaspoon
	bedtime		necessary	Tbsp	tablespoon
IM	intramuscular	pt	pint (or patient)	ung or ungt	ointment
IU	international units	pulv	powder	U	units
IV	intravenous	q	every	wt	weight

*According to the style of the American Medical Association, medical and pharmaceutical abbreviations are to be written *without* the use of periods. That is, rather than writing b.i.d. as was done in the past, you will now write bid, and so on.

tablets—Dried, powdered medications compressed into a round or disc-shaped object. Some are scored across the middle so that they can easily be broken in half.

caplets—Tablets shaped like capsules with a special coating to make them easy to swallow.

capsules—Liquid or powdered medications enclosed in a rod-shaped gelatin container.

spansules—Granules of medication enclosed in a capsule that is prepared so that the medication will be released at various times after being ingested; a sustained-release capsule, such as Dexamyl, Contac.

powders—Medications or mixtures of medications ground up into a powder.

suppositories—Molded cone-shaped mixtures of medication dispersed in a firm base, such as cocoa butter, that will dissolve and be absorbed when inserted into a body cavity such as the rectum or vagina.

Liquid State

solutions—Liquid preparations consisting of one or more substances (solutes) that are dissolved or suspended in a substance (the solvent). The most frequently used solvents are distilled water, sterile water, normal saline, and alcohol. Solutes may be (1) a 100% full-strength or pure drug in a solid, liquid, or powder form, (2) tab-

Fig. 7-2. Solid forms of drugs.

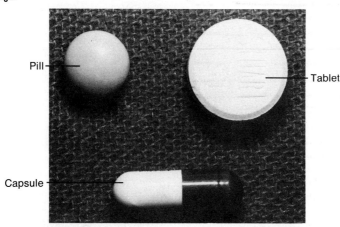

Pill

Tablet

Capsule

lets of a known specific amount of drug, or (3) stock solutions that are strong solutions of known strength used to prepare a weaker solution. To obtain a *true solution,* the solute must be completely dissolved in the solvent. If the solute is evenly dispersed throughout the solution but not dissolved, it is called a *suspension* or a *colloidal solution.* The difference between these two is determined by the molecular size of the particles of the solute, the colloidal solution containing very small particles. Drugs that are supplied in a suspension *must* be shaken before being administered and the label will bear the instruction "Shake well."

diluent—A solution that is added to another in order to reduce the strength of the initial solution or mixture. Percentages or ratios are used to describe solutions. For example, a 15% solution means that 15 parts of the solute are mixed with 85 parts of the solvent. Some solutions come prepared for immediate use; others will have to be mixed before they are suitable for use. When a solution must be prepared for use, it may be necessary to convert the apothecary system of weights and measures to the metric equivalents. Tables 7-4 and 7-5 present the equivalents for these two systems and the preparation of solutions. Some solutions may be administered by injection, by mouth, inhalation, irrigation, or lavage; others may be used topically on the skin, on dressings, or for cleansing purposes.

emulsion—An oily substance suspended in a liquid that it will not mix with or dissolve in, such as fat globules in water with an emulsifying agent; for example, various ointments, Petrogalar (a laxative), and also homogenized milk.

tincture—An alcohol solution prepared from drugs or chemicals, such as tincture of iodine, tincture of merthiolate, tincture of Zephiran (benzalkonium).

lotions—Aqueous preparations containing suspended particles used for local applications intended for soothing; for example, calamine lotion, Caladryl lotion.

elixirs—Solutions containing water, alcohol, and sugar used frequently as flavoring agents or solvents; for example, terpin hydrate elixir, phenobarbital elixir.

liniment—A liquid or soft mixture of drugs with soap, alcohol, oil, or water used for external application by rubbing it into the skin; for example, camphor liniment, chloroform liniment.

ointment—A mixture of drugs with a fatty substance used for external application; for example, A & D ointment, zinc oxide ointment, and various antibiotic ointments.

aerosol—A suspension of a drug that is administered in a fine mist or spray. It can be inhaled for treatment of respiratory conditions; others are sprayed on topically. Examples include Alevaire, Bronkosol, Mucomyst.

PROFESSIONAL RESPONSIBILITIES

Storage and Handling of Drugs

If a physician keeps medications in the office, certain rules and precautions should be followed. Ideally, all medications should be stored in a separate room in a locked cabinet and all *must* be kept in their original container. Many medications must be stored in dark containers or dark areas or refrigerated. Some *must* also be in glass containers, because the chemical composition of the drug may react with plastic. Drugs that must be refrigerated will be labeled as such. Because drugs will deteriorate, it is necessary to have a review schedule so that outdated drugs can be discarded and then replaced with a new supply. When discarding outdated drugs, you should pour liquids down a sink; drugs in the solid form should be crushed and then flushed down the sink. This method should also be used if you have taken a drug out of its original container and then are unable to use it, as it is *never* to be replaced in the container once removed. This method of disposal of medications eliminates the possible chance of drug abuse, as some people will take medications out of garbage containers and administer the drug to themselves, or dispense it to others.

To avoid medication errors, drugs for external use must be kept well separated from those to be used internally. Disinfectants, cleansing preparations, and all drugs that would be poisonous if taken internally must be stored in a location well separated from the other drugs. To facilitate easy access to the drugs, you should organize the central storage area. You may organize the drugs in an alphabetical arrangement or according to drug substance or classification, for example, antibiotics, contraceptives, diuretics, hormones, vaccines. It is also recommended to label storage areas as *external use only* and *internal use*. A further organizational system is to label areas for drugs to be used for oral administration, those for parenteral administration, and so on.

In addition, federal law requires that all controlled substances be kept in a substantially constructed, separate, securely locked cabinet or safe. Some states require that these drugs be kept in a locked cupboard in a locked room. Extra security precautions must also be taken for the needles and syringes that will be used for administering parenteral medications. Any loss or theft of controlled substances must be reported by the physician upon discovery to the DEA field office in the area. The field office will provide information on what reports are required of the physician. Also, the physician is required to notify the local police department of such theft.

Emergency Tray

A special container or tray in a readily accessible location should be kept with drugs needed for emergencies. Sterile syringes, needles, alcohol sponges, diluents, and a tourniquet should also be kept in this container. In most offices and clinics, the physician will make a checklist of the drugs and supplies to be kept in the emergency tray, varying with the need of the office and the physician's preference. The medical assistant should be familiar with these specific drugs, knowing the use, usual dosage, and method of administration for each. This container or tray must be checked frequently to replace items that have been used and to discard outdated drugs or sterile supplies.

Listed below are examples of drugs that *may* be kept on the emergency tray. These will vary according to the type of patient and possible emergency that you may encounter at your facility.

Adrenalin (epinephrine)—a vasoconstrictor and antispasmodic; used to counteract anaphylactic shock, to relieve symptoms of allergic reactions, and as an emergency heart stimulant.

Aminophylline—a bronchodilator; used to ease breathing as for asthmatic patients.

Benadryl—an antihistamine; used to relieve symptoms of allergic reactions, itching, and anaphylactic shock.

Compazine—an antiemetic; used to counteract nausea and vomiting.

Dextrose 50%—used for severe hypoglycemia.

Digoxin—a cardiac glycoside; used for congestive heart failure and certain cardiac arrhythmias.

Ipecac—an emetic; used to stimulate vomiting in some poisoning cases.

Lasix—a diuretic; used to promote the formation and excretion of urine.

Narcan—a narcotic antagonist; used in emergency situations for narcotic overdose.

Nitroglycerin—a vasodilator, used commonly for angina patients.

Pitocin—a hypothalmic hormone; stimulates uterine contractions to control postpartum bleeding in obstetric patients.

Steroids (such as hydrocortisone, Solu-Cortef, or Solu-Medrol)—used for their anti-inflammatory action.

Valium—a muscular relaxant and an antianxiety, minor tranquilizer; used to relax muscles or calm and quiet extremely anxious patients.

Additional supplies that may be kept near this tray for emergency situations include the following:

- Airway equipment (Ambu bag, and laryngoscopes and airways of different sizes)
- Defibrillator
- Intubation equipment and other related materials
- Oxygen tank, mask and/or nasal cannula
- Suction equipment

You should check the above equipment daily to make sure that it is in good working order and to ascertain that there is sufficient oxygen in the tank.

The following points must be kept in mind when oxygen is being administered:

- Do not use electrical appliances when oxygen is being administered. Do not connect or disconnect plugs when oxygen is in use.
- Do not use acetone and alcohol in the presence of oxygen.
- Do not use oil or grease on oxygen equipment. Your hands must also be free of grease when you are turning oxygen equipment on or off.
- Do not use oxygen tanks as a clothes rack.
- Keep all flammable substances away from the area where oxygen is in use.

- Post "No Smoking" signs in areas where oxygen is being used.
- Patients *should not be allowed* to have cigarettes, lighters, or matches with them while oxygen is being used. This is because they may forget that these items should not be used while oxygen is being administered and use them.
- When transporting an oxygen tank, fasten it to the platform of a carrier designed for that purpose.

Labeling

All drugs and solutions must be clearly labeled. Poisons should be clearly labeled as such and kept separate from other medications. Leave all drugs and solutions in the original labeled containers until they are administered or dispensed. Never use, but rather discard, medications or substances that are not clearly labeled or are in unlabeled containers. When pouring liquids from bottles, hold the bottle so that the label is facing the palm of your hand. Using this technique will prevent soiling or obliterating the label if any of the liquid runs down the side of the bottle (see also p. 150, Pouring Sterile Solutions). If a label becomes loose, soiled, or torn, type a new label with the exact information that was provided on the original. It is advisable to have someone else in the office check the new label for accuracy before you affix it to the container.

Controlled Substances Inventory and Prescriber's Record

A running inventory of all narcotics and controlled substances must be kept. A special record, either a card for each type of drug or a daily log book, must be maintained for 2 years (3 years in some states), during which time this record is subject to inspection and copying by authorized employees of state and federal law enforcement and regulatory agencies.

Records kept on all Schedule II controlled substances dispensed, administered, or prescribed must show the date, name and address of the patient, character and quantity of the drug provided, and pathological condition and purpose for which the drug was provided. *All records for Schedule II substances must be stored separately from other files.*

Records kept on all Schedule III, IV, and V controlled substances administered or dispensed from the office or medical bag must show the date, name and address of the patient, and the quantity of the drug dispensed or administered. Schedule III, IV, and V records may be stored separately from other files or in such form that the information is readily retrievable from the practitioner's other business and professional records.

All these records are to be kept for 2 years (3 years in some states), subject to inspection and copying by authorized employees of state and federal law enforcement and regulatory agencies.

A physician who dispenses or regularly engages in administering controlled substances and is required to keep records as stated above must take an inventory every 2 years of all stocks of the substances on hand.

All inventories and records of controlled substances in Schedule II must be maintained separately from all other records of the physician. All inventories and records of controlled substances in Schedules III, IV, and V must be maintained separately or must be in such form that they are readily retrievable from the ordinary professional and business records of the physician.

Medical assistants should play a major role in helping the physician keep all the appropriate records, guarding prescription pads, securing medication storage areas to prevent theft, ensuring the proper type of storage and correct labeling for all medications, and discarding and destroying outdated drugs.

ROUTES AND METHODS OF DRUG ADMINISTRATION

Drugs are supplied in various forms for different purposes (Table 7-3). Certain drugs can be administered in a variety of ways, and others must be administered in a specific way to be effective. Methods of administration are divided into two general categories: (1) drugs used for local effect, which are applied directly to the skin, tissue, or mucous membrane involved, and (2) drugs used for a systemic or general effect. A drug applied in this manner must be absorbed and circulate through the blood stream to produce an effect on the body cells or tissues.

Rules for Administering Medication

There are certain rules to follow when preparing and administering medications. Additional guides and rules that apply specifically to medications given parenterally (by injection) are described later in this unit.

You must know and always adhere to the *five rights* of proper medication administration, which are as follows:

- *Right* drug
- *Right* dose
- *Right* route for administration
- *Right* time
- *Right* patient

It is the patient's *right* to expect the five *rights.*

General Instructions

1. Wash your hands before preparing medications.
2. Give only medications and the correct dosage for which you have the physician's order. A safe

Table 7-3. Routes and methods used for administering medications

Routes of Administration	How Drug Is Administered	Form Drug Supplied In
Oral	The patient is given the drug by mouth to swallow. This is the simplest method and the method most desirable to patients.	Pills, tablets, capsules, spansules, or solutions. These are supplied in bulk form or as a unit dose.
Sublingual	The drug is placed under the patient's tongue and left to dissolve and be absorbed. It is *not* to be chewed or swallowed.	Tablets.
Buccal	The drug is placed between the cheek and gum to dissolve and be absorbed.	Tablets
Inhalation	The drug is given via the respiratory tract. The patient inhales the drug using a nebulizer or a special mechanical apparatus.	Aerosols, sprays, mists, or steams medicated with drugs
Rectal	The drug is inserted into the rectum. This method is used when a patient cannot tolerate the drug orally; or if unconscious; or if the drug would be destroyed by digestive enzymes. Also may be administered by proctoclysis, a drip method.	Suppositories, enemas, or other solutions
Inunction	The drug is applied or rubbed into the skin. Rubber gloves should be used when applying drugs such as nitroglycerin, or those containing mercury, to prevent absorption of the drug into your system.	Ointments, lotions, sprays, solutions, powders, tinctures, liniments
Vaginal	The drug is inserted into or applied to the vagina.	Suppository; solution, as in a douche; or liquids or ointments to be applied for local effect on the cervix or vaginal canal; also contraceptive foams and creams
Instillation	The drug is applied in drops to a membrane, as into the eye or ear.	Solutions
Irrigation	The drug is flushed through a membrane or body cavity.	Solutions
Parenteral	The drug is given by injection through a needle. Types of injections include: a. *Subcutaneous*: under the skin b. *Intramuscular*: into a muscle c. *Intradermal* or *intracutaneous*: into the upper layers of the skin. Used chiefly for skin reactions, as in allergy or tuberculosis testing d. *Intraarticular*: into a joint for local effects e. *Intraarterial*: into an artery; used in certain diagnostic procedures f. *Lumbar puncture* or *intraspinal*: into the spinal canal between two vertebrae; used to administer drugs for diagnostic techniques or for spinal anesthetics g. *Intravenous*: into a vein; used for immediate effect of a drug, for blood transfusions, or parenteral feeding	A drug solution supplied in ampules for single use; in vials for single or multiple use; and in syringes or cartridges prefilled by the manufacturer. Drugs that deteriorate in solutions may be supplied in vials in powdered form to which a specified amount of diluent is to be added when prepared for use. Sterile hypodermic tablets that are to be dissolved before the drug is administered are also available. Larger amounts of solutions for intravenous use are supplied in bottles of 250 ml, 500 ml or 1000 ml, such as dextrose in water and normal saline, to which other drugs may be added. Plasma and blood are also used for intravenous transfusions.

practice is to follow only written orders that are complete.

3. Prepare the medication in a well-lighted area away from distractions and interruptions. Give full attention to what you are doing.

4. Read the label of the medication three times:

- When removing from the storage area
- Before pouring the desired amount
- When replacing the container in the storage area

Do not use unlabeled or illegibly labeled medications.

5. Know the drug that you are giving. Check the *PDR* or other reference books if you are unsure of the usual actions, uses, dosage, route of administration, and undesirable side effects.

6. Calculate a dosage accurately, when this is necessary. Consult another competent person for verification when you doubt your answer.

7. Liquid medications (review p. 150, Pouring Sterile Solutions):
   - Shake well any medication that is in the form of an emulsion or suspension.
   - Do not use medications that have changed color, turned cloudy, or have sediment at the bottom (except suspensions).
   - Hold the bottle with the label in the palm of your hand to avoid damaging the label if the liquid runs or spills.
   - Hold the medicine or graduate at eye level so that you can measure accurately as you pour the medication (Fig. 7-3, *A*).
   - Wipe the neck of the container before replacing the cap.
   - Do not mix liquid medications unless specifically ordered to do so.

8. Tablets, pills, capsules, or spansules: Shake or drop the tablet or other preparation into the cap of the container; then drop it into a medicine cup. You must *not* handle the medication with your fingers (Fig. 7-3, *B*).

9. Do not leave poured medications unattended.

10. Do not administer medications prepared by others. If an error is made, the person administering the medication is responsible.

11. Take both the drug and container to the physician for additional identification when you have prepared the medication to be administered by the physician.

12. Know your patient. You may ask the patient to state his or her name to ensure correct identification.

13. Make sure that the patient is not allergic to the medication before you administer it.

14. Stay with the patient until you are certain that an oral medication has been swallowed.

15. Observe the patient for any unusual reactions to the drug administered.

16. Discard a medication that the patient refuses. Never replace a medication into the original container once it has been removed.

17. Report immediately to the physician if the patient refuses the medication or if an error was made so that appropriate action can be taken promptly or adjustments made for the patient's care.

18. Record as soon as possible on the correct patient's chart the date, time, drug and amount given, route of administration, and your signature. (*Errors in administering drugs must also be recorded, describing the incident in full.*) Body locations must be recorded for drugs administered parenterally. In addition, if the medication administered was a narcotic or other controlled substance, you must record this information in the physician's controlled substances records.

Dosage: Weights, Measurements, Calculations

A complete understanding of basic arithmetic is essential when preparing solutions or administering medications. A review of mathematical calculations is recommended at this time before you prepare to calculate dosages and administer medications.

The two primary systems of weights and measures used for describing dosages for medications are the apothecary system and the metric system. The *apothecary* system is our oldest system of measurement, the term being an ancient word meaning pharmacist or druggist. Today the trend is to use the *metric* system, the standard system of weights and measurements set up by the International Bureau of Weights and Measures, although it has not been completely adopted for use by everyone at this time. Therefore, it

Fig. 7-3. **A,** hold the medicine or graduate at eye level so that you can measure accurately as you pour the medication. **B,** shake or drop tablet into cap of container.

A
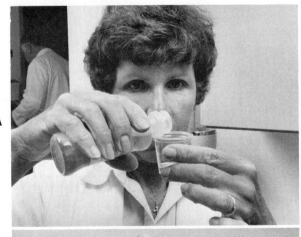

B
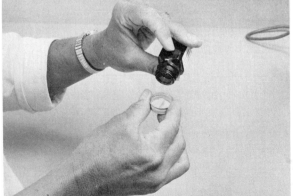

is necessary to have an understanding of both systems.

The apothecary system units of fluid measurements are the minim, fluid dram, fluid ounce, pint, quart, and gallon. The units of solid measurement are the grain, dram, ounce, and pound. Roman numerals and fractions are used with this system, for example, HCl gtt X (Hydrochloric acid drops ten); or nitroglycerin gr 1/150 (Nitroglycerin grains one/one hundred fifty).

In the metric system, the units of fluid or volume measurements are the milliliter, cubic centimeter, and liter. Units of weight or solid measurements are the milligram and gram. Arabic numbers and the decimal system are used with this system. Example: $1/1000 = 0.001$, $1/100 = 0.01$, $1/10 = 0.1$, for example tetracycline 250 mg/ml or cc.

See Tables 7-4 and 7-5 for the equivalent values of apothecary and metric measurements for liquids and solids, and the equivalents of common household weights and measurements for these systems.

At times you may be required to calculate the dose of a medication that you are to administer. A simple formula to use is

$$\frac{\text{Dose you } want}{\text{Dose you } have} = \text{Dose you give}$$

EXAMPLE: The physician has ordered 500 mg tetracycline, by mouth (po). The dose of tetracycline that you have on hand is labeled 250 mg/tablet. Therefore:

$$\frac{\text{Dose you want (500 mg)}}{\text{Dose you have (250 mg)}} = \text{Tablets to give (2)}$$

You would therefore give the patient two tablets of tetracycline 250 mg/tablet, so that the patient would receive 500 mg of tetracycline as was ordered.

The same formula can be used when preparing drugs supplied in a solution form.

Table 7-4. Metric doses with approximate apothecary equivalents*

Weights				Liquid Measures†	
Metric	Approximate Apothecary Equivalents	Metric	Approximate Apothecary Equivalents	Metric	Approximate Apothecary Equivalents
2 grams (gm) = 30 grains (gr)		15 mg = ¼ gr		1000 ml = 1 quart	
1.5 gm = 22 gr		12 mg = ⅕ gr		750 ml = 1½ pints	
1 gm = 15 gr		10 mg = ⅙ gr		500 ml = 1 pint	
0.75 gm or 750 mg = 12 gr		8 mg = ⅛ gr		250 ml = 8 fl ounces	
0.6 gm or 600 mg = 10 gr		6 mg = 1/10 gr		200 ml = 7 fl ounces	
0.5 gm or 500 mg = 7½ gr		5 mg = 1/12 gr		100 ml = 3½ fl ounces	
450 mg = 7 gr		4 mg = 1/16 gr		50 ml = 1¾ fl ounces	
300 mg = 5 gr		3 mg = 1/20 gr		30 ml = 1 fl ounce	
0.25 gm or 250 mg = 4 gr		1.5 mg = 1/40 gr		15 ml = ½ fl ounce (4 fl drams)	
200 mg = 3 gr		1.2 mg = 1/50 gr		10 ml = 2½ fl drams	
0.15 gm or 150 mg = 2½ gr		1 mg = 1/60 gr		8 ml = 2 fl drams	
120 mg = 2 gr		0.8 mg = 1/80 gr		5 ml = 75 minims (1¼ fl drams)	
0.1 gm or 100 mg = 1½ gr		0.6 mg = 1/100 gr		4 ml = 1 fl dram	
75 mg = 1¼ gr		0.5 mg = 1/120 gr		3 ml = 45 minims	
60 mg = 1 gr		0.4 mg = 1/150 gr		2 ml = 30 minims	
50 mg = ¾ gr		0.3 mg = 1/200 gr		1 ml = 15 minims	
40 mg = ⅔ gr		0.25 mg = 1/250 gr		0.75 ml = 12 minims	
30 mg = ½ gr		0.2 mg = 1/300 gr		0.6 ml = 10 minims	
25 mg = ⅜ gr		0.15 mg = 1/400 gr		0.5 ml = 8 minims	
20 mg = ⅓ gr		0.1 mg = 1/600 gr		0.3 ml = 5 minims	
				0.25 ml = 4 minims	
				0.2 ml = 3 minims	
				0.1 ml = 1½ minims	
				0.06 ml = 1 minim	

*The approximate dose equivalents in this table represent the quantities that would be prescribed, under identical conditions, by physicians trained, respectively, in the metric or in the apothecary system of weights and measures.

†A milliliter (ml) is the approximate equivalent of a cubic centimeter (cc).

Table 7-5. Equivalents of common household weights and measurements and preparation of solutions

Household	Metric	Apothecary
Liquid		
1 drop (gtts)		= 1 minim (m)
15 drops	= 1 milliliter (ml or cc)	= 15 minims
1 teaspoon (tsp)	= 4 ml	= 1 fluid dram (fl dr)
1 dessert spoon	= 8 ml	= 2 fl dr
6 teaspoons or 2 tablespoons (tbsp)	= 30 ml	= 1 fluid ounce
1 measuring cup	= 240 ml	= 8 fluid ounces
2 measuring cups	= 500 ml	= 1 pint (pt) (16 fl oz)
4 measuring cups	= 1000 ml	= 1 quart (qt) or 2 pts
1 tbsp	= 15 ml	= 4 drams (½ oz)
Dry		
⅛ teaspoon	= 0.5 gram (gm)	= 7 ½ grains (gr)
¼ teaspoon	= 1.0 gm	= 15 grs
1 teaspoon	= 4 gm	= 60 grs or 1 dram
1 tablespoon	= 15 gm	= 4 drams
2 tablespoons	= 30 gm	= 1 ounce

Preparation of solutions

Prescribed strength	Amount of full-strength drug	Fluid to be added to make up
1:1000	1 teaspoonful	1 gallon
1:1000	15 drops	1 quart
⅒ of 1%	15 drops	1 quart
1:500	2 teaspoonsful	1 gallon
1:500	30 drops	1 quart
⅕ of 1%	30 drops	1 quart
1:200	5 teaspoonsful	1 gallon
1:200	1¼ teaspoonsful	1 quart
½ of 1%	1¼ teaspoonsful	1 quart
1:100(1%)	2¼ teaspoonsful	1 quart
1:50 (2%)	5 teaspoonsful	1 quart
1:25 (4%)	2½ tablespoonsful	1 quart
1:20 (5%)	3 tablespoonsful	1 quart

EXAMPLE: The physician has ordered 500 mg of tetracycline to be given intramuscularly (IM). The bottle you have on hand is labeled tetracycline 250 mg/ml. Therefore:

$$\frac{\text{Dose you want (500 mg)}}{\text{Dose you have (250 mg/ml)}} =$$
$$\text{Dose in ml that you give (2 ml)}$$

When this formula is used, both the dose you want to give and the dose you have on hand must be expressed in the same measurements. That is, in order to give so many milligrams, the dose on hand must be in milligrams per milliliter for a solution, or in milligrams per tablet or capsule for drugs supplied in the solid form. If this is not the case, you will have to convert one measurement into the equivalent value of the other. You should be familiar with the methods used for converting one system of measurements into the other.

It is recommended that you refer to some of the many books available with practice problems in the mathematics of drugs, solutions, and dosages to gain competence in this procedure. Use the tables of weights and measurements for a reference. When you doubt your calculations, always seek help from another competent person or the physician.

FACTORS INFLUENCING DOSAGE AND DRUG ACTION

Not all individuals will respond to a given medication in the same manner. When prescribing a drug for a patient, the physician will take into account the following, as each will influence the prescribed dosage and anticipated action.

Age. Infants, young children, and the elderly will usually require a smaller dosage of a medication.

Sex. The average woman will be given a smaller dosage than the average man because of the difference in body structure and overall weight. Also, when a woman is pregnant, drugs and the dosage will be monitored very closely to prevent harmful effects to the fetus.

Weight. The usual rule is the smaller or lighter the patient, the smaller the dosage of drug. Certain medication dosages will be determined according to the weight of the patient.

Past Medical History and Drug Tolerance. If a patient has been taking a medication regularly for an extended period of time, a tolerance to the drug may have developed, and a larger dosage may be required to obtain the desired results. This is frequently seen with the use of narcotics, barbiturates, sedatives, and analgesics.

Physical or Emotional Condition of the Patient. A patient who has excruciating pain will require a larger dose of an analgesic than a patient who experiences intermittent pain. A severely depressed patient will require a larger dosage of an antidepressant than a patient suffering from mild depression.

Drug Idiosyncrasies or Allergies. At times the patient may experience an abnormal susceptibility or reaction to a drug. Alternate drugs with similar actions could then be prescribed.

Type of Action Desired or Produced. Drugs can produce local, systemic, selective, or cumulative actions. A *local action* occurs when the drug is absorbed and produces an effect at the site to which it was administered, as a local anesthetic administered to deaden sensation in the body area to be worked on. A *systemic action* occurs when the drug is absorbed and circulates in the blood stream to produce a general effect, such as central nervous system stimulants and depressants. A *selective action* is a more specific effect of a drug on one special body area than on other areas, as bronchodilators. A *cumulative* action happens when a drug accumulates in the body and exerts a greater effect than the initial dose; the drug accumulates in the body faster than it can be metabolized and excreted, such as alcohol does when a person drinks two or three drinks in 1 hour.

Route of Administration. Although there are exceptions, generally medications administered parenterally are given in smaller dosages than those given by mouth. Larger amounts of medications are used for topical application than for internal administration. Drugs administered parenterally will produce their effects much more rapidly than drugs administered orally. When a systemic effect is desired from an irritating drug, it should be given intramuscularly rather than by other parenteral routes.

Time of Administration. For optimal effects, some drugs must be taken before meals; two, three, or four times a day; or after meals to avoid irritating the lining of the stomach. Drugs will be absorbed more quickly and have a more rapid effect if taken on an empty stomach.

Interactions of Drugs. Some drugs, when taken together, may enhance or counteract the effect of the other. If the interaction is *synergistic,* one drug augments the activity of the other drug; the action of the drugs is such that their combined effect is greater than the sum of their individual effects. For example, barbiturates taken with alcohol have up to four times the depressant effect that either drug would have if taken alone. A *potentiating* interaction is a synergistic action in which one drug increases the effect of another drug when taken simultaneously, producing a combined effect that is greater than the sum of the effects of each drug taken separately. Drugs can also create an *antagonistic* interaction. This is when one drug neutralizes or counteracts the action of the other drug when they are taken together. Another type of drug interaction is termed *additive*. This is when the combined effect produced by the action of two or more drugs is equal to the sum of their separate effects.

Thus, it is vital to know if the patient is taking any other medication and, in some cases, any alcoholic beverage, before a new medication is prescribed. It is also important to know if the patient takes nonprescription drugs, for often patients do not consider drugs that they purchase over the counter as medications. Nonetheless, these drugs are medications that may possibly interact adversely with a prescription drug.

Summary

It must be remembered that drugs are potent substances that can provide individuals with extremely beneficial results when used properly and with care, but are also capable of producing hazardous or fatal results when used indiscreetly. Toxic effects, such as allergic reactions, adverse effects on the blood or blood-producing tissues, drug dependence, accidental poisoning, or drug overdose, can be the result of careless or uninformed use of any drug on the market for legal use or from illegal drugs obtained in the streets. Always handle and administer drugs with extreme care, as a life may depend on their proper use.

PATIENT EDUCATION

Patient education is a vital part of all medical care and treatment. When drug therapy is initiated, certain considerations and drug safety precautions must be brought to the patient's attention. The patient should be instructed to do the following either by the physician or medical assistant.

- Inform the physician of all drugs, either prescription or over-the-counter drugs, that you are currently taking or take periodically. If you go to more than one physician tell each of them what drugs you are taking.
- Inform each physician of any reactions or allergies that you have to drugs.
- Know the name, dosage, and purpose of each medication that you are taking.
- Know how and for how long the drug is to be taken.

Follow the instructions for taking the drug as prescribed. At times a drug should be taken with food, or before or after meals, or on an empty stomach. It is extremely important that these directions be followed precisely, as there are sound medical reasons for these directions. Some drugs should be taken with food to avoid or minimize gastrointestinal irritation and reactions. Others should be taken on an empty stomach for proper metabolism and absorption. When drugs are to be taken three or four times a day, or every 6 hours, be sure that you understand the time schedule that must be followed. Again, there is a sound scientific reason for taking drugs on a specific time schedule so that treatment will be maximized.

- If necessary, devise a calendar or diary to help you remember what drug is to be taken and when.
- Call the physician if you have any unusual reaction(s). (The patient should be informed of possible side effects.)
- Don't stop taking the medication unless directed to do so by the physician. Some drugs, such as antibiotics, must be taken for 7 to 10 days to be effective; other drugs, such as prednisone or synthroid, should be tapered off slowly under the direction of the physician.
- Be aware that some drugs may lead to a dependency if misused or abused, and understand the dangers of dependency.
- Don't save old prescriptions. Look for the expiration date on all drugs being used. Old or outdated drugs should be flushed down the sink or toilet.
- *Never* give your medications to anyone else. They are only for *your* condition.
- Don't use alcohol when taking medications until you have checked with the physician or pharmacist if this would be a safe practice.
- Avoid certain activities, such as driving a motor vehicle, when taking drugs that will cause drowsiness.
- Check with the pharmacist where to store your medications. Some drugs need to be kept in a refrigerator. Others should be kept in a dry, cool atmosphere. Usually you should not keep medications in a hot, damp bathroom cabinet.
- Don't keep medications in a bedside stand. Make sure that you are in a well-lit area when taking medications so that you can read the label to ensure that you are taking the correct medication and the correct dosage.
- *Always* read the label of the container from which you remove the medication before taking the medication. *Never* assume that you are taking the right medication without reading the label on the container.
- If you have poor vision, ask the physician or pharmacist to print the name of the drug and the treatment schedule out clearly on a separate piece of paper or card.
- Keep all drugs out of the reach of children.
- Always ask or call the physician if you have any additional questions regarding your medication therapy.
- Be aware that all of the preceding directions are vital to a successful program of medical care.

INJECTIONS

Injections are an important means of administering chemotherapy treatment. Because two foreign objects, the medication and the needle, are being introduced into the patient's body, these procedures must be performed with extreme care and excellent technique. The effectiveness of the medication is influenced by the correct choice of injection site and the use of precise technique. Any injection administered into an inappropriate body site or with incorrect technique may interfere with the body's utilization of the medication, and more important, may cause irreparable damage. The practices of aseptic (sterile) technique (see Unit V) must be observed when administering injections to minimize the danger of causing an infectious process.

Reasons Physicians Order Injections

1. To achieve a rapid response to the medication. When injected, a medication will enter the bloodstream quickly and therefore is more effective.
2. To guarantee the accuracy of the amount of medication given.
3. To concentrate the medication in a specific area of the body, such as into a joint cavity, fracture, or lumbar puncture.
4. To produce local anesthesia to a specific part of the body.
5. To administer the medication when it cannot be given by mouth or by other methods, either because of the physical or mental condition of the patient or the nature of the drug.
6. When the effect of the medication would be destroyed by the digestive tract or lost through vomiting, or when it would irritate the digestive system.

Dangers and Complications Associated with Injections

1. Injury to superficial nerves or to a vessel.
2. Introduction of infection due to the improper sterilization of the injection site, needle, or syringe, or due to an operator with unclean hands.
3. Breakage of a needle in a tissue.
4. Injecting a vein rather than a muscle.
5. Hitting a bone in a very thin patient.
6. Allergic reactions that may be mild, severe, or even fatal.
7. Toxic effects produced by the medication.
8. Too much air entering the bloodstream in a venipuncture.

Body Areas to Avoid When Administering Injections

Burned areas
Scar tissue
Edematous areas
Cyanotic areas
Traumatized areas
Areas near large blood vessels, nerves, and bones
Areas where there has been a change in skin texture or pigmentation
Areas where there are other tissue growths, such as a mole or wart

Supplies and Equipment for Administering Injections

Syringes.   Disposable plastic or glass and nondisposable glass syringes are available in several standard

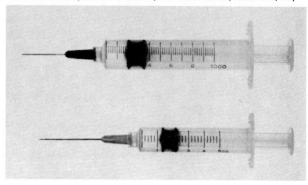

Fig. 7-5.   Syringes, 5 cc and 10 cc, with needles attached. Calibrations are marked in cubic centimeters. (Courtesy Becton-Dickinson, Division of Becton, Dickinson and Co., Rutherford, NJ)

sizes and shapes. The most common sizes used in the physician's office are 2 cc, 3 cc, 5 cc, or 10 cc. The parts of the syringe are the barrel, the outside portion; the plunger, the portion that fits inside the barrel; and the tip, the point at which the needle will be attached, which will be either a plain tip or a Luer-Lok tip (Figs. 7-4 and 7-5). Other variations of syringes include the insulin syringe (Fig. 7-6), tuberculin syringe (Fig. 7-7), Tubex metal syringe for use with a disposable needle-cartridge unit, and a disposable syringe unit-dose system. Sterile disposable syringes come supplied in a paper wrapper or a rigid plastic container. Calibrations, usually in cubic centimeters (cc) and minims, are marked on the barrel of the syringe.

Needles.   Needles come in various lengths ranging from ¼ inch to 6 inches, and with various gauges ranging from 13 to 27. The gauge of the needle and the length are indicated on the outside of the sterile protective cover or wrapper. Some manufacturers also color code the wrappers for quick and easy identification. The parts of a needle are the point, the

Fig. 7-4.   Parts of a syringe. (Courtesy Becton-Dickinson, Division of Becton, Dickinson and Co., Rutherford, NJ)

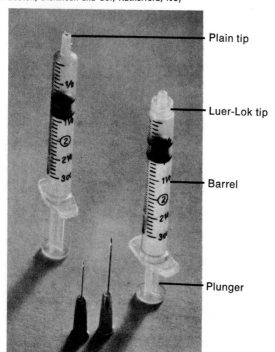

Plain tip

Luer-Lok tip

Barrel

Plunger

Fig. 7-6.   Insulin syringes. Calibrations are marked in units per cubic centimeter.

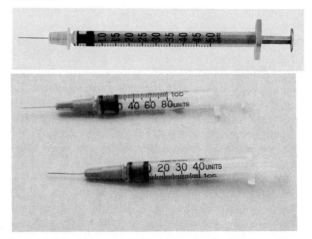

Fig. 7-7. Tuberculin syringe with fine calibrations up to 1 cc.

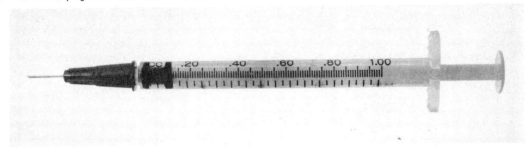

cannula or shaft, and the hub, which fits onto the tip of a syringe (Fig. 7-8). The smaller the gauge of the needle, the larger the lumen or inside diameter. For example, an 18 gauge needle has a large lumen; a 26 gauge needle has a small lumen. The size and length of a needle govern its use.

Today most practitioners use disposable needles and syringes to prevent all danger of cross-infection, although the reusable type is still available.

Skin Antiseptic.   Before an injection is administered, the skin must be cleansed with an antiseptic. The most commonly used is isopropyl alcohol placed on a sterile cotton ball, or a prepackaged sterile alcohol sponge.

Medications and Diluents.   Most medications for parenteral use are in an aqueous solution or in a suspension, although some are in an oil solution or in a suspension, and a few are in tablet or powdered form. When a sterile hypodermic tablet or powdered drug

is to be dissolved before parenteral use, sterile water or bacteriostatic normal saline will be used as the diluent. The type and amount to be used will be indicated on the container in which the drug is supplied.

Medication solutions are supplied in single or multiple dose form. Those for *single use* will be supplied (1) in syringes or cartridges that are prefilled by the manufacturer, (2) in an ampule, a small glass container with a constricted neck that is to be broken off when the drug is to be used, or (3) in a single-dose vial.

Containers with *multiple doses* of a medication are called vials. These are small bottles containing from 10 to 50 ml of a drug solution. Vials are usually covered with a soft metal cover and have a rubber, self-sealing stopper. At the time of use, this rubber stopper is cleansed with an alcohol sponge and then punctured with the needle to inject air and withdraw an equal amount of drug (Fig. 7-9). Procedures to withdraw solutions from an ampule and vial are discussed under the procedure ''Administration of an Intramuscular Injection.''

Fig. 7-8.   **A,** various sized needles with parts labeled. (Courtesy Becton-Dickinson, Division of Becton, Dickinson and Co., Rutherford, NJ). **B,** needle point and bevel.

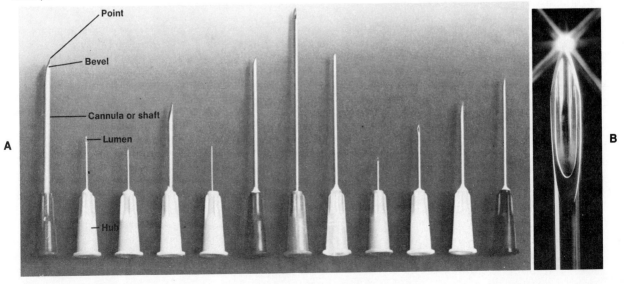

Fig. 7-9. Drugs supplied in liquid form. *Left to right,* cartridge; vial; ampule.

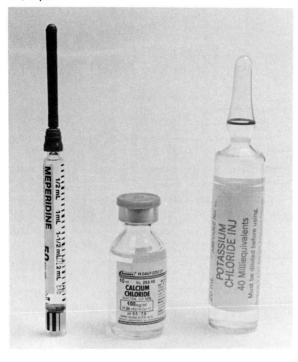

Selection of Syringe and Needle Size

The smaller the amount of medication to be given, the smaller the size of syringe to use. In special circumstances, such as the administration of insulin, it is essential that an insulin syringe be used. For measuring a very small amount of drug, use a tuberculin syringe.

Needles with large lumens are required when the medication to be injected is oily or very thick. Needles with small lumens are used for aqueous solutions. Shorter needles with a large gauge number may be used on children and very thin patients; longer needles may be required for obese patients to ensure that the needle reaches muscular or subcutaneous tissue.

Common sizes of syringes and needles used for various injections are shown in Table 7-6.

Anatomical Selection of the Injection Sites

Intramuscular Injections. The main objective when administering an intramuscular medication is to inject it deep into the muscle for gradual and optimal absorption into the bloodstream. The usual amount of solution to be given by this method is 2 to 5 ml. It is recommended to divide a 4- or 5-ml dose in half, using two different sites for injecting the medication. Identification of suitable sites for an injection is based on the use of definite anatomical landmarks, located by palpation. Four anatomical sites commonly used follow.

Gluteus Medius. The most common site for intramuscular injections, this is located in the upper outer quadrant (UOQ) of the buttock. Have the patient assume a prone position, toes pointed inward, and the buttock clearly exposed. This position allows for best relaxation of the muscles and best exposure of the area. Injecting a needle into a tense muscle causes pain. Undergarments must be completely removed. Under no circumstances must you deviate from using the correct technique. Palpate for and then draw a diagonal line from the greater trochanter of the femur to the posterior superior iliac spine. The injection is to be given well above and outside of this diagonal line. Extreme care must be taken to locate the correct site to avoid hitting the sciatic nerve or the superior gluteal artery (Fig. 7-10).

Middeltoid Area. This site is located on the upper, outer aspect of the arm, below the lower edge of the

Table 7-6. Common sizes of syringes and needles

Types of Injection	Size of Syringe	Size of Needle	Example for Use
Subcutaneous	2, 2½, or 3 cc	½ in. or ⅝ in., 25 to 26 gauge	Immunizations, heparin
Intramuscular	2 to 5 cc	1½ in. (1 in. for thin or small patients, 2 in. for obese patients), 21 or 22 gauge	Analgesics, vitamins, various antibiotics, and hormones
		1½ in., 20 gauge	Penicillin and thick solutions
Intradermal	1 cc	¼ in., ½ in., ⅜ in., or ¾ in., 26 or 27 gauge	Schick, Dick, tuberculin, and allergy skin tests
Insulin	1 cc calibrated in units	½ in. or ⅝ in., 25 gauge	Insulin
Intravenous	10, 20, or 50 cc	1¼ in., 1½ in., 22 gauge	Penicillin IV drip, transfusions
		1 to 1½ in., 18, 19, 20, or 21 gauge	Glucose, blood tests

Fig. 7-10.   Gluteus medius IM injection site. (Courtesy Wyeth Laboratories, Philadelphia, PA)

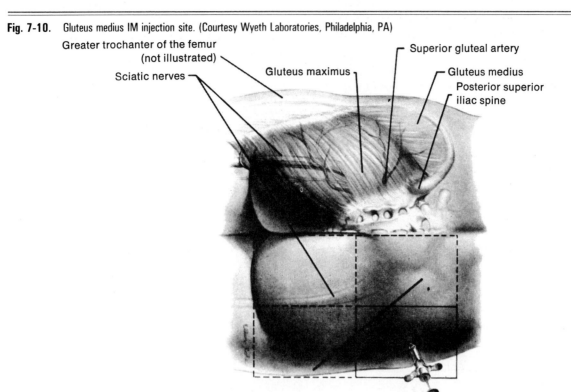

Greater trochanter of the femur
(not illustrated)

Sciatic nerves

Gluteus maximus

Superior gluteal artery

Gluteus medius
Posterior superior
iliac spine

acromion and above the axilla. Although there is easy access to this site when the patient is standing, sitting, or in a prone or supine position, the actual area that can be used for the injection is limited, as there are major vessels, nerves, and bones to be avoided in the upper arm. It is therefore recommended to limit the use of this site for injections, because of the small area available, which can tolerate only small amounts of medication and infrequent injections. In addition, patients often experience more pain and tenderness in this area (Fig. 7-11).

Ventrogluteal Area (von Hochstetter's Site).   Growing in recognition for use, this site is removed from major blood vessels and nerves. To locate this site, have the patient in a supine or side position. Palpate for the greater trochanter of the femur, the iliac crest, and the anterior superior iliac spine. Then place the palm of your right hand on the patient's left greater trochanter, your index finger on the anterior superior iliac spine, and move your middle finger posteriorly along the iliac crest as far as possible. (Do this with your left hand when injecting into the patient's right side.) A **V** space is now formed between your index and middle finger. The injection is to be given in the middle of this **V** space (Fig. 7-12 and 7-13).

Vastus Lateralis*.   This thick muscle on the upper side of the leg is also being used more frequently, as it is

*When intramuscular injections are administered to children, both the ventrogluteal and the vastus lateralis sites are recommended.

free of major blood vessels and nerves. With the patient in a supine position, locate this site by palpating the greater trochanter of the femur and the lateral aspect of the patella. Divide the distance between these two landmarks into thirds. The needle is to be inserted into the middle third of this area (Figs. 7-14 and 7-15).

Subcutaneous Injections.   The objective of a subcutaneous (sc) injection is to deposit a relatively small amount of an aqueous solution under the skin for rapid absorption into the bloodstream. The amount of the solution given by this method should not exceed 2 ml. To avoid overdistention of the tissues, the medication should be administered slowly. The most common and preferred sites for a subcutaneous injection are these:

- Outer surface of the upper arm, usually halfway between the shoulder and elbow
- Lateral aspect of the thigh
- Upper two thirds of the back

Additional sites that may be used, especially when the medication is self-administered, as a diabetic may do, include

- Areas on the abdomen
- Front aspect of the thigh

When frequent subcutaneous injections are given, sites of administration should be rotated to

(Text continues on p. 256)

Fig. 7-11. Middeltoid IM injection site. (Courtesy Wyeth Laboratories, Philadelphia, PA)

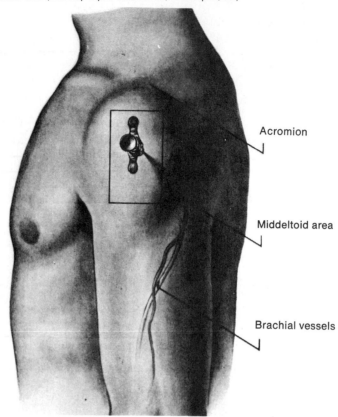

Acromion

Middeltoid area

Brachial vessels

Fig. 7-12. Ventrogluteal IM injection site. (Courtesy Wyeth Laboratories, Philadelphia, PA)

Ventrogluteal area
(in triangle)

Anterior superior
iliac spine

Iliac crest
(not illustrated)

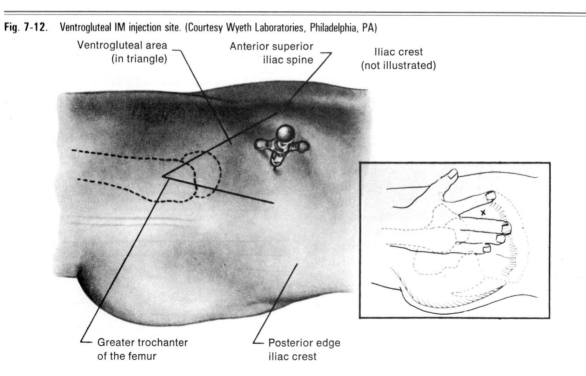

Greater trochanter
of the femur

Posterior edge
iliac crest

Fig. 7-13.   **A,** ventrogluteal area on a 100-pound woman. **B,** ventrogluteal area on a 130-pound man. (Courtesy Wyeth Laboratories, Philadelphia, PA)

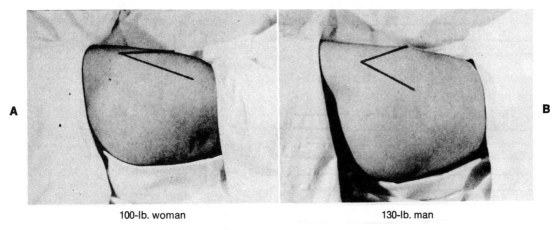

100-lb. woman   130-lb. man

Fig. 7-14.   Vastus lateralis IM injection site. (Courtesy Wyeth Laboratories, Philadelphia, PA)

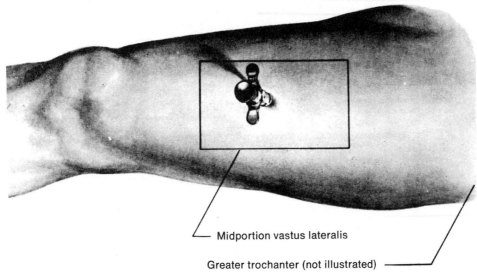

Midportion vastus lateralis

Greater trochanter (not illustrated)

Fig. 7-15.   **Left,** vastus lateralis area on 135-pound woman. **Right,** vastus lateralis area on 180-pound man. (Courtesy Wyeth Laboratories, Philadelphia, PA)

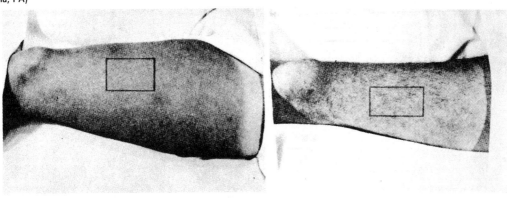

135-lb. woman   180-lb. man

prevent the damage of a tissue, excessive pain, and possible disfigurement (Fig. 7-16).

Intradermal Injections. The objective of the intradermal injection is to inject a minute amount of solution between the layers of the skin. The amount of drug given by this method is usually 0.1 ml to 0.3 ml. A tuberculin syringe (see Fig. 7-6) is used because of the fine calibrations, which provide the best means for measuring minute amounts of a drug. Drugs must be administered slowly in this method; they produce a small pale bump on the skin when given correctly.

The most common and preferred site for intradermal injections is the dorsal surface of the forearm, about 4 inches below the elbow. The lateral and posterior sides of the arm can also be used if and when required. These sites are used because they can be easily observed for reactions resulting from the drug injected and also can be kept free of irritation from clothing. Intradermal injections are used for various skin tests to determine allergies (sensitivities) to drugs and various other foreign substances, such as food substances, dust, and grass; to determine the patient's susceptibility to an infectious disease, such as tuberculosis (the Mantoux test) and diphtheria (the Schick test); or to aid in the diagnosis of infectious diseases. In addition to their frequent use for these tests, intradermal tests are used in the diagnosis of parasitic infections such as schistosomiasis and fungal diseases.

Because intradermal injections are utilized for skin tests, the procedure for administering the injection is discussed and outlined on pp. 400–401. Preparation of the syringe and needle and withdrawal of the drug into the syringe are the same as for the IM and sc injections, except that a ⅜ or ½ inch, 26 or 27 gauge needle, and a tuberculin syringe are used.

Instructions for Administering Injections

In addition to the rules listed on pp. 243–245, the following apply to injections.

1. Select the injection site carefully. You must avoid major blood vessels, nerves, and bones.
2. Use only sterile, preferably disposable, syringes and needles.
3. Select the correct size of syringe according to the amount of medication to be given and the appropriate size and length of needle, depending on the type of solution to be given and the size and condition of the patient.
4. Insert the needle using the correct angle (Fig. 7-17).
5. After inserting the needle, but before injecting the medication, always pull the plunger back to determine if you have entered a blood vessel.
6. If you have entered a blood vessel, withdraw the needle a bit, redirect and again insert the needle. Pull the plunger back to determine if you have entered a second blood vessel.
7. If a large amount of blood returns in the syringe when you pull back on the plunger, remove the needle and begin the procedure again using new medication, syringe, and needle.
8. Rotate injection sites on patients receiving frequent injections.

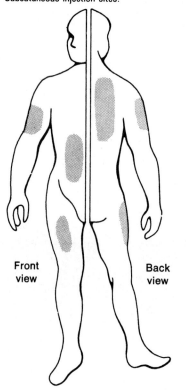

Fig. 7-16. Subcutaneous injection sites.

Front view   Back view

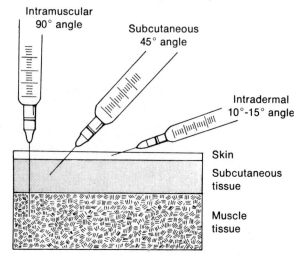

Fig. 7-17. Angles of insertion for parenteral injections.

Intramuscular 90° angle

Subcutaneous 45° angle

Intradermal 10°–15° angle

Skin

Subcutaneous tissue

Muscle tissue

9. Aseptic technique *must* be used when administering all injections.

ADMINISTRATION OF AN INTRAMUSCULAR INJECTION

Equipment

Appropriate size sterile needle and syringe, depending on amount and type of drug to be given (usually a 2 cc or 3 cc syringe, and a 21 or 22 gauge, 1½ inch needle) *or* hypodermic metal syringe when the medication is supplied in a prefilled sterile cartridge-needle unit, such as a Tubex hypodermic metal syringe.

- A 23 gauge 1 inch needle may be used when administering the drug into the deltoid muscle.

Sterile alcohol sponges
Medication ordered
Small tray

Procedure	Rationale
1. Wash your hands.	
2. Assemble the equipment.	
3. Prepare the syringe and needle for use. When using a separate syringe and needle, remove them from the wrappers, and leave the cover (sheath) on the needle intact. Grasping the hub of the needle and the barrel of the syringe, attach the hub of the needle to the tip of the syringe. Secure by turning the hub ¼ inch clockwise.	Avoid touching the tip of the syringe and the open end of the hub of the needle with your fingers. These parts are to remain sterile.
4. Compare the physician's order with the label on the medication.	These must be the same. At times you may have to calculate the dosage to be given.
5. Check the label of the medication three times during the preparation of the medication to ensure that you have the correct medication and strength.	Check the label three times: • When removing the medication from storage area • When filling the syringe • When replacing the medication in the storage area The same medication is often supplied in different strengths.
6. Take an alcohol sponge to cleanse the rubber stopper of the vial or the neck of the ampule; then discard this sponge. Withdraw medication into the syringe. *If an ampule is used:* a. Tap the tip of the ampule to dislodge any medication there. b. Cleanse the neck at the marked line. c. File across this line. d. Hold the ampule; with your other hand, cover the top end with a sponge, and break the top off going away from you (Fig. 7-18). The medication is now ready for use. e. Remove the needle cover (sheath). f. Insert the needle into the ampule (Fig. 7-19). g. Pull back on the plunger of the syringe to withdraw the required amount of medication. h. Remove the needle from the ampule. i. Replace the needle cover (sheath) over the needle. j. Place this unit on a small tray.	Cleansing helps prevent the introduction of microorganisms into the vial and prevents contamination of the needle. Files are supplied with ampules. The sponge is used to protect your fingers when the top is broken off. Do not touch the opening of the ampule with the needle. The needle is contaminated if it touches the outside or entrance of the ampule. In this instance, you must obtain another sterile needle for use.

Administration of an Intramuscular Injection (*continued*)

Procedure	Rationale
k. Check the label, and then discard the ampule.	
l. Proceed to the patient, carrying this medication and a sterile alcohol sponge on the small tray.	
If a vial is used:	
a. Take the syringe and pull the plunger back to obtain a measured amount of air equal to the amount of medication to be withdrawn from the vial.	
b. Remove the needle cover.	
c. Insert the needle through the cleansed rubber stopper, keeping it above the solution.	
d. Push the plunger of the syringe down to the bottom of the barrel.	This gives air replacement, which prevents the creation of a vacuum in the vial when the medication is withdrawn. If a vacuum is created, it makes it difficult to withdraw the medication. Do not inject more air than is required, as the pressure in the vial will then force the solution into the syringe, making it difficult to obtain an accurate dosage.
e. Invert the vial; have the vial and syringe at eye level.	Keep the vial and syringe at eye level to ensure correct measurement of the drug withdrawn.

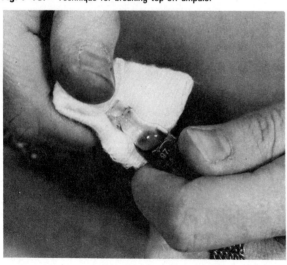

Fig. 7-18. Technique for breaking top off ampule.

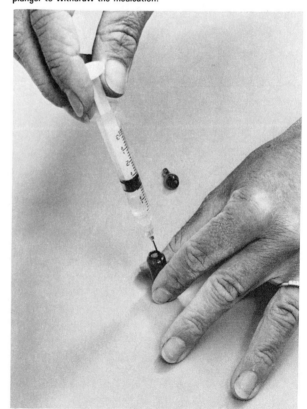

Fig. 7-19. Insert needle into ampule and pull back on syringe plunger to withdraw the medication.

Procedure	**Rationale**
f. With the needle opening in the solution, pull the plunger of the syringe back gently until the required amount of medication has been obtained (Fig. 7-20).	
g. Remove the needle from the vial.	
h. Replace the needle cover over the needle.	
i. Place the filled syringe with the covered needle on a small tray.	
j. Check the label on the vial, and replace it in the correct storage area.	Ensure that the correct medication will be administered.
k. Proceed to the patient, carrying the medication and a sterile alcohol sponge on the small tray.	
7. Identify the patient, and explain the procedure.	Correct patient identification is crucial. Explanations help gain the patient's cooperation and relaxation.
8. Select the injection site and position the patient accordingly, exposing the site clearly.	Refer to pp. 252–256, Anatomical Selection of Injection Sites. Your view and accessibility to the injection site must not be obstructed by the patient's clothing or any drape sheet. Be sure that you have ample lighting when administering the injection.
9. With the alcohol sponge, cleanse the injection site, starting at a central point and moving out to an area approximately 2 inches square; allow it to dry.	
10. Remove the needle cover.	
11. Hold the syringe with the needle facing upward; slowly push on the plunger until a tiny drop of medication comes to the needle tip.	This helps get rid of air bubbles, which must be expelled from the syringe before injecting the medication. Also, the tiny drop of medication obtained at the top of the syringe ensures that the needle is clear and not plugged.
12. Using the index finger and thumb of your nondominant hand, spread or tense the skin around the injection site.	

Fig. 7-20.   Withdrawing medication from vial. Hold syringe at eye level to ensure correct measurement of medication.

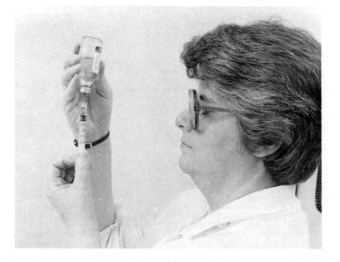

Administration of an Intramuscular Injection (*continued*)

Procedure	Rationale
13. Using your dominant hand, hold the syringe and needle as if you were holding a pencil, with the bevel of the needle facing up.	Your index finger and second finger may surround the top part of the needle hub with your thumb placed on the end of the syringe; or all three fingers may surround the bottom end of the syringe near the needle, but not touching the needle.
14. With a quick thrust, insert the needle at a 90 degree angle to about three fourths of the needle length. Do not hit the skin with the hub of the needle (Figs. 7-21 and 7-22).	Hold the needle perpendicular to the skin, and insert quickly in a dartlike thrust.
15. Steady the syringe with your dominant hand. Using your other hand, pull back on the plunger to see if any blood can be aspirated into the syringe.	Aspiration must be done to check if you have entered a blood vessel. If a blood vessel is entered, withdraw the needle slightly, redirect, and reinsert; then pull back on the plunger again to check for blood. Some recommend completely withdrawing the needle if a blood vessel is entered, then beginning the procedure again with a new needle.
16. Continue to steady the syringe with your dominant hand. With your other hand push on the plunger slowly to inject the medication.	Injection of the medication slowly allows the solution to disperse into the tissues. Discomfort caused by pressure will result if the medication is injected too quickly.
17. Using your nondominant hand, apply pressure at the injection site with the alcohol sponge, and quickly remove the needle with your dominant hand (the hand that has constantly been on the syringe and needle unit.) NOTE: By keeping your dominant hand in constant contact with the syringe and needle unit, rather than switching hands after inserting the needle (that is, some suggest inserting the needle with your dominant hand, then changing hands and steadying the syringe with your nondominant hand, then using your dominant hand to aspirate and push on the plunger), you help prevent further discomfort to the patient and tissue irritation that may occur if the syringe is jiggled or moved during a hand change.	Applied pressure and the quick withdrawal of the needle reduces discomfort and the risk of medication leaking into the subcutaneous tissues and possibly forming abscesses.
18. Massage the injection site. Move the tissue as you massage, not merely the sponge (Fig. 7-23).	Massaging the area helps spread the medication in the tissue. If rapid absorption is desired, continue to massage the area for about 2 minutes.
19. Help the patient assume a comfortable and safe position.	
20. Observe the patient for any unusual reactions, such as a rash or shock.	
21. Inform the patient if he or she is free to leave or if the physician requires additional consultation time.	
22. Place a disposable needle and syringe in a puncture resistant container without breaking or recapping the needle. The needle box should be in the room or as close as possible to the area of use (Figure 7-24).	

Procedure

Guidelines for Preventing Needlesticks

a) Slow down and *think* when using or disposing of needles.

b) DO NOT *recap* needles unless absolutely necessary. If necessary, place cap on table top before inserting needle (insert needle into cap without holding cap).

c) Never put a needle down—dispose of it promptly in approved container.

d) Never put needles or other sharp instruments in trash cans.

e) Never leave needles or other sharp instruments on counter tops, examination tables, or disposable procedure trays.

f) Never push a needle into the red plastic needle disposable box with your hand. If the needle does not go into the opening easily, use a large syringe to push it in.

g) Never try to remove a needle or syringe from the red plastic box.

After using a reusable syringe and needle, flush tap water through both until clean. Separate the needle, barrel, and plunger, and place each in a designated cleansing solution until ready to prepare all for sterilization.

23. Wash your hand.

24. Record the procedure on the patient's chart.

Dispose of both in the designated container for used syringes and needles.

Rationale

Charting example:
June 3, 19_____, 4 PM
   Penbritin-S 500 mg IM in ROQ [right outer quadrant] of buttock, for respiratory tract infection.
   Brook Thomas, CMA

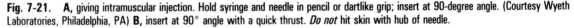

Fig. 7-21.   A, giving intramuscular injection. Hold syringe and needle in pencil or dartlike grip; insert at 90-degree angle. (Courtesy Wyeth Laboratories, Philadelphia, PA) **B,** insert at 90° angle with a quick thrust. *Do not* hit skin with hub of needle.

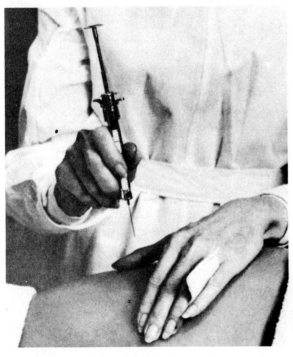

A

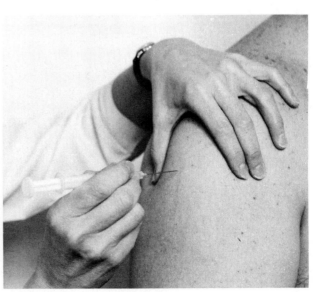

B

Fig. 7-22. Giving an intramuscular injection. Insert needle with quick thrust. Do not hit skin with hub of needle. (Courtesy Wyeth Laboratories, Philadelphia, PA)

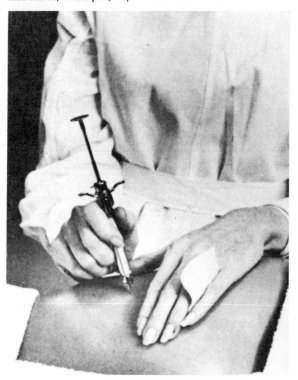

Fig. 7-23. Intramuscular injection technique. After the injection has been administered, massage and cleanse injection site with sponge to remove any blood or medication that might be present. (Courtesy Wyeth Laboratories, Philadelphia, PA)

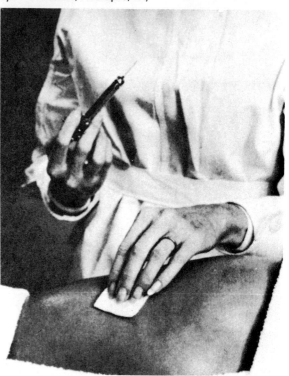

If a metal syringe and medication in a prefilled sterile cartridge-needle unit are used, the method for giving the medication is basically the same as when using a disposable or reusable syringe. After use, you should clean the metal syringe with an antiseptic solution. Sterilization is not required, as the syringe does not come in direct contact with the patient.

Loading Tubex Closed Injection System

Equipment

Tubex hypodermic syringe
Prefilled sterile cartridge-needle unit

Fig. 7-24. Puncture-resistant containers marked, "Biohazard" should be used to dispose of used syringes.

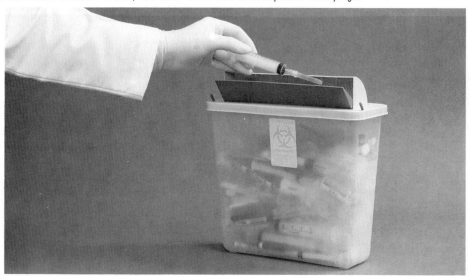

Procedure for Loading Tubex Closed Injection System

Procedure	Rationale
1. Hold the barrel of the metal syringe in your nondominant hand.	
2. Using your other hand, pull the plunger back and swing the entire handle section downward so that it locks at a right angle to the barrel (Fig. 7-25, *A*).	
3. Insert the sterile cartridge-needle unit into the barrel, needle end first (Fig. 7-25, *B*).	
4. Rotate the cartridge clockwise until a slight clicking sound is heard.	The clicking sound indicates that the cartridge is threaded correctly into the front end of the syringe.
5. Swing the plunger back into place.	
6. With your dominant hand, rotate the plunger clockwise until both ends of the cartridge-needle unit are fully engaged and another slight clicking sound is heard (Fig. 7-25, *C*).	Your nondominant hand should be holding the barrel of the metal syringe—*not* the glass cartridge.
7. Leave the rubber cover (sheath) over the needle until just before use.	This maintains the sterility of the needle.
8. After use, replace the rubber cover over the needle; rotate the plunger counterclockwise, open the syringe, and remove the cartridge-needle unit (Fig. 7-25, *D*).	
9. Dispose of both in the designated container for used syringe and needles.	

Fig. 7-25. **A** to **C**, technique for loading a Tubex Hypodermic syringe. **D**, technique for removing empty Tubex after use. (Courtesy Wyeth Laboratories, Philadelphia, PA)

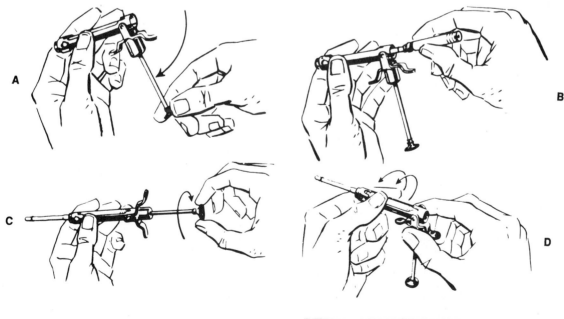

Procedure for Using the Tubex Fast-Trak Syringe

For the procedure for using this newer type of syringe and sterile cartridge-needle unit, see Figure 7-26.

Intramuscular Z-Tract Technique

The alternate intramuscular injection technique is called the Z-tract technique. It may be used for medications such as Imferon, which may cause irritation of subcutaneous tissue and discoloration from leaking medications, or when complete absorption of the medication by the muscle tissue is crucial. The preferred site for this technique is the upper outer quadrant of the buttock.

In this technique the tissue is pulled down and toward the median before, during, and after the injection. When the tissue is released the needle track that is created is a Z pattern rather than the straight needle track that is created in other intramuscular injections. The Z pattern tract keeps the medication deep in the muscle and prevents seepage up through the tissues.

Use a 2 inch needle if the patient weighs approximately 200 pounds. If you don't use a needle this long on a patient of this weight, you will need to insert the needle its full length and then indent the tissue with the hub of the needle to ensure deep muscle penetration.

Use a 1¼ to 1½ inch needle if the patient weighs around 100 pounds. Us a ¾ to 1 inch needle on children weighing around 50 pounds.

Follow steps 1 through 11 as outlined on pp. 257–259, under "Administration of an Intramuscular Injection," with the **exception** that you should change needles after you have drawn the medication into the syringe. This eliminates the chance of medication left in the needle leaking into the tissue during the injection or of an extra "needle's worth" of medication being given. This minute extra amount of drug is of less concern with adult patients than it is with children for whom even minute quantities of drug may be significant. Now proceed as follows:

Fig. 7-26. Directions for using Tubex Fast-Trak syringe. (Courtesy Wyeth Laboratories, Philadelphia, PA)

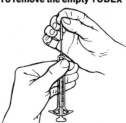

Wyeth®
TUBEX®
Fast-Trak®
Syringe

QUICK-LOADING
1 and 2 mL sizes

DIRECTIONS FOR USE
Note: The TUBEX Fast-Trak Syringe is reusable: do not discard after use.

To load the TUBEX Fast-Trak Syringe

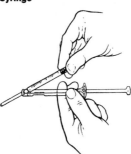

1. With plunger rod fully withdrawn, insert TUBEX Sterile Cartridge-Needle Unit, needle end first, into the barrel. Rotate the cartridge clockwise to engage the threads on the needle hub with the threads at front end of syringe (a clicking sound will be heard when fully engaged).

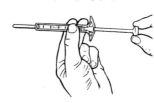

2. After engaging the TUBEX cartridge in the TUBEX Fast-Trak Syringe, thread the plunger rod to the rubber plunger by gently rotating the plunger rod clockwise until the cartridge turns with the plunger.

To maintain sterility, leave rubber needle sheath in place until just before use. Then grasp it securely at the tip and pull firmly to remove.

To Administer
Method of administration is the same as with conventional syringe. Remove rubber sheath, introduce needle into patient, aspirate by pulling back slightly on the plunger, and inject.

To remove the empty TUBEX

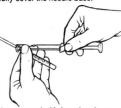

With syringe in vertical position, replace rubber sheath by holding tip between thumb and forefinger while guiding sheath over the tip of the needle. Drop the sheath over the needle and shake the syringe gently; gravity will cause the sheath to slip into place. Then carefully pull down on the bottom of the sheath to fully cover the needle base.

Unscrew and withdraw the plunger rod. Rotate cartridge counterclockwise to disengage at front end of syringe. Remove and discard only the used TUBEX Cartridge-Needle Unit. (Before discarding, the sheath-covered needle should be bent to seal the lumen in order to discourage pilferage or reuse.)

Used TUBEX Cartridge-Needle Units should not be employed for successive injections or as multiple-dose containers. They are intended to be used only once and discarded.

Note: Any graduated markings on TUBEX Sterile Cartridge-Needle Units are to be used only as a guide in mixing, withdrawing, or administering measured doses.

Wyeth does not recommend and will not accept responsibility for the use of any cartridge-needle unit other than TUBEX® in the TUBEX® Fast-Trak® Syringe.

Procedure	Rationale
12. Move the skin downward and toward the median.	The skin and subcutaneous tissue of an average adult will move about 1 to 1.6 inches. The underlying muscle within the selected injection site remains stationary.
13. Insert the needle at a 90 degree angle while maintaining traction on the tissue.	
14. Extend the thumb and index finger of the hand that is displacing the tissue to support the base of the syringe and aspirate by pulling back on the plunger using your other hand.	

Procedure	**Rationale**
Maintain traction on the tissue. If blood appears, select a new site and use a new needle.	You may damage subcutaneous tissue and cause pain if traction is released while the needle is in place.
15. Inject slowly and smoothly while maintaining traction on the tissue.	
16. Wait 10 seconds, then withdraw the needle and immediately release the skin, creating a Z pattern, which blocks any infiltration of the medication into the subcutaneous tissue.	Waiting provides time for the medication to disperse into the muscle and gives the muscle time to relax.
17. DO NOT MASSAGE THE INJECTION SITE. If bleeding occurs, gently wipe the area with a dry sterile cotton ball or gauze.	
18. Advise the patient not to exercise or wear tight clothing immediately after the injection.	This will minimize the chance of the medication spreading into other layers of tissue.
19. Continue with steps 19 through 24 under the procedure "Administration of an Intramuscular Injection."	

ADMINISTRATION OF A SUBCUTANEOUS INJECTION

Equipment

Sterile needle and syringe; usually a 2 cc syringe, ½ or ⅝ inch, 25 gauge needle

Sterile alcohol sponges

Medication ordered

Small tray to transport prepared medication to the patient

Preparation of the needle, syringe and medication follows the same procedure that was outlined under "Administration of an Intramuscular Injection." Remember to wash your hands before beginning the procedure, check the medication label three times, measure dosage accurately, identify your patient and explain the procedure, position the patient, and select the injection site correctly before administering the medication.

Follow steps 1 through 11 as outlined under the intramuscular injection technique, then do the following:

Procedure	**Rationale**
12. Grasp the skin surrounding the injection area between your thumb and index finger, *or* spread the skin and hold it taut.	The decision of which method to use will depend on the size of the patient and the size of the needle. Grasping the skin may be done on small, very thin, or dehydrated patients; spreading the skin may be used on large, well-nourished patients. Whichever method you use, be sure that you enter subcutaneous tissue when inserting the needle.
13. Hold the barrel of the syringe between your thumb and other fingers of your dominant hand, letting the hub of the needle rest on your index finger. The bevel of the needle should be facing upward.	
14. Insert the needle at a 45 degree angle into the skin using a quick, forward thrust (Fig. 7-27).	The needle should be inserted almost to its full length. Do not touch the skin with the hub of the needle.
15. Release the skin.	
16. Keep your dominant hand on the syringe for support. With your other hand, pull back on the plunger to see if you aspirate any blood.	Refer to steps 15 through 22 as outlined in the procedure for administering an intramuscular injection for full explanations of the remaining steps.

Administration of a Subcutaneous Injection (*continued*)

Procedure	Rationale
17. Inject the medication slowly.	
18. With an alcohol sponge, apply pressure to the injection site, and quickly remove the needle.	
19. Massage the injection site with the alcohol sponge, and observe the patient for any unusual reaction.	
20. Leave the patient safe and comfortable, providing any further instructions.	
21. Remove and dispose of used equipment properly.	See No. 22, pp. 260–261.
22. Wash your hands.	

23. Record the procedure on the patient's chart.	Charting example:
	June 2, 19_____, 2 PM
	  Thiomerin [a diuretic] 1 ml, sc in left upper arm.
	    Kathy Kron, CMA

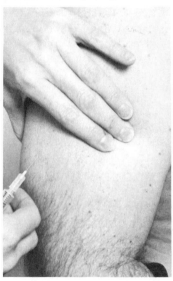

Fig. 7-27. Technique for administering a subcutaneous injection. Insert needle at a 45-degree angle.

CONCLUSION

Having completed this unit, you should be able to discuss the laws regulating the distribution and administration of medication, in addition to the responsibilities and rules governing the administration of all types of medication. Certain legal stipulations are set forth that a physician must meet before using narcotics. You should be familiar with the special laws of your state of practice and know how you can best help your physician comply with the state and federal laws applying to the dispensing, administering, and prescribing of medications, including narcotics and controlled substances. Knowledge of and familiarity with resource reference books on drugs are necessary to ensure adequate knowledge of any medication you are required to administer. There are numerous references providing information on improved medication techniques and current pharmacological products. Check with your instructor for additional assignments and reference sources in areas of your own particular interest and need.

A variety of ways in which medications may be administered has been discussed in this unit. You must be able to describe all nine routes of administration and demonstrate your ability to administer an intramuscular and a subcutaneous injection. When you feel competent in this knowledge and these two techniques, arrange with your instructor to take the performance tests. You will be expected to accurately demonstrate your ability to prepare for and administer subcutaneous and intramuscular injections to a patient, in addition to identifying the equipment used and the care of such equipment after use.

REVIEW OF VOCABULARY

Read and define the italicized terms, which have been presented in this unit.

Addiction and *habituation* of many drugs are major health problems in present-day society. To add to this problem, many use *crude drugs* rather than *pure drugs*, which may exert increasing *toxicity* in those who partake. Many individuals are unaware of the many *side effects* that drugs may produce, such as drug *tolerance* or the more severe reaction of *anaphylactic shock*. *Chemotherapy* used correctly in medical situations can produce marvelous results. At times there are *contraindications* when certain medications should not be *administered* to a patient. *Drug idiosyncrasies or side effects* may occur in patients receiving certain drugs. It is vital that this information be reported to the physician so that this particular *prophylactic* treatment may be altered.

A *cumulative action of a drug* may be desired at times and at other times *contraindicated;* thus any prolonged drug therapy must be monitored closely for various medical reasons.

The *HHS, FDA,* and *DEA* are all governmental agencies involved with the regulations controlling the commerce and *administration of drugs.*

Useful *pharmacology* book resources include the *PDR* and *USP–NF.* Familiarity with these sources is vital when knowledge of approved drugs, their dosages, actions, and contraindications is sought.

When an inventory is taken of the *stock supply of drugs* in the office, it is necessary to discard *outdated drugs* and reorder a new supply. At times you may receive medications in a *unit dose.* An accurate inventory of all medications on hand is the responsibility of the medical assistant. Always know the drug before administering it to a patient. It is also important for a medical assistant to be familiar with drugs that have been *dispensed, administered,* or *prescribed* to the patient by the physician.

REVIEW QUESTIONS

1. Explain what a drug is; list three uses and four sources from which drugs are derived.
2. Describe the difference between the trade name and the generic name of a drug, and give two examples of each.
3. Describe the difference between the following three classifications of drugs: (a) controlled substances, (b) prescription drugs, (c) nonprescription drugs.
4. List one use for each of the following: (a) analgesics, (b) anticoagulants, (c) antidotes, (d) antiseptics, (e) bronchodilators, (f) diuretics, (g) emetics, (h) hemostatics, (i) miotics, (j) narcotics, (k) tranquilizers, (l) vasodilators.
5. List seven parts of a prescription.
6. Drugs are supplied in either a solid or liquid form. List five types of solid preparations and five types of liquid preparations.
7. Describe how and where medications should be stored.
8. When the label of a medication is torn and soiled so that the name of the drug cannot be clearly identified, what should you do with it?
9. List the information that must be kept on the office record for Schedule II controlled substances after they have been administered to a patient in the office.
10. List and briefly describe ten routes by which medications can be administered.
11. List the five rights of proper medication administration.

12. When preparing medication to be administered, the label should be checked three times. List the three times when you should read the label of the medication.
13. Discuss at least ten rules and responsibilities that you must be concerned with when administering medications.
14. Discuss five factors that will influence dosage and drug action.
15. List six reasons for administering a medication by injection.
16. Discuss dangers involved and areas to avoid when giving medication by injection.
17. When asked to give a patient a subcutaneous injection, what size needle and syringe will you use? What sizes would be used for an intramuscular injection? Into which body sites would you administer each of these injections?
18. You have inserted the needle into the patient's right gluteus medius. As you withdraw the plunger of the syringe, a large amount of blood returns. What does this indicate, and what would be your next action?
19. The following orders have been written by the physician for patients. Using the abbreviation lists, transcribe these orders into English.
    a. Compazine 15 mg × 12 caps
       Sig ī cap po, tid, ac & hs, prn
    b. Digitoxin 0.1 mg × 30 tabs
       Sig ī cap po, od
    c. Digoxin 0.25 mg × 30 tabs
       Sig ī tab po, bid for 10 days, then ½ tab bid po for 10 days
    d. Benadryl 50 mg × 8 caps
       Sig ī cap po, qid for 2 d
    e. Dramamine 25 mg × 30 tabs
       Sig 25 mg, po, tid, ac, prn
    f. Vitamin B_{12}, 2 mcg, IM, qd
    g. Ampicillin 500 mg × 28 caps
       Sig 500 mg po, q6h for 7 days
    h. Streptomycin 3 gm, qd, IM for 7 days
    i. Tetracycline 250 mg × 28 caps
       Sig ī po, 1 hr ac c̄ H_2O
    j. Keflin 0.5 gm IM stat and then q6h for 7 days
    k. Plain insulin 1 vial 40 IU/cc
       Sig 20 IU sc, ac and 40 IU, hs, sc
    l. Demerol 100 mg IM stat
    m. Seconal 50 mg po, hs, may repeat ×1, prn
20. Solve the following problems to determine the amount of drug that is to be administered.
    a. Give ASA gr 10 po; bottle reads 5 gr/tablet
    b. Give Compazine 10 mg IM; ampule reads 5 mg/ml
    c. Give Digitoxin 0.4 mg po; bottle reads 0.2 mg/tablet
    d. Give ascorbic acid 0.5 gm po; bottle reads 500 mg/tablet
    e. Give Kantrex 15 gr IM; bottle reads 1 gm = 3 ml
    f. Give Maalox 1 ounce. How many ml do you give?
    g. Give tetracycline 500 mg, po; bottle reads 250 mg/capsule
    h. Give Valium 5 mg po; bottle reads 10 mg/tablet

PERFORMANCE TEST

In a skills laboratory, a simulation of a joblike environment, the medical assistant student will demonstrate skill in preparing for and administering medication safely and efficiently by accomplishing the following:

1. Intramuscular injection in one of the four sites discussed in this unit; IM injection using the Z-Tract technique.
2. Subcutaneous injection in the upper, outer part of the arm.
3. Loading and using a metal syringe with a prefilled sterile cartridge-needle unit for an IM injection.

These procedures are to be performed without reference to source materials. For these activities, the student will need a person to play the role of the patient to demonstrate the correct positioning of the patient and to locate the correct anatomical site to be used for the injection. An artificial limb may be used for performing the actual injection. Time limits for the performance of the above procedures are to be assigned by the instructor (see also pp. 32 and 35).

The student is to perform the above and record the procedures on the patient's chart with 100% accuracy.

PERFORMANCE CHECKLIST

Prepare and Administer an Intramuscular Injection

1. Wash your hands.
2. Assemble equipment.
3. Prepare syringe and needle for use.
4. Check physician's medication order with the label on the medication container.
5. Check the medication label three times as you are preparing the medication for administration.
6. Calculate the correct dosage, if applicable.
7. Take an alcohol sponge to cleanse ampule or vial.
8. *For an ampule*:
   • Tap the tip, cleanse the neck, file, and break the top off.
   • Remove the needle cover.
   • Insert the needle into the vial, and withdraw the required amount of drug.
   • Remove the needle from the ampule, and replace the cover over the needle.
   • Place the syringe with the needle and the alcohol sponge on a tray.
   • Check the label on the ampule, discard the ampule, and proceed to the patient.
9. *For a vial*:
   • Pull the plunger of the syringe back to obtain a measured amount of air equal to the amount of medication to be withdrawn from the vial.
   • Remove the needle cover, and insert the needle through the cleansed rubber stopper of the vial, keeping the needle above the solution level.

   • Push the plunger to the bottom of the barrel of the syringe.
   • Invert the vial, and with the needle opening in the solution, pull the plunger back to withdraw the required amount of medication.
   • Remove the needle from the vial and replace the cover over the needle.
   • Check the label on the vial and replace it in the storage area.
   • Proceed to the patient.
10. Identify and explain the procedure to the patient.
11. Select the injection site, and position the patient accordingly.
12. Cleanse the injection site.
13. Remove the needle cover, and expel air bubbles.
14. Insert the needle at a 90 degree angle with a quick thrust.
15. Pull back on the plunger; if no blood is aspirated, inject the medication slowly.
16. Apply pressure to the injection site with an alcohol sponge, withdraw the needle quickly, and massage the injection site.
17. Assist the patient as required, observe for any reactions, and leave the patient with further instructions, if applicable.
18. Remove used equipment and dispose of properly as indicated by the type of supplies used.
19. Wash your hands.
20. Record the procedure on the patient's chart: date, time, name of medication, dosage, route used, site of injection, reason if applicable, and your signature.

Prepare and Administer a Subcutaneous Injection

1. Wash your hands.
2. Assemble the equipment.
3. Prepare the syringe and needle for use.
4. Check the label of medication three times as you are preparing the medication.
5. Calculate dosage, if applicable.
6. Cleanse the ampule or vial with an alcohol sponge.
7. Insert the needle into the ampule or vial, and withdraw the required amount of the drug.
8. Check the label, and replace the vial in storage; or discard the ampule.
9. Identify and explain the procedure to the patient.
10. Select the injection site, position the patient, and cleanse the injection site.
11. Expel air bubbles from the syringe, and insert the needle at a 45 degree angle.
12. Pull back on the plunger; inject the medication slowly.
13. With an alcohol sponge, apply pressure to the injection site, and remove the needle quickly. Massage the injection site, and observe the patient for any reactions.
14. Leave the patient safe and comfortable, providing any further instructions.
15. Remove and dispose of equipment as indicated by the type used.

16. Wash your hands.
17. Record the procedure.

Injections Using a Tubex Hypodermic Syringe and Prefilled Sterile Cartridge-Needle Unit

The method for administering the injection is basically the same as when using disposable or reusable syringes and needles. To load and unload the Tubex hypodermic syringe with the prefilled sterile cartridge-needle unit:

1. Hold the barrel of the syringe, and with the other hand, pull the plunger back, swinging the entire handle section down to lock it at a right angle to the barrel.
2. Insert the cartridge-needle unit into the barrel, needle end first.
3. Rotate the cartridge clockwise until a slight clicking is heard.
4. Swing the plunger back into place, and rotate clockwise until both ends are fully engaged and another clicking sound is heard.
5. After use, replace the cover over the needle, rotate the plunger counterclockwise, open the syringe and remove the cartridge-needle unit.
6. Break the needle off, and dispose of both needle and cartridge in a designated container for used supplies.
7. Wash your hands.

Prepare and Administer an Intramuscular Injection Using the Z-Tract Technique

1. Follow steps 1 through 13 as listed under the checklist ''Prepare and Administer an Intramuscular Injection'' with the *exception* that you change needles after you have drawn the medication into the syringe.
2. Move the skin downward and toward the median.
3. Insert the needle at a 90 degree angle while maintaining traction on the tissue.
4. Pull back on the plunger; if no blood is aspirated, inject the medication slowly and smoothly while maintaining traction on the tissue.
5. Wait 10 seconds, then withdraw the needle and immediately release the skin.
6. DO NOT MASSAGE THE INJECTION SITE. If bleeding occurs, gently wipe the area with a dry sterile cotton ball or gauze.
7. Advise the patient not to exercise or wear tight clothing immediately after the injection.
8. Continue with steps 17 through 20 as given under the checklist ''Prepare and Administer an Intramuscular Injection.''

Unit VIII

Instillations and Irrigations of the Ear and Eye

COGNITIVE OBJECTIVES

On completion of Unit VIII, the medical assistant student should be able to apply the following cognitive objectives.

1. Define and pronounce the terms listed in the vocabulary.
2. Describe how to instill drops into the ear and eye, and explain the reason for the actions taken.
3. Describe how to irrigate the ear and eye, and explain the reasons for the steps taken.
4. Explain the difference between an irrigation and an instillation.
5. List

Two purposes for an ear instillation
Four purposes for an eye instillation
Four purposes for an ear irrigation
Four purposes for an eye irrigation

TERMINAL PERFORMANCE OBJECTIVES

On completion of Unit VIII, the medical assistant student should be able to do the following terminal performance objectives:

1. Demonstrate the proper procedure for performing an ear instillation and irrigation.
2. Demonstrate the proper procedure for performing an eye instillation and irrigation.

The above activities are to be performed with 100% accuracy 95% of the time.

Vocabulary

auricle (aw'rĭ-kl)—The outer projection of the ear; also known as the pinna (pin'nah).
canthus (kan'thus)—The inner canthus is the angle of the eyelids near the nose; the outer canthus is the angle of the eyelids at the outside corner of the eyes.

cerumen (sĕ-roo'men)—Ear wax secreted by the glands of the external auditory meatus.
conjunctiva (kon"junk-tī'vah)—The delicate membrane lining the eyelids and reflected onto the front of the eyeball.
external ear—Includes the auricle, or pinna, and the external auditory meatus.
external auditory meatus (me-ā'tus)—The canal or passage leading from the outside opening of the ear to the eardrum. Also called the external acoustic meatus.
miotic (mī-ot'ik)—A medication that causes the pupil of the eye to contract.
mydriatic (mid"rē-at'ik)—A medication that causes the pupil of the eye to dilate.
ocular (ok'ū-lar)—Pertaining to the eye.
ophthalmic (of-thal'mik)—Pertaining to the eye.
ophthalmology (of"thal-mol'ō-jē)—The study and science of the eye and its diseases.
otic (ō'tik)—Pertaining to the ear.
otology (ō-tol'ō-je)—The study and science of the ear and its diseases.
otoscope (ō'tō-skōp)—An instrument used for visual inspection of the ear.
tympanic (tim-pan'ik) **membrane** (abbreviated **TM**)—The eardrum; it serves as the membrane that separates the external auditory meatus from the middle ear cavity.

The medical assistant may be asked to perform ear and eye instillations and irrigations. These procedures differ slightly. An instillation is the dropping of a fluid into a body cavity; an irrigation is the flushing or washing of a body cavity with a stream of fluid. Practices of medical asepsis (as outlined in Unit IV) are to be observed when performing these procedures. However, if there is an open wound in the area being treated, sterile technique must be used.

To understand ear and eye instillations and irrigations and to be of most help to the patient and physician, the medical assistant should be familiar with the anatomy and physiology of these two special sense organs. It is suggested that these topics be reviewed before studying and practicing the procedures in this unit. A diagram of the ear is given in Fig. 8-1; the eye is diagrammed in Fig. 8-2.

Fig. 8-1. Diagram of ear. (From Anthony, C.P.: Text of anatomy and physiology, ed. 9, St. Louis, 1975, The C.V. Mosby Co.)

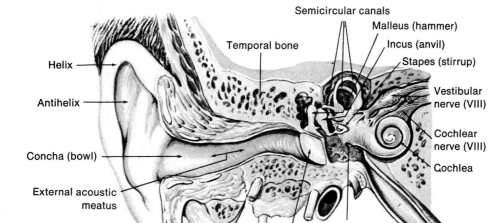

Fig. 8-2. Diagram of eye. (From Anthony, C.P., and Thibodeau, G.A.: Textbook of anatomy and physiology, ed. 10, St. Louis, 1979, The C.V. Mosby Co.)

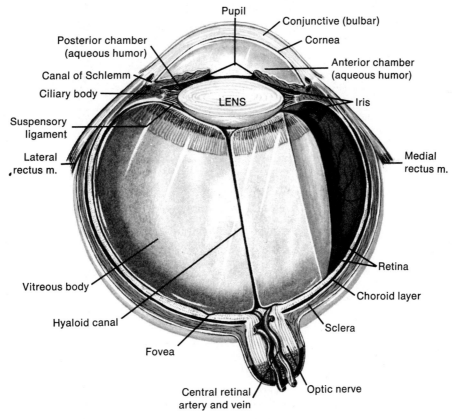

EAR INSTILLATIONS AND IRRIGATIONS

When solutions are instilled into the ear, keep in mind that the direction of the external ear canal in adults differs from that in children. To straighten the ear canal in both age groups so that the medication will be effective, slightly different techniques are used for each.

Medical aseptic technique is used when instilling solutions into the ear, as the outer ear is not sterile. However, if the tympanic membrane is not intact, sterile technique must be used. To lessen discomfort for the patient, the medications used should be warmed slightly before using. Solutions that are either too cold or too hot may cause a feeling of dizziness in addition to pain. One may warm a bottle of ear drops by placing the bottle in a plastic bag to protect the label, and then placing the bag and bottle in a basin of warm water for a few minutes. The temperature of the medication can be checked by placing a drop or two on your inner wrist; it should feel warm, not hot.

Ear Instillation

Ear instillations are performed to

1. Soften cerumen (ear wax) so that it can be removed easily later
2. Instill an antibiotic solution to combat an infection in the ear canal or eardrum.

Equipment

Prescribed medication and ear dropper
Cotton balls

Procedure	Rationale
1. Check the medication order carefully; that is, the name and amount of medication and which ear requires treatment.	Avoid medication errors.
2. Wash your hands.	
3. Assemble supplies.	
4. Read the medication label carefully three times, and check with the order. Warm the solution.	The label must be checked to avoid the possibility of any mistake.
5. Identify the patient, and explain the nature of the procedure and the purpose.	Prevent giving a drug to the wrong patient. Explanations help gain the patient's full cooperation.
6. Place the patient in a sitting or side-lying position.	
7. Instruct the patient to tilt the head toward the unaffected side.	
8. Stand at the patient's head.	
9. Withdraw the medication into the dropper, and examine the dropper for any defects.	A safe vehicle must be used to administer the medication.
10. Straighten the external ear canal. For adults, gently pull the top of the earlobe upward and backward (Fig. 8-3). For children, gently pull the bottom of the earlobe downward and backward.	The direction of the external ear canal differs in adults and children.
11. Place the tip of the dropper just slightly inside the external meatus (external ear canal), and instill the correct amount of medication.	
12. Instruct the patient to keep the head tilted or to remain on the unaffected side for a few minutes.	This position will prevent leakage of the medication from the ear.
13. Place a cotton ball over the opening of the ear only if ordered.	A cotton ball is placed over the ear opening only when ordered, as it may absorb some of the medication and prevent the desired action on the ear tissue. Also, cotton balls may prevent drainage from escaping when present.
14. Discard unused medication, and replace the dropper into the bottle, avoiding contamination.	When the dropper is contaminated, it must be replaced with a clean dropper.
15. Provide for the patient's safety and comfort. Give further instructions as required.	
16. Return supplies to designated area.	
17. Wash your hands.	

Procedure	Rationale
18. Record the procedure on the patient's chart.	Charting example: October 10, 19____, 11 AM 5 gtt Cerumenex instilled to left ear. Cotton ball placed in external ear canal and left for 15 minutes, then left ear irrigated with warm normal saline. Large amount of cerumen returned. Sarah Dolan, CMA

Fig. 8-3. Instillation of ear drops.

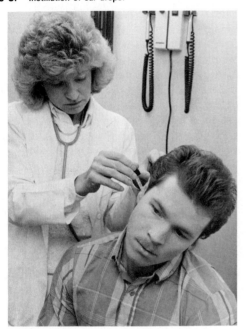

Ear Irrigation

An ear irrigation is the washing out of the external auditory canal with a stream of fluid. This procedure is done to

1. Cleanse the external auditory canal (external acoustic meatus)
2. Relieve inflammation of the ear
3. Dislodge impacted cerumen or foreign bodies from the external auditory canal
4. Apply antiseptics to combat infection
5. Apply heat to the tissues of the ear canal

Before an irrigation is done, all patients must be asked if they have a history of drainage from the ears, and if they have ever had a perforation or other com-plications from a previous irrigation. If the answer to either question is "yes," notify the physician before giving this treatment. Also, before the irrigation, a visual examination of the ear canal is done with an otoscope. When the purpose of the irrigation is to cleanse the ear canal or to remove cerumen or foreign bodies, a visual examination must also be performed after the irrigation to determine if the results are satisfactory.

When this procedure is done, extreme care must be taken to prevent injury to the tympanic membrane and the spread of any infection to the mastoid cavity.

Equipment

Drapes: towel, and a small rubber sheet if available
Kidney or ear basin for drainage
Syringe — either a metal ear syringe (such as a Pomeroy syringe), an Asepto bulb syringe (Fig. 8-4), or a rubber bulb syringe
Warm sterile solution/medication as ordered by the physician, in a container; solutions commonly used include:
Normal saline
Sterile water
Antiseptic solutions
Amount: 500 to 1000 ml, as ordered
Temperature: 100°F (approximately 38°C) (near body temperature)
Sterile cotton balls
Sterile applicators

Fig. 8-4. Asepto bulb syringe. (Courtesy Becton-Dickinson, Division of Becton, Dickinson and Company, Rutherford, NJ)

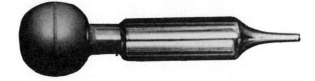

Procedure for Ear Irrigation

Procedure	Rationale
1. Follow the procedure as outlined for an ear instillation in steps 1 through 5: • Check the medication order • Wash your hands • Assemble the supplies • Check the solution/medication label three times; warm solution • Identify the patient, and explain the procedure and purpose	
2. Position the patient sitting with the head slightly tilted toward the affected side.	This position allows gravity to help the irrigating solution to flow from the ear to the basin.
3. Place a small rubber sheet (when available) and a towel over the patient's shoulder.	Protect the patient's clothing from any drainage.
4. Instruct the patient to hold the kidney or ear basin under the ear and firmly against the neck (Fig. 8-5).	The basin provides a receptacle to receive the irrigating solution and to prevent it from running down the patient's neck.
5. Cleanse the outer ear and external auditory meatus as necessary (to remove any discharge or debris present) with the irrigating solution or normal saline.	Cleansing the outer parts of the ear is necessary to prevent the introduction of foreign materials into the ear canal during the irrigation.
6. Test the temperature of the solution by putting a few drops on the inner aspect of your wrist. The solution should feel warm.	Warm solutions are more comfortable for the patient. Cold or too hot solutions may cause more discomfort and a feeling of dizziness.
7. Fill the syringe with the irrigating solution; expel any air present.	Air forced into the ear produces excessive discomfort for the patient.
8. Straighten the ear canal by gently pulling the earlobe downward and backward for infants and children; upward and backward for adults.	Straightening the ear canal allows the irrigating solution to reach all areas of the canal.
9. Place the tip of the syringe at the opening of the ear. With the tip pointing upward and toward the posterior end of the canal, gently direct a steady slow stream of solution against the roof of the canal. Use only enough force to accomplish the purpose of irrigation (Fig. 8-5).	Direct the solution at the roof of the canal to prevent injury to the tympanic membrane, to prevent pushing material further into the canal, and to facilitate directing the inflow and outflow of the solution.
10. Do not obstruct the opening of the ear canal with the syringe tip.	The solution must be able to flow freely in and out of the ear canal.
11. Observe the returning solution to see if anything is removed such as cerumen, a foreign object, or discharge.	
12. Observe the patient for any signs of discomfort or dizziness.	If these occur, discontinue irrigation and report to the physician.
13. Continue the irrigation until the desired results appear or the prescribed amount of solution has been used.	
14. On completion of the treatment, dry the external ear with a cotton ball; dry the neck when required.	
15. Have the patient keep the head tilted toward the affected side or lie on the affected side for a few minutes.	This allows any remaining solution in the ear canal to escape from the ear.
16. Remove the soiled towel and rubber sheet (if used). Provide for the patient's safety and comfort. Give further instructions as indicated.	

Procedure	**Rationale**
17. Return supplies to designated area. **18.** Wash your hands. **19.** Record the procedure on the patient's chart.	Charting example: October 11, 19_____, 12 PM Left ear irrigated with normal saline. Large amount of cerumen returned. Patient stated that he felt much relief on completion of the irrigation. Jane Evans, CMA

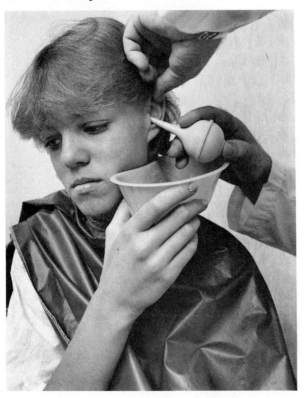

Fig. 8-5. Ear irrigation. Have patient hold kidney or ear basin under ear and against the neck. Pull earlobe up and backward. Place tip of syringe in ear pointing up and back, and gently direct a steady slow stream of solution against the roof of ear canal.

Eye Instillations

Eye instillations are performed to

1. Dilate the pupil of the eye.
2. Constrict the pupil of the eye.
3. Relieve pain in the eye.
4. Treat eye infections; relieve inflammation.
5. Anesthetize the eye.
6. Stimulate circulation in the eye.

Medications instilled into the eye are supplied either in a sterile liquid form as eyedrops or in a sterile ointment form.

Instillation of Eye Drops

Equipment

Sterile eye dropper
Sterile medication, *or*
Sterile medication in bottle with sterile eye dropper
Cotton balls or tissue

Procedure	**Rationale**
1. Check the medication order carefully, that is, the name and amount of medication and which eye requires medication.	Avoid medication errors. Know the abbreviations: OD — right eye OS — left eye OU — both eyes
2. Wash your hands. **3.** Assemble supplies. **4.** Read the medication label carefully three times, and check with the order.	The label must be checked to avoid the possibility of any mistake, because an error could have serious results.

Instillation of Eye Drops (*continued*)

Procedure	Rationale
5. Identify the patient, and explain the procedure and the purpose. Warn the patient that the medication may feel cold and to avoid flinching or squeezing the eye when it is instilled.	The patient must be identified to avoid giving the drug to the wrong patient. Explanations help gain the patient's full cooperation.
6. Have the patient assume a supine or a sitting position with the head tilted slightly backward.	
7. Stand at the patient's head.	
8. Withdraw medication into the dropper. Examine the dropper carefully for any defects.	A safe vehicle must be used for administering the medication.
9. Using the index and middle finger over a tissue, draw the lower lid down gently, *or* draw the lower lid down with index finger, and the brow up with the middle finger; have the patient look up (Fig. 8-6).	The tissue prevents your fingers from slipping when instilling the drops. Do not touch any part of the eye during the procedure except the lower lid — especially in patients who have had eye surgery.
10. Hold the dropper parallel to the eye about ½ inch away from the inner canthus (the inner angle of the eyelids near the nose), and instill the drop(s) into the center of the conjunctival sac of the lower lid (Fig. 8-6).	To avoid injuring the eye, never point the dropper toward it; never allow the dropper to touch the eyeball or the eyelids. Be extremely careful to support the head well if the patient is restless or jerking the head.
11. Instruct the patient to close the eyelids and move the eye, but not to squeeze the eyelids.	This movement helps distribute the medication over the eyeball; squeezing would cause some of the medication to be forced out.

Fig. 8-6. Instilling eye drops. Hold eye dropper parallel to eye to avoid injury to eye of patient.

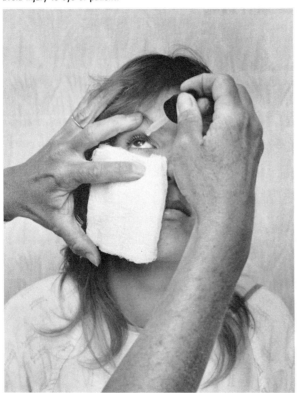

Fig. 8-7. Application of eye pad.

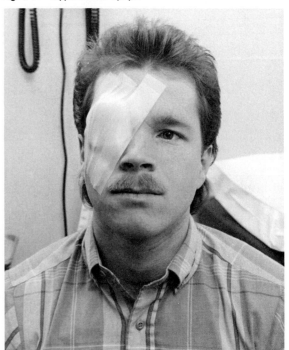

Procedure	Rationale
12. Wipe off the excess medication that overflows onto the cheek or eyelids with cotton balls or tissue.	
13. Discard the unused solution, and replace the dropper into the bottle without touching the sides or outside of the bottle with the dropper.	Avoid contaminating the dropper. When the dropper is contaminated, a new bottle of eyedrops must be ordered.
14. Provide for the patient's safety and comfort. Give further instructions as required.	At times an eye pad may be applied as a dressing over the eye for protection (Fig. 8-7).
15. Return supplies to designated area.	
16. Wash your hands.	
17. Record the procedure on the patient's chart.	Charting example: Oct. 9, 19_____, 10:30 AM 　　Neosporin Ophthalmic Solution 2 gtts given in OD. 　　　Nancy Brown, CMA

Instillation of Eye Ointment

Equipment

　Sterile eye ointment in tube
　Cotton balls or tissue

Procedure	Rationale
Same as for instilling eye drops *except:* 10. Gently squeeze a thin strip of ointment from the tube along the lower lid without touching the lid. 　NOTE: When instilling eyedrops and ointment at the same time *instill the eye drops first*, ointment last. 　If the patient's eyedropper or tube touches the eyelid and is contaminated, do not use it again until it is resterilized. 　Discard the contaminated tube unless it is being used by only one patient.	

Eye Irrigation

Eye irrigations are performed to

1. Relieve inflammation of the conjunctiva
2. Remove inflammatory secretions
3. Prepare the eye for surgery
4. Wash away foreign material or injurious chemicals
5. Provide antibacterial and antifungal effects

Equipment

Towel
Sterile eye dropper for small amounts of solution; rubber bulb or Asepto syringe for larger amounts of solution; sterile eye cup for home use
Small basin for solution
Sterile cotton balls
Kidney basin to catch the solution
Sterile solution as ordered by the physician, usually boric acid or normal saline, 30 to 240 ml (2 to 8 ounces) at 98.6°F (37°C), that is, near body temperature

Procedure	Rationale
1. Check the medication order carefully, that is, the name and amount of solution to be used and which eye is to be treated.	Know the abbreviations: OD—right eye OS—left eye OU—both eyes
2. Wash your hands.	
3. Assemble supplies.	
4. Check the label of the solution three times.	Prevent drug errors (see Unit VII).
5. Identify the patient, and explain the procedure and the purpose of the irrigation. Instruct the patient not to squeeze the eyes during the treatment.	Gain the patient's cooperation by providing an explanation and adequate instructions.
6. Have the patient assume a lying or sitting position with the head tilted backward and toward the side being treated.	The head is tilted to the side so that the solution does not run toward the inner canthus of the eye or over to the unaffected eye, which could then result in cross-infection (when the eye treated is infected).
7. Place or have the patient hold the kidney basin in position to receive the solution from the eye. Place a towel under the basin to avoid getting the solution on the patient or on the examining table when the patient is lying down (Fig. 8-8).	
8. Stand in front of or at the side of the patient.	
9. Cleanse the eyelid with a cotton ball moistened with the irrigating solution. Start at the inner canthus and wipe towards the outer canthus.	All materials (crusts, discharge, and so on) on the lids or lashes must be washed away before exposing the conjunctiva.
10. Fill the irrigating dropper or syringe with the solution.	Warm solutions are most comfortable to the patient; that is, the solution temperature should be close to normal body temperature.
11. Pull the lower lid down gently, and instruct the patient to look up, but not to squeeze the eyelids (Fig. 8-8).	If the patient has had intraocular surgery, do not ask the patient to look up, because this may cause injury.
12. Holding the dropper or syringe parallel to the eye, squeeze the solution into the eye, allowing it to flow away from the nose. Hold the dropper or syringe ½ inch from the eye, and allow the solution to flow in a steady stream, but at low pressure (Fig. 8-8).	The solution is directed away from the nose so that it does not enter the nasolacrimal duct or spill over into the unaffected eye, which could result in transmission of an infection, if it is present. Too much pressure may be injurious to the eye tissues.
13. Do not allow the dropper or syringe to touch the eye or eyelids.	Injury to the eye must be prevented.
14. Continue the procedure until the eye is free of secretions, or the desired results occur, or the prescribed amount of solution has been used.	
15. Gently dry the eye and cheek with cotton balls; discard the cotton balls in designated container.	
16. Provide for the patient's safety and comfort; provide further instructions as indicated; allow the patient to rest for a few minutes.	
17. Observe the drainage in the basin, then discard. Discard soiled disposable items; return reusable items to designated area for used supplies.	
18. Wash your hands.	

Procedure	Rationale

19. Record the procedure and results on the patient's chart.	Charting example:
	October 11, 19_____, 1 PM
	  OD irrigated with 100 ml 5% boric acid.
	    Redness in OD has markedly decreased. Patient stated that the treatment felt soothing. Patient instructed to continue treatments at home for 1 week, as ordered by Dr. McArthur, and then to return for examination.
	    Connie Bell, CMA

Fig. 8-8. Eye irrigation. Hold dropper or syringe parallel to eye, squeeze solution into eye at inner canthus, allowing it to flow away from the nose.

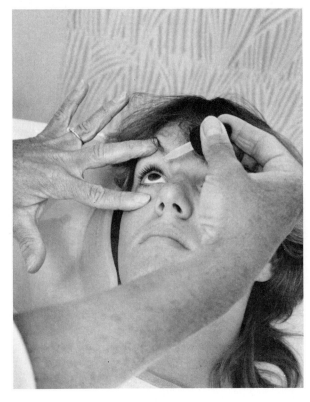

CONCLUSION

When you have practiced the procedures outlined in this unit and feel competent with your knowledge and skills, arrange with your instructor to take the performance test. You will be expected to prepare for and perform ear and eye instillations and irrigations.

When treating the eye, keep in mind that it is a delicate sense organ that must be treated gently. Solutions and medications instilled into the eye should be applied to the lower conjunctiva and *not* on the corneal surface.

When irrigating the ear, you must gently direct a steady slow stream of solution against the roof of the canal to prevent injury to the tympanic membrane, to prevent pushing material further into the canal, and to permit the solution to flow in and out of the ear freely.

REVIEW OF VOCABULARY

Using the information presented in this unit and other reference sources of your own choice, define the following terms.

Terms Pertaining to the Ear

1. Auricle
2. Cerumen
3. External acoustic meatus
4. Semicircular canals
5. Pinna
6. Tinnitus
7. Otopyorrhea
8. Otitis media
9. Audiometer
10. Meniere's syndrome
11. Tympanic membrane (TM)
12. Otoscope
13. Otology
14. Myringoplasty

Terms Pertaining to the Eye

1. Canthus
2. Cataract
3. Pupil
4. Conjunctivitis
5. Mydriatic
6. Miotic
7. Presbyopia
8. Glaucoma
9. Hyperopia
10. Errors of refraction

11. Ophthalmoscope
12. Lacrimal duct
13. Intraocular
14. Cornea

REVIEW QUESTIONS

1. Explain the difference between an instillation and an irrigation.
2. State the reason for pulling an adult's earlobe upward and backward when giving an ear instillation or irrigation.
3. List three reasons why an ear irrigation is done with a steady slow stream of solution and not a fast, high-pressure flow.
4. Explain how cerumen can be softened for later removal.
5. Explain to Mrs. Sanson how she should instill ear drops into her 5-year-old son's left ear.
6. Describe the position you would have Mr. John Rogan assume for an ear irrigation. Explain the reason for your answer.
7. The physician has asked you to prepare Nancy Lilly for an eye irrigation. List the supplies you would need, and explain how you would prepare and position Nancy for this procedure.
8. List four purposes for which an eye irrigation may be performed.
9. Explain how you would put eye ointment into Connie Hepworth's eye.
10. When eye drops and eye ointment are both ordered for the patient at the same time, which agent would you instill into the eye first?
11. Name the region of the eye into which eye drops should be instilled.

PERFORMANCE TEST

In a skills laboratory, the medical assistant student, with a partner, will assemble supplies and demonstrate with 100% accuracy the correct procedure for the following, without reference to source materials. Time limits for the performance of each procedure are to be assigned by the instructor (see also pp. 32 and 35).

1. Ear instillation
2. Ear irrigation
3. Eye instillation
4. Eye irrigation

PERFORMANCE CHECKLISTS

Ear Instillation

1. Check the medication order.
2. Wash your hands.
3. Assemble supplies.
4. Read the medication label three times.
5. Identify the patient; explain the nature and purpose of the procedure.
6. Position the patient in a sitting or side-lying position.
7. Instruct the patient to tilt the head toward the unaffected side.
8. Stand at the patient's head.
9. Withdraw the medication into the dropper; examine the dropper for defects.
10. Straighten the patient's external ear canal.
11. Place the tip of the dropper slightly inside the ear canal and instill the medication.
12. Instruct the patient to keep the head tilted (or remain lying on the side) for a few minutes.
13. When ordered, place a cotton ball over the ear opening.
14. Discard unused medication before replacing the dropper in the bottle.
15. Attend to the patient; provide further instructions when required.
16. Replace supplies.
17. Wash your hands.
18. Record the procedure on the patient's chart.

Ear Irrigation

1. Check the medication order.
2. Wash your hands.
3. Assemble supplies.
4. Check the solution label three times; warm the solution.
5. Identify the patient; explain the nature and purpose of the procedure.
6. Position the patient with the head slightly tilted toward the affected side.
7. Drape the patient's shoulder.
8. Have the patient hold the basin under the ear and against the neck.
9. Cleanse the outer ear and external auditory meatus as necessary.
10. Test the temperature of the solution.
11. Fill the syringe with irrigating solution and expel air, if present.
12. Straighten the patient's ear canal.
13. Place the tip of the syringe at the ear opening; gently direct a steady, slow stream of solution against the roof of the canal.
14. Observe the returning solution.
15. Observe the patient for pain and/or dizziness.
16. Continue until the desired results are obtained.
17. Dry the external ear with a cotton ball.
18. Have the patient maintain the position for a few minutes.
19. Remove soiled drapes; provide for the patient's safety and comfort; provide further instructions as indicated.
20. Return supplies.
21. Wash your hands.
22. Record the procedure on the patient's chart.

Instillation of Eye Drops and Ointment

1. Check the medication order.
2. Wash your hands.
3. Assemble supplies.
4. Check the medication label three times.
5. Identify the patient; explain the procedure and purpose.
6. Position the patient in a supine or sitting position with the head tilted slightly backward.
7. Stand at the patient's head.
8. Withdraw solution, and examine the dropper for defects.
9. With fingers over a tissue, draw the lower lid down gently, and have the patient look up.
10. Hold the dropper parallel to the eye; instill the correct amount of medication into the middle of the conjunctival sac of the lower lid. To instill ointment, gently squeeze a thin strip of ointment from the tube along the lower lid. Do not touch the eye or the lid.
11. Instruct the patient to close the eyelids and move the eyeball, but not to squeeze the eyelids.
12. Wipe excess solution off the cheek or eyelids.
13. Discard unused solution before replacing the dropper into the bottle, avoiding contamination of the dropper.
14. Leave the patient safe and comfortable; provide further instructions.
15. Replace supplies.
16. Wash your hands.
17. Record the procedure on the patient's chart.

Eye Irrigation

1. Check the medication order.
2. Wash your hands.
3. Assemble supplies.
4. Check the label of the solution three times.
5. Identify the patient; explain the nature and purpose of the procedure. Instruct the patient not to squeeze the eyes during the treatment.
6. Position the patient sitting or lying with the head tilted backward and toward the side being treated.
7. Position the basin to receive the irrigating solution; place a towel under the basin.
8. Stand in front of or to the side of the patient.
9. Cleanse the eyelid.
10. Fill the dropper or syringe with solution.
11. Gently pull the lower lid down; instruct the patient to look up and not to squeeze the eyelids.
12. Allow the solution to flow in a steady stream at low pressure across the eye, away from the nose.
13. Do not touch the eye or the eyelid with the syringe or dropper.
14. Continue until desired results are obtained or until all the solution has been used.
15. Gently dry the eye and cheek with a cotton ball.
16. Leave the patient safe and comfortable; provide further instructions.
17. Observe the drainage in the basin.
18. Discard the drainage and soiled disposable items; return reusable supplies to the designated area.
19. Wash your hands.
20. Record the procedure on the patient's chart.

Unit IX

Laboratory Orientation

COGNITIVE OBJECTIVES

On completion of Unit IX, the medical assistant student should be able to apply the following cognitive objectives:

1. State the importance of the information gathered from clinical laboratory tests.
2. List and discuss three formats that may be used to organize the recordings of various diagnostic procedures.
3. State the reason why most laboratory tests are performed in a commercial clinical laboratory rather than in a physician's office or in a health care agency.
4. List six types of workers in a clinical laboratory, indicating the basic functions/responsibilities of each.
5. List six specialized departments common to all clinical laboratories and describe the function of each department.
6. List five additional special departments that may be part of some clinical laboratories and describe the function of each department.
7. Discuss the medical assistant's responsibilities when dealing with a clinical laboratory.
8. List seven items that are to be included on a laboratory requisition that accompanies a specimen to the laboratory.
9. List three reasons for the performance of diagnostic studies.
10. Discuss the organization of diagnostic reports that are to be placed in the patient's chart.
11. Discuss the purpose of quality control in the laboratory.
12. List 20 safety rules that should be followed when using laboratory equipment and chemicals, and when around specimens.

TERMINAL PERFORMANCE OBJECTIVES

On completion of Unit IX, the medical assistant student should be able to do the following terminal performance objectives:

1. Demonstrate safe practices when working with laboratory equipment and specimens.
2. Demonstrate proficiency in using a microscope.
3. Identify by name the parts of a microscope.
4. Demonstrate proficiency in using a clinical centrifuge.

The above activities are to be performed with 100% accuracy 95% of the time.

Vocabulary

Vocabulary terms are presented in the specific sections to which they apply throughout this unit.

Medical practice is based on information obtained from various sources. Unit II discussed information obtained from a patient history and from a general or specific physical examination. Another important source of information to help diagnose and treat disease processes is gathered from clinical laboratory tests. It is important to remember that the physician evaluates all data gathered before a diagnosis is made or treatment initiated. Frequently, information from a combination of sources is required, as one source may not be sufficient. Repeat tests may be needed to confirm initial findings and establish the progress of a disease process or the elimination of it.

Scientific and technological discoveries have aided medicine tremendously by making accessible abundant data on numerous types of body specimens with a speed and accuracy that previously were not available. Laboratory medicine can determine changes in the chemical or physical characteristics of body fluids, excretions, and tissues, and in turn reflect changes in the anatomy and physiology of various organs. Changes noted may indicate a disease process at the site from which the specimen was obtained; for example, a wound culture may identify the presence of bacteria and an infectious process. At other times, the changes in the characteristics of the specimen may indicate a disease process in another part of the body: for example, the presence of excessive sugar in the urine may indicate diabetes mellitus, a disorder in carbohydrate metabolism, and not a disorder of the urinary system; elevated levels of certain blood enzymes may indicate a heart attack or a liver disease.

Thus, with laboratory techniques, specific data concerning the status of certain body functions and conditions may be determined. Normal values for the physical and chemical characteristics of body substances have been predetermined; each technique used has its own normal value ratio. Deviations from these set norms aid in the diagnosis and treatment of abnormal disturbances in body function and structure.

THE TYPICAL LABORATORY

Initially, many clinical laboratory procedures were performed in the physician's office. Over the years, as numerous tests were developed that were more time-consuming and required more specialized equipment, specially trained personnel became necessary. As a result, most laboratory procedures were transferred from the physician's office to a hospital, or a private or public health department laboratory. However, many physician's offices still perform basic routine tests, but find it more economical, efficient, and accurate to have most tests performed by the trained personnel of a larger clinical laboratory.

There are various types of workers in a clinical laboratory. These may include a physician who is certified as a pathologist acting as the director of the laboratory; medical technologists, who are trained at a college for 4 years and are able to perform specialized tests; medical technicians, trained for 2 years at a junior or community college, who assist and perform tests under the supervision of the medical technologist. A cytotechnologist, trained for 2 years at a college, is a highly specialized worker who examines cells and tissues microscopically for the presence of cancer. A histological technician, trained for 1 or 2 years in a technical training program, is also a specialized worker who is involved with the preparation of various types of tissues for microscopic examinations performed by the pathologist. The clinical laboratory assistant, usually trained at a technical level or below that of a 2 year college program, performs basic and routine tests under the direct supervision of the medical technologist or the director of the laboratory. Frequently, medical technologists become specialized in one or two fields in the clinical laboratory and devote all their working time to the area of their expertise.

All clinical laboratories have certain specialized departments in common. They are divided into areas based on function and types of tests performed. These areas usually include hematology, urinalysis, serology, blood banking, medical microbiology, and clinical chemistry. Parasitology and examination of feces may be special departments or they may be included in one of the other departments. Some laboratories may also have special areas for histology, mycology, immunochemistry, and cytology.

Hematology deals with the study of blood. Examination for the total cell number, the types and number of different cells, cell morphology (shape and size), and the important aspects of the functions of blood in addition to coagulation studies are all part of hematology.

Urinalysis deals with the examination of the physical, chemical, and microscopic properties of urine.

Serology involves laboratory tests that examine blood serum. Reactions involving antibodies and antigens are observed and used to determine various types of infections, such as tests for infectious mononucleosis. The tests for pregnancy and syphilis are also serology tests, as they involve immunological reactions.

Blood banking deals with the processing of blood and blood products that will be used for transfusions. It is also known as immunohematology because antigen-antibody reactions are involved in the typing of blood.

Medical microbiology deals with isolation and culture, microscopic identification, and biochemical tests to detect microorganisms that cause disease. Depending on the classification of the microorganism under investigation, the field of medical microbiology is generally divided into areas of specialization that include the following:

> **bacteriology** (bak-te"-re-ol'o-je)—The study of bacteria.
> **virology** (vi-rol'o-je)—The study of viruses.
> **mycology** (mĭ-kol'o-je)—The study of fungi.
> **rickettsiology** (rĭ-ket"sĭ-ol'o-je)—The study of rickettsiae.
> **protozoology** (pro"to-zo-ol'o-je)—The study of protozoa, the simplest forms of animals.
> **phycology** (fi-kol'o-je)—The study of algae.
> **parasitology** (par"ah-si-tol'o-jē)—The study of parasites. These may be protozoans or even larger organisms that have microscopic stages in their development.

Parasitology may be an area apart from microbiology. Stool and blood specimens are examined for the presence of eggs or parts of a variety of roundworms, tapeworms, and flukes.

Clinical chemistry examines body fluids, such as blood, urine, and cerebrospinal fluid, for any change in their chemical content. Glucose and electrolyte levels are determined, as well as the presence of uric acid or urea in the urine or blood.

Histology involves the study of specimens of tissue from any source in the body. Form and structural changes are observed microscopically.

Immunochemistry is the study of the chemistry involved with immunity.

Cytology involves the microscopic study of cells shed from a body surface to detect any malignant change.

Cost Containment

Cost containment is a factor that must be considered when ordering or performing laboratory tests. Generally speaking, it is less expensive for the patient if simple routine laboratory tests are performed in the physician's office or health care agency. There are two reasons for this. First, you can collect and perform simple laboratory tests with relative ease on samples collected at the time the patient is at your facility. Second, the physician or health care agency can avoid the costs of extensive laboratory equipment and the high salary of laboratory technicians or technologists. The next less expensive situation for patients is when you obtain the sample in your facility and forward it to a commercial laboratory or when you refer patients directly to a commercial laboratory to have the test performed. The larger the laboratory or organization, the less expensive the procedure is for the patient, because large laboratories perform tests on a large volume of samples using more sophisticated equipment. The specialized instruments available in large laboratories can perform multiple tests at the same time, thereby reducing the cost to each patient. The most expensive situation for patients is when you refer them to a hospital laboratory to have the required test performed. This cost results from the general high cost of operating a hospital, which must be shared by all departments. An example to illustrate this follows. When a laboratory test is performed in the physician's office or in a health care agency, it may cost the patient $5. When the same test is performed at a commercial clinical laboratory it may cost the patient $7, and when the test is performed at a hospital laboratory it may cost $12. Thus when laboratory tests other than the very simple procedures that you can easily perform in your facility are ordered, it is suggested that you refer patients to a commercial laboratory that is qualified and with which you have established a business relationship. This is the most cost-efficient procedure to follow.

LIAISON OF THE MEDICAL ASSISTANT WITH LABORATORIES

Because the information obtained from laboratory tests is an important source of data for the physician when treating a patient, it is essential that the medical assistant have an understanding of and establish a good communication with this branch of clinical medicine.

The medical assistant has certain responsibilities when dealing with a laboratory. These include a basic knowledge of the various tests available, proper collection and handling of specimens that are to be forwarded to a laboratory, instructions to the patient when preparing for certain tests (see Units VI and XI), and the handling of completed reports as they return to the office. To help prevent errors, good communication among all parties involved is vital. When you are not sure of the procedure for collecting or handling a specimen or what instructions are to be given to the patient, never hesitate to contact the laboratory for this information. By doing this, you avoid errors and inconvenience to the patient, who would have to return to give another specimen if the initial procedure had been performed incorrectly.

Correct labeling of the specimen and completing the laboratory requisition are other important responsibilities of the medical assistant. The container in which the specimen has been collected should always be labeled with the date, the patient's name, and the source of the specimen. The items to be indicated on the laboratory requisition that accompanies the specimen include the following:

- The patient's full name, age, sex, and address
- The physician's full name (also address when sending specimens to outside laboratories)
- Date the specimen was collected; date the specimen was sent to the laboratory if this differs from the date of collection; time the specimen was collected
- Source of the specimen
- Test(s) required
- Possible diagnosis when feasible, as this will alert the laboratory for specifics to watch for
- Medications or treatments the patient is receiving that may interfere with test results

Most laboratories will provide specific requisitions for the various types of tests that will be performed in different areas of the laboratory (see sample requisitions in Units VI and XI). Be certain that you use the correct requisition for the test(s) requested on the specimen. EXAMPLES: A blood specimen will be sent to the hematology department when the test ordered is a complete blood count; therefore, you must complete the hematology laboratory requisition. A cytology requisition is sent with a cervical smear for a Pap test.

Medical assistants should know the normal ranges of test results so that when abnormal results are reported, they can be brought to the physician's attention immediately. Depending on the office or health agency's policies, you may circle or underline abnormal results in red. This helps to bring it to the physician's attention quickly. Frequently, physicians will sign or put a check on a laboratory report after reviewing it. This gives you an indication that it may then be filed in the patient's chart. *Never* file a report before it has been reviewed by the physician. To hasten the physician's awareness of abnormal test results, many laboratories will report these by telephone immediately, then forward the written report later, signed by the laboratory worker who performed the test. Accuracy in reporting test results cannot be stressed enough, because frequently the diagnosis and treatment for a patient are contingent on these reports.

DIAGNOSTIC AND THERAPEUTIC PROCEDURES

Earlier in this book it was stated that the physician arrives at a diagnosis by employing and reviewing multiple factors and information obtained on the patient's condition; that is, the physician utilizes various studies to arrive at a diagnosis. Three reasons for diagnostic studies follow.

1. To determine (diagnose) the condition from which the patient is suffering, so that treatment, if feasible, may be initiated.
2. To discover disease in its early stage before the patient experiences any signs or symptoms. This is called screening. Screening for disease often permits the cure of the disease, because treatment can be started in the early stages of the disease process (for example, cancer), or early treatment can delay the progression of the disease (for example, hypertension).
3. To evaluate past or ongoing treatment received by the patient.

As the field of medical science continues to expand, newer and more accurate and sophisticated techniques are continually made available to help physicians diagnose disease processes. Diagnostic procedures and studies include, but are not limited to, physical examinations, surgical intervention, and laboratory technology. Other procedures utilized when diagnosing and treating disease processes require some elaboration. These involve the areas of radiology (roentgenology), the specialized field of nuclear medicine, special skin tests, physical medicine and physiotherapy, and electrocardiography.

To completely understand all these diagnostic and therapeutic procedures, special courses of study are necessary. Nevertheless, the following units give the medical assistant an exposure to various additional tests that the physician may order for a patient. (Physical examinations and minor surgery are discussed in preceding units of this book.) It is hoped that the descriptions of the following diagnostic and therapeutic studies and procedures will help the medical assistant understand the nature and purpose(s) of the numerous clinical entities available to health care practitioners for the treatment and care of patients.

Various studies, related vocabulary and procedures are presented along with special patient preparation when it is required. It is important to remember that the medical assistant is not expected to also be a laboratory, x-ray, nuclear medicine, or electrocardiography technician, or a physical therapist, but is expected to be familiar with the vocabulary and the nature and purpose(s) of diagnostic or therapeutic procedures and studies performed by these specialists. At times the medical assistant may be called upon to assist with procedures performed by these medical specialties or to perform the more routine and simplified procedures, such as routine urinalysis, skin tests, the application of heat or cold, and electrocardiograms. Additional medical assistant responsibilities may be to explain the nature and purpose of the procedure to the patient, to record the procedure on the patient's record, and to file or store the reports and films received after the test or treatment has been completed.

This unit and Units XII and XIV now present an opportunity for students to design their own step-by-step procedures and performance checklists. *Appendix B* gives a summary of studies used for diagnosing conditions affecting body organs and systems.

Organizing the Recordings of Diagnostic Procedures

A patient's medical record should be maintained in an organized manner to facilitate easy accessibility to the information. Regular-sized paper or preprinted forms are customarily used when recording all information relevant to the patient's care. If you receive reports on small sheets, affix them to standard-sized sheets before filing them in the patient's record.

There are various methods employed when filing laboratory reports in a patient's chart. Some office or health agencies have certain ways for compiling charts, so that the laboratory report papers follow or precede other entries. One common method utilizes a special standard-size sheet of paper designated specifically for these reports. The first report is placed on the lower portion of this sheet, and each additional report is placed on top of the preceding one, allowing the bottom one-half inch or so of each report to be visible, as this is where the date of the test is recorded. With this method, the most recent report is on top, which allows for a quick review of current information (Fig. 9-1).

One of three formats can be used for recording and organizing information and test results in the patient's record: the source-oriented format, the integrated format, or the problem-oriented format.

In the *source-oriented record*, all reports are filed chronologically according to their specialty. That is, all laboratory reports are filed together, x-ray reports

Fig. 9-1. Laboratory report records. Place the first report on the lower portion where indicated. Place each additional report on top of the preceding one, allowing the bottom one-half inch of each report to be visible, as this is where the date is recorded. The most recent report will be on top, allowing for quick review of current information.

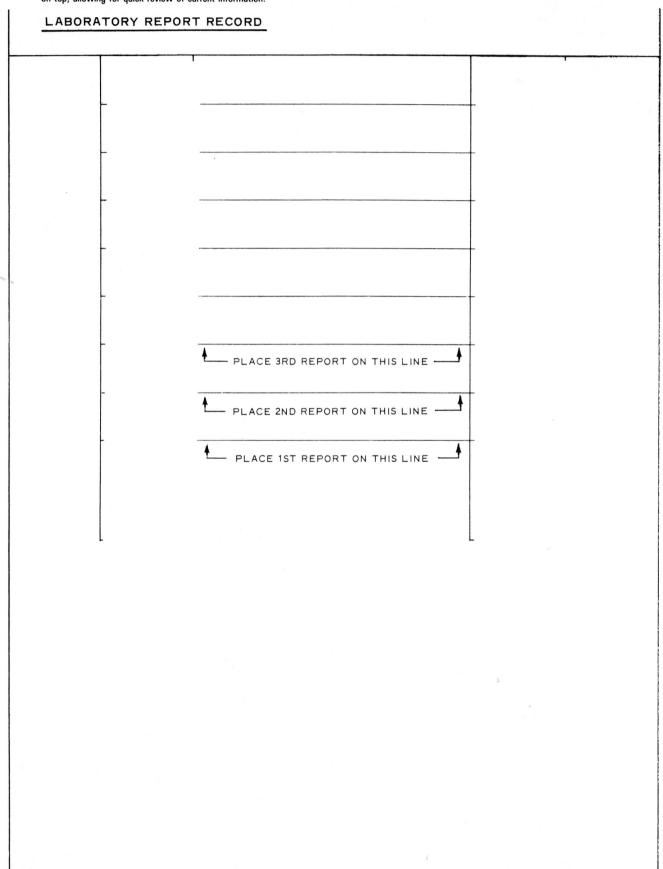

LABORATORY REPORT RECORD

PLACE 3RD REPORT ON THIS LINE

PLACE 2ND REPORT ON THIS LINE

PLACE 1ST REPORT ON THIS LINE

LABORATORY REPORT RECORD

PLACE 3RD REPORT ON THIS LINE

MICROBIOLOGY	GL 404	ST	BD

DRAWN BY	REMARKS:	DATE/TIME OF COLLECTION
		5/17

ROUTINE REQUEST

IF REQUEST IS OTHER THAN ROUTINE, PLACE STICKER WITH APPROPRIATE INSTRUCTIONS IN THIS SPACE

DATE	VERIFYING NURSE	DIAGNOSIS

LAST NAME	FIRST NAME
ADDRESS	
BIRTHDATE	AGE	SEX	CLASS
PHYSICIAN	ROOM NO.	HOSP. NO.
DATE	PHONE

CIRCLE CODE NO.	INDICATE SOURCE	SMEAR RESULT:

CULTURES

604	BLOOD	☐ EYE
600	ROUTINE	☐ EAR
607	ANAEROBIC	☐ CSF
(620)	URINE	☐ NASOPHARYNX
606	CAMPYLO-BACTER	☐ THROAT
618	AFB (SMEAR INCLUDED)	☐ SPUTUM
612	FUNGUS	☒ URINE
616	GRAM STAIN	☐ STOOL
601	ANTIBIOTIC SENSITIVITY	☐ CERVIX

CULTURE RESULT:

SCREENS

625	BETA STREP	☐ VAGINA
632	NEISSERIA	☐ WOUND
		☐ ASPIRATE
		☐ ABSCESS

INDICATE SITE:

TIME IN	TECHNOLOGIST	TIME CALLED OR TELETYPED	TIME OUT
3³⁰ pm May 17		MEDICAL RECORD	4 pm May 18

TIME IN	TECHNOLOGIST	TIME TELEPHONED OR TELETYPED	TIME OUT
1 pm - May 18		MEDICAL RECORD	3 pm May 18

are filed together, electrocardiogram records are kept together, and so on. The latest information is placed on top, as it is the most important for the patient's current care and treatment.

In the *integrated record,* all information is recorded in strict chronological order as the physician sees the patient, gives care, and orders various tests. That is, the physician dates and enters the patient's history, physical examination results, and the treatment given and ordered. The laboratory, electrocardiogram, and x-ray reports are then filed in the record immediately following the physician's notes for this particular situation. Progress notes and future laboratory or x-ray reports continue to be entered in strict chronological order.

In the *problem-oriented medical record* (review pp. 50–52), all test results (laboratory, x-ray, and physical) are entered and recorded in the Objective part of the progress notes, preceded by the number and title of the particular problem.

At times, a radiologist's office, an outside laboratory, or hospital will telephone test results before mailing a written report. The information received in this manner should be labeled as a verbal report, recorded accurately and attached to the patient's record until the actual report is received.

The medical assistant must ensure that all reports are received for diagnostic tests performed on the patient outside the physician's office. Only after they are reviewed by the physician should they be filed in the patient's record.

Develop a follow-through procedure for pending reports from outside sources. Usable methods include the following:

1. Use individual sheets for laboratory tests, x-ray reports, electrocardiograms, and consultations from outside sources; they can be kept in separate files or in a binder. Each entry should be made on a separate line giving the date, patient's name, and the test(s) ordered. As the reports are received, enter the date, and check off the entry to indicate that it has been received.
2. Keep the patient's record in a special file until all outstanding reports have been received.
3. Place the patient's record back in the usual file with a colored flag attached to indicate that reports are yet to be received.

Regardless of the method, use a *consistent* follow-through procedure to ensure that all test results are received on a regular basis.

The next two units are devoted to information on urinalysis and hematology, because urine and blood, being the two most abundant body fluids, provide a wealth of information on the health status of an individual. Reference tables for various urine and blood tests with related information and the normal evaluation ranges for their results are also presented.

No attempt will be made in this book to give detailed instructions for the procedures involved when performing all of these laboratory tests, *as most **must** only be performed by certified laboratory personnel or physicians.* The purpose of the following information and Units X and XI is to prepare the medical assistant for performing basic routine procedures that may be done in the physician's office or health care agency, and to make the medical assistant aware of some of the many laboratory tests, special equipment, and supplies that are available, along with the normal ranges for test results. The medical assistant is expected to know how to collect and handle specimens, the special instructions, when applicable, to give to the patient before the collection of a specimen, and the normal test results. By attaining this knowledge and these skills, patient care can be enhanced, and the medical assistant's value to the physician, patient, and laboratory is vastly increased.

The remainder of this unit is devoted to a discussion on quality control and laboratory safety, and on two major pieces of laboratory equipment, the microscope and centrifuge. The medical assistant should be familiar with this information and equipment if simple laboratory procedures are performed in the physician's office or health care agency, and also when specimens and blood samples are to be prepared for transport to a commercial laboratory.

QUALITY CONTROL AND LABORATORY SAFETY

Quality Control

Quality control and laboratory safety are vitally important aspects of laboratory technology. They are directly related to the collection, handling, processing, and testing of all specimens. *Quality control* involves methods used to ensure the reliability of the tests performed and test results obtained. This begins with the proper care and handling of specimens as discussed in Unit VI, in addition to evaluating the techniques and equipment used to perform the tests. Controls provide the laboratory worker with the capability to evaluate the changes and/or errors that are commonly associated with routine clinical chemistry. The controls should be used to establish confidence that the variables that cause errors are in check or within a range of acceptability as established by the laboratory. Guidelines have been established to aid the laboratory to initiate a quality control program using solutions of known values. By understanding the trends established by responsible interpretation of control values, better results are obtained with clinical procedures. Controls are tested often, usually in duplicate, to control laboratory error. By realizing that quality control assesses the sources of variables, from specimen transporting to recording of results, better values are obtained—with a high degree of confidence in the procedures used. An example of controls used for routine urinalysis is given in Unit X, "Urinalysis."

Laboratory Safety

Laboratory testing involves certain hazards to safety such as exposure to strong chemicals and infectious materials. Thus it is most important that laboratory workers use safe and good techniques when around and using laboratory equipment, chemicals, and specimens. The following *safety rules* are to assist you to work in a safe manner.

General:

- Do not eat, drink, or smoke in the laboratory.
- Use protective equipment, such as rubber gloves, when required.
- Keep pens, pencils, and fingers away from your mouth.
- Wash your hands *frequently* and *thoroughly*.
- If you are pregnant you should not be exposed to potential or known pathogenic agents.
- If you are inexperienced you should be well supervised.
- When you have an open wound or an eczematous condition you should not handle pathogenic material unless the risks involved can be obviated by protective equipment.
- Process specimens from known infectious material separately from other specimens. Disinfect equipment used for these specimens after use.
- Clean your work area with a disinfectant at the end of the day and at least one other time during the day.

Chemicals and Reagents:

- Current inventory control is important. Discard chemical reagents in accordance with their expiration dates.
- Store labeled chemicals and reagents under nonreactive conditions with respect to light, moisture, and temperature. Follow the manufacturer's recommended storage procedures.
- Avoid pipetting by mouth. Use a commercial pipetting device.
- Use disposable gloves when handling disinfectants and when cleaning automatic blood-analyzing equipment.

Equipment:

- Clean automatic blood- and serum-analyzing systems after each use according to the manufacturer's directions.

- Discard materials used to wipe machine parts during operation and cleaning with other pathological waste.
- Do not wear loose-fitting clothing when working around a bunsen burner.
- Do not use bunsen burners near areas where oxygen is in use or where flammables are stored.
- Know emergency fire procedures if use of a bunsen burner is required.
- Do not leave bunsen burners unattended when they are lit.
- Position centrifuges in areas where their vibrations will not cause items to fall off nearby shelves.
- Always balance the load in a centrifuge to avoid damage to the equipment and injury to yourself.
- Cover centrifuges when in use.
- Take care when loading and unloading a centrifuge to avoid spilling the specimens.
- Turn the centrifuge off before opening the lid (if it is not equipped with an interlocking device).

Glassware:

- Take a regular inventory of all glassware. Discard all chipped or cracked pieces.
- Handle and store all glassware carefully to avoid breakage.

Identification of Materials (Chemicals and Reagents):

- Label *all* materials clearly. Replace soiled labels immediately.
- Do not use, but discard any unlabeled item.
- When affixing a label, moisten it with a damp sponge. Do not lick the label.
- Make sure that poisons, corrosives, and flammable materials are labeled as such. Have a proper storage area for these items away from other solutions that you may have in the office or clinic.

THE MICROSCOPE

The microscope (Fig. 9-2) is a precise scientific instrument used in the laboratory when an enlarged image of a small (microscopic) object is required. When using the microscope, details of structure not otherwise distinguishable are revealed. Microscopes vary greatly in quality. For maximum efficiency the operation of a microscope must be studied carefully. Complete instructions for assembling and using the microscope are provided by each manufacturer. Read these instructions completely before you use the microscope for laboratory procedures.

Fig. 9-2. **A,** Nikon Labophot microscope. **B,** Nikon Optiphot microscope. (Courtesy Nikon Inc., Instrument Division, Garden City, NY)

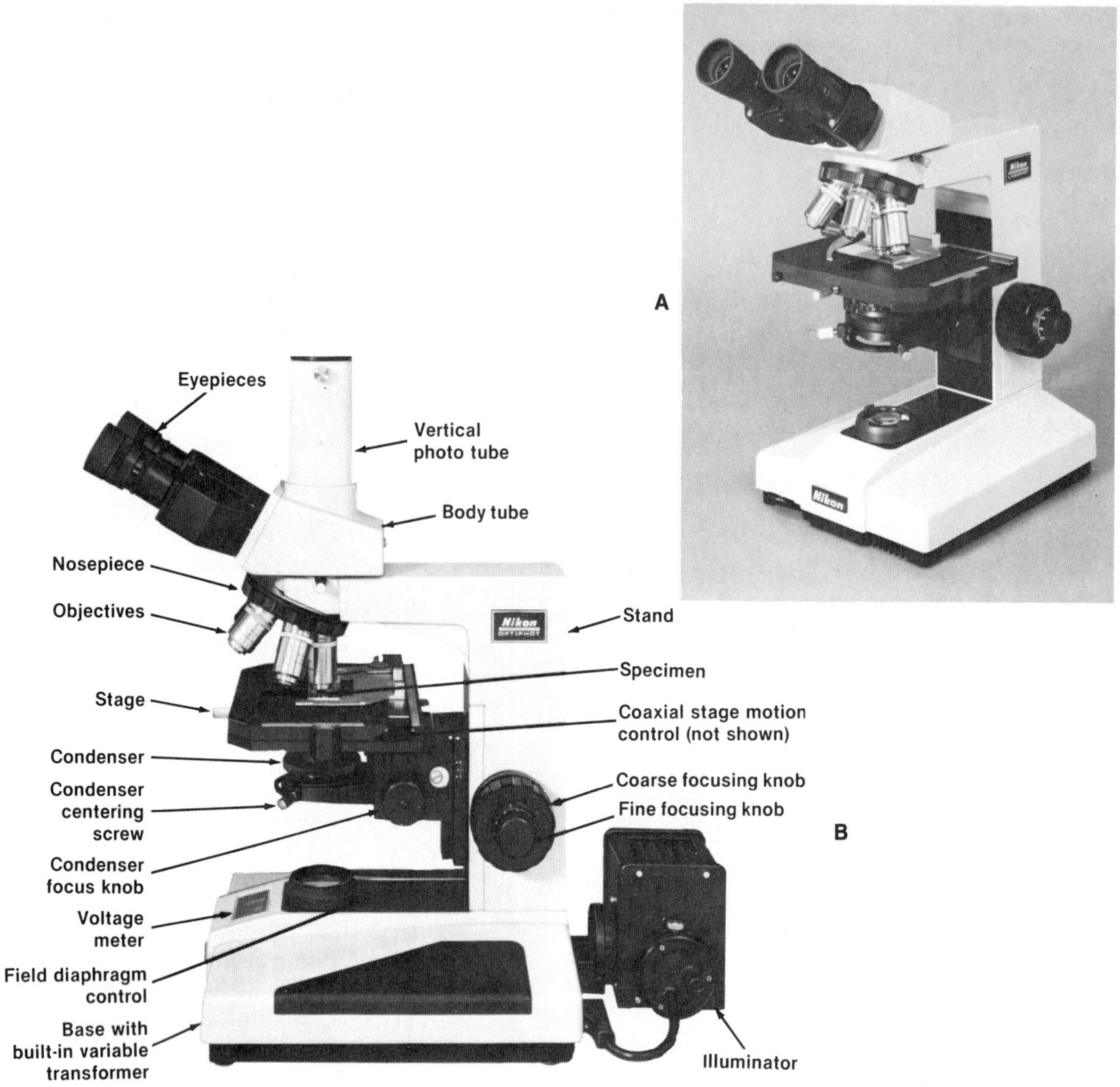

Parts of the Microscope

Eyepieces. Eyepieces fit into the eyepiece tubes. The eyepieces in common use today are marked 5×, 6×, or 10×. The latter has the greatest magnifying power. Because the exterior surface of the eyepiece is exposed, it is likely to become dusty; therefore it should be carefully cleaned before use. This cleaning can be done with a special lens paper or with a soft cloth.

Nosepiece and Objectives. The microscope is provided with a revolving nosepiece into which the various objectives are screwed. Care must be used in properly attaching the objectives to the nosepiece. Follow the procedure provided by the manufacturer of the microscope. The objectives make up the lens system on the nosepiece. *Never* at any time force the objec-

tive or allow its lower end (the lens) to touch the metal stage. Lenses are very expensive and are easily damaged by contact with any other objects—slides, cover glasses, specimens.

Objectives have different magnifying powers. The following are commonly used:

- The lowest power objective, marked 16 mm or 10×
- The intermediate power (frequently called the high dry power) marked 4 mm, 43×, or 45×
- The highest power, the oil-immersion objective, marked 1.8 mm, 97× or 100×

In becoming familiar with the different objectives, remember that the low power is the shortest of the three objectives, whereas the oil immersion is the longest of the three. Another point of differentiation is the size of the opening in the smaller end of the objectives. The objective with the widest lens is the lowest power, and conversely the one with the smallest lens is the highest power, the oil-immersion lens. Some examples of magnification power are as follows.

Eyepiece	Objective	Magnification
5×	10×	50
10×	10×	100
5×	45×	225
10×	45×	450
5×	100×	500
10×	100×	1000

Arm or Stand.   The arm or stand (Fig. 9-2) is used for carrying the microscope. When carrying the microscope, place one hand on the arm and support the base of the microscope with your other hand.

Body Tube.   The body tube directs the path of light from the light source to the eyepieces.

Stage.   The stage is the flat heavy part on which slides are placed for examination. On the stage are found two slide clips. In place of these clips, it is more convenient to apply an attachable mechanical stage, which is used to move the slides more precisely. This mechanical stage is almost indispensable in laboratory work, especially when the work requires high-power magnification.

Substage.   Fitting into the opening on the stage, and immediately below it, is the substage. This part holds the substage condenser, a necessity in microscopic work. Its purpose is to condense the light upon the object under examination. For best results you should focus the proper amount of light onto the object by lowering and raising the substage by means of the pinion adjustment (or condenser focus knob). On the lower part of the substage will be found the shutter or diaphragm. This shutter is to close off light or to admit more light. Since the amount of light required varies, adjustment of the substage in connection with specific uses of the microscope will be described.

Other Parts of the Microscope.   The *pinion head* or *coarse-focusing knob,* the larger one, is used for coarse adjustment of the microscope. The *fine-focusing knob,* the smaller one, is used in fine adjustment and focusing. These two knobs are important because they must be used every time the instrument is used. When you are looking for the field, it is always necessary to lower the head of the microscope by means of the coarse adjustment. After this is accom-

plished, the fine adjustment is then used. This is absolutely essential when using high-power magnification. Another part is the *light source* or *illuminator.*

Care, Cautions, and Maintenance

1. When carrying the microscope, hold it by the arm with one hand, supporting the bottom of the microscope base with the other.
2. Handle the microscope gently, taking care to avoid sharp knocks.
3. Do not try to adjust the microscope yourself if you do not fully understand its mechanism. You may throw the instrument out of balance and adjustment or damage the lens by hitting it on the stage.
4. Never force the adjustment knobs if they do not turn easily. They may need oiling or simple adjustment.
5. Never force a high-powered objective on a microscope slide. Doing so may break the slide, scratch the objective, or damage the lens.
6. Be sure that the lens of the objective is clean before attempting to do microscopic work. Do not leave dust, dirt, or finger marks on the lens surfaces. To clean the lens surfaces, remove dust using a soft-hair brush or gauze. Only for removing finger marks or grease should a soft cotton cloth, lens tissue, or gauze lightly moistened with absolute alcohol (methanol or ethanol) be used. For cleaning the objectives and immersion oil, use only xylene. For cleaning the surface of the entrance lens of the eyepiece tube, use absolute alcohol. Observe sufficient caution in handling alcohol and xylene.
7. Avoid the use of any organic solvent (for example, thinner, ether, alcohol, or xylene) for cleaning the painted surfaces and plastic parts of the instrument.
8. Avoid the use of the microscope in a dusty place or where it is subject to vibrations or exposed to high temperatures, moisture, or direct sunlight.
9. Never attempt to dismantle the instrument, in order to avoid the possibility of impairing its operational efficiency and accuracy.
10. Attention must be given to protect the objective lenses. Never leave immersion oil on the objective when the instrument is not being used. Before you put the microscope away, rotate the nosepiece so that the low-power objective is in position.
11. Remove the eye lens at regular intervals to clean out the dust and dirt particles that may have collected there.
12. When the microscope is not in use, cover it with the accessory vinyl cover and store it in a place free from moisture and fungus. It is especially recommended that the objectives and eyepieces

be kept in an airtight container containing desiccant.

13. Contact the salesperson for any serious problems you may have with the instrument.

Space for Using the Microscope

The microscope should be kept set up and ready for use. However limited the office laboratory area is, sufficient space must be allotted exclusively for the use of the microscope. It need be no more than a shelf wide enough to accommodate the equipment. Added to this should be a convenient seat *of proper height.* A kitchen stool will suffice. Attempting work with the microscope handicapped by improper relationship between the height of the worktable and stool is fatiguing and may lead to unreliable work.

Use of the Microscope (Fig. 9-3)

The material to be examined under the microscope will be placed on a glass slide. The slide is then placed on the microscope stage and fastened with the clips or held in place by the mechanical stage. Using the lowest power objective and a 10× eyepiece, slowly lower the microscope head by using the coarse-focusing knob. When you find the field, adjust the light by raising or lowering the pinion attached to the substage. Next, open or close the diaphragm to admit just the proper amount of light to give a clear, distinct field. To make the field of vision clear, use the fine-

Fig. 9-3. Technologist using microscope.

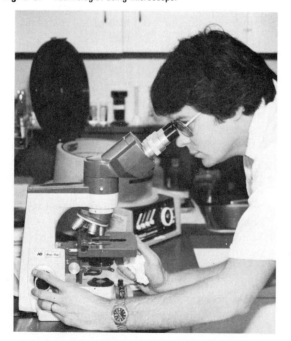

adjustment knob. From this point on, you can obtain a higher power of magnification by changing the objective.

Proper Adjustment of Illumination

The problem of obtaining maximum efficiency of illumination remains. Two factors enter into this problem: the light itself and the manipulation of the diaphragm, which controls the amount of light admitted to the condenser.

To know when the illumination has been properly adjusted, place a slide on the microscope and focus the low-power lens upon it. Remove the ocular and look down the tube of the microscope at the lenses of the objective. If shadows appear in this field, try to eliminate them by raising and lowering the condenser.

The most difficult part of illumination seems to be the proper manipulation of the iris diaphragm. Two cardinal principles should be remembered. *First,* the lower the power of the objective used, the more the light should be cut. In using the 16 mm lens to examine urine sediment or to count leukocytes, close the diaphragm almost completely; when the 4 mm objective is brought into play, the opening should be slightly increased; and when using the oil-immersion objective, the diaphragm may be opened wide. *Second,* the more brilliantly stained the object being viewed, the more light you can admit. As an example, if a differential blood count is being made with the 4 mm lens (the high dry power), the diaphragm may be at least half open, whereas during the examination of urinary sediment, especially if seeking hyaline casts, the light should be cut almost completely off. If this is not done, these hyaline structures will not be seen. *The diaphragm should be constantly adjusted while an examination is being made to get the most revealing picture. It is controlled by a little lever below the condenser. You should learn to seek this out and manipulate it subconsciously, as the fine adjustment is kept in constant use while focusing. If you are having trouble with an examination and things are not seen as clearly as they should be, examine the amount of light being admitted. The trouble is not infrequently caused by improper adjustment of the diaphragm.*

Focusing

In the microscopes illustrated in Figure 9-2, a coarse- and fine-adjustment control will be seen, the coarse adjustment being the larger knob placed behind the smaller, which is for fine adjustment. The coarse adjustment is for finding the relative focus; the fine adjustment is for bringing out the details clearly. *Do not use these interchangeably.* Using the coarse adjustment for fine focusing will result in broken cover glasses and slides; *trying to find a field with the fine adjustment will place too much strain on it and quickly wear it out.*

Place a slide on the stage and bring the low or high dry power objective down until it almost touches. Then, while looking into the microscope, slowly raise it with the coarse adjustment until the image is seen. Then, using the fine adjustment, bring out the details as described. It is a good plan never to turn the fine adjustment more than two thirds of one revolution. It is frequently desirable to keep the slide moving on the stage while attempting to focus. If this is not done, you may find that you are trying to focus on a spot where there is no material.

If it is found impossible to obtain a clear image although the illumination has been found satisfactory, the eyepiece should be rotated. If the blur is seen to rotate, the eyepiece is the source of the trouble. Remove it and wipe it thoroughly. The upper portion should be frequently cleaned, as it becomes soiled from contact with the eyelashes. In the event that the difficulty is not in the ocular, it is possible that the back of the objective has become fogged. This is not an infrequent occurrence if the instrument has been brought into a warm room from a cold one. Again, it is possible that the objective has been dipped into some fluid — immersion oil or water — and this has dried and caused fogging. Water can be removed with moistened lens tissue, and the lens can then be polished dry. If oil has dried on the lens, it must be cautiously removed with the smallest possible amount of xylene and the excess of this reagent wiped away with lens tissue.

Never focus down while looking through the microscope. This is inviting disaster to slides and cover glasses as well as possible damage to the lens. Observe from one side when you do focus down.

Use of Objectives

Of the three objectives, which are designated 16 mm, 4 mm, and 1.8 mm respectively, the 16 mm is the shortest in length and has the widest lens. The objective is used for low-power work, principally examining urine sediment, counting leukocytes, and inspecting the counting chamber of red cells for irregularity of distribution *(but only an expert should use it for counting these cells).* The 4 mm lens, the high dry, is mostly used for close inspection of the urinary sediment, counting red blood cells, and making routine differential blood cell counts.

Always use a cover glass when using the high dry power objective for examining urinary sediment. Do not dip the lens into the fluid without this protection. When using the 4 mm objective for differential blood counts, spread a thin film of immersion oil on the slide, over the stained blood, before making the examination.

The oil-immersion lens (1.8 mm) is used for obtaining the highest magnification in a conventional light microscope. Used with the eyepiece that gives a magnification of 10 diameters (marked 10×) the object as seen is about 1,000 times its actual size. To use this lens, place a drop of oil (such as Nujol) on the slide and focus down with coarse adjustment until the tip of the lens just touches the oil. Now, look through the microscope and focus upward very slowly with the coarse adjustment. When the object is seen, bring it into proper detail by use of the fine adjustment. This lens is used for all types of bacteriological work, for seeking malarial parasites, and for all other purposes demanding high magnification.

Practical Pointers for Microscope Use

If a single-tube microscope is used, learn to work with both eyes open. Squinting or closing one eye causes unnecessary strain. If much work is done, frequently shift from one eye to the other.

If you wear glasses, learn to do microscopy without them if possible. The instrument will focus to compensate for your visual defects if you are nearsighted or farsighted. On the other hand, if astigmatism is your difficulty, glasses will have to be worn, as this difficulty cannot be corrected by the microscopic lens.

CENTRIFUGES

Centrifuges are motorized devices that rotate at a high speed (Figures 9-4 and 9-5). The speed is stated

Fig. 9-4. Centrifuge used for blood and urine separations.

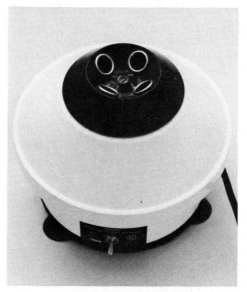

Fig. 9-5. **A** and **B,** centrifuges used for microhematocrit applications. **C,** view inside TRIAC centrifuge. Capillary tubes will be placed inside the numbered columns.

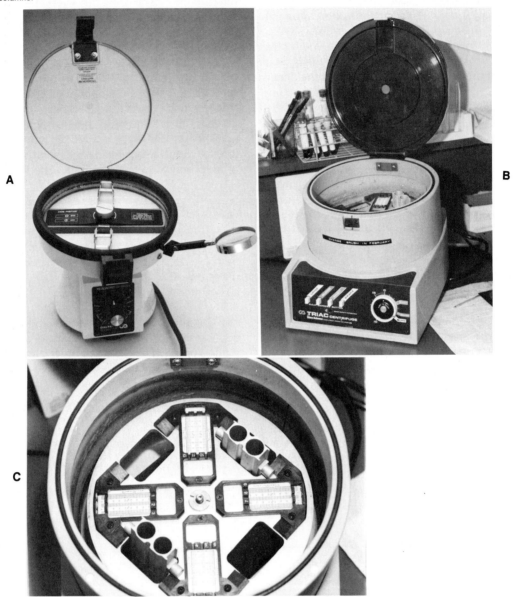

as *revolutions per minute (rpm)*. Centrifuges are used to separate components of varying densities contained in liquids by spinning them at high speeds. Through centrifugal (moving away from a center) force, heavier or solid components move to the lower part of the container, and the lighter substances move to the upper part of the container. By this process the two substances, solid material and fluid supernatant, are separated.

Centrifuges are used in every department of a clinical laboratory. In a physician's office or health care agency, centrifuges will be used if a microscopic analysis of urine is performed and also when serum is required for hematology or blood chemistry laboratory tests.

There are numerous types of centrifuges available. Each must be selected according to the intended use. Centrifuges commonly used in a physician's office or clinic are table models. One type is used for routine blood and urine separations (Figure 9-4), and another type is used for microhematocrit applications (Figure 9-5). The speed at which these centrifuges operate varies from 3200 rpm for the routine blood and urine separations to 11,500 to 15,000 rpm for the microhematocrit centrifuges. Special centrifuge tubes should be used in the centrifuges for serum or urine separations. These tubes are either conical or round-bottomed and made of a special quality glass. Some Vacutainer tubes used for blood collection may also be put into the centrifuge. Capillary tubes are to be used in the microhematocrit centrifuges. It is important that you always use tubes that are the correct size and strength for the required application.

In the centrifuge there are special centrifuge cups with rubber cushions that are used to hold the tubes containing the blood or urine samples. Be certain that the cushions are at the bottom of the holders before you place the tubes into them.

Placement of Tubes in the Centrifuge

When you place a tube containing a specimen into the centrifuge you must counterbalance it with a tube of similar design and weight. This other tube must be placed directly opposite the tube containing the specimen and should contain a liquid of equal weight. Water can usually be used for this purpose (Fig. 9-6). If you do not balance the load in a centrifuge, severe vibration of the centrifuge may occur and you may possibly lose the specimens. *Do not* use tubes that are cracked or badly scratched, because they may break under the stress of the centrifugal force. If breakage does occur, immediately turn the centrifuge off. Don rubber gloves and clean the centrifuge cushion and cup. You must clean these areas before using the centrifuge again to avoid additional breakage of tubes.

Operating the Centrifuge

When you operate the centrifuge you must close the cover. (Many newer models will not work if you do not close the cover.) If you are using an older model centrifuge, *do not* open the cover until the rotor has completely stopped. *Do not* brake sharply when using centrifuges that operate with hand brakes. Always use tubes that are the correct size and strength for the required application. Electrical appliances such as the centrifuge should have three-pronged grounding plugs, and there should be sufficient grounded outlets available. Frequent lubrication, calibration, and cleaning are required for the proper operation of all centrifuges. Specific instructions for operating each centrifuge are provided by the manufacturer. Read these instructions completely and carefully before you operate any centrifuge.

CONCLUSION

With the advances in the knowledge of physiology and improved technology, scientific, diagnostic and therapeutic procedures have increasingly become valuable aids to the physician and the patient. From

Fig. 9-6. Placing specimen tubes in centrifuge. When you place only one specimen tube into the centrifuge, you must place another tube of similar design and weight containing a liquid of equal weight (water can be used) directly opposite the specimen tube.

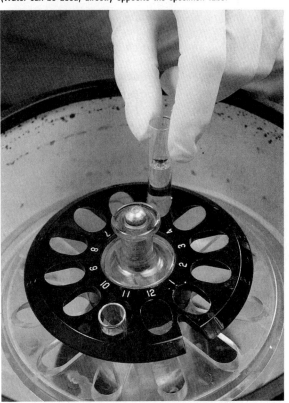

all the diagnostic and therapeutic procedures presented in the preceding units and Units X through XV, it can be readily seen that modern medicine offers many methods to physicians for arriving at a diagnosis and treating disease processes. The functional and structural alterations of body tissues, organs, and systems in disease can be studied and treated. Great strides have been made, and even greater achievements are expected as the mysteries of scientific research continue to unfold. At the opposite end of the spectrum from the concept of disease is health. For the body to remain healthy, the functions of the body systems must be normal. A primary requirement for survival of the human organism is the maintenance and safeguarding of the anatomical and physiological equilibrium of the individual cells that make up the sum of the body and its parts.

There are numerous sources you may refer to for expanding your knowledge on the topics discussed in the following units. Check with your instructor for additional enrichment assignments and references in areas of your own particular need and interest.

REVIEW OF VOCABULARY

Using the information presented in this unit and other reference sources of your own choice, read and define the italicized terms.

All clinical laboratories have certain specialized departments in common. They are divided into areas based on function and types of tests performed. These areas usually include *hematology, urinalysis, serology, blood banking, medical microbiology,* and *clinical chemistry. Parasitology* and examination of feces may be special departments or they may be included in one of the above. Some laboratories may also have special areas for *histology, mycology, immunochemistry,* and *cytology.*

Correct labeling of a *specimen* and completing a *laboratory requisition* are important duties of the medical assistant when sending *specimens* to *outside laboratories.*

One of three formats can be used for recording and organizing information and test results in the patient's record: the *source-oriented format, the integrated format,* or *the problem-oriented format.*

Special care must be given to the *microscope* and *centrifuge* when you use these pieces of equipment for laboratory work.

REVIEW QUESTIONS

1. State the importance of the information gathered from clinical laboratory tests.
2. List six specialized departments common to all clinical laboratories. Describe the function of each department.
3. Describe the medical assistant's responsibilities when dealing with a commercial clinical laboratory.
4. List seven items that are to be included on a laboratory requisition that accompanies a specimen to the laboratory.
5. Describe how reports would be filed in the source-oriented record.
6. List seven safety rules that should be adhered to when working with laboratory equipment and specimens.
7. State how you should carry a microscope.
8. State what type of tubes should be used in a centrifuge.

PERFORMANCE TEST

In a skills laboratory, a simulation of a joblike environment, the medical assistant student is to demonstrate the correct procedure for the following without reference to source materials.

1. Demonstrate proper use and care of a microscope.
2. Demonstrate proper use and care of a centrifuge.
3. Given sample laboratory requisitions and physician's orders, correctly complete each requisition to be sent to the laboratory along with a specimen.
4. Demonstrate the use of safety rules when working with laboratory equipment and specimens.

PERFORMANCE CHECKLISTS

The medical assistant students are to design their own step-by-step procedures and performance checklists for the performance test in this unit.

Unit X

Urinalysis

COGNITIVE OBJECTIVES

On completion of Unit X, the medical assistant student should be able to apply the following cognitive objectives:

1. Define and pronounce the vocabulary terms listed.
2. Briefly describe the formation of urine, list the main normal components of urine, and give a description of normal urine.
3. Define "routine urinalysis," listing the three basic categories into which it is divided, along with the major observations and examinations made in each category.
4. Describe the fourth category of tests that may now be included in a routine urinalysis.
5. Describe the standard procedure to follow when performing a routine urinalysis.
6. Identify normal and abnormal findings obtained on a complete urinalysis. Relate the abnormal findings to the most probable or possible causes.
7. Describe a reagent strip that is used for doing chemical tests on a urine specimen.
8. Explain how reagent tablets are to be stored.
9. Discuss the advantage and use of the Tek-Chek and Chek-Stix quality control systems for the chemical analysis of urine.
10. List the organized and unorganized sediment that may be present in a urine specimen, indicating if they are normal or abnormal findings.
11. Identify urine tests, other than those performed on a routine urinalysis.

TERMINAL PERFORMANCE OBJECTIVES

On completion of Unit X, the medical assistant student should be able to do the following terminal performance objectives:

1. Demonstrate the correct procedure for performing a physical and chemical analysis of a urine specimen.
2. Demonstrate the correct procedure for preparing a urine specimen for a microscopic examination.

3. Demonstrate the correct procedure for testing a urine specimen for the presence of glucose, acetone, and bilirubin using the Clinitest, Acetest, and Ictotest reagent tablets.
4. Demonstrate the correct procedure for testing a clean-catch midstream urine specimen for bacteriuria using the Microstix-3 reagent strip.
5. Demonstrate the correct procedure for testing a urine specimen for the presence of glucose using the Tes-Tape.
6. Demonstrate the correct methods for using the Tek-Chek and Chek-Stix quality control systems.

The student is expected to perform the above activities with 100% accuracy.

Vocabulary

acetonuria (as'ĕ-tō-nu'rē-ah) or **ketonuria** (kē"tō-nu'rē-ah)—The presence of acetone or ketone in the urine.

albuminuria (al-bū"mi-nu'rē-ah)—The presence of serum albumin in urine.

anuria (ah-nu'rē-ah)—The absence of urine.

bacteriuria (bak-te"rē-u'rē-ah)—The presence of bacteria in urine.

dysuria (dis-u'rē-ah)—Painful or difficult urination.

glucosuria (gloo"kō-su'rē-ah) or **glycosuria** (gli"kō-su'rē-ah)—Abnormally high sugar content in urine.

hematuria (hēm"ah-tu"rē-ah)—The presence of blood in urine.

oliguria (ol"i-gu'rē-ah)—Scanty amounts of urine.

polyuria (pol"ē-u'rē'ah)—Excessive excretion of urine.

proteinuria (pro"te-in-u'rē-ah)—An abnormal increase of protein in urine.

pyuria (pī-u'rē-ah)—The presence of pus in the urine.

qualitative tests—Used for screening purposes. These tests provide an indication as to whether or not a substance is present in a specimen in abnormal quantities. A qualitative test does not determine the exact amount of a substance present in a specimen. Color charts are usually used to interpret qualitative tests. *Sometimes* they are called semiquantitative tests. Results are reported in terms such as trace, small amount, moderate, large amount, or 1+, 2+, 3+, and so on, or simply as positive or negative.

quantitative tests—More precise tests. They determine accurately the amount of a specific substance that is present in a specimen. A high level of skill is required to perform these tests on sophisticated equipment. Results are reported in units such as grams (gm) per 100 milliliters (ml), or milligrams (mg) percent, or milligrams per deciliter (dl).

URINARY SYSTEM: FORMATION AND COMPONENTS OF NORMAL URINE

The organs of the urinary system include the two kidneys, two ureters, one bladder, and one urethra. Urine is formed in the kidneys, and passes through the ureters into the bladder, where it remains until the individual voids, and then it is excreted through the urethra. The kidneys, located in the retroperitoneal cavity (which means they lie behind the peritoneum), lie anterior and lateral to the twelfth thoracic and first three lumbar vertebrae; they are relatively small, approximately 4½ inches long, 2 inches wide, and 1¼ inches thick. Being highly complex and discriminatory organs, they help maintain the state of homeostasis in the internal environment by selectively excreting or reabsorbing various substances according to the needs of the body. You should recall from your studies in anatomy and physiology the nephron unit, which is the functional unit of the kidney. Each kidney has approximately 1,000,000 nephron units working together to selectively retain or excrete the substances passing through them. Blood, entering the kidneys by way of the renal arteries, eventually reaches the nephron unit for this process to occur. Approximately 1200 ml (30 ml = 1 ounce) of blood flows through the kidneys each minute. This represents about one fourth of the total blood volume in an adult. As blood enters the glomerulus of the nephron, water and the low molecular weight components of the plasma filter through to Bowman's capsule, then to Bowman's space, and on through the various parts of the tubules. It is in the tubules that reabsorption of some substances, secretion of others, and the concentration of the urine occur as mechanisms for conserving body water. Many components of the plasma filtrate, such as water, glucose, and amino acids, are partially or completely reabsorbed, and potassium, hydrogen ions, and other substances are secreted. On the average, nearly all the water that passes through this network is reabsorbed; approximately 1 liter (1000 ml) or so is secreted as the largest component of urine (Fig. 10-1). The main normal components of urine follow:

1. Water — about 95% of urine is water.
2. Nitrogenous waste substances or the organic compounds, that is, urea, uric acid, and creatinine.
3. Mineral salts or the inorganic compounds, such as sodium chloride, sulfates, and phosphates of different kinds.
4. Pigment — derived from certain bile compounds, it gives color to the urine.

Many physiological changes in the body can lead to an upset in the normal functions carried out by the kidneys. Urine, which is continuously formed in and excreted from the body, provides important information with regard to many diseases and disorders. Accordingly, it is widely studied as an aid in diagnosis, in monitoring the course of treatment of disease, and also in providing a profile of the patient's health status. Urine has been referred to as a mirror that reflects activities within the body and as such provides much varied information as a result of many chemical, physical, and microscopic measurements. The analysis of urine can provide information on the whole body as well as its many parts. Kidney disorders modify the composition of urine and may also affect many other body functions. The study of urine may also reflect the situation in which kidney function is normal but other parts of the body are functioning incorrectly.

ROUTINE URINALYSIS

TURBIDITY - CLOUDINESS

A routine urinalysis, or basic urinalysis as it is often called, can be easily and quickly performed. It is a basic test, but it provides the physician with a tremendous amount of information when a disease process is present. This test can help confirm or rule out a suspected diagnosis. All patients having a physical examination or entering the hospital for treatment will have a urinalysis performed. Frequently it is a routine test for many patients seen in the physician's office or clinic and will be repeated annually or as frequently as is necessary to evaluate the patient's health status.

A routine urinalysis is divided into three basic categories. (A fourth category — detection and semiquantitation of bacteriuria — can now also be done easily in the microbiology and urinalysis laboratories.) These categories, the major observations, and examinations for each follow.

1. General physical characteristics and measurements
   a. Appearance
   b. Color
   c. Odor
   d. Quantity
   e. Specific gravity

Fig. 10-1.   **A,** Coronal section through right kidney. **B,** Nephron unit with its blood vessels. Blood flows through nephron vessels as follows: intralobular artery → afferent arteriole → glomerulus → efferent arteriole → peritubular capillaries (around tubules) → venules → intralobular vein. (From Anthony, C.P.: Textbook of anatomy and physiology, ed. 9, St. Louis, 1975, The C.V. Mosby Co.)

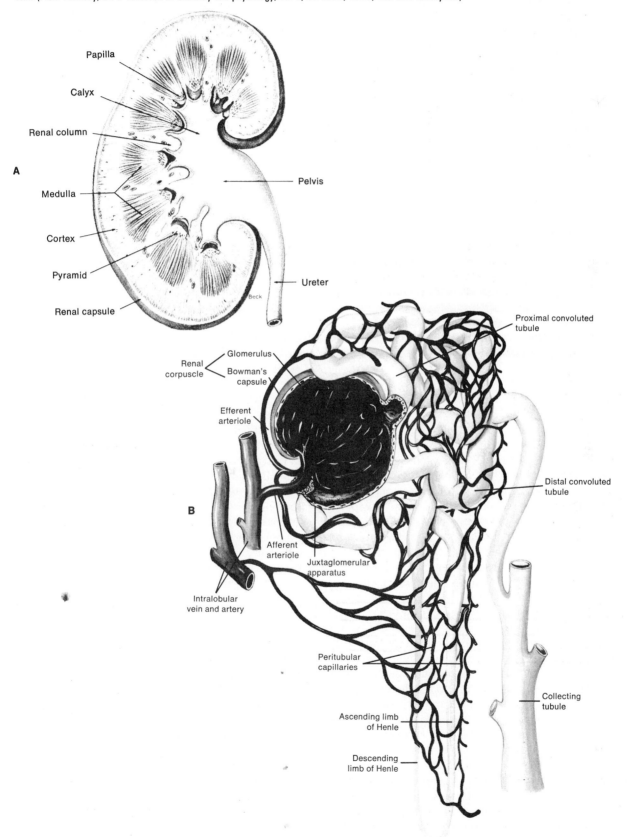

Papilla

Calyx

Renal column

A

Pelvis

Medulla

Cortex

Pyramid

Ureter

Renal capsule

Beck

Glomerulus

Renal
corpuscle

Bowman's
capsule

Proximal convoluted
tubule

Efferent
arteriole

B

Distal convoluted
tubule

Afferent
arteriole

Juxtaglomerular
apparatus

Intralobular
vein and artery

Peritubular
capillaries

Collecting
tubule

Ascending limb
of Henle

Descending
limb of Henle

2. Chemical examinations
   a. Reaction (pH)
   b. Protein
   c. Glucose
   d. Ketone
   e. Bilirubin
   f. Blood
   g. Nitrite
   h. Urobilinogen
   i. Special tests when indicated, such as for pregnancy, phenylketonuria, and porphyrinuria.
3. Microscopic examination of centrifuged sediment
   a. Cells (epithelial, red blood cells, and white blood cells)
   b. Casts
   c. Bacteria
   d. Parasites and yeasts
   e. Spermatozoa
   f. Crystals
   g. Artifacts and contaminants
4. Detection and semiquantitation of bacteriuria
   a. Culture plate methods — this requires the special facilities and personnel of a microbiology laboratory. Tests should be done immediately, or the specimen should be refrigerated.
   b. Nitrite test and culture strip methods — this can now be done in the urinalysis laboratory.

Standard Procedures

A freshly voided random urine specimen is collected in a dry, clean container. (Review types of urine specimens outlined in Unit VI, Collecting and Handling Specimens; also review Unit IX, Laboratory Orientation). This specimen should be examined within 1 hour to avoid changes or deterioration to the contents. If the examination cannot be performed within this time, the specimen should be refrigerated at 5°C (41°F) to preserve the specimen.

When you are doing the examination, the *first* procedure is to note the physical characteristics of the urine; the *second* is to measure the specific gravity; the *third* is to perform the series of chemical tests; and the *fourth* is to prepare the specimen for the microscopic examination. This fourth step is accomplished by centrifuging 10 to 12 ml of a thoroughly mixed urine specimen; then the residual sediment is resuspended in 0.25 to 1 ml of urine on a slide for the microscopic examination. The remainder of the urine specimen should be kept until all the procedures are completed, in case any of the tests have to be repeated, or if other special tests have to be performed, when indicated.

Tests performed on a random specimen of urine are *qualitative*. Only the concentration of a substance in this particular specimen can be measured. The total amount of a substance excreted can be mea-sured only when urine is collected over an accurately measured period of time, such as when collecting a 24 hour specimen.

General Physical Characteristics and Measurements

Appearance.   The appearance is generally the first observation made on a urine specimen by virtue of just handling the specimen.

Normal, fresh urine is usually transparent or clear. If the specimen is alkaline, it may appear white and cloudy because of the presence of carbonates and phosphates, but will clear when a small amount of acid is added to the urine. Urate crystals may be present in an acid urine, giving the specimen a pinkish, cloudy appearance, which usually clears on heating to 140°F (60°C). Both of these appearances are normal.

Abnormal cloudiness in urine may be seen in patients who have a urinary tract infection. This may be caused by the presence of pus cells, leukocytes, and bacteria, or by the alkalinity of the urine. Also important to note when observing the appearance of urine is the presence of any sediment (solid particles) in the urine. When red blood cells, white blood cells, or casts are present in large amounts, this could indicate renal disease or bladder or urinary tract infection.

Color.   Normal fresh urine color ranges are described as straw-colored, yellow, or amber, the result of the presence of the yellow pigment, urochrome. The concentration of normal urine determines the degree of the color: highly concentrated urine is dark; dilute urine is pale. Various other factors affect the color of urine, for example, medications, dyes, blood, and food pigments. In many disease states color changes are caused by the presence of pigments that normally do not appear.

Medications such as multivitamins may make the urine a very pronounced dark yellow; nitrofurantoin (Furadantin) (used in the treatment of urinary tract infections) may make the urine brown; and phenazopyridine (Pyridium) (an analgesic used for relief of pain, frequency, urgency, and other discomforts arising from irritation of the lower urinary tract mucosa) produces a reddish orange discoloration of the urine. The presence of hemoglobin in the urine may make it reddish brown; bile pigments may turn urine yellow to yellow-brown or greenish. Melanins (dark pigments that occur abnormally in certain tumors), when excreted in urine, cause it to turn brown-black if left standing. If the patient is eating large amounts of carrots, the urine may turn a bright yellow. In hepatitis the urine may be a pronounced orange (when the urine is shaken, even the bubbles will be orange if the patient has hepatitis). Also when an individual eats a fair amount of rhubarb, the urine may be red to red-brown.

Odor.   Normal urine has a characteristic aroma that is thought to be caused by the presence of certain acids. An ammoniacal odor will develop when urine is left standing for any length of time, due to the decomposition of urea in the specimen.

Urine containing acetone, as seen in patients with diabetes mellitus, may have a fruity odor. Urinary tract infections may cause the urine to be foul-smelling or putrid.

Although you will usually record the odor of urine when performing a routine analysis, it is generally thought to be of little significance in diagnosing a patient's condition.

Quantity.   The normal quantity of urine voided by an adult in a 24 hour period varies somewhat, depending on the individual's fluid intake, the temperature and climate, the amount of fluid output through the intestines (as in diarrhea), and the amount of perspiration. The average quantity is about 1500 ml and ranges from 750 to 2000 ml. The quantity voided by children is somewhat smaller than the amounts excreted by adults, but the total volume is greater in proportion to body size.

To measure the quantity of urine, pour the specimen into a large graduated cylinder, and record the quantity in cubic centimeters or milliliters. The amount recorded is reported as urine quantity per unit of time (usually 24 hours). Measuring the quantity of urine output is an important aid in diagnosing conditions or diseases related to polyuria, oliguria, or anuria.

Anuria is the absence of urine. At times it may be described as the diminution of urine secretion to 100 ml or less in 24 hours. This may be seen in shock, severe dehydration, and urinary system disease.

Oliguria is the diminution of urinary secretions to between 100 and 400 ml in 24 hours, more commonly defined as scanty amounts of urine. This is seen in drug poisoning, deep coma, cardiac insufficiency, after profuse bleeding, vomiting, diarrhea, and perspiration. Oliguria is also present with decreased fluid intake and with an increased ingestion of salt.

Polyuria is an excessive excretion of urine. This occurs in diabetes mellitus, diabetes insipidus, chronic nephritis, and following the ingestion of diuretic medications or an excessive intake of fluids. It also may be present during periods of anxiety or nervousness.

Dysuria is painful or difficult urination, symptomatic of many conditions such as cystitis, prolapse of the uterus, enlargement of the prostate, and urethritis.

Specific Gravity.   The specific gravity of urine is its weight compared with the universal standard weight of an equal amount of distilled water (expressed as 1.000). This measurement indicates the relative degree of concentration of dilution of the specimen, which in turn helps determine the kidney's ability to concentrate and dilute urine.

Normal specific gravity of urine is generally between 1.010 and 1.025, although it may range from 1.005 to 1.030, depending on the concentration of the urine. The first morning specimen has the highest specific gravity, generally being greater than 1.020. It will then vary throughout the day, depending largely on the individual's fluid intake.

Abnormally low specific gravity values may be seen in patients who have diabetes insipidus, pyelonephritis, glomerulonephritis, and various kidney anomalies. In these conditions, the kidneys have lost effective concentrating abilities.

Abnormally high values will be seen in patients with diabetes mellitus, congestive heart failure, hepatic disease, and adrenal insufficiency. The specific gravity will also be elevated when the patient has lost an excessive amount of water through the gastrointestinal tract, as with diarrhea and vomiting, or through the skin during excessive perspiration. High amounts of glucose and protein in the urine, as seen in patients with diabetes mellitus, will also increase this value.

There are several methods by which the specific gravity of urine can be measured. The newest and easiest method is by using one of three of the Ames Company's Multistix reagent strips. The strip is dipped into a urine specimen and then is compared with the color chart. The test strip will reflect specific gravity as it changes color from blue (low specific gravity) through shades of green to yellow (high specific gravity). (See also *Chemical Examinations of Urine Using Reagent Strips*.)

Specific gravity can also be measured by using a refractometer — Total Solids (TS) Meter — a delicate, hand-held instrument that requires calibration daily. Only one to two drops of urine are required when using this meter. The procedure for use is as follows (Fig. 10-2):

1. Clean and dry the surface of the prism and cover, and close the cover.
2. Using an eye dropper, place a drop of urine at the notched end of the cover. The urine should be drawn over the prism by capillary action.
3. Pointing the meter toward a light source, rotate the eyepiece to focus on the calibrated scale. You will observe a light and a dark area (Fig. 10-2).
4. Read the results on the specific gravity scale at the line that divides the light and dark areas (Fig. 10-2).
5. Record the results.
6. Clean the prism with a damp cloth and then dry it.

The specific gravity of urine can also be determined by using an urinometer, a weighted bulb-

Fig. 10-2. **A,** using a refractometer to determine the specific gravity of urine. **B,** Point meter toward light source, rotate eyepiece to focus on calibrated scale, and read the results on the specific gravity scale at the line that divides the light and dark areas. The specific gravity of this specimen is 1.020.

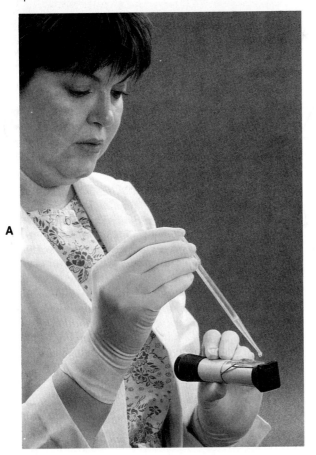

A

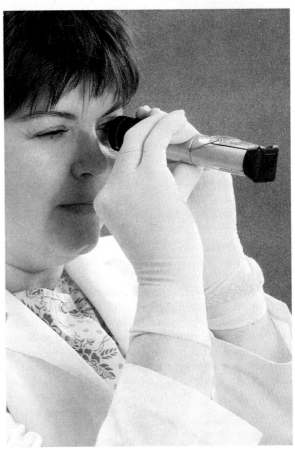

B

shaped instrument that has a stem with a scale calibrated from 1.000 to 1.040. The procedure for using the urinometer follows.

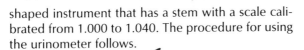

Procedure for Determining the Specific Gravity of Urine Using the Urinometer (Fig. 10-3)

Equipment

One 5 inch high glass cylinder
One urinometer

Procedure	Rationale
1. Wash your hands and assemble the equipment.	
2. Pour well-mixed urine into the cylinder to the three-quarter mark.	
3. Place the urinometer in the urine, and spin it gently.	The urinometer will float in the urine. When there is insufficient urine to float the urinometer, the specific gravity cannot be read. You would then simply record "Quantity insufficient."
4. Place the cylinder so that the lower line of the meniscus is at eye level.	The meniscus is a crescent-shaped structure appearing at the surface of a liquid column.
5. Read the specific gravity by noting the point where the lower middle part of the meniscus crossed the urinometer scale. Do not allow the urinometer to touch the sides of the cylinder.	An inaccurate reading results if the urinometer touches the sides of the cylinder.

Procedure	Rationale
6. Record the reading. **7.** Discard the urine. Rinse the urinometer and cylinder with water. Wipe the urinometer dry before using it again. **8.** Wash your hands.	

The urinometer should be placed in distilled water and checked daily to test its reliability. If it does not read 1.000 when in the distilled water, the urinometer must be replaced. Also, if an unusually high reading is found when testing a urine specimen, remove the urinometer and rinse it under cool water to remove all urine residual; test in distilled water, and then retest the urine specimen. These extra steps are important in case someone had previously left an unclean urinometer, which would lead to abnormal testing results when used again.

Chemical Examinations of Urine Using Reagent Strips

Chemically impregnated reagent strips have virtually replaced older, more cumbersome methods for performing a urinalysis. They provide an easy and rapid method for obtaining the results of tests done in a routine or basic urinalysis, thus are especially practical and convenient for use in a physician's office or clinic. In addition to these strips, other special paper tapes, chemical tablets, selectively treated slides, and simplified culture tests are available for special examinations.

The pH of urine and several other components can be easily and rapidly determined with the use of a variety of specially prepared reagent strips and a color chart. The reagent strip is a clear plastic strip with up to ten pieces of colored filter paper attached, each used to identify different components in the urine. Every piece of filter paper is impregnated with various chemicals and will change color when dipped in the urine. Color changes on the filter papers will depend on the presence and amount of the substance that is being measured.

The most complete reagent strip is the Multistix 10 SG,* which is used for determining the pH and specific gravity, and the presence and amount of urobilinogen, nitrite, blood, bilirubin, ketone, glucose, protein, and the presence of intact and lysed leukocytes (white blood cells) in urine. There are various other Multistix reagent strips available. The Multistix product name includes a number suffix that indicates the number of urine tests on the strip. In addition, strips that test specific gravity have an SG suffix.

Reagent strips are supplied in plastic bottles containing 100 strips with directions for use. The color chart and specified times used to read the results of the tests are presented on the sides of the bottle. Both open and unopened product expiration dates are established for these strips to ensure maximum product quality.

*Ames Co., Division of Miles Laboratories, Inc.; Elkhart, IN.

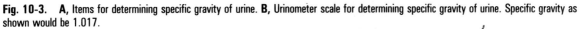

Fig. 10-3. A, Items for determining specific gravity of urine. **B,** Urinometer scale for determining specific gravity of urine. Specific gravity as shown would be 1.017.

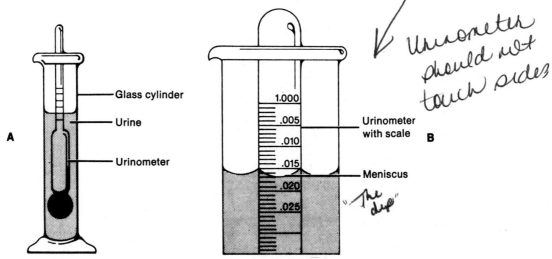

Because the pH of urine is usually determined as part of a complete urinalysis, it is desirable to use a multiple reagent strip such as one of the Multistix or one of the other reagent strips. Table 10-1 shows the wide range of Ames reagent strips and tablets that are readily available for use.

Procedure for Using a Reagent Strip

1. Dip the test areas of the strip into a freshly voided urine specimen; remove immediately and tap to remove excess urine (Fig. 10-4, *A* and *B*).
2. Compare the test areas to the appropriate color chart on the bottle at the specified times (Fig. 10-4, *C*).
3. Record the results.

For best results, reading urine tests at the proper time is critical. Multistix reagent areas are designed to be read from the bottom up. After removing the Multistix 10 SG reagent strip from the urine, read the results at the following specified times (Fig. 10-5):

glucose—read at 30 seconds
bilirubin—read at 30 seconds
ketone—read at 40 seconds
specific gravity—read at 45 seconds
blood—read at 50 seconds
pH—read at 60 seconds
protein—read at 60 seconds
urobilinogen—read at 60 seconds
nitrite—read at 60 seconds
leukocytes—read at 2 minutes

Table 10-1. Rapid reagent tests for routine and special urinalyses*

Reagent test	Substances determined	Technique†
N-Multistix	pH, protein, glucose, ketones, bilirubin, blood, nitrite and urobilinogen	Use fresh, uncentrifuged urine. Preservatives may be added. Dip reagent strip in specimen, remove, and compare each reagent area with corresponding color chart on bottle label at the number of seconds specified.
Multistix	pH, protein, glucose, ketones, bilirubin, blood, and urobilinogen	As above
Multistix 10 SG	Glucose, bilirubin, ketone, specific gravity, blood, pH, protein, urobilinogen, nitrite, leukocytes	As above
Multistix 9	Glucose, bilirubin, ketone, blood, pH, protein, urobilinogen, nitrite, leukocytes	As above
Multistix 9 SG	Glucose, bilirubin, ketone, specific gravity, blood, pH, protein, nitrite, leukocytes	As above
Multistix 8	Glucose, bilirubin, ketone, blood, pH, protein, nitrite, leukocytes	As above
Multistix 8 SG	Glucose, ketone, specific gravity, blood, pH, protein, nitrite, leukocytes	As above
Multistix 7	Glucose, ketone, blood, pH, protein, nitrite, leukocytes	As above
Uristix 4	Glucose, protein, nitrite, leukocytes	As above
Multistix 2	Nitrite, leukocytes	As above
N-Multistix SG	Glucose, bilirubin, ketone, specific gravity, blood, pH, protein, urobilinogen, nitrite	As above
Bili-Labstix	pH, protein, glucose, ketones, bilirubin, and blood	As above
Labstix	pH, protein, glucose, ketones, and blood	As above
Hema-Combistix	pH, protein, glucose, and blood	As above
Combistix	pH, protein, and glucose	As above
N-Uristix	Protein, glucose and nitrite	As above
Uristix	Protein and glucose	As above
Clinistix	Glucose	As above
Albustix	Protein	As above
Hemastix	Blood	As above
Microstix-nitrite	Nitrite	As above

Table 10-1 (*continued*)

Reagent test	Substances determined	Technique†
Urobilistix	Urobilinogen	As above, but preferably using a 2 hour urine specimen collected in early afternoon (between 2 and 4 PM).
Microstix-3	Bacteriuria	Dip culture-reagent strip in specimen for 5 seconds, remove, read nitrite test area after 30 seconds. Insert and seal strip in sterilized plastic pouch provided, incubate for 18 to 24 hours. Compare color densities on total and Gram-negative culture pads with chart provided, without removing strip from pouch. Incinerate pouch with strip still sealed inside.
Ictotest	Bilirubin	Place 5 drops of urine on the special mat. Cover with the reagent tablet. Flow 2 drops of water onto tablet. Compare the color reaction with the color chart.
Diastix	Glucose	Use fresh, uncentrifuged urine. Do not use preservative containing formaldehyde. Dip reagent strip in specimen, remove, and compare with color chart on bottle label.
Ketostix	Ketones (principally acetoacetic acid)	As above, but urine must be at least at room temperature at the time of testing.
Keto-Diastix	Glucose and ketones (principally acetoacetic acid)	As above for Diastix and Ketostix.
Clinitest	Reducing substances, including sugars	Add Clinitest tablet to test tube containing mixture of 5 drops of urine and 10 drops of water. Spontaneous boiling occurs; after it stops, compare color in tube with color chart.
Phenistix	Phenylpyruvic acid (phenylketonuria, or PKU)	Use fresh, uncentrifuged urine. Dip reagent strip in specimen, remove, and compare with color chart on bottle label.

*Courtesy Ames Co., Division Miles Laboratories Inc., 1986.
†See package inserts for proper procedures.

For screening positive from negative specimens only, all reagent areas except leukocytes may be read between 1 and 2 minutes.

The addition of a leukocyte test to dry reagent strips may reduce the need for microscopic analysis. Chemical testing for leukocyte esterase detects lysed white blood cells that cannot be detected microscopically. Since leukocyte esterase will be present hours after sample collection, false negatives are reduced.

Microscopic analysis of urine is not indicated when negative findings are obtained for leukocytes, nitrite, protein, and occult blood. Time-consuming microscopics can be reduced to those specimens where positive chemical results suggest that more specific information is needed.

Urine Chemistry Analyzers For Use With Reagent Strips

The Ames Multistix reagent strips are also designed for use with instrumentation, such as with the Ames Clinitek 200 urine chemistry analyzer for moderate to large volume urine testing, or the Clinitek 10 urine chemistry analyzer for small to medium volume urine testing (Fig. 10-6). These instruments are semi-automated and are designed to *read* the reagent strips. Readings are standardized for improved precision through the elimination of visual color discrepancies and operator and environmental variables. Both of these analyzers are easy to use. Directions for use are supplied with the instruments, and they must be followed explicitly.

Fig. 10-4. Using a reagent strip. **A,** Dip test areas into urine. **B,** Remove immediately and tap to remove excess urine. **C,** Comparing results of chemical analysis of urine when using reagent strip. (Courtesy Ames Co., Inc., Elkhart, IN)

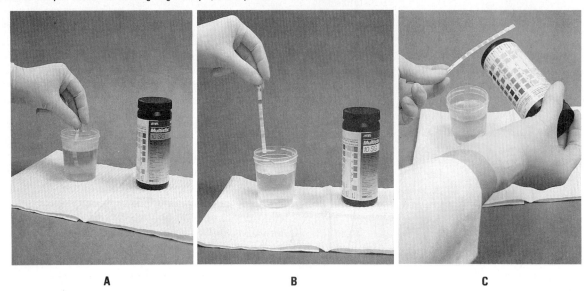

A   B   C

Clinitek 10

When the Clinitek 10 analyzer is turned on, the feed table automatically moves out to the *load* position; then the instrument goes through a self-test cycle. After this cycle is completed, the name of the Ames strip programmed to be read is displayed (see Fig. 10-6).

After properly immersing the reagent strip in urine and removing the excess urine by blotting, slide the strip onto the feed table, pad-side up, within 10 seconds after pressing the *Start* button. Be sure that the tip of the strip lies flat on the table and is touching the end stop of the feed table insert.

Record the test results shown on the display panel; then remove and discard the used reagent strip.

Significance of Test Results (Table 10-2)

Multistix 10 SG reagent strips may provide diagnostically useful information about the status of carbohydrate metabolism, kidney and liver function, acid-base balance, bacteriuria-pyuria, and many other conditions as follows:

Reaction (pH)

pH is the symbol for the hydrogen-ion concentration that expresses the degree of acidity or alkalinity of a solution. The pH is measured on a scale ranging from 0 to 14, with 7 being neutral; 0 to 7 is acidic, and 7 to 14 is alkaline. Usually freshly voided normal urine from patients on normal diets is acidic, having a pH of 6.0, although normal kidneys are capable of secreting urine that may vary in pH from 4.5 to slightly higher than 8.0.

Excessively acid urine may be obtained from patients on a high protein diet or who are taking certain medications such as vitamin C or ammonium chloride, and from patients who are retaining a large amount of sodium. In the conditions of uncontrolled diabetes mellitus and acidosis, you will also find the patient's urine to be very acidic.

Alkaline urine is seen in patients who have ingested a large meal, and in those who consume a diet high in milk and other diary products, citrus fruits, and vegetables. Certain medications, such as sodium bicarbonate, will help produce alkaline urine. Urinary tract infections, specimens contaminated by bacteria, and specimens left standing for any length of time will also produce highly alkaline urine.

Protein

Normal urine may contain protein, mostly albumin, after exposure to cold, excessive muscular activity, or ingestion of large amounts of protein.

Albuminuria (al-bu-mĭ-nu-re-ah) is the presence of serum albumin or serum globulin in the urine. It is usually a sign of renal impairment; however, it can also occur in healthy individuals following vigorous exercise.

(Text continues on p. 310)

Fig. 10-5.   Multistix 10 SG chart used for determining amounts of ten factors when performing urinalysis. (Courtesy Ames Co., Inc., Elkhart, IN)

ames   **COLOR CHART**

Multistix®

10 SG

Reagent Strips for Urinalysis
For In Vitro Diagnostic Use

READ PRODUCT INSERT BEFORE USE.
IMPORTANT: Do not expose to direct sunlight.
          Do not use after 11/90.

MILES

TESTS AND READING TIME

Test							
LEUKOCYTES 2 minutes	NEGATIVE		TRACE	SMALL +	MODERATE + +	LARGE + + +	
NITRITE 60 seconds	NEGATIVE		POSITIVE	POSITIVE	(Any degree of uniform pink color is positive)		
UROBILINOGEN 60 seconds	NORMAL 0.2	NORMAL 1	mg/dL 2	4	8	(1 mg = approx. 1 EU)	
PROTEIN 60 seconds	NEGATIVE	TRACE	mg/dL 30 +	100 + +	300 + + +	2000 or more + + + +	
pH 60 seconds	5.0	6.0	6.5	7.0	7.5	8.0	8.5
BLOOD 50 seconds	NEGATIVE		NON-HEMOLYZED TRACE	HEMOLYZED TRACE	SMALL +	MODERATE + +	LARGE + + +
SPECIFIC GRAVITY 45 seconds	1.000	1.005	1.010	1.015	1.020	1.025	1.030
KETONE 40 seconds	NEGATIVE	mg/dL	TRACE 5	SMALL 15	MODERATE 40	LARGE 80	LARGE 160
BILIRUBIN 30 seconds	NEGATIVE		SMALL +	MODERATE + +	LARGE + + +		
GLUCOSE 30 seconds	NEGATIVE	g/dL (%) mg/dL	1/10 (tr.) 100	1/4 250	1/2 500	1 1000	2 or more 2000 or more

©1988 Miles Inc., Diagnostics Division, Elkhart, IN 46515 USA   Rev. 11/88   0401032

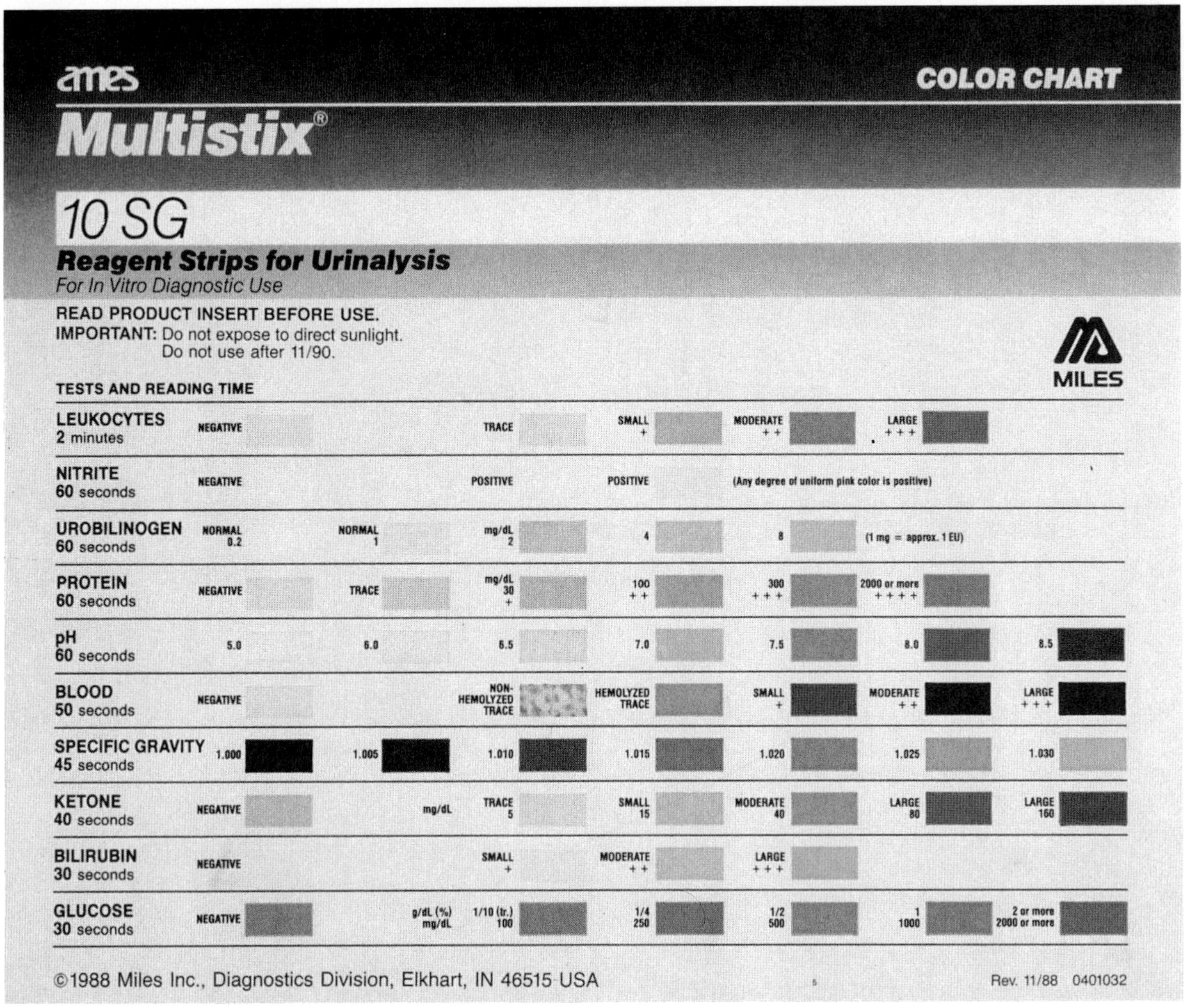

Fig. 10-6.   Clinitek 10 urine chemistry analyzer. A semi-automated instrument designed to read the reagent strip. Results show up on the display panel. (Courtesy Ames Co., Inc., Elkhart, IN)

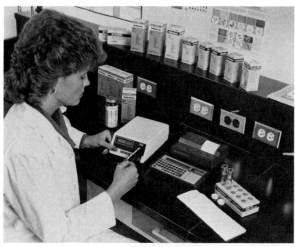

Table 10-2. Urine profile of differential disease findings*

N = Normal   I = Increased   D = Decreased

Multistix Urine Reagent Strip Tests	Hepatic	Renal	Pancreatic	Gastrointestinal	Cardiovascular	Other
pH		Renal tubular acidosis—I Bacterial infections—I Chronic renal failure—I	Diabetic acidosis—D	Diarrhea—D Pyloric obstruction—I Vomiting—I Malabsorption—N or D	Congestive heart failure—N	Dehydration—D Starvation—D Low-carbohydrate diets—I Acetazolamide therapy—I Metabolic acidosis—D Metabolic alkalosis—I Emphysema—D
Protein		Nephrotic syndrome—I Pyelonephritis—I Glomerulone-phritis—I Kimmelstiel-Wilson syndrome—I Malignant hypertension—I			Benign hypertension—I Congestive heart failure—I Subacute bacterial endocarditis—I	Toxemia of pregnancy—I Gout—I Brown-spider bite—I Acute febrile state—I Carbon tetrachloride poisoning—I Electric-current injury—I Potassium depletion—I Orthostatic proteinuria—I
Glucose		Lowered renal threshold—I Renal tubular disease—I	Pancreatitis—I Diabetes mellitus—I	Alimentary glycosuria—I	Coronary thrombosis—I	Pheochromo-cytoma—I Hyperthyroidism—I Acromegaly—I Shock—I Pain—I Excitement—I
Ketones	von Gierke's disease (glycogen storage disease)—I		Diabetic acidosis	Vomiting—I Diarrhea—I		Starvation—I Low-carbohydrate diets—I Eclampsia—I Trauma—I Chloroform or ether anesthesia—I Hyperthyroidism—I

Parameter					
Specific gravity	Glomerulonephritis—D Pyelonephritis—D	Hepatic disease—I	Vomiting—I Diarrhea—I	Congestive heart failure—I	Diabetes insipidus—D Fever—I
Nitrite	Urinary tract infection				
Bilirubin	Complete and partial obstructive jaundice—I Viral and drug-induced hepatitis—I Cirrhosis—I	Carcinoma of the head of the pancreas—I	Choledocholithiasis—I	Congestive heart failure in the presence of jaundice—I	Recurrent idiopathic jaundice of pregnancy—I Noxious fumes—I Chlorpromazine hepatitis—I
Blood	*Hematuria in:* Acute nephritis Passive congestion of the kidneys Calculi Malignant papilloma Renal carcinoma Nephrotic syndrome Polycystic kidneys	*Hematuria in:* Cirrhosis (impaired prothrombin function)	*Hemoglobinuria in:* Kimmelstiel-Wilson syndrome	*Hematuria in:* Diverticulosis of the colon	*Hematuria in:* Bacterial endocarditis *Hemoglobinuria in:* Intravascular hemolysis Hypertension with renal involvement
					Hematuria in: Chronic infections Chronic phenacetin ingestion Sulfonamide therapy Sickle-cell disease *Hemoglobinuria in:* Severe burns Hemolytic anemias Transfusion reaction Sudden cold Eclampsia Allergic reactions Multiple myeloma Alkaloids—poisonous mushrooms
Urobilinogen	Obstruction of the bile duct—D Liver cell damage—I Cirrhosis—I	Carcinoma of the head of the pancreas—D	Suppression of the gut flora—D (antibiotic therapy)	Congestive heart failure—I Extravascular hemolysis—I.	Noxious fumes—I Hepatitis associated with infectious mononucleosis—I Thalassemia—I Pernicious anemia—I Hemolytic anemias—I Chlorpromazine hepatitis—D

*These findings are characteristic of the conditions listed, but are not necessarily found consistently in all cases. Definitive diagnosis must rely upon clinical acumen and the results of other indicated procedures. (Courtesy Ames Co, Inc., Division of Miles Laboratories, Inc., Elkhart, IN)

Proteinuria (prō'te-in-u're-ah) is an abnormal increase of protein in the urine. This is an important indicator of renal disease. Also it is seen in congestive heart disease, constrictive pericarditis, multiple myeloma, and toxemia of pregnancy. Functional proteinuria is seen in fever, excessive exercise, emotional stress, exposure to heat or cold, and fad diets.

Glucose

Normal urine does not contain any detectable glucose unless the concentration of blood glucose exceeds 160 to 180 mg/100 ml; at that point, glucose begins to spill into the urine.

Glucosuria (Gloo'kō-su're-ah) or **glycosuria** (gli"kō-su're-ah) is abnormally high sugar content in the urine. The major cause of this is diabetes mellitus. Other common causes of glucosuria include an excessive carbohydrate intake, pain, excitement, liver damage, shock, and sometimes general anesthesia. Ingestion of large amounts of vitamin C may interfere with glucose testing and produce a false positive result.

Ketone

Normally, ketone bodies do not appear in urine unless the patient is on a carbohydrate-deficient diet or a diet that is extremely rich in fat content.

Acetonuria (as"ĕ-tō-nu're-ah) or **ketonuria** (kē"tō-nu're-ah) is the presence of acetone or ketone bodies in the urine. This is an important symptom in diabetes mellitus. Ketonuria is also seen in patients whose carbohydrate intake is decreased, such as with fasting or anorexia, in gastrointestinal disturbances, and following general anesthesia.

Bilirubin

Normally, no bilirubin appears in the urine.

Bilirubinuria (bĭl"ĭ-roo"bĭ-nu're-ah) is the presence of bilirubin in the urine. This occurs in liver disease, bile duct obstruction, and cancer of the head of the pancreas.

Blood

A few red blood cells noted in urine when examined under the microscope are normal. The Multistix 10 SG does not determine the number of red blood cells present, but provides an indication of the presence of occult blood conditions.

Hematuria (hēm"ah'tu-rē-ah) is the presence of blood in the urine. The urine may be slightly blood-tinged, grossly bloody, or a smoky brown color. This is symptomatic of injury, disease, or calculi in the urinary system. Certain drugs, such as anticoagulants or sulfonamides, may also cause hematuria.

Nitrite

Normal urine should yield negative results; a positive result is a reliable indication of significant bacteriuria.

Bacteriuria (bak-te"rē-u're-ah) is the presence of bacteria in the urine. A positive nitrite test is indicative of a urinary tract infection.

Urobilinogen

Normal urine contains a small amount of urobilinogen. Biliary obstruction leads to the absence of urobilinogen in the urine; reduced amounts are seen during antibiotic therapy; and increased amounts of urobilinogen in the urine are present in liver tissue damage and in congestive heart failure.

Leukocytes

Positive results are clinically significant. Positive and repeat trace results indicate that further testing of the patient and/or sample is needed, according to the medically accepted procedures for pyuria.

Specific Gravity

See page 301.

Tests for Glucose, Acetone, and Bilirubin Using Chemical Reagent Tablets

Clinitest*. When the presence of glucose is determined by use of a reagent strip, a more quantitative

*Ames Co.; Elkhart, IN.

Fig. 10-7. Clinitest procedure. **A,** Place 10 drops of water into test tube containing 5 drops of urine. **B,** Add one Clinitest tablet to test tube. **C,** Compare contents in test tube with color chart.

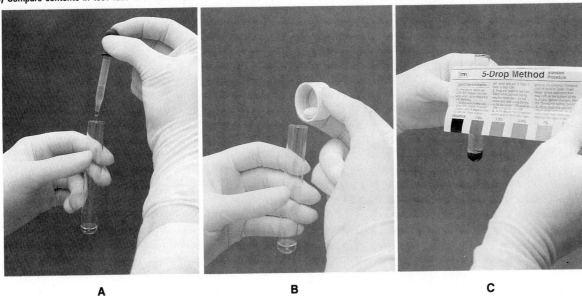

A   B   C

determination may be required. This can be accomplished by using the Clinitest reagent tablet 5-drop method (Fig. 10-7).

1. Place 5 drops of urine into a test tube.
2. Rinse dropper; add 10 drops of water to the test tube.
3. Add one Clinitest tablet to the test tube.
4. Wait 15 seconds while the spontaneous boiling occurs; this is the normal action seen when the tablet is added to the urine and water mixture. Do not touch the bottom of the test tube, as intense heat is generated during this reaction.
5. Once the boiling stops, shake the tube gently and compare the color of the contents with the color chart that accompanies the bottle of tablets. Do not wait longer than 15 seconds to compare the

colors, as results seen after this period are invalid. There are six color blocks ranging from dark blue (indicating a negative reading) through green and tan up to orange, which is read as 2% or 4+, indicating the presence of large amounts of sugar. The results are interpreted and recorded as negative, trace, 1+ 2+, 3+, or 4+, *or* 0%, ¼%, ½%, ¾%, 1%, or 2%.

Observe the solution in the test tube carefully during the reaction and the 15 second waiting period to detect rapid, pass-through color changes due to large amounts of sugar (over 2%). Should the color *rapidly* pass through green, tan, and orange to a dark greenish brown, record as over 2% (4+) sugar without comparing the final color development with the color chart.

6. Record the results.

Test Result	Color change	Interpretation
Negative (0%)	Dark blue	No glucose present
Trace (¼%)	Green	250 mg/dl*
1+ (½%)	Olive green	500 mg/dl
2+ (¾%)	Greenish-brown	750 mg/dl
3+ (1%)	Tan	1000 mg/dl
4+ (2%)	Orange	2000 mg/dl

*1 deciliter (dl) = 100 milliliters (ml)

NOTE: The use of this method is not advisable for patients receiving the drugs nalidixic acid (NegGram), cephalothin (Keflin), cephalexin monohydrate (Keflex), cephaloridine (Loridine), probenecid (Benemid), or large amounts of ascorbic acid, as they may cause a false positive. The preferred method in these situations is testing the urine by the Tes-Tape method. This will be discussed later in this unit.

A modification of the above standard (5-drop) procedure is the Clinitest reagent tablet 2-drop method, also used for quantitative determination of reducing sugars, generally glucose, in urine. Directions for use are identical to the standard procedure *except* use 2 drops of urine and 10 drops of water. For this specific tablet, the results are identified by comparing the contents in the test tube with a color chart having seven color blocks ranging from dark blue through green and tan up to orange. The results are interpreted and recorded as 0, trace, ½%, 1%, 2%, 3%, or 5% or more.

Acetest*. To detect the presence of acetone and acetoacetic acid in urine, you may use the Acetest reagent tablet.

1. Place one tablet on a clean piece of paper, preferably white.
2. Place 1 drop of urine on the tablet.
3. At 30 seconds, compare the test results with the color chart. Colors will range from buff to lavender to purple. The four color blocks indicate negative, small, moderate, or large concentrations being present.
4. Record the results.

NOTE: This tablet may also be used to test serum, plasma, or whole blood. Serum or plasma ketone readings are made 2 minutes after application of the specimen to the tablet. When testing whole blood for ketones, apply the specimen to the tablet, wait 10 minutes, then remove clotted blood and read the results immediately.

Ictotest**. To detect liver function, a simple test on urine to determine the presence of bilirubin may be done with the use of the Ictotest reagent tablet.

1. Place 5 drops of urine on the piece of special mat that is provided with the tablets.
2. Place a tablet in the center of the wet area.
3. Put 2 drops of water onto the tablet.
4. Determine any color change on the mat around the table within 30 seconds, and compare with the color chart. The presence of a blue or purple color indicates a positive reaction.
5. Record the results.

Summary. These three reagent tablets and the reagent strips must be kept in the bottles that they are supplied in with the cap secured tightly. Exposure to the air or moisture for any length of time will cause them to deteriorate, and they would then be unfit to use for testing urine. Do not remove the desiccants from the bottles. Store at temperatures under 30°C (86°F). Do not store in a refrigerator. Do not use after the expiration date indicated on the bottle.

CONTROLS FOR ROUTINE URINALYSIS

The various qualitative (or semiquantitative) tests for urinary pH, protein, blood, glucose, ketones, bilirubin, nitrite, urobilinogen, and specific gravity should be checked from time to time using solutions containing known quantities of these substances. Two convenient quality control systems to help determine if Ames urinalysis tests are properly performed and interpreted are available. These control systems are called Tek-Chek and Chek-Stix. They are particularly valuable in instituting a quality control system, or making an existing system more convenient by the use of ready-made controls. There are four different Tek-Chek packages, each consisting of four vials which provide different controls (results). When purchased, each package comes supplied with a summary of the Tek-Chek system, instructions for use, and the expected values that should be obtained when using the control vials. Table 10-3 shows the table of expected values that should be obtained when using Tek-Chek #1 - No. 1301, a summary of the system, and instructions for use. Table 10-4 provides a summary and explanation of the Chek-Stix urinalysis control strips.

TEST FOR GLUCOSE USING THE TES-TAPE*

The Tes-Tape is a roll of paper that is treated specifically for the analysis of glucose in urine. It comes packaged in a small plastic dispenser, with directions for use and a color chart for comparing the test results printed on the sides.

Instructions for Use:

1. Tear off 1½ inches of Tes-Tape paper (Fig. 10-8,A).
2. Dip one end of tape into the urine specimen, and remove (Fig. 10-8,B).
3. Wait 1 minute, then compare any color change on the tape with the color chart on the dispenser (Fig. 10-8,C). If the tape indicates 3+ or higher, make a final comparison 1 minute later.
4. Record the results.

*Ames Co.; Elkhart, IN.
**Ames Co.; Elkhart, IN.

*Eli Lilly and Co.; Indianapolis, IN.

Table 10-3. Tek-Chek® Controls for routine urinalysis

SUMMARY AND EXPLANATION:

TEK-CHEK® Controls for Routine Urinalysis are lyophilized human urine specimens, designed for use with Ames Reagent Strip and Tablet Tests in routine urinalysis.

TEK-CHEK is reconstituted by the addition of 15 ml of water. Specific chemical additions are made to the pooled urines prior to lyophilization so that, when reconstituted, each of the two TEK-CHEK Control Urines will react to one or more of AMES Reagent Strips or Tablets to yield the results listed in the Table of Values in this insert. The bottles are designated as No. 1 and No. 4. TEK-CHEK No. 4 contains a combination of natural and artificial ingredients to give positive results with Ames products.

Major areas of use of TEK-CHEK Control Urines in a quality control program to upgrade urinalysis are,

Knowns:

1. For demonstration and teaching purposes.
2. To determine if the test reagents are reacting properly.
3. To confirm the user's ability to properly perform and reliably interpret the Ames tests.

Unknowns:

1. To develop proficiency in routine urinalysis performed in the laboratory, from sample handling through test procedures to reporting of results.
2. To provide confidence in obtaining good results in routine urinalysis.

Each laboratory should define its own standards of acceptable performance after a period of routine use of an established quality control program. Quality control has become an integral part of several sections of the clinical laboratory and should be more widely used in routine urinalysis.[1,2] Establishment of quality control programs as a means of helping to assure good results has been recommended by the accreditation groups involved with the Clinical Laboratories Improvement Act of 1967 and by scientific associations involved with clinical laboratory personnel such as the CAP, ASCP, AACC and ASMT.

REAGENTS:

TEK-CHEK Control Urines are of two kinds, each with specific characteristics. After reconstitution of the lyophilized material with 15 ml of water, results may be expected as follows:

TEK-CHEK 1: Normal urine with negative reactions for glucose, protein, ketone, bilirubin, occult blood, and nitrite, with normal urobilinogen, and defined pH and specific gravity.

TEK-CHEK 4: Composite positive with positive reactions for glucose, protein and occult blood; normal urobilinogen; negative ketone, bilirubin, and nitrite; and a defined pH and specific gravity.

WARNINGS AND PRECAUTIONS: TEK-CHEK Control Urines are for *in vitro* diagnostic use. Improper storage may cause TEK-CHEK to become darkened or discolored. Such material may give misleading results and should not be used.

INSTRUCTIONS FOR RECONSTITUTION: Remove cap from vial, add 15 ml of water and swirl gently to reconstitute lyophilized urine. Do not shake solution as shaking will denature protein.

STORAGE: TEK-CHEK 1 should be stored at temperatures under 30°C. TEK-CHEK 4 must be stored under refrigeration (2°-8°C). TEK-CHEK 1 and 4 must be used within the expiration date and are stable for 5 days after reconstitution if stored under refrigeration (2°-8°C). Allow to warm to room temperature before use. Do not mix controls or make any chemical additions. Chemical additions to reconstituted controls may seriously affect results due to chemical interference, dilution or both.

PROCEDURE: Each laboratory should define its own quality control program utilizing control urines in the routine urinalysis schedule. Controls should be used as knowns to check procedure and technique, to check product reactivity and for teaching and demonstration purposes. Unknowns should be hidden in each series of specimens and tested with the regular urine specimens, using the same reagents, personnel and handling procedure. A typical routine urinalysis quality control program has been described[1] as follows:

Quality Control Supervisor: 1.) Reconstitute one bottle of TEK-CHEK Urine Control #1 (negative) and one bottle of TEK-CHEK Urine Control #4 (composite positive). 2.) Place the negative and the composite positive control into the same type of urine specimen container used in the laboratory and place one or both of these controls as "hidden" specimens in each batch of specimens tested on all shifts. Retrieve controls before specimens are centrifuged for microscopic examination and reuse at random in each series making sure to check them each time to make sure no change in reactivity has occurred. 3.) At intervals during the day, or at the end of the day, tabulate the "hidden control" results obtained on a quality control chart which can be maintained a month at a time as charts are for blood chemistries.

(Table 10-3 continues)

Table 10-3 (*continued*)

Analyst: 1.) Test, as knowns, the negative specimen and the composite positive and record the results in the laboratory urinalysis record book as "tests on reference specimens." 2.) Record results on unknowns or "hidden" specimens in the laboratory notebook and/or on the request slip as for any routine urine.

RESULTS: Results using TEK-CHEK Control Urines either as knowns or as hidden unknowns should be recorded in the same terms used for routine testing.

EXPECTED VALUES: Table of Values   For use only with Control No 0001022

Test	Expected Results with TEK-CHEK No. 1301	Ames Reagent Strips and/or Tablets
pH	5	COMBISTIX® HEMA-COMBISTIX®, LABSTIX®, BILI-LABSTIX®, MULTISTIX®, N-MULTISTIX®, N-MULTISTIX®-C, MULTISTIX® SG, N-MULTISTIX® SG
Protein	Negative	ALBUSTIX®, URISTIX®, N-URISTIX®, COMBISTIX, HEMA-COMBISTIX, LABSTIX, BILI-LABSTIX, MULTISTIX, N-MULTISTIX, N-MULTISTIX-C, MULTISTIX SG, N-MULTISTIX SG
	Negative	BUMINTEST®
Blood	Negative	HEMASTIX®, HEMA-COMBISTIX, LABSTIX, BILI-LABSTIX, MULTISTIX, N-MULTISTIX, N-MULTISTIX-C, MULTISTIX SG, N-MULTISTIX SG
Glucose	Negative	DIASTIX®, KETO-DIASTIX®, URISTIX, N-URISTIX, COMBISTIX, HEMA-COMBISTIX, LABSTIX, BILI-LABSTIX, MULTISTIX, N-MULTISTIX, N-MULTISTIX-C, MULTISTIX SG, N-MULTISTIX SG
	Negative	CLINISTIX®
	Negative	CLINITEST®
Ketone	Negative	KETOSTIX®, KETO-DIASTIX, LABSTIX, BILI-LABSTIX, MULTISTIX, N-MULTISTIX, N-MULTISTIX-C, MULTISTIX SG, N-MULTISTIX SG
	Negative	ACETEST®
Bilirubin	Negative	BILI-LABSTIX, MULTISTIX, N-MULTISTIX, N-MULTISTIX-C, MULTISTIX SG, N-MULTISTIX SG
	Negative	ICTOTEST®
Nitrite	Negative	N-URISTIX, MICROSTIX®-NITRITE, N-MULTISTIX, N-MULTISTIX-C, N-MULTISTIX SG
Phenylketones (PKU)	Negative	PHENISTIX®,
Urobilinogen	0.1 to 1.0 EU/dL	UROBILISTIX®, MULTISTIX, N-MULTISTIX, N-MULTISTIX-C, MULTISTIX SG, N-MULTISTIX SG
Specific Gravity*	1.015 to 1.020	MULTISTIX SG, N-MULTISTIX SG
	1.015	(T.S. Meter)

*Because of the manner in which TEK-CHEK 4 Control is processed and the constituents added to the Control, specific gravity values determined using Ames Reagent Strips are approximately 0.007 higher than values determined using the T. S. Meter. Equivalent results are obtained using both methods with TEK-CHEK 1.

BIBLIOGRAPHY:

1. Free, H. M. and Free, A. H.: Quality control of urinalysis in large hospitals and small laboratories. In *Progress in Quality Control in Clinical Chemistry, Transactions of 5th International Symposium,* Aneido, G., VanKampen, E. J. and Rosalki, S. B. Eds., Hans Huber, Bern, 1973, p. 332.
2. Becker, S. T., Ramirez, G., Pribor, H., and Gillen, A. L.: A quality control product for urinalysis. *Amer. J. Clin. Path.,* 59:185, 1973.

(Courtesy Ames Co., Division of Miles Laboratories, Inc., Elkhart, IN)

Fig. 10-8. **A, B,** and **C,** Test for glucose in urine using Tes-Tape. (Courtesy Eli Lilly and Co., Indianapolis, IN)

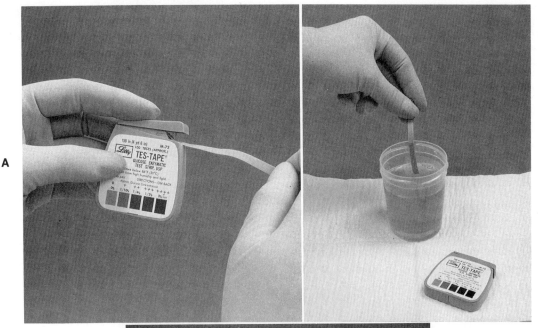

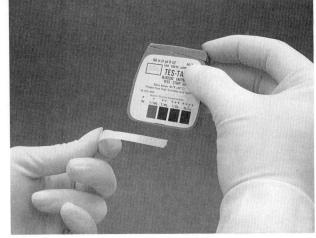

MICROSCOPIC EXAMINATION OF CENTRIFUGED URINE SEDIMENT

The third part of the routine urinalysis is the microscopic examination of the sediment present in the urine. The purpose of this examination is to identify the type and the approximate number of formed elements present, which in turn helps the physician determine the presence of a disease process. The sediment in urine is usually classified as organized or unorganized sediment. *Organized sediment* includes red blood cells, white blood cells, epithelial cells, casts, bacteria, parasites, yeast, fungi, and spermatozoa. *Unorganized sediment* is usually chemical and includes crystals of various components and other amorphous (having no definite shape) material. The urine specimen to be used in the microscopic examination must be freshly voided, preferably a clean-catch voided specimen, and examined without excessive delay so that cellular deterioration is prevented. Microscopic examination of urine is performed after the urine is centrifuged. Centrifugation produces a solid portion called sediment.

Preparation and Microscopic Examination of Specimen

Equipment

Fresh urine specimen
Conical centrifuge tubes
Clinical centrifuge
Droppers
Glass slides
Cover glass
Microscope

Table 10-4. Chek-Stix® urinalysis control strips

Reactive Controls for Specific Gravity, pH, Protein, Glucose, Ketone (Acetoacetic Acid), Bilirubin, Blood, Nitrite and Urobilinogen for Use with Ames Visual Reagent Strips.

SUMMARY AND EXPLANATION: Each CHEK-STIX® Urinalysis Control Strip is a firm plastic strip to which are affixed six separate analyte areas. These each contain one or more natural or synthetic ingredients which, when dissolved out of the analyte areas in a measured quantity of distilled or deionized water, provide positive or defined results with Ames Visual Reagent Strips used in urinalysis.

CHEK-STIX control solution is prepared by reconstituting one strip in 12 mL of distilled or deionized water in a URIN-TEK® or similar tube. This control solution will react with Ames Reagent Strips to yield the results listed in the Table of Values in this insert.

Major areas of use of CHEK-STIX in a urinalysis quality control program are:

When used as a known positive solution:
1. To determine if Ames Reagent Strips are reacting properly.
2. To confirm the user's ability to properly perform and reliably interpret the reagent strip tests.
3. For demonstration and teaching.

When used as a blind or unknown solution:
1. To develop proficiency in routine urinalysis performed in the laboratory from sample handling through test procedures to reporting of results.
2. To provide confidence in obtaining good results in routine urinalysis.

REAGENTS: Each CHEK-STIX Control Strip is to be reconstituted in 12 mL of distilled or deionized water. Results should be as shown in the Table of Values on reverse side. Reactive ingredients are:

    Protein — bovine serum albumin
    Glucose — glucose
    Ketone — methylacetoacetate
    Bilirubin — crystalline bilirubin
    Blood — bovine hemoglobin
    Nitrite — sodium nitrite
    Urobilinogen — p-phenylenediamine dihydrochloride

WARNINGS AND PRECAUTIONS: CHEK-STIX Control Strips are for *in vitro* diagnostic use.

INSTRUCTIONS FOR PREPARATION:
1. Place 12 mL of distilled or deionized water in a URIN-TEK tube or a tube of similar size (approximately 16 × 100 mm). *Do not use tap water.*
2. Remove a CHEK-STIX Control Strip from the bottle and replace the cap promptly and tightly.
3. Place the strip in the tube. Cap tightly.
4. Gently invert the tube back and forth for 2 minutes.
5. Allow the tube to stand for 30 minutes at room temperature.
6. Invert one more time.
7. Remove and discard the strip.

See Unit IX for information on microscopes and centrifuges.

Procedure

1. To obtain the sediment, place 10 to 15 ml of thoroughly mixed urine in a centrifuge tube and centrifuge for 5 minutes at the standard speed of 1500 rpm (revolutions per minute).
2. Pour off the supernatant fluid.
3. Allow the several drops of urine that remain along the side of the tube to flow back down into the sediment, then tap the tube with your finger to mix the contents.
4. Place a drop of this sediment on a slide, and cover with a cover glass. The slide is now ready to be examined.
5. Position the slide on the microscope stage.
6. Adjust the low-power objective of the microscope and examine the slide for casts in at least ten different fields; then examine for other elements that are present in just a few fields. Reduce the light to a minimum by almost completely closing the diaphragm beneath the stage on the microscope, and scan the entire slide to obtain an overall picture of the sediment. It is necessary to vary the intensity of the light source on the microscope so that correct identification of the various components may be obtained.

Table 10-4 (*continued*)

STORAGE AND STABILITY: Store CHEK-STIX Control Strips in original, tightly capped bottle at temperatures under 30°C (86°F). Do not store in refrigerator. Do not remove desiccant from bottle. CHEK-STIX control solution should be stored at temperatures under 30°C and is stable for 8 hours after preparation, except for bilirubin which has limited stability in aqueous solution. Ketone reactivity will increase with time due to continued hydrolysis of the reactive ingredient. Do not make any chemical additions to the CHEK-STIX control solution. They may seriously affect results due to chemical interference and/or dilution.

PROCEDURE: After reconstituting a CHEK-STIX Control Strip with 12 mL of distilled or deionized water, the control solution should be treated and tested in the same manner as a urine specimen. Do not dip more than 12 Ames Reagent Strips into a single tube of control solution, as expected values may change.

RESULTS: CHEK-STIX control solution provides results with Ames Reagent Strips in the same manner as urine specimens. The values to be expected are given in the following table:
EXPECTED RESULTS: Table of Values   For use only with Control No. 9002111

TEST	EXPECTED RESULTS WITH AMES VISUAL REAGENT STRIPS
pH	8.5
Protein	Trace — 30 mg/dL (SI Units: Trace — 0.3 g/l)
Glucose	1/10 g/dL* (SI Units: 0.0056 mmol/l)
Ketone	Moderate — Large
Bilirubin	Positive
Blood	Moderate — Large
Nitrite	Positive
Urobilinogen	Positive Colors may be atypical.
Ascorbic Acid	Negative** Colors will be atypical.
Specific Gravity	1.000 — 1.005 Not adjusted for pH.
Phenylketones	Negative

*Expected glucose result with all Ames Reagent Strips *except* CLINISTIX® Reagent Strips. Expected result with CLINISTIX is "Dark."

**Color will be atypical due to the alkalinity, high concentration of bilirubin, and color of CHEK-STIX control solution.
LIMITATIONS OF PROCEDURE: CHEK-STIX Control Strips are for use only with Ames Visual Reagent Strips. The use of CHEK-STIX with Ames Reagent Tablets is not recommended.
AVAILABILITY: CHEK-STIX is available in bottles of 25 strips (#1360K).

Courtesy Ames Co., Division of Miles Laboratories, Inc., Elkhart, IN)

7. Next adjust the microscope to the high-power objective in order to identify the specific types of cells, such as red blood cells, white blood cells, crystals, and other elements present in the sediment. Further identification of the various types of casts should also be done at this time.

8. Estimate the approximate number of the various structures identified. Casts are counted per low-power field; epithelial cells, white blood cells, and red blood cells are reported in terms of cells per high-power field (hpf), for example, 10 to 15 WBC/hpf. To determine the number of elements present, count the number of each type seen in at least ten fields. The average of this number is then used for the reported value. The other elements (crystals, bacteria, parasites, and spermatozoa) are reported as none, rare, occasional, frequent, many, or numerous.

There is no easy way to learn how to identify these structures (Fig. 10-9). A great deal of practice and training is required to master this skill. Reference charts and books should always be used without hesitation. Usually this examination is performed by laboratory personnel; on occasion the physician may do it in the office or clinic laboratory. It is not commonly a responsibility of the medical assistant to do the actual examination, although there may be instances when you may be required to prepare the slide for the examination.

Fig. 10-9. Atlas of urine sediment. (Courtesy Ames Co., Inc., Elkhart, IN)

Crystals found in acid urine (×400)

Uric acid   Amorphous urates and uric acid crystals   Hippuric acid   Calcium oxalate   Tyrosine needles / Leucine spheroids / Cholesterin plates   Cystine

Crystals found in alkaline urine (×400)

Triple phosphate Ammonium and magnesium   Triple phosphate going in solution   Amorphous phosphate   Calcium phosphate   Calcium carbonate   Ammonium urate

Sulfa crystals

Sulfanilamide   Sulfathiazole   Sulfadiazine   Sulfapyridine

Cells found in urine

RBC and WBC   Renal epithelium   Caudate cells of renal pelvis   Urethral and bladder epithelium   Vaginal epithelium   Yeast and bacteria

Casts and artifacts found in urine (×400)

     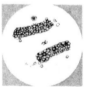

Granular casts fine and coarse   Hyaline cast   Leukocyte cast   Epithelial cast   Waxy cast   Blood cast

   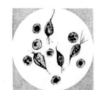

Cylindroids   Mucous thread   Spermatozoa   *Trichomonas vaginalis*   Cloth fibers and bubbles

Significance of Microscopic Test Results

Normal urine sediment contains a limited number of formed elements. The presence of one or two white blood cells and red blood cells and a few epithelial cells per high-power field is usually not considered abnormal. At times an occasional hyaline cast may also be considered as a normal finding. Mucous threads in moderate amounts are normal.

Organized Sediment

1. Cells
   a. Red blood cells (RBC): The presence of more than one or two RBC per high-power field is an abnormal finding. This may be caused by a variety of kidney and systemic diseases, as well as from trauma to the urinary system, violent exercise, or possible contamination from menstrual blood. Hemorrhagic diseases such as hemophilia may also produce hematuria. The presence of red blood cells in the urine must always be reported, as this is a significant finding.
   b. White blood cells (WBC): The presence of large numbers of WBC in the urine usually indicates the presence of a bacterial infection in the urinary tract, and/or pyuria. Pyuria (pī-u′rē-ah) is the excretion of urine containing pus. This indicates renal disease that may be either infection or lesions in the bladder, urethra, ureters, and kidneys.
   c. Epithelial cells: The presence of large numbers of renal epithelial cells and bladder-type epithelial cells is abnormal and should always be reported. The presence of a large number of renal epithelial cells may indicate degeneration of the renal tubules. Proteinuria and casts are frequently seen in this condition.
2. Casts:
   It is essential that casts be correctly identified, as the presence of these structures is a most significant laboratory finding. Inflammatory disorders or damage to the glomerulus, tubules, or general renal tissue are usually associated with the presence of casts and are usually accompanied by albuminuria.

   The various types of casts include red blood cell casts, white blood cell casts, epithelial cell casts, hyaline casts, granular casts, and waxy and fatty casts.
3. Bacteria:
   Normal urine does not contain bacteria unless the specimen was contaminated by improper collection techniques and handling, or by vaginal secretions in the female. The presence of numerous bacteria in the urine may indicate a urinary tract infection. A true infection can be differentiated from contamination if the specimen also contains white blood cells.
4. Yeasts and parasites:
   Yeast may be seen as a contaminant in the urine of females who have vaginal moniliasis, or it may indicate a urinary moniliasis, especially in patients who have diabetes mellitus.

   Parasites seen in the urine are usually contaminants from vaginal or fecal excretions.
5. Spermatozoa:
   Spermatozoa may appear as contaminants in the urine. They frequently are present in urine after sexual intercourse or nocturnal emissions.

Unorganized Sediment

1. Crystals:
   The type and quantity of crystals in the urine vary with the pH of the specimen. Normally, most crystals are of little importance and will form in urine as it cools.

   Crystals seen in normal acid urine are uric acid, amorphous urates, hippuric acid, and calcium oxalate. Crystals seen in normal alkaline urine include triple phosphate, ammonium, magnesium, calcium phosphate, calcium carbonate, and ammonium urate. Abnormal crystals found in acid urine include cholesterin, cystine, leucine, and tyrosine.
2. Artifacts and contaminants:
   These include hair, cloth fibers, mucous threads, and other contaminants. It is important to differentiate these structures from other elements in the sediment that may indicate the presence of a disease process.

DETECTION AND SEMIQUANTITATION OF BACTERIURIA

When obtaining a urine specimen for bacteriological examination, you should collect a clean-catch midstream specimen in a sterile container (refer to Unit VI for this procedure). The first voided specimen of the day should be used whenever possible because bacteria will be more numerous. The examination should be done within 1 hour from the time of collection. When this is not possible, refrigerate the specimen to prevent the growth of microorganisms, and test the specimen within 8 hours. *Never* add a preservative to a urine specimen that is to be used for bacteriological culture tests, as the preservative will destroy the viability of most of the bacteria that may be present.

Culture Plate Methods

This technique requires the special facilities and trained personnel of a microbiology laboratory.

There the identification and precise quantitation of bacterial species will be ascertained. If the specimen is not cultured immediately, refrigeration is mandatory.

Nitrite Test and Culture Strip Methods

A chemical test using a reagent strip, as discussed under the chemical examination of urine, is used for the nitrite test. The culture strip method, a simplified semiquantitative culture test, provides greater precision than is possible with the nitrite test. Frequently used are the Microstix-3 reagent strips. This is a three-way bacteriuria test. The strip contains three pads: (1) a nitrite reagent pad, (2) a dehydrated culture media pad that favors the growth of all types of bacteria commonly seen in urinary tract infections, and (3) a dehydrated culture media pad that supports growth of only gram-negative bacteria. A thermostatically controlled incubator specifically designed for use with the Microstix-3 is available. It is small, about the size of an average textbook, and relatively inexpensive; therefore, it is very practical for use in a urinalysis laboratory in a physician's office or clinic.

Procedure for Using the Microstix-3 Reagent Strip

1. Remove the strip from the wrapper; avoid contact of the test areas with anything.
2. Dip the strip in the urine specimen for 5 seconds and remove.
3. Read the nitrite test area 30 seconds later. Any degree of a pink color indicates the presence of 10^5 or more organisms per ml of urine.
4. Insert the strip in the sterile plastic pouch provided, and seal.
5. Incubate the pouch for 12 to 18 hours.
6. Read the results without removing the strip from the transparent pouch. Compare the color densities on both culture pads with the chart provided. Magenta spots on the pads indicate bacterial locations.
7. Record the results and dispose of the still-sealed pouches by incineration.

OTHER URINE TESTS

Protein Determinations

Bence Jones protein is the name of an abnormal protein in the urine that is frequently seen in patients who have multiple myeloma and a few other abnormalities. This protein is characterized by the fact that during special testing methods (the Bence Jones Protein Test) it precipitates when urine is heated, but

disappears once the urine is cooled. Many feel that this is not a very sensitive test, because it can miss detecting small amounts of the Bence Jones protein or other similar types of abnormal protein. Thus, many laboratories have discontinued using this test and are now doing the urine-protein electrophoresis. This test determines the relative concentration and also the type of abnormal protein present in the urine. It can be performed on a random urine specimen, although it is preferable to collect a 24 hour specimen in most cases.

Hormone Determinations

These urine tests help detect metabolic and endocrine conditions or disorders. One common test performed is the pregnancy test in which urine is tested for the presence of the human chorionic gonadotropin (HCG) hormone. There is a wide range of tests on the market that are used for this purpose. Many are slide tests that provide results within a few minutes. Complete instructions for use are provided with the test equipment when purchased. Although these are highly reliable tests, incorrect results may be obtained at times because of the presence of protein or blood in the urine, or when the urine is too dilute. For most reliable results, the urine should have a specific gravity of at least 1.015. The first morning specimen is preferred for testing.

Multiple-Glass Test

The multiple-glass test is performed on men to evaluate a lower urinary tract infection. See page 195 in Unit VI for the procedure used to collect three specimens for this test.

CONCLUSION

Numerous other tests can be performed on urine to aid the physician when diagnosing and treating a patient's condition. It is not within the scope of this book to discuss all of them in detail. *Most must be performed in a laboratory by qualified personnel.* For a reference, see Table 10-5 for additional urine tests, the average normal values, and the type of specimen that is required for testing.

Having completed the unit on Urinalysis, practice the procedures. When you feel that you know the equipment and steps of the procedures, arrange with your instructor to take the performance tests. You will be expected to demonstrate accurately your ability to prepare for and perform all of the procedures that have been presented.

Table 10-5. Average normal values for urine determinations*

Test	Average normal value	Type of specimen
Addis Count	WBC 1,800,000 RBC 500,000 Casts 0-5,000	12-hour
Albumin		
Qualitative	Negative	Random
Quantitative	10-100 mg/24 hr	24-hour
Aldosterone	2-23 μg/24 hr	24-hour, refrigerated
Amino acid nitrogen	100-290 mg/24 hr	24-hour, refrigerated, collected in thymol
Ammonia	20-70 mEq/24 hr	24-hour
Ammonia nitrogen	0.14-1.47 gm/24 hr	24-hour
Bence Jones Protein	Negative	First morning specimen
Bilirubin	Negative	Random
Blood, occult	Negative	Random
Calcium		
Sulkowitch	Positive 1+	Random
Quantitative	100-250 mg/24 hr on an average diet	24-hour
Catecholamines	100-230 μg/24 hr	24-hour, preserve with 1 ml concentrated H_2SO_4
Chloride	110-250 mEq/24 hr	24-hour
Concentration test	Specific gravity of 1.025 or higher	Withholding fluids for the day before the test
Coproporphyrin	20 μ/100 ml	Random
Random	Adults: 50-200 μg/24 hr	24-hour, preserve with 5 gm Na_2CO_3
24-hour	Children: 0-80 μg/24 hr	
Creatine	Men: 0-40 mg/24 hr Women: 0-100 mg/24 hr Higher in children	24-hour
Creatinine	Men: 1.0-1.9 gm/24 hr Women: 0.8-1.7 gm/24 hr	24-hour
Dilution test	Specific gravity of 1.001 to 1.003	After 1200 ml water load
Estrogens	Men: 4-25 μ/24 hr Women: 4-60 μg/24 hr	24-hour, refrigerate
Glucose		
Qualitative	Negative	Random
Quantitative	130 mg/24 hr	24-hour
Hemoglobin	Negative	Random
17-hydroxycorticosteroids	Men: 5.5-14.5 mg/24 hr Women: 5-13 mg/24hr	24-hour, tranquilizers interfere
17-ketosteroids	Men: 8-15 mg/24 hr Women: 6-11.5 mg/24 hr Children: 5 mg/24 hr	24-hour, tranquilizers interfere
Ketones	Negative	Random
Lead	100 μg/24 hr	24-hour, collect in lead-free bottle
Osmolality		
Normal fluid intake	500-800 mOsm/kg water	Random
Full range	38-1400 mOsm/kg water	Random
pH	4.6-8.0	Random
Phenylpyruvic acid	Negative	Random
Phosphorus	0.9-1.3 gm/24 hr	24-hour
Porphobilinogen	Negative	Random
Potassium	25-100 mEq/24 hr	24-hour
Pregnanediol	Men: 0-1 mg/24 hr Women: 1-8 mg/24 hr Children: Negative	24-hour, refrigerate
Pregnanetriol	Men: 1.0-2.0 mg/24 hr Women: 0.5-2.0 mg/24 hr Children: <0.5 mg/24 hr	24-hour, refrigerate

(Table 10-5 continues)

Table 10-5 (*continued*)

Test	Average normal value	Type of specimen
Protein		
Qualitative	Negative	Random
Quantitative	10-150 mg/24 hr	24-hour
Bence Jones	Negative	First morning specimen
Sodium	110-260 mEq/24 hr	24-hour
Specific gravity		
Random	1.002-1.030	Random
24-hour	1.015-1.025	24-hour
Sugars	Negative	Random
Titratable acidity	200-500 ml of 0.1 NaOH/24 hr	24-hour, preserve with toluene
Urea nitrogen	6-17 gm/24	24-hour
Uric acid	250-750 mg/24 hr	24-hour
Urobilinogen		
Semiquantitative	0.3-1.0 Ehrlich units/2 hr	2-hour afternoon specimen
Quantitative	1.0-4.0 mg/24 hr	24-hour, collect in dark bottle with 5 gm Na_2CO_3, refrigerate
Uroporphyrin	10-30 μg/24 hr	24-hour, collect in dark bottle with 5 gm Na_2CO_3
VMA (Vanilmandelic acid)	1-8 mg/24 hr	24-hour, preserve in 3 ml 25% H_2SO_4; no coffee or fruit for 2 days before test
Volume Adults	600-1500 ml/24 hr	24-hour

*Courtesy Ames Co., Division of Miles Laboratories, Inc., Elkhart, IN, 1986. After Davidson, I. and Henry, J. B.: Todd-Sanford clinical diagnosis by laboratory methods, Philadelphia, 1969, W. B. Saunders Co., and Goodale, R. H. and Widmann, F. K.: Clinical interpretation of laboratory tests, Philadelphia, 1969, F. A. Davis Co.

REVIEW OF VOCABULARY

The following is a sample of recorded patient information using words that have been presented in this unit. Read this and define the italicized terms.

    This patient, a 45-year-old man, was first seen in my office today with the chief complaint of *dysuria* for the past month. The patient stated that this was associated with *polyuria*, gross *hematuria*, weakness, back pain, and a high fever. He has never experienced *oliguria*, and stated that he drinks copious amounts of water daily. One week ago he had an attack of dyspnea and coughing. The urinalysis today revealed marked *proteinuria, glycosuria,* and *ketonuria; specific gravity* of 1.030. *Microscopic examination* revealed *white cells* of 15 to 20/high-power field (hpf) and *red cells* of 10-15/hpf. *Pyuria* was also detected in large amounts. Further study and examination were recommended for this patient. He will be admitted to the hospital at the end of this week.

                          M. Crossett, M.D.

REVIEW QUESTIONS

1. List the four major components of normal urine.
2. Why and when is a routine urinalysis performed?
3. List five physical characteristics of urine and eight chemical examinations that are part of a routine urinalysis.
4. List and classify urine microscopic sediment as either organized or unorganized sediment.
5. Indicate if the following urinalysis results are normal or abnormal findings:
   a. Specific gravity of 1.035
   b. Red
   c. Glucose 4+
   d. Acetone, negative
   e. Numerous bacteria
   f. Foul odor
   g. Cloudy
   h. Quantity, 3500 ml in 24 hours
   i. pH 6.5
   j. Protein, trace amounts
   k. Ketones, large amount
   l. Blood, negative

m. Urobilinogen 0.1 to 1, small amount
n. Nitrite, positive

6. For each of the following, list two conditions or diseases in which each may be detected:
   a. Albuminuria
   b. Glucosuria
   c. Acetonuria
   d. Bilirubinuria
   e. Hematuria
   f. Bacteriuria
   g. Polyuria
   h. Oliguria
   i. Anuria
   j. Dysuria
   k. Excessively acid urine
   l. Excessively alkaline urine
   m. Very low specific gravity
7. Name three items used for measuring the specific gravity of urine.
8. Differentiate between normal and abnormal sediment and contaminants that may be observed during a microscopic examination of urine.
9. You are asked to perform the chemical analysis on a urine specimen and find the bottle of reagent strips on the refrigerator with the cap removed. Is this the proper storage method for these reagent strips? Would you use one of these strips to perform the tests? Explain the reason for your answer.
10. A urine specimen that was collected at 10 AM for a microscopic examination was placed in your laboratory on the shelf. It is now 3 PM. What would you do with this specimen? Explain the reason for your answer.
11. Describe two tests for determining bacteriuria and three tests for determining glucosuria.
12. To determine if a woman is pregnant, urine may be tested to detect the presence of which hormone?

PERFORMANCE TEST

In a skills laboratory, a simulation of a joblike environment, the medical assistant student is to demonstrate skill in performing the following procedures without reference to source materials. For these activities the student will require a fresh urine specimen or a synthetic preparation of the same. Time limits for the performance of each procedure are to be assigned by the instructor. (See also pp. 32 and 35.)

1. Given a fresh urine specimen and the required supplies, perform a routine physical and chemical analysis on the specimen and record the results, then prepare the specimen for a microscopic examination.

2. Given a fresh urine specimen and the required supplies, perform a Clinitest, Acetest, and Ictotest, and record the results.
3. Given a fresh urine specimen and Tes-Tape, test the urine for the presence of glucose, and record the results.
4. Given a fresh clean-catch midstream urine specimen and a Multistix-3 reagent strip, perform a semiquantitative culture test, and record the results.
5. Given a Chek-Stix urinalysis control strip or a Tek-Chek system, determine if the test reagent strips are reacting properly.

The student is expected to perform the above activities with 100% accuracy.

PERFORMANCE CHECKLISTS

Routine Urinalysis

1. Wash your hands.
2. Obtain a urine specimen from the patient, and assemble the required equipment.
3. Observe the specimen for the physical characteristics of appearance, color, and odor. Record your observations.
4. Pour the specimen into a graduated cylinder if the amount is to be recorded, and measure the quantity.
5. Pour well-mixed urine into the 5 inch cylinder provided with the urinometer.
6. Place the urinometer into the urine, and spin it gently.
7. Read the specific gravity value by noting the point where the lower middle part of the meniscus crosses the urinometer scale. Record the reading.
8. Using the Multistix 10 SG, dip the test areas of the strip into the urine specimen, and remove immediately.
9. Tap the strip against the side of the bottle to remove excess urine.
10. Compare the test areas with the appropriate color chart on the Multistix 10 SG bottle at the specified times.
11. Record the results accurately and promptly.
12. Pour 10 to 15 ml of thoroughly mixed urine into a centrifuge tube and centrifuge for 5 minutes at the standard speed of 1500 rpm.
13. Pour off the supernatant fluid.
14. Allow urine drops along the side of the tube to flow back into the sediment, and tap the tube with your finger to mix the contents.
15. Place a drop of the sediment on a glass slide and cover with a coverglass.
16. Place the slide on the microscope stage, and adjust the low-power objective to examine the slide for casts; scan the entire slide for an overall

picture of the sediment after reducing the microscope light to a minimum.*

17. Adjust the microscope to the high-power field and examine the slide for specific cells and crystals.
18. Estimate the approximate number of the various structures identified.
19. Record your findings promptly and accurately.

Clinitest

1. Wash your hands.
2. Assemble required supplies, and obtain a urine specimen from the patient.
3. Place 5 drops of urine into a test tube.
4. Rinse dropper and add 10 drops of water to test tube.
5. Place Clinitest tablet in this test tube.
6. Wait 15 seconds while boiling occurs.
7. Shake tube gently and compare color of the contents with color chart.
8. Read and record the results.
9. For the 2-drop method, use 2 drops of urine and 10 drops of water, and proceed as above.

Acetest

1. Wash your hands.
2. Assemble required supplies and obtain a urine specimen from the patient.
3. Place one tablet on clean, preferably white, paper.
4. Place 1 drop of urine on the tablet.
5. At 30 seconds, compare the test results with the color chart.
6. Read and record the results.

*Frequently the actual examination of the slide will be done by a laboratory technician or the physician. The medical assistant may be required only to prepare the specimen for the examination, which would then include just steps 1 through 16, and 19.

Ictotest

1. Wash your hands.
2. Assemble required supplies, and obtain a urine specimen from the patient.
3. Place 5 drops of urine on special mat provided with tablets.
4. Place one tablet in the center of wet area on mat.
5. Put 2 drops of water onto the tablet.
6. At 30 seconds, determine any color change on mat around the tablet, and compare with color chart.
7. Read and record the results.

Testing for Glucose Using the Tes-Tape

1. Wash your hands.
2. Assemble required supplies, and obtain a urine specimen from the patient.
3. Tear off 1½ inches of Tes-Tape paper.
4. Dip one end of tape into urine and remove.
5. Wait 1 minute, then compare color changes with color chart on dispenser.
6. Record the results.

Multistix-3 Culture Strip Method

1. Wash your hands.
2. Assemble required supplies and obtain a clean-catch midstream urine specimen from the patient.
3. Remove strip from wrapper.
4. Dip strip in urine for 5 seconds, then remove.
5. Read nitrite test area 30 seconds later.
6. Insert strip into the sterile plastic pouch provided and seal.
7. Incubate pouch for 12 to 18 hours.
8. Read results without removing strip from plastic pouch.
9. Record the results.
10. Dispose of the still-sealed plastic pouch by incineration.

Unit XI

Hematology

COGNITIVE OBJECTIVES

On completion of Unit XI, the medical assistant student should be able to apply the following cognitive objectives.*

1. Define and pronounce the listed vocabulary terms, and define the listed laboratory abbreviations.
2. List the components of blood; state where each is formed in the body and the functions of each.
3. Differentiate between granulocytes and agranulocytes.
4. List body sites used for obtaining capillary and venous blood for testing. List body sites to avoid when obtaining blood samples.
5. Explain the difference between a collection tube with an additive and one without an additive, indicating the preferred use for each.
6. List seven factors that should be considered before performing a venipuncture.
7. List the general order of draw when more than one tube of blood is to be obtained during a venipuncture for various different tests.
8. Discuss how a blood specimen should be handled after collection.
9. List at least five blood tests that require the patient to be in a fasting state before having a blood sample drawn.
10. Given the laboratory results on blood tests that are presented in this unit, determine if they represent normal values, and relate the abnormal findings to the most probable or possible causes.
11. List six blood tests that are performed for a complete blood count (CBC) and the normal values for each.
12. List blood tests that would be listed under the following classifications: hematology, chemistry, serology, thyroid function tests.
13. Explain the terms multiphasic tests, test panels, and profiles.
14. Discuss automation in the clinical laboratory and the advantages this provides.
15. Discuss the advantages of the Accu-Chek II and Glucoscan 2000 and 3000 blood glucose meters used in monitoring blood glucose levels.

*It is suggested that you review Unit IX before proceeding with this unit.

TERMINAL PERFORMANCE OBJECTIVES

On completion of Unit XI, the medical assistant student should be able to do the following terminal performance objectives:

1. Demonstrate the correct procedure for obtaining a blood sample from a patient by performing a skin puncture using (1) a lancet and (2) a Penlet.
2. Demonstrate the correct procedure for obtaining a blood sample from a patient by performing a venipuncture using (1) a syringe and needle and (2) using a vacutainer needle and holder, and vacuum tube.
3. Demonstrate the correct procedure for obtaining multiple blood samples using the vacutainer holder and needle, and evacuated blood collection tubes.
4. Demonstrate the correct procedure for using (1) the Unopette system and (2) the Microtainer capillary whole blood collector.
5. Demonstrate the correct procedure for performing (1) a copper sulfate relative density test used for screening anemia and (2) a hematocrit on capillary blood.
6. Demonstrate the correct procedure for determining the presence of glucose in blood by using a (1) Dextrostix, (2) the Accu-chek II and bG Chemstrip, and (3) a Glucoscan Blood Glucose meter and Glucoscan test strip.
7. Demonstrate the correct method for recording information relevant to the above procedures and findings.

The student will be expected to perform the above activities with 100% accuracy.

Vocabulary

agglutination (ah-gloo"tĭn-nā'shun)—A clumping together of cells, as of blood cells or bacteria. An example is when red blood cells (RBC) clump together as a result of an incompatible blood transfusion.

agranulocyte (a-gran'ū-lō-sīt")—A white blood cell (WBC) with a clear or nongranular cytoplasm. There are two types, monocytes and lymphocytes.

anemia (ah-nē′mē-ah)—There is a variety of forms of anemia, but broadly speaking it is a lack of red blood cells in the circulating blood or a reduction of hemoglobin or both. Anemia is thought of as a symptom of a disease or disorder; it is not a disease.

anisocytosis (an-i″-sō-sī-tō′sis)—A state of abnormal variations in the size of red blood cells in the blood.

blood dyscrasia (dis-krā′zē-ah)—An abnormal or diseased condition of the blood.

electrolyte (e-lek′tro-līt)—Substances that separate into their component atoms when dissolved in water. They play an important part in maintaining fluid balance and a normal acid-base balance and in the functions of cells in the body. EXAMPLES: sodium, potassium, calcium, magnesium, chloride, and bicarbonate.

electrophoresis (e-lek″tro-fo-re′sis)—A laboratory method used to diagnose certain diseases by analyzing the plasma protein content.

erythrocytosis (ĕ-rith″rō-sī-tō′sis)—Increased numbers of red blood cells (erythrocytes).

granulocyte (gran′ū-lō-sit″)—A white blood cell having granules in its cytoplasm. These types of WBCs are neutrophils, basophils and eosinophils.

   band-form granulocyte—A granular WBC in a stage of development.

hemoglobin (hē″mō-glō′bin)—A protein in an RBC that carries oxygen and carbon dioxide. The pigment in hemoglobin is what gives the blood its red color. The protein in hemoglobin is globin; the red pigment is heme. For the body to make hemoglobin, it must have iron, which is derived from the food we eat.

hemolysis (hē-mol′ĭ-sis)—The destruction of red blood cells with the release of hemoglobin into the plasma.

hyperbilirubinemia (hī″per-bil″i-roo″bĭ-nē′mē-ah)—Increased or excessive levels of bilirubin in the blood.

hypercalcemia (hī″per-kal-sē′mē-ah)—Increased or excessive levels of calcium in the blood.

hypercholesterolemia (hi′per-kō-les″ter-ol-ē′mē-ah)—Excessive levels of cholesterol in the blood.

hyperchromia (hi′per-kro′me-ah)—An abnormal increase of the hemoglobin levels in red blood cells.

hypercythemia (hy′per-sī-thē′mē-ah)—An excessive number of red blood cells in the circulating blood.

hyperemia (hi′per-ē′mē-ah)—An excessive amount of blood in a part.

hyperglycemia (hī″per-glī-sē′mē-ah)—Excessive amounts of glucose in the blood.

hyperkalemia (hī″per-kah-lē′mē-ah)—An excessive level of potassium in the blood.

hypernatremia (hī′per-na-trē′mē-ah)—An excessive amount of sodium in the blood.

hyperoxemia (hī″per-ok-sē′mē-ah)—A condition in which the blood is excessively acidic.

hyperproteinemia (hī″per-prō″tē-ĭ-nē′mē-ah)—An excessive amount of protein in the blood.

hypo (hī′pō)—A word part meaning an abnormal decrease or deficient amounts. If you replace this word element and definition for the word element "hyper" in all of the preceding terms (except in hyperemia and hyperoxemia), the correct meaning will be defined.

hypoxemia (hī′pok-sē′mē-ah)—A deficient amount of oxygen (O_2) in the blood.

ischemia (is-kē′mē-ah)—A deficient amount of blood in a body part due to an obstruction or a functional constriction of a blood vessel.

isocytosis (ī″sō-sī-tō′sis)—A state in which cells are equal in size, especially equality of size of red blood cells.

leukemia (lū-kē′mē-ah)—A malignant disease of various types that is classified clinically as acute or chronic, depending on the character and duration of the disease; myeloid, lymphoid, or monocytic, depending on the cells involved. This disease affects the tissues of the lymph nodes, spleen, and/or bone marrow. Symptoms include an uncontrolled increase of white blood cells, accompanied by a decrease in red blood cells and platelets. This results in anemia and an increased tendency to infection and hemorrhage. Other classical symptoms include pain in bones and joints, fever, and swelling of the liver, spleen, and lymph nodes. The precise cause is unknown.

leukocytosis (lū″kō-sī-tō′sis)—An increased number of circulating white blood cells.

leukopenia (lū″kō-pē′nē-ah)—A deficient number of circulating white blood cells.

macrocyte (mak′rō-sīt)—The largest type of red blood cell; seen in cases of pernicious anemia (vitamin B_{12} deficiency) and folic acid deficiency.

microcyte (mī′krō-sīt)—An abnormally small red blood cell, found in cases of iron deficient anemia and thalassemia.

mononucleosis (mon″-ō-nū″′klē-ō′sis)—An abnormal increase of the mononuclear white blood cells in the blood.

   infectious mononucleosis—also called glandular fever, is an acute infectious disease, caused by the Epstein-Barr virus.

phagocytosis (fag″ō-sī-tō′sis)—The process by which white blood cells destroy and engulf or ingest harmful microorganisms.

poikilocytosis (poi"kĭ-lō-sī-tō'sis)—The presence of red blood cells in the blood that show abnormal variations in shape.

polycythemia (pol"ē-sī-thē'mē-ah)—An abnormally increased amount of red blood cells or hemoglobin.

reticulocyte (rĕ-tik'ū-lō-sīt)—A nonnucleated immature red blood cell. Generally, of all the red blood cells in the circulating blood, less than 2% are reticulocytes.

septicemia (sep"tĭ-sē'mē-ah)—A condition in which there are toxins or bacteria in the blood.

serum (se'rum)—The clear, straw-colored liquid portion obtained after blood clots; it consists of plasma minus fibrinogen, which is removed in the process of clotting.

thrombocyte (throm'bō-sīt)—A blood platelet.

thrombocythemia (throm"bŏ-sī-thē'mē-ah)—An increased number of platelets in the circulating blood.

thrombocytopenia (throm"bo-si"to-pe'ne-ah)—A decreased number of platelets in the circulating blood.

uremia (ū-rē'mē-ah)—A toxic condition in which there are substances in the blood that should normally be eliminated in the urine.

venipuncture (vēn"ĭ-pungk'tur)—Puncturing a vein to collect a blood specimen or to administer a medication.

vitamin K—A vitamin that is essential for the formation of prothrombin and the normal clotting of blood. A deficiency may result in hemorrhage because of a prolonged prothrombin time.

Hematology, the study of blood, covers vast areas and numerous tests. Today, in the physician's office or health care facility, most of the tests will be performed by a trained laboratory worker, or blood samples will be obtained and then sent to a larger clinical laboratory for testing. At other times, the patient will be sent directly to the laboratory to have the blood sample drawn. Most laboratories use automated equipment when performing many of the tests. These modern advances in laboratory technology have made it possible to obtain quick and accurate results on a relatively small sample of blood.

For the most part, it will not be a duty of the medical assistant to perform blood tests, other than a few simple ones. Depending upon the laws of the state in which you practice, you may be called upon to perform a skin puncture or a venipuncture to obtain blood samples for testing at a clinical laboratory. Even though you may not do these procedures, it is important that you be familiar with the equipment and supplies that are needed, so that you are capable of assisting the physician as required or explaining the procedure to a patient. These procedures, supplies, and some of the routine and basic blood tests will be discussed in this unit.

BLOOD COMPONENTS, FUNCTIONS, AND FORMATION

Blood, a type of connective tissue, is composed of a clear yellow liquid portion, the plasma, in which the cellular or formed elements are suspended. Plasma makes up about 55 percent of the blood by volume. The remaining 45 percent consists of the formed elements, which are red blood cells (RBC), white blood cells (WBC), and platelets. The average adult has approximately 5 to 6 quarts of blood.

Blood has at times been referred to as the "river of life," because it is by way of this special tissue that numerous substances are transported to all the cells in our body for nourishment and function, and waste products are in turn carried to certain body systems for disposal. It is a transportation system in our body, helping also in the maintenance of acid-base, electrolyte, and fluid balance of the internal environment.

Plasma, which is 90 percent water, acts as the carrier for the formed elements and other substances, which include blood proteins, carbohydrates, fats, amino acids (proteins), mineral salts (the electrolytes), hormones, enzymes, gases, antibodies, and waste products, such as urea and uric acid.

The formed elements all have special functions. The red blood cell's or erythrocyte's prime function is to transport oxygen from the lungs to the body cells and carbon dioxide from the cells back to the lungs to be exhaled. Each RBC contains a protein substance, hemoglobin (Hgb, Hg, or Hb), which gives red color to blood, and also transports the oxygen and carbon dioxide to and from the body cells. Anemia is the result of too few RBCs in the circulating blood, or RBCs with reduced amounts of hemoglobin, or both.

The five types of white blood cells or leukocytes are classified into general groups, the granular and agranular. *Granular* WBCs, sometimes called polymorphonuclear leukocytes, include the eosinophils, basophils, and neutrophils. They are characterized by their heavily granulated cytoplasm and segmented nuclei. The *agranular* leukocytes are the monocytes and lymphocytes, both having a solid nucleus and a clear cytoplasm. The prime function of WBCs is to protect the body against infection and disease; some fight invading bacteria by their phagocytic activity (destroying and ingesting harmful microorganisms), and others play an important role in producing immunity to disease. Infection in the body is indicated when there is a marked rise in the WBC count. Also, in leukemia, the WBC count is greatly increased.

Platelets (thrombocytes), the smallest of the formed elements in blood, play a vital role in initiating the clotting process of blood. Thrombocytopenia may be accompanied by bleeding.

All blood cells are produced in hemopoietic (blood-forming) tissue. The agranular WBCs are produced mainly in lymph nodes and other lymphoid tissues. Granular WBCs, RBCs, and platelets are produced in the red bone marrow or myeloid tissue of bones such as the femur, humerus, sternum, vertebrae, and cranial bones.

OBTAINING BLOOD SAMPLES

Types and Sources

For most routine hematological studies, there are two sources of blood for testing. Capillary or peripheral blood is obtained by performing a skin puncture on the palmar surface of the fingertip or on the ear lobe. For infants, the skin puncture is done on the plantar surface of the great toe or heel. You *must* avoid areas that are cyanotic, scarred, traumatized, edematous, and heavily calloused. A minimal amount of blood, just a few drops, is obtained by this method, but it is sufficient to perform some of the routine tests, such as the complete blood count (CBC), some coagulation studies, and some of the chemistry tests.

The second source for obtaining blood is a vein. This is called venous blood, and the procedure by which it is obtained is called a venipuncture. The most common sites for obtaining blood by this method are the basilic and cephalic veins located in the antecubital area of the arm, which is at the inner aspect of the arm opposite the elbow. This is the more common method for obtaining a blood sample, and also is the method that must be used when larger amounts of blood are needed to perform several different tests. When one cannot obtain blood from a vein in the antecubital space because of stenosed or collapsed veins or if the patient has plaster casts on both arms, alternative sites to use are the veins on the top of the hand, in the wrist, or even in the foot. In extreme situations, blood may be obtained from the femoral vein. This site must be used *only* by physicians.

At times special blood studies, such as blood gases, will be ordered. In these circumstances, arterial blood (blood from an artery, usually the brachial or femoral) rather than venous blood is required. A physician or qualified laboratory personnel *must* obtain this blood sample. A situation in which this may be necessary in the physician's office is when an emphysemic patient has an acute episode of shortness of breath. The physician may draw arterial blood for blood gases while the patient is still breathing room air; then if oxygen is administered to the patient, the physician would draw another arterial blood sample for examination. In the latter case, it is important to indicate on the laboratory requisition how many liters of oxygen were administered to the patient so that this can be considered when the test results are interpreted.

COLLECTION TUBES AND PROPER HANDLING OF A VENOUS BLOOD SAMPLE

Because of the multitude of tests that can be performed on a blood sample, there are certain requirements that must be met when collecting and handling the sample. Using excellent technique, you will collect the samples in either a plain tube without additives or in a tube that contains anticoagulant additives. *The type of test to be performed as well as the laboratory's preference will govern this choice.*

Tubes Without Additives

Generally speaking, a tube without an additive added is used when you want a clot to form to obtain serum for testing. Once collected, the blood is left standing in an upright position at room temperature, usually for 30 to 60 minutes, to allow a clot to form. To separate the serum from the clot, the sample is then centrifuged for 10 minutes. After this, serum is removed from the tube and is ready for testing.

A more convenient method used when serum is required for testing is the use of a serum separator tube to collect the blood sample (Fig. 11-1). Once collected, the sample is left standing at room temperature for 30 to 60 minutes and then centrifuged for 10 minutes. After centrifugation, a jelly-like substance will be between the clot and the serum in the tube. The sample can then be sent to the laboratory in this tube. This sample is used most frequently for most blood chemistries (varying with the laboratory's preference), serology tests, and for Rh factor testing.

Tubes with Additives

Tubes containing EDTA anticoagulant additive are recommended for use when doing hematology studies. The white blood cells and platelets are best preserved in this type of tube, and better red cell morphology results will be obtained. The additive has no adverse effects on the blood sample when a sufficient quantity of blood is obtained. Problems will arise if too little blood is drawn into tubes containing anticoagulant additives. Misleading results and therefore incorrect diagnoses will occur; for example, the hematocrit is lowered and poor red blood cell morphology results, because the red blood cell shrinks and produces a false appearance. All tubes with anticoagulant additives must be filled with blood.

Fig. 11-1. **A,** Vacutainer evacuated blood collection system. **B,** serum separation tube (SST) used for various tests performed on serum. **C,** sterile Vacutainer serum tubes of various sizes without additives, used for chemistry tests, serology tests, blood typing, and other tests. (**B** and **C,** courtesy Becton-Dickinson, Division of Becton, Dickinson and Co., Rutherford, NJ)

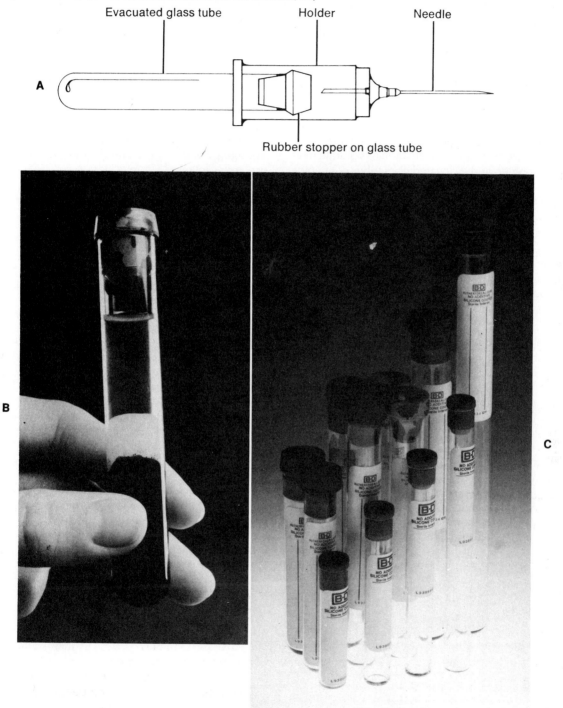

Evacuated glass tube   Holder   Needle

Rubber stopper on glass tube

A tube containing an anticoagulant additive, such as heparin, prevents the blood from clotting. Depending on methods utilized by the laboratory when performing certain tests, this is generally the preferred tube to use when collecting a sample for blood chemistries, and especially for potassium levels. Do not use this tube for hematology studies, as the heparin additive will distort the cells and lead to false results.

There are several other additives used in tubes for collecting venous blood. It is important that the correct tube, plain or with an additive, be used. Most laboratories will supply these tubes with directions indicating which to use for various tests. *They are not interchangeable and must not be confused.*

Vacutainer System

Rather than using the conventional syringe, needle, and test tube when obtaining blood samples, newer, more convenient systems consisting of a disposable needle, a holder, and vacuum tubes are available. One such unit is the Vacutainer system, which consists of a holder-needle combination or separate needle and holder, and evacuated glass tubes containing a premeasured vacuum to provide a controlled amount of blood draw. The tubes have color-coded rubber stoppers that indicate the type of test that they are best suited for, and are supplied plain or with additives, sterile or nonsterile. (The trend today is to use sterile tubes for all collections.) All are available in a variety of sizes, the most common being 3, 5, 7, 10, and 15 ml capacities. Vacutainers are supplied in packages with labels that indicate the additives present in the tubes, the expiration date, and the approximate draw amount (see Fig. 11-1).

The most frequently used vacuum tubes classified according to the tube top color, additive content, average amount of blood drawn, and recommended use are as follows:

Tube Top Color	Additive	Average Amount of Blood Drawn	Common Blood Determinations
Red (most common)	No additive	10 ml	Used for tests done on serum — Blood bank tests, e.g., blood typing (ABO and Rh factor) and cross-matching; serology tests; serum pregnancy test; most blood chemistries; immunology tests; viral studies; AIDS antibody (HTLV-III antibody)
Lavender	EDTA (Ethylenediamine tetraacetic acid, an anticoagulant)	5ml	Used for tests done on whole blood or plasma — hematologic tests including a CBC, WBC, RBC, hematocrit, hemoglobin, platelet count, reticulocyte count, and sedimentation rate
Blue	Sodium citrate (an anticoagulant)	5ml	Used for tests done on whole blood — coagulation studies including prothrombin time (PT), partial thromboplastin time (PTT), and thrombin time (TT)
Green	Sodium heparin	5ml	Used for tests done on whole blood or plasma — blood chemistry tests especially potassium levels; electrolytes; blood gases
Gray	Potassium oxalate and sodium fluoride	5ml	Used for tests done on whole blood or plasma — blood glucose; blood alcohol; the coagulation study activated clotting time (ACT)
Gray and red (mottled top; serum separation tube)	Silicone serum separation material	5ml	Used for tests done on serum — can be used for every test where you want the blood to clot **DO NOT USE FOR BLOOD BANK TESTS**

When you are to draw more than one tube of blood the general order of draw is as follows:

- First draw — blood culture tubes (for example, sterile tubes with no additive, then blood should be transferred to a culture medium within 5 minutes)
- Second draw — tubes with no additives (for example, red tops)
- Third draw — coagulation tubes (for example, blue tops)

- Last draw — tubes with additives (for example, lavender, green, and gray tops)

After the blood has been drawn, the tubes without an additive are *not* to be inverted or shaken, but are to be centrifuged as was discussed previously. Tubes that contain an additive should be gently inverted 8 to 10 times to mix the blood with the additive. *Do not shake these tubes,* as vigorous mixing may cause hemolysis. The amount of blood drawn will vary according to the size of the tube used.

Amount and Handling the Specimen

The amount of venous blood to be drawn is 3 to 30 ml, varying with the test(s) to be performed. Consult your laboratory for the exact amounts that are needed for each specific test that is to be performed. Frequently 1 to 2 ml more blood than is required is drawn to avoid having a patient return for a second collection if the first battery of tests does not turn out.

A blood specimen must be tested on the same day of collection. Depending on the test(s) to be performed, blood should be examined within 8 hours or less from the time it was collected, and preferably within 2 to 4 hours from the time that it was drawn. Blood for bacteriological studies must be collected in special containers and must not sit around. These specimens must be examined as soon as possible. Blood drawn for an electrolyte panel should be refrigerated if it is not tested immediately. Other blood samples may be left standing on the counter for 2 to 4 hours before testing, although some results may vary if the blood is left standing for 2 or more hours. On request, your laboratory will provide schedules that list specific sample requirements for each test they perform. The quality of a test is diminished if a blood sample stands for a long time before being tested; for example, glucose levels will decrease within a couple of hours, and potassium levels will rise if serum is left standing on the cells; the sedimentation rate will be lowered if left standing for over 2 hours, and the bacteria count will increase.

As with all specimens, blood samples must be accurately identified and labeled, and adequate amounts are to be forwarded to the laboratory as soon as possible. The time the sample was drawn should also be indicated on the laboratory requisition. To prevent errors, patient identification on the collection tube must be identical to that on the requisition. Correct patient preparation must be adhered to when required. Some tests (or the physician's preference) require the patient to fast 8 to 14 hours before having blood collected, such as for a fasting blood sugar. Other tests require timed samples; that is, samples may be collected every hour for 3 consecutive hours, as in a glucose tolerance test. Proper recording on the patient's chart is essential. This includes the date, time, sample(s) obtained, test(s) to be performed, and when the sample was sent to the laboratory. (see also *Care, Handling, Transporting, and Storing Specimens*, in Unit VI.)

VENIPUNCTURE TECHNIQUE

Venipuncture is the preferred method for obtaining blood samples and must be used when a larger amount of blood is required for testing. From 3 to more than 30 ml may be drawn by this method. To spare the patient the pain of unsuccessful punctures, consider the following before doing a venipuncture:

1. Ask the patient if he or she has any preference as to which vein you should puncture. Patients often know where their better veins are and which sites should be avoided.
2. Palpate the vein before inserting the needle to determine if the vein is patent.
3. Use a sturdy-walled vein for the puncture. The walls of sturdy veins will feel firm when you touch them, and they will exhibit elasticity and resilience when pressure is carefully applied.
4. Fragile veins are usually narrow veins. If you must puncture these veins, use a 23 gauge needle rather than a 21 gauge needle.
5. Do not use a weak-walled vein. These veins are soft to the touch and lack the elasticity of a sturdy vein.
6. Do not use sclerosed veins. These veins will be resistent to pressure, even if they do look like good veins.
7. Do not use vacuum apparatus to draw blood from a small or constricted vein because this will cause the vein to collapse.

Equipment

70% alcohol and sterile cotton sponges; or disposable alcohol sponges
Sterile cotton sponges
Tourniquet
Sterile disposable needle, usually 1 inch, 1¼ inch, or 1½ inch, 21 gauge
Sterile disposable syringe, either 5, 10, 20, or 30 cc size, depending on the amount of blood to be obtained
Test tube(s) with proper patient identification, with or without an additive, depending on the test that is to be performed; *or a vacuum tube (rather than the syringe and test tube, or vacuum tube, you may use the Vacutainer system with appropriate tube[s], needle and holder; see Fig. 11-1)*
A Band-Aid

Venipuncture Using a Syringe and Needle

Procedure	Rationale
1. Wash your hands.	
2. Assemble required equipment.	

Venipuncture (*continued*)

Procedure	Rationale
3. Identify the patient, and explain the procedure.	Explanations help gain the patient's cooperation.
4. Have the patient sit with the arm well supported in a downward position (Fig. 11-2).	This avoids movement by the patient.
5. Prepare equipment for use: attach the needle to the syringe (or to the Vacutainer holder [Fig. 11-1,A]) leaving the needle shield in place. Label the collection tube with the patient's name, the date, and time (Fig. 11-3).	If you are drawing blood from more than one patient, it is best to label the tubes after you have drawn the blood. Often when tubes are prelabeled, people have a tendency to use the wrong tube if they are in a rush or under pressure.
6. Select the site for venipuncture by palpating the antecubital space.	This site is located on the inner aspect of the arm, opposite the elbow. You must *avoid* the artery. At the antecubital site, the basilic and cephalic veins are used for drawing blood samples.
7. Apply the tourniquet around the patient's arm 3 to 4 inches above the elbow. Palpate the vein again (Figs. 11-4 and 11-5).	You may ask the patient to open and close the hand several times to help produce engorgement of the vein in the arm.
8. Swab the venipuncture site with an alcohol sponge.	**Do not palpate the venipuncture area after cleansing with alcohol.**
9. Remove the needle shield.	
10. Using your nondominant hand, draw the skin over the puncture site until tense. Gently and slowly insert the needle at a 15 degree angle through the skin into the vein (Fig. 11-6).	Countertension immobilizes the vein and exerts tension in the opposite direction to that of the needle. Thus the needle goes in more easily and less painfully. You will retain better control over the needle when the vein is immobilized by the countertension. The bevel of the needle should be facing upwards, because by doing this, the sharpest point of the needle is inserted first.

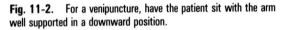

Fig. 11-2. For a venipuncture, have the patient sit with the arm well supported in a downward position.

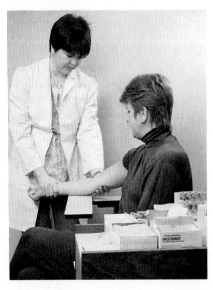

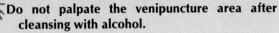

Fig. 11-3. Label the collection tube with the patient's name, the date, and the time.

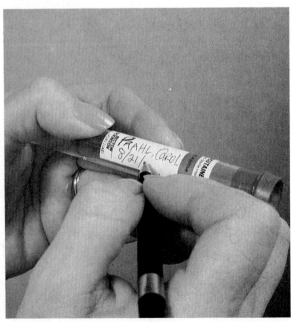

Procedure	**Rationale**
11. Having entered the vein using your dominant hand, now use your nondominant hand to slowly pull on the plunger of the syringe to withdraw blood. As soon as blood starts to flow into the syringe, release the tourniquet (Fig. 11-7 and see Fig. 11-9).	Make sure that you do not move the needle and syringe after entering the vein. If you withdraw the blood too rapidly, you may cause the vein to collapse, and thus will be unable to obtain the required sample. Keep in mind that a nontraumatic venipuncture produces the most reliable results, because any tissue injury can falsely elevate some results, such as enzyme levels.
12. When you have obtained the required amount of blood, place a dry sterile sponge over the puncture site, and withdraw the needle, using a straight downward motion.	✱ **The tourniquet must be off before the needle is withdrawn.**
13. Apply pressure with a sterile sponge over the puncture site for a few minutes; you may have the patient elevate the arm at this time.	You may ask the patient to hold the sponge over the puncture site and apply the pressure. Elevation prevents oozing of blood at the puncture site.
14. Remove the needle from the syringe and inject blood into the test tube(s) (Fig. 11-8). NOTE: When injecting blood into a vacuum tube from a syringe and needle system, leave the needle on the syringe, and *gently* insert the needle through the rubber stopper on the tube. The vacuum inside will draw the required amount of blood into the tube.	When using different tubes for multiple samples, first inject blood into the tubes that do not contain any additives, then inject blood into the coagulation tubes, then into tubes containing an additive.
15. Cap the tubes. Those that contain an additive should be *gently* inverted 8 to 10 times to mix the blood with the additive. *Do not shake these tubes.* Do not mix blood in the plain tubes (that is, tubes without an additive).	Vigorous mixing may cause hemolysis.
16. Apply a Band-Aid to the puncture site if desired.	
17. Destroy and discard disposable syringe and needle in containers designated for disposal. (If you have used a nondisposable glass syringe rather than a disposable one, rinse it with cold water, separate the barrel and plunger, and soak in soap and water.)	

[handwritten annotations: "pressure" repeated multiple times; "(– destruction – breakdown hemolysis.)"]

Fig. 11-4. A, apply the tourniquet around the patient's arm 3 to 4 inches above the elbow. Cross the ends of the tourniquet and pull the ends away from each other to create tension. **B,** secure the tourniquet by tucking the upper end into the band to form a half-bow. The tourniquet must be tight enough to obstruct venous blood flow.

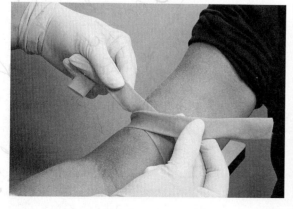

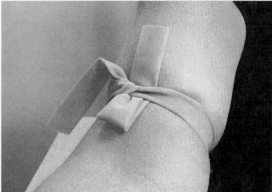

Venipuncture (*continued*)

Procedure	Rationale
18. Wash your hands.	
19. Complete the laboratory requisition, and send it to the laboratory with the blood sample(s) obtained.	

20. Record on patient's chart.	Charting example:
	May 18, 19_____, 1 PM
	  Venipuncture done on left arm.
	  Two samples sent to lab for
	  a CBC and blood chemistries.
	    Charles Rubin, CMA

Fig. 11-5. Palpate the vein once again after the tourniquet has been positioned.

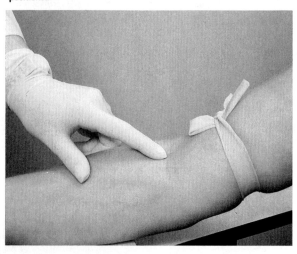

Fig. 11-6. Gently and slowly, insert the needle at a 15 degree angle through the skin into the vein.

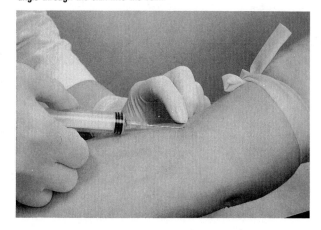

Fig. 11-7. After entering the vein, use your nondominant hand to slowly pull on the plunger of the syringe to withdraw blood. Release the tourniquet as soon as blood starts to flow into the syringe.

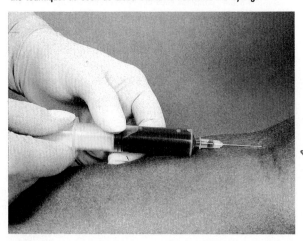

Fig. 11-8. After obtaining the required amount of blood and removing the needle from the vein, inject the blood into the tube. When using a vacuum tube, leave the needle on the syringe, and gently insert the needle through the rubber stopper on the tube.

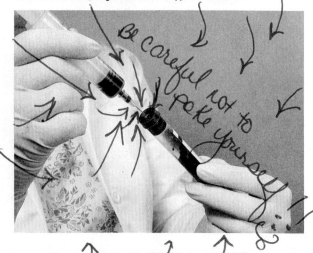

Fig. 11-9. Correct position of patient's arm and tube assembly to prevent possibility of backflow. Tourniquet is released as soon as blood begins to flow. (Courtesy Becton-Dickinson, Division of Becton, Dickinson and Co., Rutherford, NJ)

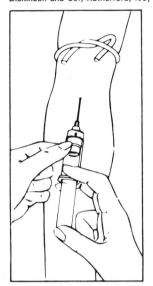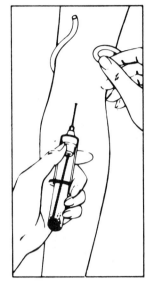

Venipuncture Using the Vacutainer Evacuated Blood Collection Tube(s) For Drawing Single and Multiple Blood Samples (Figs. 11-1, A, and 11-9)

1. Complete steps 1 through 5 as described in Venipuncture Technique Using A Syringe and Needle.
2. Select the correct tube for the type of sample required, and label it. Gently tap tubes that contain additives to dislodge any additive that may be trapped around the stopper.
3. Insert the tube into the holder up to the guideline; push the tube stopper onto the needle inside the holder.
4. Perform the venipuncture in the usual manner (steps 6 through 10 in venipuncture technique using a syringe and needle).
5. Place two fingers at the end of the holder; with your thumb, push the tube onto the needle to the end of the holder (Fig. 11-9).
6. Release the tourniquet as soon as blood begins to fill the tube (Fig. 11-9). Do not allow contents of tube to contact the stopper or the end of the needle during the procedure. NOTE: If blood doesn't flow into the tube or if the blood flow ceases before an adequate amount is collected, take the following steps:
   a. Check to see that the needle cannula is in the correct position in the vein.
   b. If a multiple sample needle is being used, remove the tube and place a new tube into the holder.
   c. Remove the needle and tube and discard. Start the procedure over again.

Single Sample Collection

7. Remove the needle from the vein when the vacuum is exhausted and blood stops flowing into the tube (Fig. 11-10).
8. Apply pressure with a sterile sponge to the puncture site, and have the patient elevate his or her arm for a few minutes to prevent oozing of blood (Fig. 11-10).
9. Remove the tube of blood from the holder.
10. For tubes that contain additives, *gently* invert eight to ten times to mix blood thoroughly with the additive. *Do not shake.*
11. Apply a Band-Aid to the puncture site if required.
12. Discard the needle in a designated container; complete the laboratory requisition and forward with the blood sample to the laboratory.
13. Wash your hands.
14. Record on the patient's chart.

Multiple Sample Collection

7. Remove the tube from the holder when the vacuum is exhausted and the blood stops flowing. Keep the needle holder steady.
8. Place the second and succeeding tubes into the holder, puncturing the diaphragm of the stopper to initiate the blood flow. Keep the needle holder steady. Tubes without additives are drawn first, then coagulation tubes, and then tubes with additives.
9. While blood is flowing into succeeding tubes, gently invert previously filled tubes that contain additives 8 to 10 times to mix the additive with the blood. *Do not shake.* Vigorous mixing may cause hemolysis.
10. Remove the needle from the vein when blood stops flowing into the last tube (Fig. 11-10).

Fig. 11-10. Remove needle from vein when vacuum is exhausted and blood stops flowing into tube. Apply pressure with a sterile sponge to the puncture site.

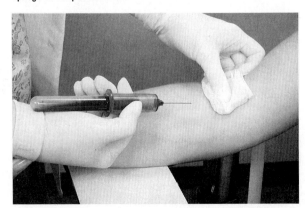

11. Apply pressure with a sterile sponge to the puncture site (Fig. 11-10), and have the patient elevate the arm for a few minutes to prevent oozing of blood.
12. Remove the tube of blood from the holder. _Gently_ invert the tube 8 to 10 times if it contains an additive. _Do not shake._

13. Apply a Band-Aid to the puncture site if required.
14. Discard the needle in a designated container; complete the laboratory requisition and forward it with the blood sample to the laboratory.
15. Wash your hands.
16. Record on the patient's chart.

FINGERTIP SKIN PUNCTURE TECHNIQUE USING A LANCET

Equipment

A sterile disposable lancet
70% alcohol and cotton sponges; or disposable alcohol sponges
Clean blood pipette _or_ capillary tube _or_ Unopette _or_ Microtainer (this piece of equipment will vary with your agency's preference, with the test(s) to be performed on the blood sample, and with the methods used by the laboratory)

_or_

A reagent strip if you are doing a simple test for blood glucose (see p. 344).

Procedure	Rationale
1. Wash your hands.	
2. Assemble equipment and supplies.	
3. Identify the patient and explain the procedure.	Explanations help gain the patient's cooperation.
4. Have the patient seated with the arm well supported.	This avoids movement by the patient.
5. Select the lateral part of the tip of a finger or the earlobe for the puncture site; use the heel or great toe for an infant.	Avoid the thumb and index finger as they are usually more calloused than the other fingers. Using the lateral part of a fingertip rather than the palm side will lessen discomfort for the patient.
6. "Milk" or gently rub the finger along the sides.	This promotes circulation. If the patient's fingers are cold, you may rub them or apply a warm pack to promote circulation. You may also instruct the patient to dangle his or her hand toward the floor to help force blood into the finger.
7. Clean the puncture site with an alcohol sponge; allow the area to dry.	Do not blot or blow on the puncture site. Allow it to air-dry.
8. Grasp the patient's finger on the sides near the puncture site with your nondominant thumb and forefinger.	
9. Hold the lancet with your dominant fingers and make a quick in-and-out puncture on the patient's fingertip. Hold the lancet at a right angle to the lines on the patient's finger (Fig. 11-11).	Lancets are usually designed so that you can make a puncture to a depth of 3 to 4 mm., which is sufficient to obtain drops of blood.
10. Wipe away the first drop of blood with a clean cotton sponge.	The first drop of blood is not a desirable sample, as it will contain tissue fluid.
11. Apply gentle pressure above the puncture site to cause the blood to flow freely.	Do not squeeze the finger, as this liberates tissue fluid, which in turn dilutes the blood and causes inaccurate results.
12. Obtain the blood sample as required by the test to be performed. You may: • Use the pipette to take up the blood sample. Take up the blood sample to the desired level in the pipette. _or_	

Procedure	Rationale

- Lightly touch the blood drop to the test pad on the reagent strip, and continue the test according to the individual test directions.

13. When more than one sample is needed, wipe the finger with a clean cotton sponge and obtain fresh drops of blood in each pipette.

You may have to apply gentle pressure to the finger to obtain more blood.

14. When using bulb pipettes and Unopettes, make dilutions according to instructions for the specific test to be performed.

Blood collected in Microtainers and capillary tubes is not to be diluted, but is sent directly to the laboratory for testing.

15. Apply pressure to the puncture site with a dry cotton sponge.
16. Label the blood samples and laboratory requisition correctly, and forward to the laboratory for testing.
17. Wash your hands.
18. Record on the patient's chart.

Charting example:

April 21, 19_____, 11 AM

Finger puncture done on second finger, left hand. Blood sample sent to laboratory for a CBC (complete blood count).

Ann Patterson, CMA

Fig. 11-11. Fingertip skin puncture technique using a lancet.

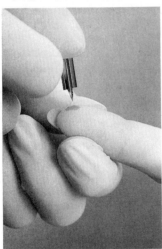

FINGERTIP SKIN PUNCTURE USING THE PENLET* BLOOD SAMPLING PEN (Fig. 11-12)

Equipment

Penlet with disposable caps (Fig. 11-12, *A*)
Sterile lancet
70% alcohol and cotton sponges *or* disposable alcohol sponges

*Lifescan Inc., Mountain View, CA.

Procedure

1. Wash your hands.
2. Assemble equipment and supplies.
3. Identify the patient and explain the procedure.
4. Have the patient seated with the arm well supported.
5. Load the Penlet with a sterile lancet.
   Remove the clear plastic cap and press the lancet straight into the lancet holder until it comes to a firm stop. This will leave the device cocked. *Do not twist* the lancet into position (Figs. 11-12, *B* and 11-12, *C*).
6. Select the lateral part of the tip of a finger for the puncture site.
7. "Milk" or gently rub the finger along the sides.
8. Clean the puncture site with an alcohol sponge; allow the area to dry.
9. Hold the end of the Penlet firmly with one hand and with the other hand twist off the lancet protective disk (Fig. 11-12, *D*).
10. Replace the Penlet cap.
11. Grasp the patient's finger on the sides near the puncture site with your nondominant thumb and forefinger.
12. Position the opening of the Penlet's transparent cap over the skin area that will be punctured (Fig. 11-12, *E*).
13. Press the trigger button. The depth of penetration of the lancet will depend on the amount of pressure with which the Penlet is held against the

Fig. 11-12. **A,** Penlet automatic blood sampling pen to use for obtaining a skin puncture blood sample. **B, C, D,** and **E,** technique for using the Penlet puncture device. (Courtesy Lifescan Inc., Mountain View, CA)

A

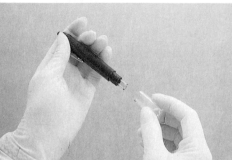

B

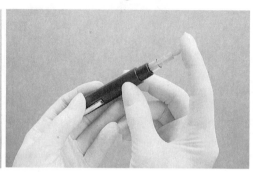

C

D

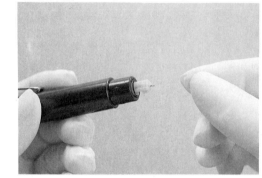

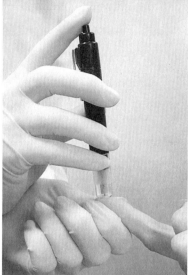

E

skin. The greater the pressure, the deeper the puncture will be (Fig. 11-12, *E*).

14. Complete this procedure by following steps 10 through 18 in the fingertip skin puncture technique using a lancet.

15. To remove the lancet from the Penlet, take the cap off and insert the inside rim of the cap into the notched side of the lancet and pull the lancet out. Dispose of in a container for used sharp instruments.

16. Put a clean cap on the Penlet and replace in the proper storage area.

UNOPETTE SYSTEM

The Unopette system consists of a disposable self-filling diluting pipette and a plastic reservoir prefilled with a precise amount of diluent. These systems serve as a collection and dilution unit for microblood samples. There are various types of Unopette systems available that contain the appropriate diluting substances required for hematology and chemistry tests (Fig. 11-13).

Fig. 11-14 shows the **MICROTAINER CAPILLARY WHOLE BLOOD COLLECTOR.**

BLOOD TESTS

The results obtained from laboratory examinations performed on blood samples, combined with other clinical information, help the physician in various aspects of patient care, such as screening for or diagnosing a condition, evaluating body functions, therapeutic decision-making, and monitoring therapy provided.

There are numerous blood tests that can be performed to aid the physician when diagnosing, treating, or evaluating a patient's condition. Some of these tests are performed on whole blood, whereas others are performed on blood serum. A few simple procedures that may be performed in the physician's office or health agency, and a table of many common tests done frequently in laboratories by certified personnel with the aid of automated equipment follow on pp. 341–354 and 359–363. The actual performance of these tests is usually not a responsibility of the medical assistant, because in general *most state laws require that individuals performing laboratory procedures must be certified laboratory technicians or technologists, or physicians, certified or licensed in the state of their practice.* Nonetheless, it is important for

Fig. 11-13. Techniques for using the Unopette system for laboratory procedures. (Courtesy Becton-Dickinson, Division of Becton, Dickinson and Co., Rutherford, NJ)

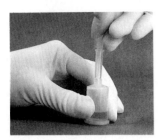

1. Puncture diaphragm

Using the protective shield on the capillary pipette, puncture the diaphragm of the reservoir as follows:
a. Place reservoir on a flat surface. Grasping reservoir in one hand, take pipette assembly in other hand. Push tip of pipette shield firmly through diaphragm in neck of reservoir, then remove.

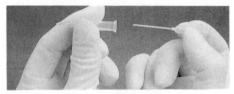

b. Remove shield from pipette assembly with a twist.

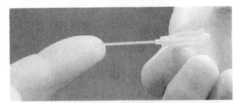

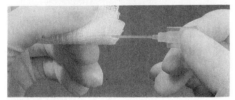

2. Add sample

Fill capillary with sample and transfer to reservoir as follows:
a. Holding pipette *almost* horizontally, touch tip of pipette to sample. (See alternate methods in illustrations above.) Pipette will fill by capillary action. Filling is complete and will stop automatically when sample reaches end of capillary bore in neck of pipette.

b. Wipe excess sample from outside of capillary pipette, making certain that no sample is removed from capillary bore.

c. Squeeze reservoir slightly to force out some air. Do not expel any liquid. Maintain pressure on reservoir.

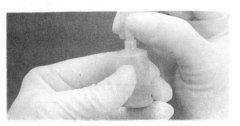

d. Cover opening of overflow chamber with index finger and seat pipette *securely* in reservoir neck.

e. Release pressure on reservoir. Then remove finger from pipette opening. Negative pressure will draw blood into diluent.

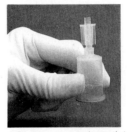

f. Squeeze reservoir *gently* two or three times to rinse capillary bore, forcing diluent into, *but not out of,* overflow chamber, releasing pressure each time to return mixture to reservoir.

CAUTION: If reservoir is squeezed too hard, some of the specimen may be expelled through the top of the overflow chamber.

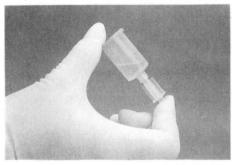

g. Place index finger over upper opening and gently invert several times to thoroughly mix sample with diluent.

(*Fig. 11-13 continues*)

Fig. 11-13 *(continued)*

3. Count cells (option 1)
Mix diluted blood thoroughly by inverting reservoir (see 2g) to resuspend cells immediately prior to actual count.

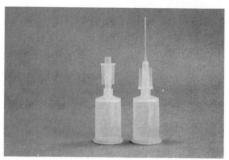

a. Convert to dropper assembly by withdrawing pipette from reservoir and reseating securely in reverse position.

b. Invert reservoir, gently squeeze sides and discard first three or four drops.

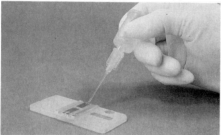

c. Carefully charge hemacytometer with diluted blood by gently squeezing sides of reservoir to expel contents until chamber is properly filled.

OR

3. Transfer contents (option 2)
Transfer thoroughly mixed contents of each reservoir to appropriately labeled test tubes or corresponding cuvettes as follows:

a. Convert reservoir to dropper assembly by withdrawing pipette and reseating securely in reverse position as shown above.

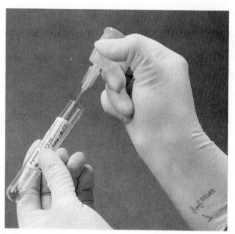

b. Place capillary tip into appropriately labeled test tube or cuvette which will accommodate 5.0 ml of reagent and squeeze reservoir to expel entire contents.

OR

3. Store diluted specimen (option 3)

Cover overflow chamber with capillary shield or remove capillary and insert tip of shield firmly into reservoir opening. (Note time for which diluted specimen remains stable for each test.)

Fig. 11-14. Microtainer Brand capillary whole blood collector. (Courtesy Becton-Dickinson, Division of Becton, Dickinson and Co., Rutherford, NJ)

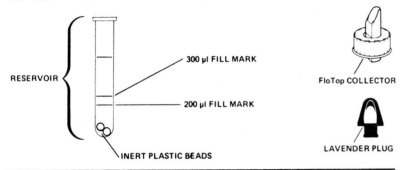

B·D MICROTAINER Brand
Capillary Whole Blood Collector

0.39 mg. DISODIUM EDETATE per reservoir

FOR LABORATORY USE ONLY · NON—STERILE · STORE BELOW 25ºC

THE FOLLOWING COMPONENTS ARE USED WITH THIS PROCEDURE:

RESERVOIR

300 µl FILL MARK

200 µl FILL MARK

INERT PLASTIC BEADS

FloTop COLLECTOR

LAVENDER PLUG

The MICROTAINER System for capillary whole blood samples provides a method for collecting, anticoagulating, storing and identifying the capillary blood sample. . . all in one unbreakable plastic tube.

ANTICOAGULANT

Each MICROTAINER Tube contains sufficient EDTA Na_2 (disodium edetate) to anticoagulate 300 microliters of capillary blood.

MIXING BEADS

Each MICROTAINER Tube contains two (2) inert plastic beads which aid in the dispersion of blood and anticoagulant for proper mixing of sample.

MICROTAINER Tubes for whole blood collections are to be used to collect and store capillary blood samples for outline hematological use. This system is composed of a one piece FloTop collector; a plastic tube containing an anticoagulant, EDTA Na_2 (disodium edetate), two (2) inert plastic mixing beads, and a lavender plug.

USERS SHOULD BE THOROUGHLY FAMILIAR WITH THE CONTENTS OF THIS PACKAGE INSERT PRIOR TO USE.

The FloTop collector directs the free flowing blood directly into the unbreakable plastic MICROTAINER tube. The tubes are marked at the 200 and 300 microliter (µl) levels which indicate the desired filling range.

When the appropriate sample has been collected, the FloTop collector is removed from the tube and is replaced with the lavender plug and gently inverted, 8 to 10 times, to insure adequate anticoagulation of the specimen. The stoppered tube is now provided with protection against contamination, evaporation and spillage.

The anticoagulated whole blood samples can be directly pipetted from the MICROTAINER Tube and assayed for routine hematological parameters.

NON-INTERFERENCE WITH HEMATOLOGICAL DETERMINATIONS

Parallel comparisons of samples collected with the MICROTAINER Brand Capillary Whole Blood Collector and routine microcollection techniques have shown no significant differences for the following determination.[1]

WBC	MCH
RBC	MCHC
HGB	MCV
HCT	Platelets
Reticulocytes	
White Cell Differentials	

(Fig. 11-14 continues)

the medical assistant to be familiar with the type of tests available and the normal values for each, and to have an understanding of the significance of normal and abnormal results. When aware of this information, the medical assistant has greater understanding and appreciation for the diagnosis, treatment, and evaluation of patients under the physician's care, in addition to being of greater value to the patient, physician and laboratory.

At times, basic screening tests will be performed in the physician's office, and then the more detailed tests and precise results will be obtained from larger laboratories using automated equipment.

All tests have predetermined normal values or ranges that establish the limits within which the results indicate the absence of any pathological condition. Normal ranges are established on the basis of the procedures and equipment used by the laboratory. It is important to keep this in mind when reviewing laboratory reports received on specimens ob-

tained from the patients under your physician's care. Often you may obtain a list of normal blood values from the laboratory that performs the procedures.

Generally speaking, hematology tests are done on whole blood, and serological tests and blood chemistries are done on serum or sometimes on plasma. Blood banking and transfusion services use cells as well as serum for testing.

A conscientious medical assistant should be alert for new techniques that may be valuable to the physician in the office. Manufacturers provide brochures and catalogues with information on the latest developments. Medically oriented magazines are another good source for obtaining this information.

Patient Preparation for Blood Tests

There are very few blood tests that require any special preparation of the patient. Generally, special preparation means that the patient should fast, that is,

Fig. 11-14 *(continued)*

DIRECTIONS FOR CAPILLARY BLOOD COLLECTION
Please read complete directions for use before performing procedure

PREPARATION FOR SPECIMEN COLLECTION

The following materials needed for micro sample collection should be assembled beforehand and placed where they will be readily accessible.

1. Properly identified MICROTAINER Tubes

NOTE: If plastic bead(s) adheres to bottom of tube, gently tap to dislodge prior to initiating collecting procedure.

2. Lavender plugs

3. Antiseptic Swab

4. Dry Sterile Swab (gauze pad)

5. Sterile MICROLANCE Lancet

Pre-assemble MICROTAINER Tube by removing lavender plug and replacing with FloTop collector.
DO NOT DISCARD PLUG.

1. Select puncture size, cleanse with appropriate antiesptic.

2. Wipe away excess antiseptic with sterile swab (gauze pad) until site is dry.

3. Puncture skin with sterile lancet.

4. Wipe away first drop of blood.

5. Hold MICROTAINER Tube with FloTop Collector at an angle below horizontal with vent hole in upward position.

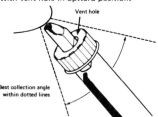

Vent hole

Best collection angle within dotted lines

6. Touch tip of the FloTop collector to under side of drop as shown. Blood will flow freely through the FloTop collector and down the tube wall. Do not scrape up blood sample.

7. Upon termination of collecting procedure, treat wound in a normal manner.

8. Twist off FloTop collector from tube and discard.

9. Seat lavender plug securely in tube opening and gently invert tube eight (8) to ten (10) times to insure proper mixing of sample. Send specimen to laboratory.

10. Carton platform may be used for storage of tubes.

STABILITY

This product is stable if used prior to the expiration date under the conditions stated on the carton and case.

COMPONENTS OF SYSTEM

1. MICROTAINER Tube containing anticoagulant (disodium edetate) and two (2) inert plastic mixing beads.

2. One piece plastic FloTop collector.

3. Lavender plug.

NON-STERILITY OF COMPONENTS

The MICROTAINER Capillary Whole Blood Collector is non-sterile. Each package is clearly labeled with that information.

LIMITATIONS OF SYSTEM

1. To insure stability of capillary blood specimens for platelet determinations, mixing of samples should be done MANUALLY, both at time of collection and at time of dilution, prior to cell counting. Mechanical mixing devices (rocking or rotating types) must not be used.

Testing has demonstrated that prolonged mixing of specimens by mechanical rocking or rotating devices may result in decreased platelet counts.

2. For hematological determinations other than those listed above, for which specimens are collected using the MICROTAINER Capillary Whole Blood Collector, the user must establish to his satisfaction that the values obtained meet his criteria for clinically acceptable values.

3. Testing has shown that capillary specimens can be stored in the MICROTAINER Tube for up to 4 hours, prior to dilution, for the following parameters:[1]

    WBC,RBC,HGB,HCT,MCH,MCHC,MCV

4. Specimens for platelet counts should be mixed MANUALLY by inversion four (4) to six (6) times just prior to dilution for platelet counts. Specimens should be diluted within two hours of collection.

5. Capillary blood specimens for differential counts should be removed from the MICROTAINER tube within 1 hour.[1]

6. Capillary blood specimens for reticulocyte counts should be removed from the MICROTAINER Tube within 1 hour.[1]

REFERENCES:

1. Data on file, Becton, Dickinson and Company, Rutherford, New Jersey.

---

abstain from all solid foods and liquids for up to 14 hours before the blood sample is drawn. This is required because food substances may alter the reliability of the test results. Water may be taken before some tests. The laboratory will provide you with specific directions. Usually you are to instruct the patient to take nothing by mouth (NPO) after midnight the night before the test is to be done.

The principal tests that require the patient to fast beforehand include fasting blood sugar; glucose tolerance test; any type of lipid analysis, such as cholesterol and triglycerides; and the sequential multiple analysis (SMA-12, SMA-18, SMAC-20, and SMAC-24), a series of 12, 18, 20, and 24 blood chemistries. Some laboratories also request that the patient be fasting before all enzyme and electrolyte tests. At other times fasting tests will be done according to the individual orders of the physician. Care must be taken to provide the patient with correct and adequate instructions in these situations.

Copper Sulfate Relative Density Test for Screening Anemia and a Hematocrit

Gross screening tests to determine if a patient has a sufficient volume of red blood cells (RBCs) can be done by performing a relative density test with a few drops of blood in a copper sulfate solution. This test can indicate if a patient may have a reduced capacity to produce RBCs, a problem with any blood loss, or an insufficient diet for the adequate production and functioning of red blood cells. This test is based on the fact that red blood cells are the heaviest portion of blood. The copper sulfate solution is prepared so that the density of this solution is equal to that of blood with 37% RBCs for women and 40% RBCs for men. These two figures are the normal lower limits for the percentage of red blood cells in women and men, thus allowing you to divide all patients screened by this method into two groups—those above and those below the lower limit. When the results of this test indicate a volume of RBCs in the blood below the normal range, it should be followed by a more precise test, that is, a hematocrit. The hematocrit (Hct) represents the volume percentage of red blood cells present in whole blood. The normal ranges for a hematocrit are women, 37% to 40%; men, 40% to 54%. Both of these tests are an important aid to the physician when diagnosing and treating patients with anemia. They are relatively simple and can easily be performed in the physician's office or health agency.

Equipment

Sterile alcohol swabs
Clean gauze pads
Sterile disposable lancets
Capillary tubes (heparinized and nonheparinized)
Copper sulfate (CuS) solution for anemia testing for women and men
Clean containers to hold the copper sulfate solution
Crito-seal clay trays or other sealing compound
Microhematocrit centrifuge
Microhematocrit reading card
Capillary bulbs (small rubber bulbs that fit over the capillary tube)

Procedure	Rationale
1. Wash your hands.	
2. Assemble and prepare equipment and supplies for use. Fill a container approximately two-thirds full with the copper sulfate solution.	Cover the CuS solution when not in use; do not expose it to direct sunlight or freezing temperatures, or allow it to evaporate. When doing multiple tests, change the solution after testing 15 patients.
3. Identify the patient, and explain the procedure.	
4. Perform a skin puncture on the fingertip. (See steps 1 to 11 in Fingertip Skin Puncture Technique, p. 336).	
5. Once blood flows freely, use a nonheparinized capillary tube to receive blood.	You may hold the tube in a horizontal position or slightly lower when filling the tube.
6. Apply pressure over the puncture site with a clean dry gauze pad.	You may have the patient do this while you attend to the test.
7. Hold the capillary tube vertically over the container of copper sulfate to allow the blood to drop into the solution. If the blood does not drop into the solution, apply the capillary bulb to the tube, then squeeze the bulb to force blood into the solution.	
8. Determine the test result. One of three reactions will occur: a. Blood drops through the solution without hesitating or rising. b. Blood hesitates and then drops through the solution. c. Blood hesitates, rises to the top of the solution, and eventually drops through the solution.	*Result indication* There are enough red blood cells present in the blood. Record the result as "normal." There may not be enough red blood cells; a hematocrit should be performed. There are probably not enough red blood cells present; a hematocrit should be performed.

Copper Sulfate Relative Density Test (*continued*)

Procedure	Rationale

9. *When a hematocrit is indicated:*
 • Swab the finger with a sponge, then "milk" the finger and, using the same puncture site, obtain another blood sample in a heparinized tube.
 • Seal the dry end of the tube with clay by sticking it into the Crito-seal clay tray.
 • Place the tube into a slot in the microhematocrit centrifuge, with the sealed end down.
 • Close and secure the lid of the centrifuge.
 • Adjust the timer, and spin down for 5 minutes.
 	
 • Using the scale provided on the centrifuge or the microhematocrit card, read the results as a percentage.
 • Dispose of contaminated materials properly.
 10. Wash your hands.
 11. Record the results.
	
	 Centrifuging the blood sample causes the red blood cells to settle at the bottom of the capillary tube.
	
	 Charting example:
	 April 26, 19_____, 12 PM
	   Skin puncture done on second finger, left hand. CuS test done, and hematocrit was indicated. Hct: 34%
	     Anne Kaelberer, CMA
	 or
	 CuS test indicated need for Hct.
	 Hct: 34%

BLOOD CHEMISTRIES

Some basic blood chemistries can be performed easily in the physician's office with the use of chemically impregnated reagent strips to determine the presence of blood glucose and blood urea nitrogen (BUN). (Blood glucose testing is more accurate than urine tests for glucose and is especially valuable in the management of diabetes.) In addition, there are compact and economical instruments on the market such as the Ames Seralyzer Blood Chemistry Analyzer. This instrument is a reflectance photometer that gives accurate quantitative results from blood serum or plasma for 15 routine diagnostic tests. Blood chemistries, certain therapeutic drug assays (TDA), and electrolytes are determined using special reagent test strips. The blood chemistry analyzer is particularly useful in the physician's office when on-site testing is desirable so that test results can be viewed as an aid to prompt decision making, frequently while the patient is still in the office. Most tests require less than 15 minutes elapsed time, averaging 2 minutes of operator time. Once the test strip is placed on the specimen table you can read the test results on the digital display in less than 2 minutes. Complete instructions for specimen collection, preparation, and use are supplied with the instrument (Fig. 11-15).

Test For Blood Glucose Using Dextrostix*

The Dextrostix is a reagent strip that measures blood glucose levels over a range of 45 to 250 mg/100 ml of blood (or 45 to 250 mg/dl). It is supplied in glass bottles that have a color chart on the side that is used for determining test results. Only fresh whole blood is to be used on these strips, as plasma and serum will give false results.

*Ames Co., Inc., Elkhart, IN.

Fig. 11-15. Ames Seralyzer blood chemistry analyzer—a compact instrument that performs 15 routine diagnostic tests. (Courtesy Ames Co., Inc., Elkhart, IN)

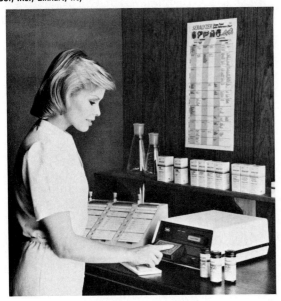

Instructions

1. Do a skin puncture on a fingertip. Allow a *large* drop of blood to form.
2. Place a large drop of blood on the test area of the strip. (This may be done by putting the strip on the blood over the puncture site.)
3. Wait 60 seconds exactly, holding the strip horizontally to avoid blood runoff from the test area.
4. Holding the strip vertically, wash the blood off, using a sharp stream of water from a wash bottle. No more than 1 to 2 seconds is required.
5. Compare the color on the test area with the color chart on the bottle. There are five color blocks representing 45, 90, 130, 175, and 250 mg/100 ml of blood.
6. Record the results.
7. Wash your hands.

NOTE: If not enough blood is used, you will obtain lower values. If you overwash the strip, you can wash color off and obtain lower values.

To obtain more precise blood glucose results, the same manufacturer has marketed an instrument, the Eyetone Reflectance Colorimeter, to be used with the Dextrostix. From a precisely calibrated meter that covers the range of 10 to 400 mg/100 ml blood glucose, rapid and accurate determination can be read. Complete instructions for use are provided with the instrument.

Test For Blood Glucose Using The Accu-Chek® II and Chemstrip® bG*

The Accu-Chek II is a battery-operated meter used to measure blood glucose (sugar). Chemstrip bG test strips are "read" by the Accu-Chek II to determine blood glucose levels. The Accu-Chek II will provide blood glucose readings between 20 and 500 mg/dl. The Chemstrip bG may also be read visually without using the Accu-Chek II. The results obtained will be very close to those you get when using the Accu-Chek II. This equipment can be used in the physician's office or by the patient at home (Fig. 11-16, A and B). The purpose of testing with Chemstrip bG at home is to measure the amount of blood glucose in the blood. The results of this test help the patient determine how much insulin, food, and exercise are needed to control diabetes.

Equipment

Accu-Chek II Blood Glucose Monitor with a "J" size battery
Vial of Chemstrip bG 50's (Cat. No. 00502)
Alcohol swab
Lancet or automatic finger pricking device
Dry cotton or rayon ball

Procedure for Programming the Accu-Chek® II

1. Open the box containing the vial of Chemstrip bGs. The box contains the package insert, a vial of 50 reagent strips, and a calibration strip that is wrapped in paper. Carefully remove the paper cover from the strip. This is the calibration strip that is used to program your Accu-Chek II meter for the new vial of strips. (Be sure that you are using Chemstrip bG 50, Cat. No. 00502.)
2. Compare the lot number on the calibration strip to the lot number on the side of the Chemstrip® bG vial. These numbers must match exactly before proceeding to the next step.
3. Now you must program the meter. This step *must* be performed whenever you open a new vial of Chemstrip bG 50 test strips. *Programming of the meter is required only once per vial of test strips.* The capacity for memory enables the meter to retain the calibration curve until it is reprogrammed for use with a different vial of strips.
4. To start, place the meter on a flat surface with the calibration slot toward you. Insert the pointed end of the calibration strip into the calibration slot until it touches the surface of the work area.

*Courtesy Boehringer Mannheim Corporation, 1986. Accu-Chek® and Chemstrip® are registered trademarks of Boehringer Mannheim GmbH, Indianapolis, IN.

Fig. 11-16. Accu-Chek II and Chemstrip bG companion system for blood glucose testing. (Courtesy Boehringer Mannheim Corp., 1986, Indianapolis, IN. Accu-Chek and Chemstrip are registered trademarks of Boehringer Mannheim GmbH)

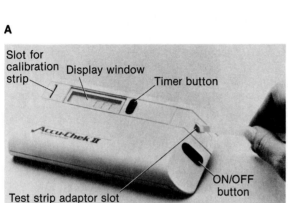

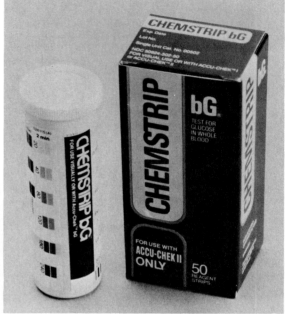

5. Press the ON/OFF button once to turn the Accu-Chek® II on.
6. Now slide the monitor toward you so that the calibration slot hangs over the edge of the work surface. Reach under the monitor and grasp the end of the calibration strip. Pull the strip through the slot with a smooth motion.
7. "CCC" should appear on the display and a beep should be heard. If not, repeat steps 4 and 6 until "CCC" appears on the display.
8. Position an unused Chemstrip bG test strip on its side with the test pads facing *away* from the ON/OFF button.
9. Insert the Chemstrip bG strip into the test strip adapter until it reaches the end of the chamber.
10. Firmly depress the TIME button until a beep is emitted. "888" will appear on the display. Repeat steps 8 and 9, if necessary, until "888" appears on the display screen. It will be followed by a three-digit code. This code number corresponds to the code printed on the Chemstrip bG vial label.
11. Remove the test strip from the test strip adapter and turn the meter off by depressing the ON/OFF button. You have programmed the meter, and it is now ready to be used to test the patient's blood for glucose.

Procedure for Testing Blood Glucose with the Accu-Chek® II

1. Turn the meter on by depressing the ON/OFF button once. The numeral "888" will appear on the display, followed by a three-digit code.

2. Lay an unused Chemstrip® bG test strip on a flat work surface with the test pads facing up.
3. Do a skin puncture on the patient's fingertip using a lancet or an automatic finger-puncture device.
4. Lightly squeeze the fingertip, let go; repeat several times until a large droplet of blood has formed.
5. Lightly touch the blood to the test pads on the Chemstrip bG strip. Make sure to cover both yellow and white squares completely. *Do not smear the blood.*
6. Immediately press the TIME button. The meter will count to 60.
7. During the displays of 57, 58, 59 the Accu-Chek II will emit three high beeps and, at 60, one low beep.
8. When the display reads 60 seconds, wipe the blood from the test pads with a clean, dry cotton ball using moderate pressure. Do not leave any blood on the test pads.
9. The Accu-Chek II will continue to count to 120 seconds. While the meter is counting, turn the test strip on its side with the test pads *facing* the ON/OFF button and insert the reacted test strip into the test strip adaptor. *The strip must be inserted before the display reads 120* (see Fig. 11-16,A).
10. When the display reads 120, a high beep will be emitted, followed by the blood sugar value displayed in mg/dl. Read the blood sugar value on the display screen.
   NOTE: If "HHH" appears on the display screen, the blood sugar level is over 500 mg/dl.

Wait an additional minute, then take the reacted test strip out of the meter and compare it to the color chart on the side of the Chemstrip® bG vial to estimate results up to 800 mg/dl.

If "LLL" appears on the display screen, the blood glucose value is lower than the reading range of the instrument (less than 10 mg/dl). Values below 20 mg/dl have not been confirmed clinically. Consult Troubleshooting Guide of Accu-Chek II manual.

11. Record the test result.
12. Press the ON/OFF button to turn the Accu-Chek® II off. Remove the test strip from the meter.

   NOTE: Accu-Chek II switches off automatically after about 5 minutes of inactivity.

How to Change the Battery in the Accu-Chek® II

1. Hold the Accu-Chek II face down in your hand.
2. Remove the battery compartment cover by placing your thumb on the grooved cover and sliding it toward you until it detaches from the instrument case.
3. Lightly press in and up on the edge of the battery to release it from the compartment. Tilt the instrument down until the battery slides out of the compartment.
4. Position the new "J" size battery with the notched corner in the upper left-hand position. Slide the battery into the compartment and push the battery in and down until it locks into position.
5. Place the battery compartment cover on the meter and snap it into place.

   NOTE: The compartment cover will not fit on the meter correctly if the battery is not inserted properly.

How to Clean the Accu-Chek® II Monitor

1. The outer casing may be wiped with a slightly dampened cloth and a *mild* household cleaning agent. Dry thoroughly. You should also clean the test strip adapter each time you calibrate the meter.
2. Remove the adapter from the meter by placing your thumb on the grooved surface above the test strip chamber and sliding the cover toward you. Slide the cover away from the meter.
3. Pinch together the two small black tabs located behind the beige chamber cover.
4. Slide the test strip adapter out of the cover.
5. Clean the inner surfaces of the channel of the test strip adapter with alcohol and a cotton swab.
6. Also clean the window surfaces on the side of the adapter. Dry all parts thoroughly.

7. To reassemble the adapter, hold the black adapter with your thumb and index finger on the small tabs. Hold the beige cover in your other hand with the metal clip facing you. Position the black adapter over the extension from the chamber cover and slide the adapter into the cover until it snaps into place.
8. Slide the reassembled adapter into position in the instrument case.

Using the Glucose Control Solution

Glucose Control Solution should be used for the following reasons:

- To practice correct technique
- To check for test strip deterioration (vial left uncapped, exposed to excessive heat or cold)
- To verify the performance of Accu-Chek® II (results are lower or higher than expected and don't agree with how the patient feels)

Instructions:

1. Place a drop of the Glucose Control Solution on the Chemstrip® bG instead of blood. *Use only Glucose Control Solution designed for use with Accu-Chek® II.*
2. Follow steps 6 through 12 of the blood-testing procedure.
3. Record your value and make sure it is within the control range listed in the package insert.

Reading the Chemstrip® bG Visually

1. Follow steps 2 through 5 of the section entitled "Procedure for testing blood glucose with the Accu-Chek® II."
2. Immediately start timing for 60 seconds.
3. At the end of the first 60 seconds, using moderate pressure, wipe blood from the test pads with a clean, dry cotton ball.
4. Now wait another 60 seconds.
5. Compare the two reacted colors on the test pads to the color chart on the Chemstrip bG vial.
6. If the test pad matches 240, wait an additional 60 seconds before making a final reading.
7. Sometimes the colors on the treated area of the test strip will match a color block on the chart exactly. Colors range from beige through various shades of blue and green. At other times, you will find that the reacted colors fall between color blocks.

   For example:

   The bottom (blue) square matches 180.
   The top (green) square matches 240.

The result would be approximately 210.

$$180$$
$$+240$$
$$420 \div 2 = 210 \text{ mg/dl.}$$

8. NOTE: If the patient has eyesight problems, this test cannot be used by the patient without the use of the Accu-Chek® II meter.

How to Avoid Inaccurate Readings

1. Always carefully place a large drop of blood onto the test pads of the Chemstrip® bG. Do not smear or rub the blood into the test pads.
2. Always use a drop of blood which is large enough to adequately cover both test pads simultaneously.
3. Always use a cotton ball to remove blood from the test pads. Wipe the pads with two or three even strokes using a clean area of the cotton ball.
4. Always use a watch with a second hand to monitor the reaction times.
5. Always discard Chemstrip bG test strips on the expiration date shown on the vial. Use of expired strips may result in inaccurate readings.
6. Always use the color chart from the vial that corresponds to the strips. Use of a different vial color chart may result in inaccurate readings.
7. Do not cut or alter the strips in any way.

Storage of the Chemstrip® bG

Chemstrip bG may be damaged if the strips are exposed to heat, light, or moisture. You should follow these suggestions:

- Keep the Chemstrip bG strips in the original vial. Do not transfer the strips into any other container.
- Store at room temperature under 86° F (30° C). Do not freeze.
- Always keep the vial capped tightly.

How to Tell If the Chemstrip bG Has Spoiled

1. Check the expiration date, which is stamped on the side of every vial.
2. Throw away any strips you still have after the expiration date.
3. If in doubt, replace the strips with a new vial of Chemstrip bG.

Test For Blood Glucose Using The Glucoscan™ 2000 and 3000 Blood Glucose Meters

LifeScan Inc. manufactures a series of two blood glucose meters, the Glucoscan 2000 Meter and the Glucoscan 3000 Meter. To the user, the Glucoscan 3000 Meter is similar to the Glucoscan 2000 Meter with the addition of a built-in memory, volume control for

audio signals and the ability to convert from mg/dl to mmol/L. Because the clinical performance characteristics are identical, the data presented below and in Figure 11-17 are applicable to both meters in this series. These meters are designed for convenience, ease of use, and accuracy.

Glucoscan blood glucose meters are portable, battery-operated reflectance photometers that are used with Glucoscan test strips to measure glucose concentrations in whole blood in a simple 60 second procedure. The meters are factory calibrated, thus eliminating the inconvenience of calibrating each test strip to the meter. However, you should check the calibration of the meter daily with a calibration checkstrip to verify meter performance. (Complete instructions for calibrating the meter are given in the owner's booklet provided with each meter.) Glucoscan test strips are individually foil-wrapped to prevent deterioration or contamination. Each test strip is ready for use when removed from the foil wrapper. Always check the expiration date printed on the foil wrapper before using a test strip. Never use an expired or a discolored test strip. A normal test strip is ivory-colored or light beige.

The Glucoscan meters measure the amount of color change that takes place when the glucose in a drop of whole blood reacts with reagents (chemicals) in the test strip reagent pad (where you put the blood). When the reacted test strip is placed in the meter and the test strip door is closed, a LED (light-emitting diode) shines light on the reagent pad. The reflected light from the reagent pad is measured electronically, and the amount of glucose in the blood is digitally displayed on the Glucoscan meter display.

The meters will automatically turn off 2 minutes after the blood glucose result has been displayed or if left on for more than 2 minutes during any part of the procedure without any further activity. To conserve the life of the batteries, turn the meter off after each test by pressing the power button.

For the procedure for using the Glucoscan 2000 and 3000 blood glucose meters see Figure 11-17. All Glucoscan meters are supplied with an owner's booklet that provides detailed information and instructions for use.

Inaccurate test results may be obtained from the meters for any of the following reasons:

1. Inadequate amount of blood placed on the test strip; the entire reagent pad must be completely covered.
2. The wrong test strips were used; *only* Glucoscan test strips can be used with the Glucoscan meters. Glucoscan test strips must not be cut or altered in any way.
3. The Glucoscan test strips used were:
   - Beyond their expiration date printed on each foil wrapper and on the outer package label

Fig. 11-17. Procedure and technique tips for using the Glucoscan 2000 and 3000 blood glucose meters. **A,** Instant start procedure. **B,** Countdown start procedure. (Courtesy Lifescan Inc., Mountain View, CA)

Instant Start Procedure and Technique Tips
GLUCOSCAN 2000 and 3000
Blood Glucose Meters

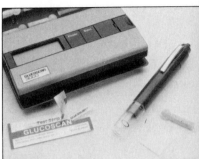
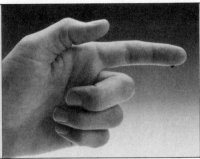
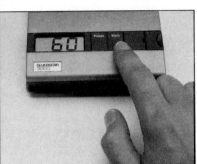

1. Choose a clean, dry work surface and assemble the following materials:
- GLUCOSCAN 2000* or 3000* Meter
- GLUCOSCAN Test Strip and Blotting Paper
- PENLET Blood Sampling Pen
- Lancet

*The test procedure and technique for the GLUCOSCAN 2000 and 3000 Meters are identical.

2. Press POWER button to turn on your Meter — Display reads 　60　.

Prick the side of your fingertip with the PENLET to obtain a drop of blood.

Turn pricked area of finger downward. Squeeze firmly until a large hanging drop of blood forms.

3a. Press START button and immediately apply the blood to the test pad.

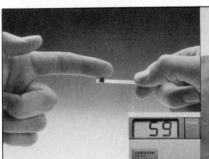
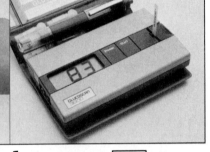

3b. Cover the entire pad with blood.

Apply the blood on the pad in a single, smooth motion. You may use the surface tension to spread the blood, but do not smear or rub blood on the pad.

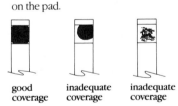

good coverage　　inadequate coverage　　inadequate coverage

4. Display reads 　23　 — Prepare to blot. Invert Test Strip with test pad over blotting paper. Do not touch the blood to the paper yet.

Display reads 　20　 — Press the pad straight down onto the blotting paper and blot for 2 seconds...release ...blot on a clean area of blotting paper for another 2 seconds.

The first blot should leave a red area and the second blot should leave a colorless wet square.

Open the Test Strip Door and insert the Test Strip into the Test Strip Holder ANY TIME before the Display counts down to 　00　. Close the Test Strip Door.

5. After Display reads 　00　 — Test result will be displayed.

IMPORTANT: Read detailed instructions in your GLUCOSCAN Owner's Booklet before doing a blood test.

A

Fig. 11-17 *(continued)*

Countdown Start Procedure and Technique Tips
GLUCOSCAN 2000 and 3000
Blood Glucose Meters

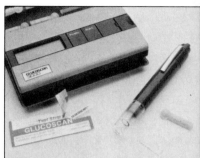

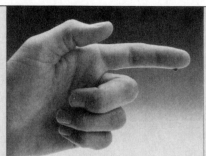

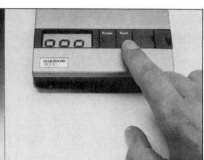

1. Choose a clean, dry work surface and assemble the following materials:
- GLUCOSCAN 2000* or 3000* Meter
- GLUCOSCAN Test Strip and Blotting Paper
- PENLET Blood Sampling Pen
- Lancet

*The test procedure and technique for the GLUCOSCAN 2000 and 3000 Meters are identical.

2. Press POWER button to turn on your Meter—Display reads [000].

Prick the side of your fingertip with the PENLET to obtain a drop of blood.

Turn pricked area of finger downward. Squeeze firmly until a large hanging drop of blood forms.

3a. Press START button.

During the countdown, Display reads [000]...[00]...[0]

Bring the Test Strip up to your finger to prepare to apply blood.

Display reads [60]

Apply the blood to the test pad.

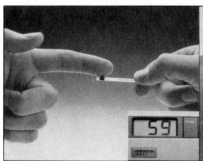

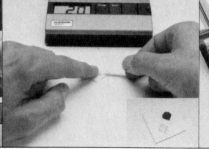

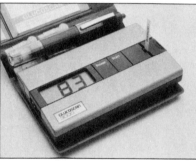

3b. Cover the entire pad with blood.

Apply the blood on the pad in a single, smooth motion. You may use the surface tension to spread the blood, but do not smear or rub blood on the pad.

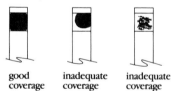

good coverage   inadequate coverage   inadequate coverage

4. Display reads [23]—Prepare to blot. Invert Test Strip with test pad over the blotting paper. Do not touch the blood to the paper yet.

Display reads [20]—Press the pad straight down onto the blotting paper and blot for 2 seconds...release ...blot on a clean area of blotting paper for another 2 seconds.

The first blot should leave a red area and the second blot should leave a pale blue or colorless wet square.

Open the Test Strip Door and insert the Test Strip into the Test Strip Holder ANY TIME before the Display counts down to [00]. Close the Test Strip Door.

5. After Display reads [00]—Test result will be displayed.

IMPORTANT: Read detailed instructions in your GLUCOSCAN Owner's Booklet before doing a blood test.

B

- Discolored before use (normal reaction pad is ivory-colored or light beige)
- Showing an abnormal color development during the test time (normal color development is blue/purple)

4. Incorrect timing; the blood must be in contact with the reagent pad for exactly 40 seconds before blotting. Blotting must begin when the display reads *20*.
5. The Glucoscan test strip holder and window area are dirty.
6. The Glucoscan meter is out of calibration; e.g., the calibration checkstrip result does not fall within the specified checkstrip range.
7. Inappropriate diagnostic use; Glucoscan test strips are for *in vitro* diagnostic use only.
8. Using the meter in intense direct sunlight may give low readings; shade the meter.

The Accu-Chek II and the Glucoscan 2000 and 3000 blood glucose meters are particularly valuable to diabetic patients who have to monitor their blood glucose levels closely. These meters can be used virtually anywhere. In many situations it is much easier for a person to obtain a small blood sample by a fingerprick than it is to obtain a urine sample. In addition a blood glucose level provides more accurate information than does a urine glucose level. Even the most accurate urine-testing method does not reflect the exact status of blood glucose at a given time. Urine tests also require you or the patient to compare colors on the test strip to colors on a color chart to determine the percentage of glucose. People with visual disturbances or color blindness cannot accurately use these methods and must rely on others to verify the results. The portable blood glucose meters eliminate these problems and accurate results can be obtained.

COMPLETE BLOOD COUNT (CBC): HEMATOLOGY TEST

Since the complete blood count is the most common laboratory procedure ordered on blood, it will be discussed more fully than other tests. A CBC gives a fairly complete look at the components in blood, providing a wealth of information on a patient's condition. The tests performed in a CBC include red blood cell count (RBC), hemoglobin (Hgb), hematocrit (Hct), white blood cell count (WBC), differential (Diff) white cell count, and a stained red cell examination (red cell morphology). The first four tests are quantitative measurements, and the last two are qualitative. All these tests are performed on whole blood (Table 11-1).

Table 11-1. Normal values for a complete blood count performed on whole blood

Test	Values
Red cell count	
Females	4,000,000 – 5,500,000/cu mm blood
Males	4,500,000 – 6,000,000/cu mm blood
Hemoglobin	
Females	12 – 16 gm/100 ml blood
Males	14 – 18 gm/100 ml blood
Hematocrit	
Females	37% – 47%
Males	40% – 54%
White cell count (females and males)	5000 – 10,000/cu mm blood
Differential	
Polymorphonuclear neutrophils	60% – 70%
Monocytes	2% – 6%
Lymphocytes	20% – 40%
Eosinophils	1% – 4%
Basophils	0.5% – 1%
Morphology (stained red cell examination)	Normal

Red Cell Count

The red cell count is the number of red blood cells found in each cubic millimeter of blood. *Manual counting in the past led to errors, thus was of questionable value. Presently with the automated counting equipment available, this determination is considered more reliable.* Elevated red cell counts indicate polycythemia, or that the patient has moved to a location with a higher altitude where the air contains less oxygen. In the latter case, the body requires more red cells to carry sufficient oxygen to meet its needs. Decreased numbers of red cells will be seen in patients with some form of anemia, after a hemorrhage, and also after the initial hemoconcentration of shock.

Hemoglobin

A hemoglobin determines the oxygen-carrying ability of the blood. It is a simple and most efficient method to detect any anemia (pernicious, iron deficiency, sickle cell) and the severity of the condition. It also helps the physician determine the effectiveness of treatments administered to the patient. A patient is considered anemic if the hemoglobin value is below 12 gm/100 ml. Low hemoglobin values will also be

Fig. 11-18.   Main types of leukocytes. **A,** *Granulocytes-neutrophils: Segmented neutrophils* are round or oval cells. The cytoplasm is a lavender or pink color, with pinkish or lavender granules. The nucleus is segmented, having from two to 12 segments, but usually three or four, and it stains a purplish or lavender color. **B,** *stab neutrophils* are round or oval, with a cytoplasm similar in color to that of the segmented neutrophils. It contains fine granules that are pinkish or reddish violet. The nucleus is one continuous piece that looks like a flexible rod. It commonly forms letter shapes, such as C, S, N, and U. The nucleus is colored a dark purple or lavender, and occupies about one fourth of the cell. **C,** *juvenile neutrophils* are round or oval, and cytoplasm is usually a bluish pink, containing granules that may be definite or fine and of a purplish or reddish color. The nucleus is bean shaped, usually purplish in color, and usually occupies about half the cell (juvenile neutrophil also appears at bottom of panel **B**). *Not shown, myelocyte neutrophils'* cytoplasm often takes an almost neutral stain, tinged with blue, and it, as well as the nucleus, is dotted with definite pinkish or purple granules. The nucleus is round or oval, ordinarily stains bluish purple, and takes up about two thirds of the cell. **D,** *granulocytes-eosinophils.* Eosinophils' cytoplasm has light blue tinges and is covered with coarse, round, or oval bright pink or red granules. The nucleus is usually segmented and stains a deep lavender to light blue. **E,** *lymphocytes'* cytoplasm is usually a bright blue and at times may be almost negligible, as the purple or lavender nucleus may take up almost the entire cell. Immature lymphocytes are larger than mature cells, having much more cytoplasm, which generally stains a very pale, glasslike blue. Occasionally, a few pink granules may appear in the cytoplasm. The nucleus is usually round or oval but may be indented as well. It stains a purple or lavender color. **F,** *monocytes* are the largest of all the white cells. Often they are quite irregular in shape and usually take a pale stain. The cytoplasm is usually a smoky blue-gray, sometimes sprinkled with a fine pink dust. The nucleus generally is kidney shaped or round, often lobulated, staining a lavender color.

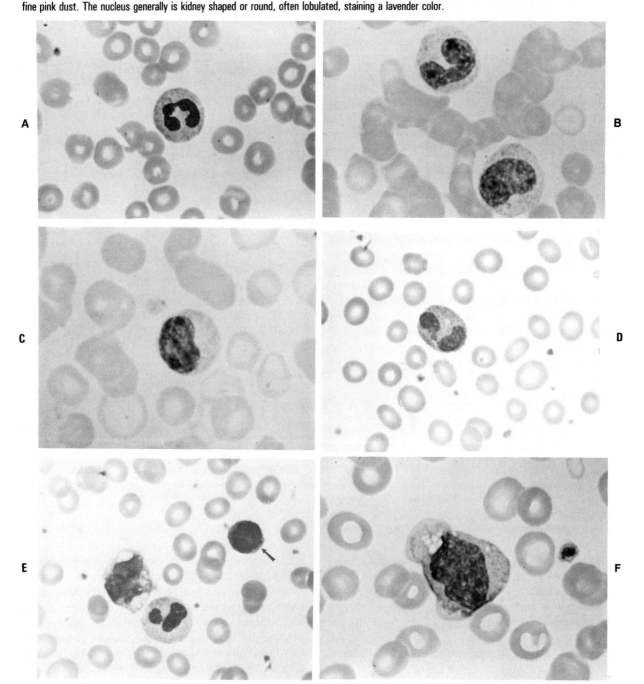

caused by hemorrhage. Elevated concentrations of hemoglobin may be seen in severely burned or dehydrated patients. This is because the body has lost considerable amounts of fluid; thus the red cells are suspended in less fluid, and more hemoglobin is present in each 100 ml of blood.

Hematocrit

The hematocrit, or packed-cell volume, represents the percentage of red blood cells in the total blood volume. Elevated hematocrits will be seen in patients with polycythemia; a low hematocrit is seen in anemia and leukemia. Generally, the hematocrit and hemoglobin concentrations are related. Each 1% hematocrit contains .34 gm of hemoglobin; the hematocrit should equal three times the hemoglobin within 3%. Thus if a patient's hemoglobin is 14 gm/100 ml, the hematocrit should fall between 39% and 45% (14 × 3.0 = 42, and plus or minus 3 = 39% to 45%). Deviations from this relationship usually indicate the presence of red cells of abnormal size or hemoglobin content.

White Blood Cell Count

The white blood cell count is the number of WBCs found in each cubic millimeter of blood. As with the red cell count, automated equipment now provides us with a more reliable count. A person's white count will vary somewhat during a day, because of exercise, emotional states, or digestion. Increases as great as 2000 WBC/cu mm may be seen in these situations. Pathologically, the WBC count will increase in infections and leukemia. Decreased WBC count may be caused by radiation therapy, immunosuppressive therapy (chemotherapy) for cancer and transplant patients, toxic reactions, measles, typhoid fever, and infectious hepatitis. This is due to a depression of the bone marrow's blood-forming centers.

Differential White Cell Count

The differential is a test that determines the percentage of each of the five different types of white blood cells in the blood. Each type of white cell has a specific function. Together, with the degree of increase or decrease in the total number of white cells and with the percentage of each type of white cell, the physician is able to make a more definite diagnosis. Characteristic abnormal numbers and types of white cells are seen in various diseases (Fig. 11-18).

Neutrophils.   The body's primary lines of defense against infection are the neutrophils. They seek and destroy any invading bacteria by the process of phagocytosis. Increased numbers of neutrophils are seen in conditions such as appendicitis, tonsillitis, pneumonia, abscesses, granulocytic leukemia, and meningitis. A decreased neutrophil count (neutropenia) is seen in mumps, hepatitis, measles, aplastic anemia, agranulocytosis, and also in patients who are taking certain drugs, such as certain antibiotics, antihistamines, anticonvulsants, and sulfonamides. In these cases the decrease in the neutrophils causes an increase in one of the other white blood cells, especially in the lymphocytes. Thus one must know the actual value for each of the five types of WBCs to determine if this is the case.

Monocytes.   The body's second line of defense against invasion by foreign substances is the monocytes. These are also phagocytes, as they ingest any foreign particles or bacteria that the neutrophils are unable to. The monocytes will also clean up any cellular debris that remains after an infection or abscess subsides. Increased numbers of monocytes will be seen in patients who have tuberculosis, amebic dysentery, typhoid fever, Rocky Mountain spotted fever, subacute bacterial endocarditis, or monocytic leukemia, or in those patients who are recovering from a bacterial infection. Conditions with decreased numbers of monocytes are difficult to indicate, since the normal count of the cells is so low.

Lymphocytes.   The lymphocytes circulate through the body to destroy the toxic products of protein metabolism and to identify and produce antibodies against foreign cells. Recent studies are identifying new roles of these cells especially in the field of immunology. Increased numbers of lymphocytes (lymphocytosis) are seen in viral diseases such as influenza, German measles, mumps, whooping cough, and infectious mononucleosis, as well as in lymphocytic leukemia. Decreased numbers are seen in patients who are taking cortisone, ACTH, and epinephrine. Other types of leukemia and radiation also cause lymphopenia.

Eosinophils and Basophils.   Little is known about the eosinophils and basophils. It is thought that the eosinophils aid in detoxification by breaking down protein material and are associated with allergic reactions and production of antihistamine. Increased eosinophil counts are seen in patients who have hay fever, allergies, skin diseases, parasite infections, and asthma. Decreased counts are seen in patients who have increased levels of insulin, epinephrine, and ACTH. Stress following surgery may also cause eosinopenia.

Basophils are thought to produce heparin and histamine; thus some believe that they help prevent blood from clotting in inflamed tissues and play a role in clot breakdown. Increased basophil counts are seen in patients who have hemolytic anemias, chronic granulocytic leukemia, and have had their spleen removed (splenectomy) and exposure to radiation. Decreased conditions have not been identified.

Abnormal White Cells

The five types of white cells just discussed are all normal cells found in peripheral blood. In some disorders and diseases immature neutrophils or atypical lymphocytes will be seen. The immature neutrophils are myeloblasts, promyelocytes, myelocytes, metamyelocytes, and band cells. You will see these terms on some laboratory reports included with a differential report.

Stained Red Cell Examination

Using the same stained slide that was used for determining the differential, the laboratory technologist will then examine the red blood cells for any variation in size, shape, structure, color, or content. Anisocytosis, macrocytosis, microcytosis, and poikilocytosis are reported as slight, moderate, or marked.

Summary

As you can see, the significant findings obtained from a complete blood count are numerous. Evaluation of these findings, along with the total clinical picture of a patient's condition, provides the physician with valuable information for screening, diagnosing, treating, or evaluating and monitoring the progress of treatment for patient care.

AUTOMATION IN THE CLINICAL LABORATORY

Within the past 15 to 20 years, clinical laboratories have been confronted with an ever-increasing work load. An answer to this problem has been sought in automated instrumentation. These specialized modular systems automate or semiautomate the time-consuming, step-by-step procedures formerly performed by manual analysis. With refinement of instrumentation, fast and accurate methods have been developed for reporting a wide variety of laboratory information on body fluids, which include whole blood, plasma, serum, urine, and cerebrospinal fluid. The human element of error is virtually eliminated, assuring the absolute objectivity of measurement so important to accurate diagnosis and

monitoring. Multiphasic tests or test panels or profiles consist of a battery of automated tests performed on the same specimen at the same time. It has been found that it is more useful and economical to subject every specimen to a battery or panel of automated tests than to limit the examination to one or two tests. Through this system of routine total blood counts and biochemical profiling, additional disease screening tests may be routinely performed. Most hematology panels in laboratories that have any volume at all are done on the Coulter systems or other systems, such as the Technicon H-I system. There are several different machines; most of them automate or at least semiautomate the whole process, using only 1 ml of blood. Test results are obtained visually on a digital display or video screen, or on a hematology printout card (Fig. 11-19 and Fig. 11-20). The latest state-of-the-art systems use laser technology. Laser counters in hematology, such as the ELT-8, perform an automated CBC. The laser looks at the cells to determine the results. Traditionally, the chemistry sections of laboratories are the most heavily automated. Most laboratories will have at least some form of automation in chemistry if not in other departments. Frequently used biochemical panels are the SMA 12/60, SMA 18, SMA 20, SMAC 20 or 24. SMA stands for sequential multiple analysis, the C indicates that it is computer-assisted, and the numbers indicate the number of tests that are performed. Another panel is simply called a Chemistry Screening Panel 12, 20 or 24. The numbers indicate how many tests are to be performed. These are general terms that are used, as the type of tests run in these panels will vary with the laboratory and how they have programmed the automated equipment for use. All of these panels are screening devices that allow the physician to focus on abnormal results for further study and investigation. Test results from the SMA systems are reported on an $8\frac{1}{2} \times 11$ inch sheet of precalibrated vertical graph paper called a SCG (serum chemistry graph), SMA 12, or on a similar horizontal graph for the other systems (Figs. 11-21 and 11-22). Rather than sending the physician this graph paper, many laboratories now have special computer printout forms that also record the results of the tests performed. The laboratory keeps the graph as its permanent record and sends the computer printout to the physician. One example of the computer forms used is a sheet divided into columns. In different columns the names of the tests, the normal values, and the results of the tests performed are recorded.

Many multiphasic tests, panels, or profiles are devised to provide information on particular body system disorders or suspected conditions and also for screening purposes, some of which include a hepatobiliary profile, diabetes profile, cardiac screening, renal function, thyroid function, and arthritis. The grouping of specific tests provides the physician with

Fig. 11-19. **A,** Coulter S-Plus for automated cell counting. **B,** Coulter diff3 system for automating complete differential.

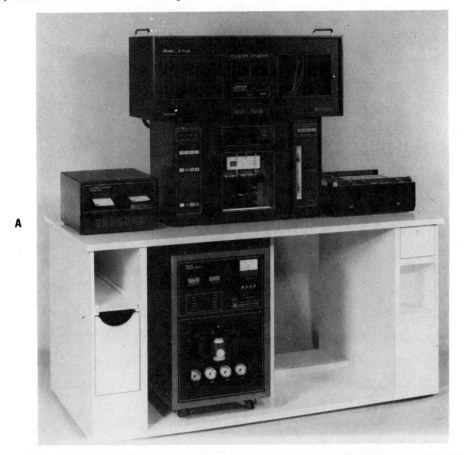

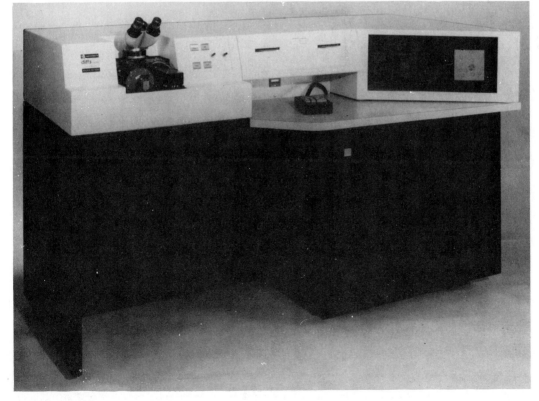

(Fig. 11-19 continues)

Fig. 11-19. **C,** Coulter Counter ZBI 6 System for semiautomated hematology profiles. It will determine red blood cell count, white blood cell count, hemoglobin, hematocrit, mean corpuscular volume, and platelet count. Test results are obtained from digital readouts on equipment. **D,** Hematology printout card that shows results of tests performed on Coulter S-Plus and on Coulter diff3 system. (Courtesy Coulter Electronics, Inc., Hialeah, Fla.)

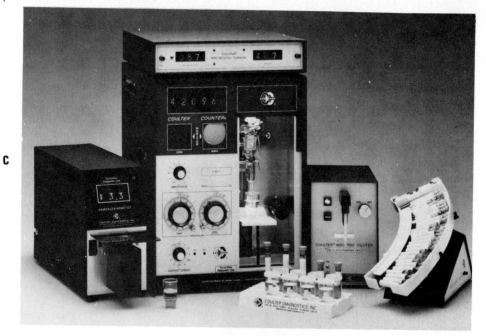

C

D

Fig. 11-20. The compact Technicon H.1 system provides accurate, comprehensive information on all cell types of clinical interest. It offers the choice of: CBC with platelets; CBC and full Diff plus RBC morphology; and Lymphocyte subset analyses from a single aspiration of blood. Multiple report formats let the operator review a variety of results on the video screen, and any CRT data can be printed out on a graphic printer. The Technicon H.1 provides a standard computer interface. Results may be automatically transmitted "live" to a remote laboratory computer, thus reducing data handling, transcription effort, and potential errors. (Courtesy Technicon Instruments Corp., Tarrytown, N.Y.)

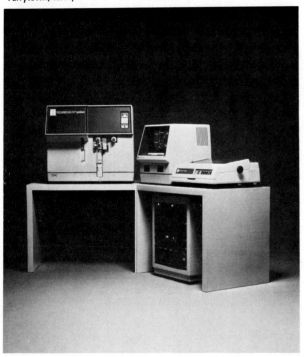

Fig. 11-21. Technicon RA-2X system is a chemistry analyzer that can be preprogrammed with 100 different tests. For chemistry profiles, one can select up to 27 tests at a time from this extensive menu, including immunoassays and electrolytes. Results are displayed on the computer screen and printed out on the printer. (Courtesy Technicon Instruments Corp., Tarrytown, N.Y.)

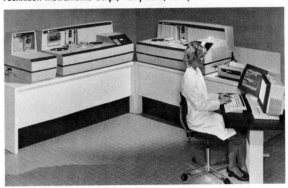

and perform all the procedures that have been presented.

REVIEW OF VOCABULARY

The following are samples of patient information from medical charts. In each, terms that have been presented in this unit are used. Read these and define the italicized terms. When laboratory values are given, determine if these are normal or abnormal results.

PATIENT NO. 1:

This patient has a history of various *blood dyscrasias:*
  1984—*anemia* and *anisocytosis*
  1986—both *hypernatremia* and *hypoglycemia* in different months
  1987—*septicemia* from undetermined causes
Present symptoms indicate *uremia* and *infectious mononucleosis.* Blood samples were obtained by *venipuncture* and sent to the laboratory for *multiphasic* tests.

PATIENT NO. 2:

Liver function studies showed minimal elevations of the *SGOT* at 49.6 and 62 and then 41 units. *LDH* was not elevated, ranging at 100, 130, and 115. *Hypercholesterolemia* was revealed. *Serum electrolytes* showed slight *hypokalemia* of 3.4. With the use of potassium supplementation, the potassium rose to 4.1. The patient manifested some peripheral edema, which ultimately required the use of small doses of diuretics (Lasix 20 mg per day). This was felt to probably be the result of *hypoproteinemia. Serum albumin* was 3.0; total protein 6.4. *Bilirubin* remained minimally elevated at 1.4 and 1.2. *Alkaline phosphatase* was elevated at 278 and 288 IU/L (normal to 90). *CBC* showed a *hemoglobin* of 12.9 gm, *hematocrit* of 37.6%, with *leukocytosis* of 15,000 and 13,500, and slight *poikilocytosis.* A *reticulocyte count* was 2.5%. *Prothrombin time* was 72%. *VDRL* was negative.

an overall view of the patient's status that a single test could not provide. An example of a cardiac profile (panel) may include an SGOT, SGPT, LDH, CPK, CBC, sedimentation rate, prothrombin time (PT), cholesterol, triglycerides, and potassium.

A kidney function profile may include total protein, albumin, globulin, A/G ratio, creatinine, BUN, BUN/creatinine ratio, sodium, potassium, chloride, uric acid, and cholesterol. A liver function profile may include alkaline phosphatase, LDH, SGOT, SGPT, total bilirubin, total protein, albumin, globulin, A/G ratio, and so on. See Table 11-2 for additional information on some of these tests and others.

CONCLUSION

You have now completed the unit on hematology. Practice the procedures, and when you feel that you know the equipment and steps of the procedures, arrange with your instructor to take the performance tests. You will be expected to demonstrate accurately your ability to prepare for

Fig. 11-22. The Serum Chemistry Graph displaying results from the SMA 12/60 on 12 biochemical tests. Results are presented in concentration terms on a precalibrated strip chart record. Normal test ranges for each parameter are printed as shaded areas; horizontal line crossing graph represents test results. Time from aspiration of given sample to finished chart is only 8 minutes—less time than it takes to complete any one of these tests by other methods. (Courtesy Technicon Instruments Corp., Tarrytown, N.Y.)

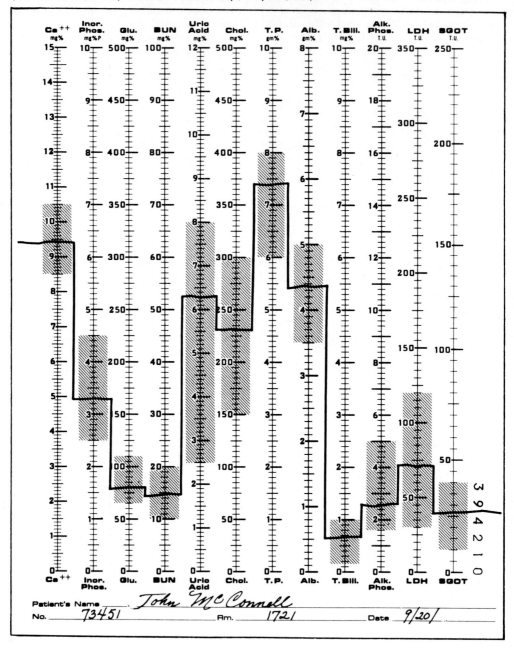

Table 11-2. Examinations made on blood

Test	Performed on	Normal Values*	Significance
Hematology blood tests			
1. Sedimentation rate (sedrate or ESR)	Whole blood	Wintrobe tubes: Female: 0–20 mm/hr Male: 0–9 mm/hr Wester: Female and male: 0–20 mm/hr	Increased in almost all infections, myocardial infarction, active rheumatoid arthritis, pulmonary infarction, shock, surgical operations, and pregnancy. Decreased in sickle cell anemia, polycythemia, cardiac decompensation, and newborn infants.
2. Microhematocrit (MCHC)	Whole blood	32%–36%	Same as for regular hematocrit.
3. Reticulocytes (immature RBCs)	Whole blood	0.5%–1.55% of all RBCs in peripheral whole blood	Increased when bone marrow is manufacturing RBCs at an increased rate. May be seen in patients with acute or chronic hemorrhage, or in sickle cell anemia. Normally elevated in infants and pregnant women. Decreased in aplastic and pernicious anemia.
4. Coagulation tests and platelets			
a. Bleeding time	Capillary whole blood	1–3 min	Increased time indicates platelet deficiency, which may be due to pernicious anemia, aplastic anemia, acute leukemias, hemorrhagic disease of the newborn, multiple myeloma, chronic lymphocytic leukemia, and Hodgkin's disease.
b. Clot retraction time	Venous blood	30–60 min	Prolonged time seen in primary or secondary thrombocytopenia due to aplastic or pernicious anemia, Hodgkin's disease, multiple myeloma, acute leukemia, and hemorrhagic disease of the newborn.
c. Coagulation or clotting time	Blood	Lee-White: 6–10 min Capillary tube: 3–7 min	Used as a measurement of the ability of blood to clot properly. May indicate that vitamin K or calcium levels are inadequate for clotting of blood.
d. Fibrinogen (quantitative)	Blood plasma	200–600 mg/100 ml	Increase seen in inflammatory processes, infections, pregnancy, menstruation, and after x-ray treatment. Decreases noted in liver diseases, anemia, and severe malnutrition.
e. Platelet count	Whole blood	200,000–400,000/cu mm blood	Decreased numbers may indicate disease of the spleen; also will cause bleeding.
f. Thromboplastin test	Whole blood	Abnormal thromboplastin formation	This test is used to differentiate blood coagulation abnormalities.

(Table 11-2 continues)

359

Table 11-2 *(continued)*

Test	Performed on	Normal Values*	Significance
5. Prothrombin time (PT or Pro-Time)	Blood serum	70%–110% of control value	Prolonged time may indicate vitamin K deficiency, liver disease, or an excessive use of dicumarol in treatment. When anticoagulation therapy used, PT kept at from 2 to 2½ times normal.
Blood chemistries			
1. Calcium (Ca++)	Blood serum	9.0–11.5 mg/100 ml or 9.0–11.5 mg/dl	Increased in chronic nephritis with uremia, bone tumors including metastatic cancer of bone, hyperparathyroidism, Addison's disease, adenoma of parathyroids, emphysema, cardiac decompensation.
2. Inorganic phosphorus (Inor phos)	Blood serum	3–4.5 mg/100 ml or 3–4.5 mg/dl	Increased in uremia, Bright's disease, excessive vitamin D intake, and hypoparathyroidism. Decreased in diabetes mellitus. Decreased in hypoglycemia and after excessive insulin.
3. Glucose	Blood serum	80–120 mg/100 ml	Increased in some kidney diseases.
4. Blood urea nitrogen (BUN)	Blood serum	10–20 mg/100 ml or 10–20 mg/dl	Increased in leukemia, gout, acidosis, toxemia.
5. Uric acid	Blood serum	2.5–8.0 mg/100 ml or 2.5–8.0 mg/dl	Increased in liver disease with obstructive jaundice, nephrosis, diabetes mellitus, hypothyroidism, and in diets too high in saturated fat or cholesterol. Decreased in anemia, malabsorption, hyperthyroidism, and hepatic failure.
6. Cholesterol	Blood serum	Up to 20 yr.: 120–230 mg/100 ml or mg/dl 30 yr.: 120–240 mg/100 ml or mg/dl 40 yr.: 140–240 mg/100 ml or mg/dl 50 yr.: 150–240 mg/100 ml or mg/dl 60 yr.: 160–240 mg/100 ml or mg/dl 100 yr.: 160–240 mg/100 ml or mg/dl	
7. Total protein (TP)	Blood serum	6.0–8.0 gm/100 ml or 6.0–8.0 gm/dl	Increased in dehydration, malignancy, hepatic disease, infection. Decreased levels in overhydration, hepatic insufficiency, burns, malnutrition, nephrosis.
8. Albumin (Alb)	Blood serum	3.5–5.5 gm/100 ml or 3.5–5.5 gm/dl	Increase seen in dehydration. Decreased in overhydration, hepatic insufficiency, malnutrition, burns, nephrosis.
9. Total bilirubin (indirect)	Blood serum	0.2–1.2 mg/100 ml or 0.2–1.2 mg/dl	Increase seen in hemolysis, hepatic disease, obstructive jaundice, pulmonary infarct.
10. Alkaline phosphatase (Alk phos)	Blood serum	2–4.5 Bodansky units 4–13 King Armstrong units 20–90 IU/L	Increased in children and in women in the third trimester of pregnancy; in hepatic disease, obstructive jaundice, bone growth, osteoblastic bone tumors, peptic ulcer, and colitis. Decreased in hypothyroidism, anemia, malnutrition, pernicious anemia.

Test	Specimen	Normal value	Clinical significance
11. LDH (Lactic dehydrogenase)	Blood serum	90–200 IU/L	Increased in myocardial infarction, muscle necrosis, hemolysis, kidney infarct, liver disease, and cerebral damage.
12. SGOT (Serum glutamic oxaloacetic transaminase)	Blood serum	10–40 units/L	Very high levels seen 24 hr after a myocardial infarction, in liver disease, complete biliary obstruction and jaundice with hepatic cirrhosis. Increased in skeletal trauma, hemolysis, cerebral damage. Lower levels seen in pregnancy, chronic dialysis, beri beri.
SMA 12/60 includes the preceding 12 chemistry tests			
13. Triglycerides	Blood serum	40–140 mg/100 ml or 40–140 mg/dl	Increased in diets too high in saturated fat or cholesterol. High level is a risk factor for heart attack. Decreased in anemia.
14. CPK (Creatine phosphokinase)	Blood serum	1–10 units 0.2 to 1.42 units (two methods)	Increased in myocardial infarction, pulmonary edema, pulmonary infarction, DTs, and muscular dystrophy.
15. Creatinine	Blood serum	0.7–1.7 mg/dl	Increased in nephritis and impaired kidney function.
16. Icterus index	Blood serum	3–8 units	Used to discover early jaundice and for a liver function test.

Serology (*Certain special blood tests are covered in this item*)

Test	Specimen	Normal value	Clinical significance
1. STS (serological test for syphilis) includes			
a. Fluorescent treponemal antibody (FTA)	Blood serum	Negative	Used to confirm diagnosis of syphilis if VDRL or RPR is positive.
b. Rapid plasma reagin (RPR)	Blood serum or plasma	Negative	Both are screening tests for syphilis. Sometimes false positive results are obtained.
c. VDRL (Venereal Disease Research Laboratory)	Blood serum	Negative	Positive results confirmed with the FTA.
2. Special human antibodies			
a. Coombs direct	Blood serum	Negative	Used to test newborn's blood for erythroblastosis fetalis. Also used in blood cross matching.
b. Coombs indirect	Blood serum	Negative	Used to detect blood incompatibilities when cross matching; also to detect Rh incompatibility in maternal blood before delivery by demonstrating anti-Rh antibodies.
c. Heterophil antibody (MonoSpot test)	Blood serum	Concentrated to 1/28	Elevated in infectious mononucleosis and serum sickness.
d. LE test (lupus erythematosus)	Whole blood	Negative	A slide test for antinucleoproteins found in systemic LE.
3. Bacterial and viral antibodies			
a. ASO (antistreptolysin) titer	Blood serum	To 400 units/ml	Increased values seen in rheumatic fever, and acute glomerulonephritis caused by hemolytic streptococcus.

(Table 11-2 continues)

Table 11-2 *(continued)*

Test	Performed on	Normal Values*	Significance
b. Bacterial agglutinations Dysentery Brucellosis Paratyphoid A & B Typhoid O & H Typhus fever Leptospirosis	Blood serum	No agglutination	Certain infections caused by viruses, bacilli, rickettsiae, and spirochetes produce antibodies in the serum, which in turn cause agglutination (clumping) of these organisms.
c. Widal test	Blood serum	Negative	A test to diagnose typhoid and paratyphoid fevers.
4. Rheumatoid factors			
a. Latex slide agglutination	Blood serum	1:40 is uppermost serum dilution	Positive in rheumatoid arthritis and in some connective tissue diseases.
b. RA (rheumatoid arthritis) test	Blood serum	Negative	Results positive in 85%–90% of patients with rheumatoid arthritis.
Thyroid function			
1. T_3 uptake (resin uptake/radioassay)	Blood serum	25%–35%	Increased in hyperthyroidism; decreased in hypothyroidism.
2. T_4 total thyroxin radioimmunoassay (T_4/RIA)	Blood serum	5.2–12.2 μg/dl	Decreased level of T_3 and increased level of T_4 if a woman is taking birth control pills. The free thyroxin index is done in this case to confirm normal thyroid function.
3. $T_3:T_4$ ratio	Blood serum		
4. Free thyroxin index (includes total T_4)	Blood serum	0.5–1.7	
Other tests			
1. Glucose tolerance test (standard test)	Blood serum	(Results per 100 ml blood) *Fasting blood glucose: 80 mg— 120 mg* *After ingesting test dose of glucose:* 30 min — 150 mg 60 min — 135 mg 2 hr — 100 mg 2½ hr — 80 mg	Used to detect abnormalities in carbohydrate metabolism such as occur in diabetes mellitus, hypoglycemia, and adrenocortical and liver dysfunction. In diabetes, fasting blood sugar (FBS) is around 120 mg/100 ml or higher. After 1 hr, level rises over 180 mg/100 ml, and does not return to normal in 2 and 3 hr specimens. Normally blood sugar will return to normal after 2 hr.
2. Glucose tolerance sum (GTS)			In older patients, diabetes is sometimes hard to diagnose. Some physicians will use the GTS. They will add the FBS, ½ hr, 1 hr, and 2 hr values obtained from the glucose tolerance test. If the sum of these values is less than 500 mg, the patient is not considered diabetic. When the sum is over 800 mg, the

patient is considered diabetic. Various other tests will be done to confirm this diagnosis and rule out liver disease, chronic diseases, or potassium depletion.

	Test	Specimen	Normal Values	Significance
3.	Blood culture	Sample of blood grown on culture media	No growth after incubation period	Growth on culture media indicative of blood stream infection or septicemia.
4.	Bone marrow	Marrow aspirated from iliac crest or sternum, then placed on a slide and stained for examination	Various primitive cells are found	Abnormal cell findings may indicate a blood disorder such as leukemia.
5.	Blood typing	Whole blood or blood serum	*One of the following:* Type O—45% of the population (Universal donor) Type A—40% of the population Type B—10% of the population Type AB—5% of the population (Universal recipient) And either: Rh positive—85% of population Rh negative—15% of population	Must be done before a patient receives a blood transfusion, to ensure a compatible transfusion; also important in pregnancy to help prevent erythroblastosis fetalis.
6.	Radioimmunoassay for serum pregnancy *or* HCG Beta subunit for pregnancy	Serum	Quantitative results: 1st wk: 20–60 mIU/ml 2nd wk: 60–200 mIU/ml 3rd wk: 200–2000 mIU/ml 2nd or 3rd mo: 20,000–200,000 mIU/ml 2nd trimester: 12,000–60,000 mIU/ml 3rd trimester: 10,000–30,000 mIU/ml	Results reported as either positive or negative for pregnancy. A result of 5–15 mIU/ml *may* indicate an ectopic pregnancy. A result of less than 5mIU/ml would be considered negative for an ectopic pregnancy.
7.	HTLV III antibody for AIDS NOTE: In many states it is a state regulation that the patient must sign a consent form before this test is performed.	Serum or plasma	Negative	A negative result indicates that the antibody is not in the blood. A positive result indicates that the antibody is in the blood.

NOTE: For many years laboratories have reported a number of their test results in milligrams (mg) percent, or milligrams (mg) per 100 milliliters (ml), or 100 cubic centimeters (cc). A newer method, utilized by many, is the use of a deciliter (dl); 1 dl = 0.10 L or 100 ml or 100 cc. Thus in a report, mg/dl is the same as mg% or mg/100 ml. Keep in mind that test values may differ, depending on the methods and procedures used by the laboratory.

REVIEW QUESTIONS

1. Define blood.
2. List the white blood cells that are classified as granulocytes and those that are classified as agranulocytes.
3. When asked to obtain a blood sample for a battery of 12 blood chemistry tests, what method and body site would you use to obtain this sample?
4. You have obtained a skin puncture blood sample. What tests might you perform in the office on this sample?
5. The following blood report has been sent to your office. Indicate which test results are normal and which are abnormal.

   White blood cells — 15,000/cu mm
   Red blood cells — 5.6 million/cu mm
   Diff
      Lymphocytes — 55%
      Eosinophils — 8%
      Neutrophils — 65%
   SGOT — 65 units/ml
   Alkaline phosphatase — 85 IU/L
   Prothrombin time — 90% of control
   Hematocrit — 45%
   Uric acid — 13 mg/100 ml
   BUN — 18 mg/100 ml
   Cholesterol — 160 mg/100 ml
   VDRL — negative
   Coomb's indirect — negative
   Latex slide agglutination — positive

6. The physician has ordered a VDRL, a CBC, SMA-12, and a triglyceride test for J.D. Would you give this patient any special instructions before having a blood sample drawn? Could you collect one sample of blood in one tube? Would you use plain tube(s) or tube(s) with an anticoagulant additive? Explain the reasons for your answers.
7. The physician suspects that a patient may have hypothyroidism. What blood tests might be ordered to help diagnose this patient's condition?
8. What simplified tests might you do in the office to determine the presence of sugar in the blood?
9. Sexually transmitted diseases are on a constant rise at the present time. Frequently a physician will order a blood test to detect the presence of syphilis or use one of these tests as a screening purpose for unsuspected cases. List three blood tests that may be performed to detect the presence of syphilis in a patient.
10. List the blood test(s) that a physician may order to help diagnose the following conditions or diseases:
    Liver disease
    Infectious mononucleosis
    Myocardial infarction
    A diet too high in fat content
    Kidney disease
    Leukemia
    Chronic or acute infections
    Anemia
    Diabetes
    Rheumatoid arthritis
    Septicemia

11. List the tests performed when a CBC is ordered.
12. Define: multiphasic tests, test panel, and profile.
13. List three blood tests that require a patient to fast before the blood sample is drawn.
14. List the two most common veins used to obtain a blood specimen by venipuncture. State/describe the anatomical location of these veins. State how much blood may be drawn from the patient by this method.
15. List three blood tests that would usually require you to use a collection tube without an additive. State the color of the rubber stopper of the vacuum tube that you would use for this. Explain what you would do with this specimen after collection is completed (2 steps).
16. State when you would use a collection tube with the additive EDTA. What color is the rubber stopper on this vacuum tube?
17. State when you would use a collection tube with the additive heparin. State the reason why you would not use this tube for hematology studies.
18. State four reasons why it is vital that the ordered blood test be performed within 8 hours or less once the blood sample has been drawn.
19. State when you would release the tourniquet on the patient when performing a venipuncture.
20. Describe what may happen if you withdraw blood too quickly when using a standard syringe and needle when performing a venipuncture.
21. State why you do not shake tubes containing an additive and blood specimen, and why you should just gently invert them 8 to 10 times.

PERFORMANCE TEST

In a skills laboratory, a simulation of a joblike environment, the medical assistant student is to demonstrate the correct procedure for the following without reference to source materials. For these activities, the student will need a person to play the role of a patient; *or* an artificial appliance representing a human arm and hand, and a blood sample. Time limits for the performance of each procedure are to be assigned by the instructor. (See also pp. 32 and 35.)

1. Given the required supplies and equipment, obtain blood samples from the patient by performing a fingertip skin puncture and a venipuncture. Then record these procedures on the patient's chart.
2. Having obtained a capillary blood sample in a nonheparinized capillary tube, perform a copper sulfate relative density test, and record the results on the patient's chart.
3. Having obtained a capillary blood sample in a heparinized capillary tube, perform a hematocrit test using the microhematocrit centrifuge, and record the results on the patient's chart.
4. Given a blood sample and a Dextrostix, test the sample for the presence of glucose, and record the results on the patient's chart.

5. Having obtained a blood sample by performing a fingertip skin puncture, test the blood for the presence and amount of glucose using an Accu-Chek II and a Chemstrip bG; using a Glucoscan blood glucose meter and a Glucoscan test strip.

The student is expected to perform the above procedures with 100% accuracy.

PERFORMANCE CHECKLIST

Fingertip Skin Puncture to Obtain Blood Sample

1. Wash your hands.
2. Assemble the required equipment and supplies.
3. Identify the patient, and explain the procedure.
4. Select the correct site on fingertip.
5. ''Milk'' the finger gently along the sides.
6. Clean the puncture site with alcohol swab.
7. Allow the area to air dry.
8. Grasp the patient's finger on the sides near the fingertip.
9. Take the lancet to make a quick in-and-out puncture on the patient's fingertip. (Hold the lancet at a right angle to the lines on the patient's finger.)
10. Wipe off the first drop of blood with a clean sponge.
11. Using gentle pressure above the puncture site, allow the blood to flow freely.
12. Collect a blood sample in a pipette.
13. When more than one sample is required, wipe the finger with a clean cotton sponge between each sample collected to obtain fresh drops of blood each time.
14. Apply pressure to the puncture site with a dry cotton sponge.
15. Label the specimen(s) obtained; forward to the laboratory with a correct requisition.
16. Wash your hands.
17. Record on patient's chart.

Venipuncture to Obtain Blood Sample

1. Wash your hands.
2. Assemble the required equipment and supplies.
3. Identify the patient, and explain the procedure.
4. Have the patient seated with the arm well supported in a downward position.
5. Prepare equipment for use: attach the needle to the syringe, and label the tube(s) with the date and the patient's name.
6. Select the site for the venipuncture, and palpate the anterior cubital space.
7. Apply the tourniquet around the patient's arm, above the elbow. Palpate the vein again.
8. Cleanse the skin site with an alcohol sponge.
9. Draw skin over the puncture site until tense.
10. Gently and slowly insert the needle into the vein.
11. Slowly pull on the plunger of the syringe to withdraw blood; release tourniquet as soon as blood flows into the syringe.

12. When the sample has been drawn, place a dry sterile sponge over the puncture site and withdraw the needle.
13. With this sponge, apply pressure over the puncture site for a few minutes. (You may have the patient do this.)
14. With the sponge in place and still applying pressure, have patient elevate the arm for a few minutes more.
15. Remove the needle from the syringe and place the blood in the collection tube.
16. Cap the tubes, then gently invert tubes that contain an additive 8 to 10 times. *Do not shake these tubes.*
17. Apply a Band-Aid to the puncture site if required.
18. Destroy and discard disposable syringe and needle in designated containers.
19. Wash your hands.
20. Complete the laboratory requisition, and send with sample(s) drawn to the laboratory.
21. Record on patient's chart.

Copper Sulfate Relative Density Test

After obtaining the capillary blood sample in a nonheparinized capillary tube:

1. Hold capillary tube vertically over the container of copper sulfate solution, allowing blood to drop into this solution.
2. If blood does not drop freely into the solution, apply the bulb to the capillary tube, then squeeze the bulb to force blood into the solution.
3. Determine the results.
4. Record the results on the patient's chart.

Hematocrit

After obtaining a capillary blood sample in a heparinized capillary tube:

1. Seal the dry end of the tube by sticking it into the Crito-seal clay tray.
2. With the sealed end down, place the tube into a slot in the microhematocrit centrifuge.
3. Close and secure the lid of the centrifuge.
4. Adjust the timer, and spin down for 5 minutes.
5. Read the results using the scale provided on the centrifuge, or use the microhematocrit card to read the results.
6. Wash your hands.
7. Record the results as a percentage.

Test for Blood Glucose Using a Dextrostix

Given a blood sample and a Dextrostix:

1. Place a large drop of blood on the test area of the strip.
2. Holding the strip horizontally, wait exactly 60 seconds.
3. Holding the strip vertically, wash the blood off with

a sharp stream of water from a wash bottle; 1 to 2 seconds is sufficient time.

4. Compare the color on the test area to the color chart on the bottle.
5. Read and record the results in mg/100 ml of blood.
6. Wash your hands.

Test for Blood Glucose Using the Accu-Chek II and Chemstrip bG

1. Wash your hands.
2. Assemble the equipment.
3. Identify the patient and explain the procedure.
4. Turn the meter on by pressing the ON/OFF button once.
5. Lay the Chemstrip bG test strip on a flat work surface with test pads facing up.
6. Perform a skin puncture on the patient's fingertip.
7. Lightly touch the blood drop to the test pads on the Chemstrip bG strip. Do not smear the blood. Completely cover both pads.
8. Press the TIME button on the meter. The meter will count to 60.
9. When the display reads 60 seconds, wipe the blood from the test pads with a clean, dry cotton ball using moderate pressure. Do not leave any blood on the test pads.
10. While the meter is counting to 120 seconds, turn the test strip on its side with the test pads facing the ON/OFF button and insert the reacted test strip into the test strip adaptor. *The strip must be inserted before the display reads 120.*
11. When the display reads 120, a high beep will be emitted, followed by the blood glucose value displayed in mg/dl. Read the blood glucose value on the display screen.
12. Record the results.

13. Turn the meter off. Remove the test strip from the meter.
14. Attend to the patient.
15. Clean and replace equipment in storage area.

Test for Blood Glucose Using the Glucoscan 2000 or 3000 Blood Glucose Meter

1. Wash your hands.
2. Assemble required equipment and supplies.
3. Identify the patient and explain the procedure.
4. Turn the meter on.
5. Perform a skin puncture on the patient's fingertip. Turn the pricked area of finger downward. Squeeze firmly until a large hanging drop of blood forms.
6. Press START button on the meter and immediately apply the blood to the reagent pad.
7. Cover the entire pad with blood. Do not smear or rub blood on the pad.
8. Prepare to blot when the display reads 23. Invert test strip with reagent pad over the blotting paper. Do not touch the blood to the paper yet.
9. When the display reads 20 — press the pad straight down onto the blotting paper and blot for 2 seconds, then release.
10. Blot pad on a clean area of blotting paper for another 2 seconds.
11. Open the test strip door on the meter and insert the test strip into the test strip holder *any time* before the display counts down to 00.
12. Close the test strip door.
13. Test result will be displayed when the display reads 00. Record the result.
14. Attend to the patient.
15. Clean and replace equipment and supplies in the proper storage area.

Unit XII

Diagnostic Radiology, Radiation Therapy, and Nuclear Medicine

COGNITIVE OBJECTIVES

On completion of Unit XII, the medical assistant student should be able to apply the following cognitive objectives:

1. Define and pronounce the terms listed in the vocabulary and text of this unit.
2. Explain the medical specialties of diagnostic radiology, radiation therapy, and nuclear medicine, listing examples of procedures performed by each.
3. Explain the nature and purpose of the diagnostic and therapeutic procedures as outlined in this unit.
4. Define the term *contrast medium* as used in radiology; state the function of contrast media and list at least three examples of these.
5. List and explain the nature of at least 10 radiological procedures that use contrast media.
6. Discuss and distinguish between the special techniques of mammography, xeroradiography, thermography, positron emission tomography (PET), tomography, computed tomography (CT), ultrasonography, magnetic resonance imaging (MRI), digital radiography, and radiation therapy.
7. List and explain four basic positions used for proper exposure of the body part during radiography.
8. State and discuss the dangers, hazards, and safety precautions relevant to x-ray equipment and procedures.
9. List seven side effects that may be experienced by patients receiving high levels of radiation therapy.
10. List three body changes that may occur with overexposure to radiation.
11. Discuss the medical assistant's responsibilities relevant to radiological procedures.
12. List at least eight x-ray examinations that do and eight that do not require special patient preparation.
13. Describe and discuss the possession, care, and storage of reports and x-ray films received in the physician's office.
14. Describe and discuss the steps involved in the processing of x-ray films.

TERMINAL PERFORMANCE OBJECTIVES

On completion of this unit, the medical assistant student should be able to do the following terminal performance objectives.

1. Demonstrate proficiency in communicating proper preparation for x-rays to the patient.
2. Identify and demonstrate safety hazards and precautionary measures relevant to x-ray equipment.
3. Demonstrate the care and storage of the finished product when received in the physician's office.
4. Prepare and assist the patient for radiological procedures.
5. Position the patient correctly for different x-ray exposures (if licensed to do so).

The student is to perform the above activities with 100% accuracy 95% of the time.

Radiology Vocabulary

cassette (kah-set')—A light-proof aluminum or bakelite container with front and back intensifying screens, between which x-ray film is placed when used for x-ray examinations.
density—The quality of being dense or impenetrable.
detail—The sharpness of the radiograph image.
enema (en'ĕ-mah)—The introduction of a solution into the rectum; for an x-ray examination of the colon, a radiopaque solution is administered by enema.
fluoroscope (floo'or-o-skōp")—An instrument used during x-ray examinations for visual ob-

servation of the internal body structures by means of x-rays. The body part to be viewed is placed between the x-ray tube and a fluorescent screen. As x-rays pass through the body, shadowy images of the internal organs are projected on the screen.

fluoroscopy (floo"or-os'ko-pē)—Visual examination by means of a fluoroscope.

ionizing (i"on-i-zing) **radiation**—Radiant energy given off by radioactive atoms and x-rays.

irradiate (ĭ-rā'dē-āt)—To treat with radiant energy.

irradiation (i-rā"dē-ā'shun)—Exposure to radiation; the passage of penetrating rays through a substance or object.

oscilloscope (ŏ-sil'ō-skōp)—An instrument for visualizing the shape or wave form of sound waves, as in ultrasonography, or of electric currents, as when monitoring heart action and other body functions.

radiation (rā"dē-ā'shun)—Electromagnetic waves of streams of atomic particles capable of penetrating and being absorbed into matter. Examples of electromagnetic waves are x-rays, gamma rays, ultraviolet rays, infrared rays, and rays of visible light. Atomic particles are alpha and beta particles.

radiogram (rā'dē-ō-gram")—A picture of internal body structures produced by the action of gamma rays or x-rays on a special film.

radiograph (rā'dē-ō-graf") or **roentgenograph** (rent'gen-ō-graf) or **roentgenogram** (rent'gen-ō-gram")—The film or photographic record produced by radiography.

radiography (rā"dē-og'rah-fe)—The taking of radiograms.

radioisotope (rā"dē-ō-ī'so-tōp)—A radioactive form of an element consisting of unstable atoms that emit rays of energy or streams of atomic particles. Radioisotopes occur naturally, as in the case of radium, or can be created artificially, as in the case of cobalt.

radiologist (rā"dē-ol'o-jist)—A physician specialist in the study of radiology.

radiolucent (rā"dē-ō-lū-sent)—That which permits the partial or complete passage of radiant energy such as x-rays. Dense objects appear white on the x-ray film because they absorb the radiation. An example of this is bone.

radionuclide (rā"dē-ō-nū'klīd)—A radioactive substance.

radiopaque (rā-dē-ō-pāk')—That which is impenetrable by x-rays and other forms of radiant energy; matter that obstructs the passage of radiant energy, such as lead which is frequently used as a protective device.

voltage (vōl-tij)—The electromotive force measured in volts (the units of force for electricity to flow).

RADIOLOGICAL PROCEDURES

Radiology (rā"dē-ol'ō-jē) is the specialty of medical science that deals with the study, diagnosis, and treatment of disease by using x-rays, radioactive substances, and other forms of radiant energy such as gamma rays, ultraviolet rays, alpha and beta particles, and sound and magnetic waves.

The procedures involved in radiology can be divided into three specialties: diagnostic radiology, radiation therapy (radiation oncology), and nuclear medicine.

The equipment used for radiological procedures is very expensive and sophisticated; thus, most physicians requisition these examinations or therapy from outside sources, such as from a major treatment center, local hospital, or radiology office. However, some diagnostic radiology procedures, such as radiographs of the chest or skeletal fractures, may be performed in some larger offices or clinics or in physicians' offices in rural areas. It takes special training and great skill to do radiological procedures and for physicians to accurately interpret the fluoroscopic, scanning, and x-ray images formed. Skilled radiologic technologists, called radiographers, prepare and position the patient and take the x-ray images. These individuals must be registered nationally to practice. In addition, those who practice in California, New York, and 20 other states must also be licensed or certified by the state. The radiologist, a licensed physician specially trained in radiology, reads and interprets the films, scanning images, and fluoroscopic images.

For medical assistants to be well qualified and able to contribute to total patient care, it is imperative that they know the varied techniques, the purposes, and the nature of the specialized and highly technical radiology procedures. *Medical assistants are not legally allowed to perform radiological procedures (unless licensed and registered to do so).* Descriptions of various x-ray, fluoroscopic, and nuclear medicine studies follow.

X-RAYS

X-rays are also called roentgen rays, after the discoverer, Wilhelm Konrad Roentgen (1845-1923), a physicist at the University of Würzberg, Germany, in 1895. They are a form of radiation that consists of energy waves of very short wavelength. It is this extremely short wavelength that gives x-rays the special power of penetration. Although not visible to the human eye, x-rays can be captured on film as a visible image and can also be seen fluoroscopically by an image intensifier. The density of the matter at which x-rays are aimed and the voltage used determine the degree of penetration of x-rays.

X-rays, capable of penetrating the body completely or in varying degrees and also of changing the basic structure of cells of the body, are used beneficially in the diagnosis of conditions and in the treatment of tumors and other medical conditions, such as blood malignancies.

Various types of equipment are used for radiological procedures. The equipment used for diagnostic procedures is of lower voltage than that used for radiation therapy.

DIAGNOSTIC RADIOLOGY

By exposing body parts to x-rays, diagnostic radiological procedures create images on films or views on the fluoroscope and/or on videotape or videodisc that enable the physician to view the internal structures and functions of the body to pinpoint disease or anomalies. The observations made are then interpreted by the physician-radiologist, who then dictates the findings and radiologic diagnosis. The findings interpreted from these procedures help the physician make a diagnosis or evaluate ongoing treatment; they are also used to determine the effectiveness of a treatment program after therapy has been completed. In addition to the routine chest or skeletal films, there are many special diagnostic procedures and techniques that reveal more specific information about the function and structure of an organ.

Fluoroscopy: Image Intensification

Fluoroscopy, an image intensifier-television system, is an x-ray examination using an instrument that permits visual observation of deep structures of the body. X-rays from the x-ray tube pass through the patient's body and project shadowy images of organs and bones through an image intensifier. This information is fed to television monitors so that images can be readily observed during the procedure. Videotape and/or videodisc systems can record these images. This allows for playback during the procedure or after it has been completed. A permanent recording of the fluoroscopic image can be made on 35 mm film. This is called *cinefluorography* and occurs simultaneously with television monitoring and/or image recording on a videotape and/or videodisc unit.

The major advantage of the fluoroscope over the usual type of x-ray film is that the action of organs, joints, or entire body systems can be observed in motion. The use of a contrast medium during fluoroscopy may be necessary in some procedures utilizing this system.

Contrast Medium Techniques

A contrast medium is a radiopaque substance that is used in diagnostic radiology to permit a more accurate visualization of internal body parts and tissues in contrast to their adjacent structures.

Contrast media include liquids, powders, gas, air, or pills; these are administered orally, parenterally (by injection), or through an enema, each being specific for the examination of a particular organ or structure. The contrast medium opacifies the body part(s) under examination. Thus, the structure and functions of the organ(s) can be observed and studied through x-ray films or fluoroscopy. Artificial positive contrast media include barium sulfate and iodine compounds. Because these media have more density, they absorb more of the radiation. They will appear white on x-ray images. Negative contrast media include air, gas, and carbon dioxide. They appear black on x-ray images.

Barium Sulfate. This is a chalky compound, now available commercially in a premixed flavored (such as cherry) liquid or paste. Often x-ray departments will buy the powder form and mix it with water to the desired consistency.

Barium sulfate is an opaque medium used for two main types of x-ray and fluoroscopic examinations of the gastrointestinal (GI) tract. A barium meal or upper GI series is the oral ingestion of the barium mixture to outline the esophagus, stomach, and if ordered, the small intestine, depending on the physician's request. A barium enema (BE), or lower GI series, outlines the colon for study after the instillation of the barium mixture through an enema. On occasion, a third examination, a barium swallow, is done to outline the esophagus (after the oral ingestion of the barium mixture) (Figs. 12-1 and 12-2).

Iodine Compounds. Containing up to 50% and more iodine, these radiopaque contrast media are used for the following tests on various body systems. If the patient is allergic to iodine, these examinations should not be performed. Other diagnostic techniques may then be employed. The iodinated contrast media used for these procedures will interfere with thyroid studies performed by the nuclear medicine department; therefore, these procedures should not be performed when the patient is having thyroid function tests.

> **angiogram**—X-ray record of blood vessels after injecting a contrast medium through a catheter inserted in the appropriate vessel (arteriogram, lymphangiogram, phlebogram) (Fig. 12-3).
> **angiocardiogram**—X-ray record of the heart and great vessels after injecting a contrast medium into a large peripheral vein or into a chamber of the heart by direct heart catheterization.

Fig. 12-1.   Upper gastrointestinal barium study done under fluoroscopic control by radiologist and technologist. (Courtesy Picker Corporation, Cleveland, OH)

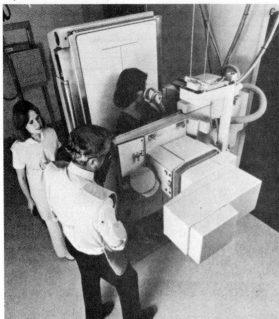

Fig. 12-2.   Physicians viewing gastrointestinal x-ray films.

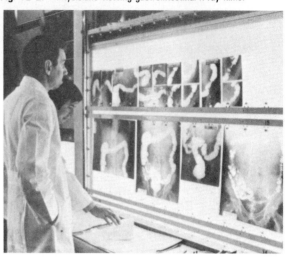

Fig. 12-3.   Vascular procedures suite. Patient is shown positioned for cerebral angiogram via femoral approach. Automatic injector and bilateral automatic film changers are employed. (Courtesy Picker Corporation, Cleveland, OH)

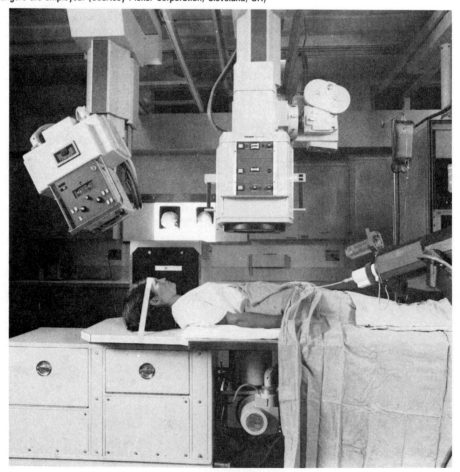

arteriogram—X-ray record of an artery or arterial system after injecting a contrast medium through a catheter inserted in an artery.

arthrogram—X-ray record of a joint after injecting a contrast medium into the joint.

bronchogram—X-ray record of the bronchial tree and lungs after instillation of a contrast medium into the bronchi via the trachea with a special instrument. This procedure is almost extinct since the introduction of the new, more sophisticated modalities.

cerebral angiogram—X-ray record of the cerebral vessels after injecting a contrast medium into the common carotid artery; for x-ray records of the vessels in the posterior fossa or the occipital lobes, the medium is injected into the vertebral artery in the neck.

cholecystogram*—X-ray record of the gallbladder after oral injestion of radiopaque granules or tablets taken the evening before the examination.

diskogram—X-ray record of the vertebral column after injecting a contrast medium into an intervertebral disk. This procedure is done infrequently.

hysterosalpingogram—X-ray record of the uterus and fallopian tubes after injecting a contrast medium through the vagina into the uterus.

intravenous cholangiogram*—X-ray record of the bile ducts after injecting a contrast medium intravenously. The contrast medium is excreted by the liver into the bile ducts; x-ray films are taken at intervals as the contrast medium is excreted through the hepatic, cystic, and common bile duct into the duodenum.

intravenous pyelogram (IVP)—X-ray records taken at intervals after intravenous injection of a contrast medium at intervals to observe the excretion rate and the concentration of the dye in the renal pelves and the outline of the ureters and urinary bladder.

lymphangiogram—X-ray record of the lymphatic vessels after the injection of a contrast medium into the lymphatic system.

myelogram—X-ray record of the spinal cord after injection of a water-soluble or an oily contrast medium into the subarachnoid space through a lumbar puncture needle.

retrograde pyelogram—X-ray record of the urinary tract after introduction of a contrast medium through a urinary catheter into the ureters and pelves of the kidneys.

urogram—X-ray record of any part of the urinary tract after intravenous injection of a contrast medium. See also intravenous pyelogram.

---

*In most facilities these procedures have been replaced by ultrasound examinations (sonography) of the gallbladder and bile ducts.

Air, Oxygen (O₂) and Carbon Dioxide (CO₂).   Since the introduction of computed tomography and magnetic resonance imaging (see pp. 373–376), the frequency with which these negative contrast media have been used for cerebral pneumography (pneumoencephalography and pneumoventriculography) in radiology departments has essentially disappeared. Still at times these negative media can be used for examination of the spinal cord, joints, and in combination with barium sulfate during a barium enema. Oxygen is rarely used. Carbon dioxide is used most frequently, as it is absorbed by the body faster than air or oxygen, thus limiting the duration of headaches that may follow a myelogram.

> **arthrogram**—X-ray record of a joint after injecting air or other gas into the articular capsule. Air can be combined with an iodine compound for double contrast studies.
>
> **myelogram**—X-ray record of the spinal cord after the injection of air or gas (carbon dioxide) into the subarachnoid space by means of a lumbar puncture.

Mammography

Mammography, an x-ray examination of the breast to identify breast lesions or tumors, involves detection of radiodense tissue or calcifications. Mammography is the most effective method for detecting early and curable breast cancer. The new dedicated mammographic units perform diagnostic x-ray examinations of the breast at radiation doses 5 to 10 times lower than the older units. Machines of this type provide enormous potential benefit for early cancer detection, and the minimal levels of radiation exposure have essentially removed any meaningful risk. Radiation physicists have estimated that the radiation risk of a low-dose mammogram may be equivalent to the lung cancer risk of smoking one cigarette. In addition, this "state-of-the-art" machine obtains magnified and grid images that can more optimally evaluate the young, dense, and small breast. Two films are taken from different angles: (1) the sitting or standing axillary, and (2) the sitting or standing craniocaudal views (Fig. 12-4).

To achieve diagnostic x-ray images of the breasts at extremely low radiation doses, the breast must be compressed firmly by a clear plastic plate. Many women find this uncomfortable but tolerable. Some women find breast compression intolerable. For women with painful, tender breasts, it is suggested that they (1) schedule the examination during the time in the menstrual cycle when the breasts are least tender. This corresponds to the first 10 days of the cycle for many women; (2) avoid caffeine-containing products such as coffee, tea, chocolate, cocoa, and soft drinks for 1 week before the examination; (3)

Fig. 12-4. **A,** technologist positioning patient for right craniocaudal view of breast for mammography. **B,** x-ray of female breast (mammography) showing entire breast back to rib cage. (Courtesy Picker Corporation, Cleveland, OH)

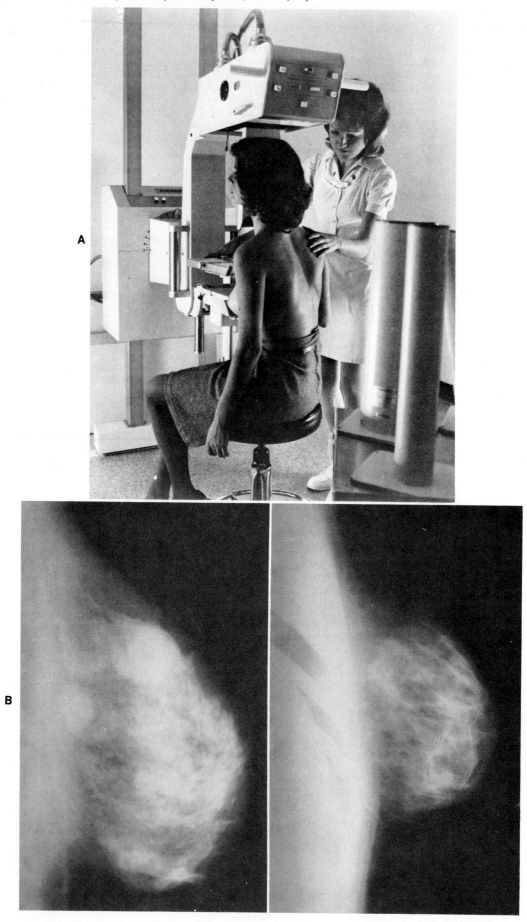

verbally cooperate with the radiographer to mutually arrive at a degree of compression that is tolerable to them and consistent with the technical requirements of the examination. The patient should be asked not to wear any powder or deodorant on the day of the examination, as these products sometimes show up as artifacts on the x-ray images.

The American Cancer Society recommends that "women without symptoms of breast cancer, ages 35 to 39, should have one mammogram for the record; women age 40 to 49 should have a mammogram every 1 to 2 years, and women age 50 and over, once a year. All women are advised that monthly breast self-examination is an important health habit." (See Unit III.)

Xeroradiography

Xeroradiography uses a dry electrophotographic technique to produce images on specially treated xerox paper. This system, used mostly for mammography, can also be used to obtain x-ray images in small areas in soft tissue and some bone. In general xeroradiography compares favorably with the radiation dose the patient receives from other film-screen recording systems. The major advantages over a conventional film-screen system is its ability to outline or enhance the edges of a density, for example, bone, tumors, or foreign bodies such as glass.

Thermography

Thermography is a heat-sensing technique used in the detection of breast tumors. Essentially, an apparatus makes a photographic image of the varying skin temperatures. Body areas that are warm appear light; cool areas appear dark; and medium temperature areas appear gray on the thermogram. Localized skin temperature elevations, such as occur over inflammatory or malignant lesions, are then sharply delineated against the temperatures of the surrounding tissues.

Though research continues, *the majority opinion is that thermography is not a sufficiently reliable procedure to use for screening or detecting breast cancer.* Thus it is *not recommended* and is *seldom used* now except in institutions continuing investigative work. X-ray mammography is the superior diagnostic tool for detecting breast cancer.

Tomography

Tomography, or sectional roentgenography, has a special ability to penetrate dense shadows. X-ray pictures are taken in sections at different depths in the patient's body, focusing on the plane of the structure

to be studied. Structures in front of and behind the plane under examination are blurred out.

Because of this, tomography can be a valuable diagnostic procedure when a definitive diagnosis cannot be made from conventional radiographs. Used to demonstrate and evaluate a number of different disease processes, traumatic injuries, and congenital abnormalities, tomography can be used in any part of the body, but is most effective in areas of high contrast, such as in the lungs and bones. One of the most frequent uses is to demonstrate and evaluate benign and malignant processes in the lungs.

Although computed tomography (CT) and magnetic resonance imaging (MRI) (see below through p. 376) have replaced the use of tomography to a great extent, there are still times when tomography is the examination of choice. Many hospitals do not have the CT and MRI units because of the high cost. Also the cost to the patient is much higher for a CT or MRI examination. Tomography can often provide a satisfying diagnosis or at least screen the patient for further evaluation by the other more sophisticated modalities.

Positron Emission Tomography (PET)

Positron emission tomography is a computerized radiographic technique that uses radiopharmaceuticals (radioactive substances) to examine the metabolic activity of various body structures. The patient either inhales or is injected with a radiopharmaceutical. The computers and electronic circuitry of the PET device detect and convert gamma rays into color-coded images which indicate the intensity of the metabolic activity of the organ involved. Patients are exposed to very small amounts of radiation because the radioactive substances used are very short-lived. Presently PET is *used predominately as a research tool* to study blood flow and the metabolism of the heart and the blood vessels, and to determine local cerebral blood flow and the local cerebral metabolic rate of glucose. PET measures regional brain function that cannot be determined by any other diagnostic method including computed tomography (CT) and magnetic resonance imaging (MRI). Current PET studies are used for patients with epilepsy, brain tumors, Alzheimer's disease, a stroke, spasmodic torticollis, and other movement disorders.

Computed Tomography (CT Scan)

The CT scanner, the developers of which were awarded the Nobel Prize for medicine in October 1979, has been a most significant breakthrough in medical technology.

Computed tomography is an advanced radiological modality that provides valuable clinical information in the early detection, differentiation, and demarcation of diseases of the head and body. It often provides diagnostic information that cannot be obtained by any other method, especially in neurological work.

Quick and noninvasive, the CT scan is particularly helpful in solving problems where there is conflicting information from other radiological or laboratory studies, and may be necessary for planning radiation therapy for certain tumor masses. Its use has frequently replaced some examinations, such as echoencephalography (see Diagnostic Ultrasound) and others, many of which carry greater risk and discomfort to the patient, such as the pneumoencephalogram and arteriogram. In addition, computed tomography does, in certain cases, replace procedures that would require the patient to be hospitalized. This technique is employed for neurological procedures;

to detect cerebral abnormalities, for example, tumors, lesions, hematomas, and bleeding in the brains of newborn infants; to search for childhood cancer; to detect masses in the chest, abdominal, and pelvic cavities; and to examine the liver, spleen, pancreas, kidneys, adrenal glands, pituitary gland, optic nerve, and for a generalized survey for lymphoma or metastases (Fig. 12-5).

Machines called scanners (such as ACTA, CT/T, Synerview, Delta, Syntex) beam x-rays to scan the body site in a series of x-rays. The scanner combines the capabilities of traditional x-ray with that of a computer, providing an image of soft tissue in three dimensions. The x-ray tube and detector source rotate 360 degrees around the patient's head or body part being studied, taking multiple "slices" — cross-sectional readings. Thus every tissue and organ is x-rayed from all sides. As they pass through the body, the absorption rates of the x-rays are detected, and the density of the tissue is relayed to the computer. From the calculations performed by the computer, densities are translated into a picture of the body as if it were neatly cut into slices, each a fraction of an inch thick. This picture is projected on a screen for the radiologist to study (Fig. 12-6).

The conventional x-ray film reveals only certain organs and tissues, and requires multiple exposures to estimate the size and location of diseased areas. The CT scanner can distinguish nearly every type of tissue and has the ability to distinguish more minute differences in the various tissues. CT can determine the size and location of any pathologic condition with great accuracy. When first developed around the midseventies, the CT scans were slow, but now many machines in use can complete a scan in 4 to 5 seconds, and a more sophisticated machine can complete a scan in 1 second. Nevertheless, one of the limitations of CT is that it takes 15 to 30 minutes or longer to complete all the slices required for a complete examination. Thus most CT scanners can only be used for 15 to 20 examinations during an 8-hour work day.

Minimal patient preparation is required for CT scans. Some facilities require the patient to have nothing by mouth for 4 hours before the examination if a contrast medium is used. For abdominal and pelvic scans the patient preparation is usually the same as the one used for a barium enema (see p. 369). When a contrast medium is not used, no patient preparation is required. A contrast medium can be administered orally or intravenously.

Research is continuing for a scanner that can make clear x-ray images of the fast-beating human heart. Some researchers are presently testing it as a noninvasive method to determine whether vein grafts installed in a coronary bypass surgery are allowing blood to flow freely or have become closed and useless. The National Aeronautics and Space Administration (NASA) is also interested in this device, as it may

Fig. 12-5. **A,** technologist positioning patient for head scan with computed tomography total body scanner. **B,** control room for the CT scanner. The x-ray generation controls, scanning control console, and viewing monitors are found here. Main computer hardware is usually located in adjacent room.

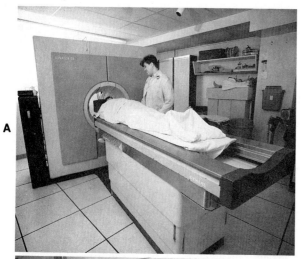

A

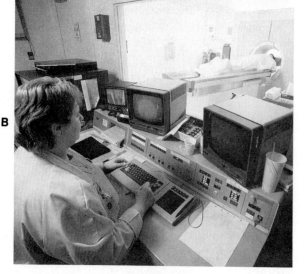

B

Fig. 12-6. Images from CT head, body, and spine scans. (Courtesy General Electric Co., Medical Systems Division, Milwaukee, WI)

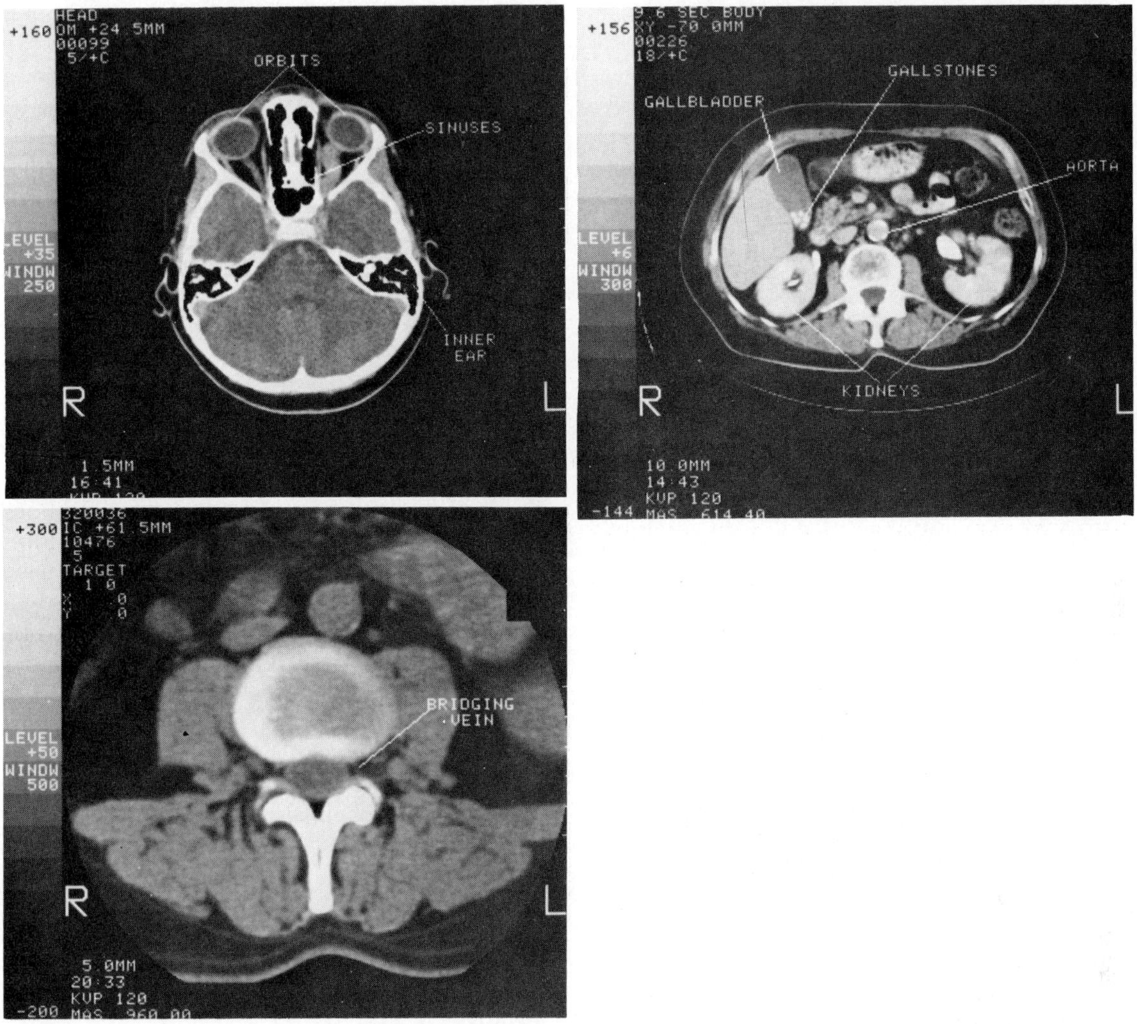

be valuable in detecting the loss of calcium in bones, a serious consequence of weightlessness in space travel.

Although the use of the CT scan is superior in numerous situations, at times the findings obtained do indicate the need for additional and invasive procedures so that a conclusive diagnosis can be established.

Magnetic Resonance Imaging (MRI)

A newer and equally exciting form of imaging technique for examining the body is the MR. Magnetic resonance is a computer-based, cross-sectional imaging modality that examines the interactions of magnetism and radio waves with tissue to obtain its images. Magnets, as the name suggests, are at the heart of this system. Many machines use superconducting magnets, as the more powerful the magnets, the clearer the images produced.

There are major advantages to the MR. It can examine properties of body tissue that have never before been visualized. Both anatomic and physiologic information can be obtained. No x-rays, that is no ionizing radiation of any kind, are used to obtain the MR image. It is a painless and noninvasive technique. There are no known harmful effects to the patient when exposed to the current levels of magnetic field strength and radiowave energy transmission.

Magnetic resonance is used to detect tumors in soft tissues because even in early stages malignant tissue responds to the magnetic pull differently from normal tissue. No other imaging technique can detect such subtle differences in soft tissues. It is also used to examine the brain (it can distinguish brain tumors from tiny blood clots and determine the chemical changes that cause dementia in the elderly); spinal cord tumors, cystic changes of the spine, and disc disease; the gastrointestinal tract; the heart muscle, septal defects and cardiac valve leaflets; the lungs; the extremities (but bone lesions and calcium within tumors are seen better with CT); tumors of the liver and spleen; pelvic structures, e.g., bladder tumors, neoplasms in the female genital tract; it may detect prostate tumors; and it can outline the kidneys, adrenal glands, and retroperitoneal structures such as lymph nodes (although there is limited evidence that MR is superior to CT in this area).

However, MRI has its limitations. It can't see the hard part of the bones, so we still need x-rays, CT, or other techniques to diagnose fractures and malformations in bones. Also the strong magnetic field is potentially dangerous to patients with cardiac pacemakers and to those patients who have any type of metallic implants in them, such as aneurysm clips on blood vessels within the skull or clips tying off other blood vessels. The pull of the magnets could slip the clips out of place, and vessels could be torn. It is therefore important to check that the patient does not have a pacemaker or metallic implants before a MR is scheduled.

The image produced by the computer can be viewed on a television monitor. If desired, the images can be photographed for further study. These images can also be stored on a computer disk temporarily and then transferred to magnetic tape for permanent storage and retrieval.

The explosion of MR technology within the last decade still leaves questions on how far-reaching its applications will be and on the proof of its superior nature over other imaging modalities.

Digital Radiography

Digital radiography is the use of the conventional image intensifier-television system (fluoroscopy) in which the television signal is first digitized (information is stored in computer units called bits) and processed by the computer before the x-ray image is displayed on a standard television monitor.

The use of digital radiography has been successful in angiography. This procedure can replace the more complex and time-consuming procedure of arterial catheterization. Four advantages of this procedure are that it is safer for the patient, less painful, uses a lower x-ray dose and a much smaller amount of contrast medium.

A contrast medium is injected through a catheter that is placed into a vein, preferably the basilic vein, or alternately in the cephalic vein or the superior vena cava. As the x-ray images are taken they are formed electronically and displayed on the television monitor. At the same time, the image is stored on a videotape, videodisc, or digital disk.

Digital angiography is used for head and neck angiograms, and images of the pulmonary arteries and cardiac structures. Hospitalization of the patient is not required.

As digital radiographic devices and procedures expand, traditional studies in which film processing has been used will gradually be replaced by digital image processing.

Diagnostic Ultrasound

Diagnostic ultrasound, sometimes called diagnostic medical sonography or ultrasonography, does not utilize ionizing radiation to diagnose or treat disease, but uses very high frequency inaudible sound waves that bounce off the body to record information on the structure of internal organs.

In this examination, the patient's skin is covered with water, oil, or a special jelly that helps conduct the sound waves into the body. A special instrument emitting sound waves is placed and moved on or near the patient's skin. Sound waves pass through the skin, strike the body tissues, and pass an echo reflection back to the instrument. These ultrasonic echoes are then recorded on the oscilloscope as a picture of a series of dots. This record produced is called an echogram or sonogram. The method of image recording in which the data is stored on film, paper, or other recording material is called the hard copy.

Ultrasound can be used to detect abnormalities in the heart (echocardiography), major blood vessels, kidneys, abdominopelvic cavity, breast, scrotum, muscles, spine, and brain (echoencephalogram [EECG], although this has now been replaced by the CT scan, when available, because of the superiority of the CT images of the entire cranial vault versus very limited knowledge available from the EECG). It is also used to determine the presence of a pregnancy if other tests are unsuccessful, to differentiate between single and multiple pregnancies, or to view placental position, various stages, and fetal positions during pregnancy, and for neonate examinations (Figs. 12-7 and 12-8). In some procedures body structures, such as the diaphragm, cardiac or fetal heart motion, or other organ structures that move with respiration, are visible as they change position in time.

Ultrasound has the advantages of being a painless, noninvasive procedure that does not expose the patient to ionizing radiation. After 30 years of use, physicians have found no evidence that diagnostic ultrasound causes any untoward biological effect. Therefore, it has generally been accepted as a safe technique.

Ultrasound is also used for treatment in physical medicine (by physical therapists) for deep muscle or tension pain. In this case a different machine with a different soundwave intensity is used. This is discussed in the physical therapy unit.

Other Diagnostic Radiological Examinations

Abdomen. A survey film (flat plate) of the abdomen is ordered without the use of a contrast medium when abnormal conditions of the abdomen are suspected.

Fig. 12-7. **A,** Sectorview ultrasound system for scanning abdominal organs. (Courtesy Picker Corp., Cleveland, OH) **B,** ultrasound system for scanning abdominal organs. (Courtesy Picker Corp., Cleveland, OH) **C,** ultrasound system for scanning abdominal organs. (Courtesy General Electric Co., Medical Systems Division, Milwaukee, WI)

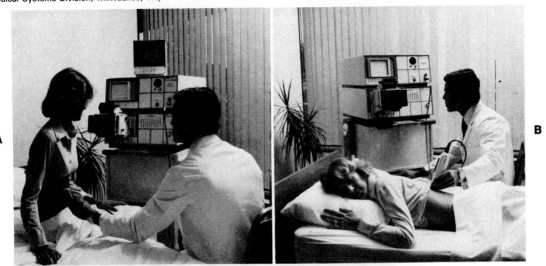

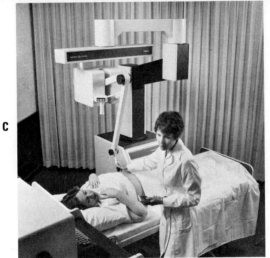

such as tumors, abscesses, enlarged or perforated organs, or hematomas.

In the plain survey, three films are often taken. The patient may be placed in the erect, supine, prone, or lateral decubitus position, depending on the suspected pathological condition to be studied (Fig. 12-9).

Routine Chest X-Ray Film. An x-ray record of the chest is obtained with the patient in the posteroanterior erect position. Generally, a lateral view is also taken (Fig. 12-10).

KUB (Kidney, Ureter, Bladder). A flat plate of the abdomen is used to study the kidneys, flank area, gas pattern, abdominal wall, bones of the pelvis, and any unusual masses.

Skull Series. A series of radiographs of the skull is used to determine cranial injuries or the effects of trauma to the head and neck. Computed tomography has replaced the use of these films except in cases of severe trauma.

Paranasal Sinuses Films. X-ray records are made of the paired sinuses within the frontal, ethmoid, sphenoid, and maxillary bones of the face.

Bone X-Ray Films. X-ray records are made of bones suspected of disease or trauma, such as tumors and fractures or displacement. X-ray studies of the vertebral column are common. Radiographs of the neck are referred to as cervical x-ray films; those of the middle back are referred to as thoracic x-ray films; and those of the lower back are referred to as lumbosacral x-ray films (Fig. 12-11).

Fig. 12-8.   Obstetrical ultrasound.

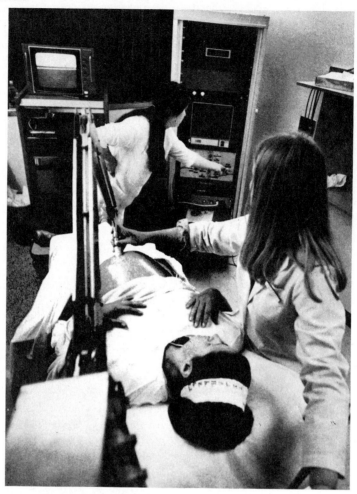

Fig. 12-9.   Radiologic technologist performing routine radiographic work (for example, pelvis or abdomen) with overhead tube mount. (Courtesy Picker Corp., Cleveland, OH)

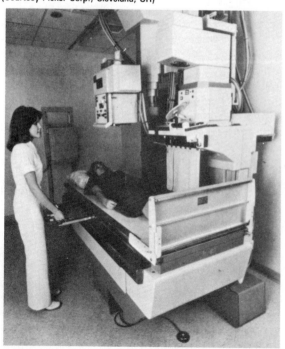

RADIATION THERAPY

It is desirable for the medical assistant to have some knowledge of radiation therapy, because patients who are to receive or have experienced this may ask questions of the medical assistant. When radiation is applied for treatment of cancer and various other conditions by x-rays, alpha, beta, and gamma rays, and other radioactive substances, it is called radiation therapy, radiotherapy, or radiation oncology, the purpose being to administer a definite amount of radiation to a specific location to irradiate diseased cells. Radiation therapy alters the diseased cell so that it cannot reproduce and will eventually age and die, leaving no new cells behind. Only the most extreme dose of radiation will kill the cells directly.

The amount of energy that is deposited within the tissue and the condition of the biologic system determine the effectiveness of ionizing radiation in living tissue. The radiosensitivity of most tissues is dependent on

• The number of undifferentiated (lack or absence of normal cell differentiation) cells in the tissue.

Fig. 12-10.   Physician interpreting and dictating the results of a chest x-ray film. (Courtesy General Electric Co., Medical Systems Division, Milwaukee, WI)

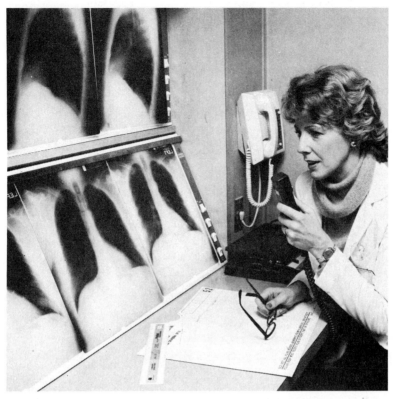

Fig. 12-11.   Pediatrics orthopedic patient having recheck film of left forearm in cast, utilizing power-driven, cordless, mobile x-ray unit. Note protective apron that technologist is wearing. (Courtesy Picker Corp., Cleveland, OH)

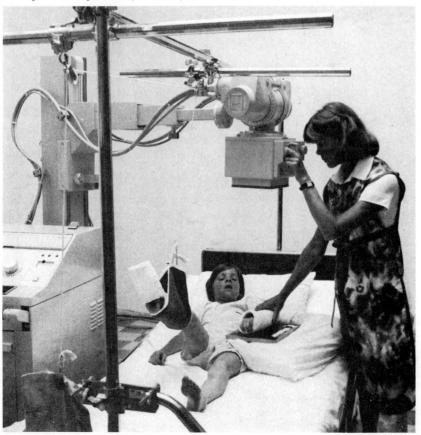

- The degree of mitotic activity (cell division that produces new cells) of the tissue. It is during mitosis that human cells are most sensitive to radiation.
- The length of time that cells of the tissue continue to reproduce.

The primary target of ionizing radiation is the DNA molecule in the human cell.

Certain tumors are more radiosensitive than others. Some that are highly radiosensitive include tumors of the ovaries and testes, lymphomas, Wilms' tumor of the kidney, retinoblastomas, and Hodgkin's disease. Those that are moderately radiosensitive include basal and squamous cell carcinomas of the skin, and adenocarcinoma of the prostate. Tumors that are relatively *radioresistant* include sarcomas of the bone, connective tissue, and muscle, and nerve tumors.

Certain sources of radioactivity are used for specific types or locations of cancer. Radium, for example, gives off rays (alpha, beta, and gamma) that affect the growth of tissue. In the form of seeds or needles (radium implants), radium can be implanted directly into a malignant tumor in the uterus or mouth for a prescribed period of time (possibly 3 to 4 days) to act on and destroy abnormal cells. This is called interstitial treatment. Permanent implant therapy may also be done using radon 222 seeds and iodine 125 seeds. These implants are left in the patient forever. Radioisotopes of cobalt can also be used for implantation in addition to teletherapy or possible surgery. Teletherapy is radiation treatment administered by a radioactive isotope, such as cobalt-60 or cesium-137, emitting high-energy gamma rays. These are housed in shielded units, similar to large x-ray units, which are placed at a distance from the patient. A beam of gamma radiation is aimed at the specific part of the body requiring treatment. Radiotherapy of this type is especially useful in the treatment of deep-seated malignancies not readily accessible for implantation. Radioisotopes are also available in a liquid form that can be used for local irradiation in the pleural or peritoneal cavities and also for the thyroid gland. The use of radiation therapy in cancer is based on the fact that cancer cells are more sensitive to x-rays and other radioactive substances than other cells in surrounding normal tissue.

Ionizing radiation affects both normal and diseased cells. The dose of radiation administered should be sufficient to treat the diseased area, but not so great that it would permanently damage the surrounding normal tissues. Treatment techniques are designed to deliver a precise dose to the tumor while limiting the amount of radiation to the uninvolved portions of the tissue. Greater damage occurs to the abnormal cells because more of these cells are undergoing mitosis and are more poorly differentiated. Normal cells have a greater capability of repairing the resulting damage than do malignant cells. Low-voltage x-rays are used to treat conditions that require only surface penetration, such as skin lesions, whereas high-voltage radiation is used to treat deep-seated malignancies.

Effective treatment of cancer with radiation therapy depends on the following:

- The extent to which the disease has progressed
- The type of cells in the tumor
- The general health of the patient
- The location of the tumor
- The radiocurability of the tumor

For definitive treatment the cancer must be in a tissue that is more radioresistant than the tumor.

Approximately 70% of all newly diagnosed cancer patients are treated with radiation therapy. Radiation therapy may be the only treatment used for some cancers, such as cancer of the larynx, skin, oral cavity, nasopharynx, cervix (although surgery may be the preferred treatment for cancer of the cervix), and Hodgkin's disease and malignant lymphoma (chemotherapy may also be used here). Frequently surgical interventions or chemotherapy, or a combination of the two, are used in conjunction with radiation therapy for the treatment of cancer of the breast, uterus, lungs, and others. Other modalities such as computed tomography and ultrasonography are used to locate the tumor(s) and to localize the boundaries of organs not involved. After therapy these modalities can be used to record tumor regression and the effectiveness of the treatment program.

The advantageous role of radiation therapy for the treatment of cancer is well documented. It appears that it will continue to play an important and expanded role in the treatment of cancer.

NUCLEAR MEDICINE

Nuclear medicine is the medical specialty that deals with the diagnosis and treatment of disease processes with the use of radioactive substances, although it is employed predominantly for diagnostic purposes (Fig. 12-12). Radioactive pharmaceuticals are thought to be radionuclides, in which the nuclei of the atoms of that particular isotope are undergoing spontaneous disintegrations. These radionuclides are administered intravenously or orally to the patient or a radioactive gas may be inhaled. Sophisticated measuring equipment and imaging devices that are interfaced with computers are used. A radiosensitive instrument known as a gamma camera or scintillation probe maps the area to be studied. To obtain the information desired, the gamma camera remains stationary over the organ of interest. This instrument records an image relating to the patterns of radioactivity concentrated within the organ being studied by this method.

Fig. 12-12. Patient having nuclear medicine scan.

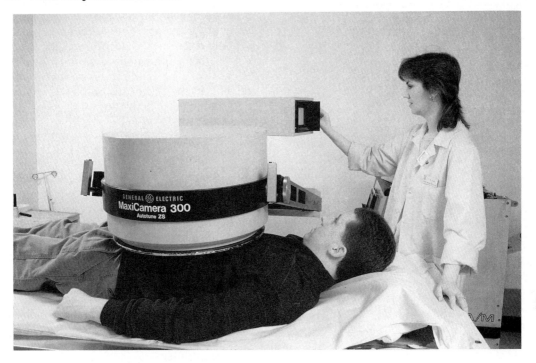

This image is called a scintigram or scintiscan and is used by the physician to diagnose tumors or other disease processes. The scintillation probe is used primarily in the evaluation of hyperthyroidism. The probe is placed in close proximity to the skin over the organ being studied and records the concentration of radioactivity within the organ by giving a numerical printout.

When a radionuclide is used to make a medical diagnosis, the physician refers to the concentration of radionuclides as being "hot spots" or "cold spots." If the radionuclide concentrates in an abnormality, it will be known as a hot spot within the scan; or, if the tumor does not concentrate the radionuclide, it will be known as a cold spot within the surrounding tissue that has concentrated the radioactive pharmaceutical. Hot spots or cold spots can both denote abnormality, depending on the organ being studied. All radionuclides used for diagnostic procedures are short-lived, which means that they remain radioactive only for a short time. Consequently, the radiation dose to the patient is small and usually does not cause any ill effects.

When radioisotopes are used in therapy doses, the effects are much like those seen when high-level radiation therapy is given to the patient. *The following are symptoms that may be seen when either radiation or radioisotope therapy is given:* loss of hair, shedding of skin, hemopoietic dysfunction, diarrhea, nausea, irritation of mucous membranes (such as in the mouth, throat, bladder, or vagina), and chromosomal changes.

Scanning Studies Used for Diagnosis

bone scan—Used to detect osteogenic sarcoma and its metastases, bone neoplasms, localized lesions for biopsy, osteomyelitis, stress fractures, and to evaluate arthritis and Paget's disease.

bone marrow scan—Used to detect hemolytic and iron deficiency, to detect decreased marrow function secondary to radiation therapy, and to measure the functional marrow reserve in patients on chemotherapy.

brain scan—Used to detect, localize, or follow the course of suspected or proved vascular malformations; inflammatory diseases, abscesses, cerebrovascular accidents, metastatic brain tumor, and subdural hematomas.

cardiac scan—Used to detect myocardial infarctions, and blood flow related to cardiac stress testing and cardiac artery stenosis. Sometimes used to evaluate pericardial effusion and localized ischemic scar damage.

hepatobiliary scan—Used to detect gallbladder patency and functioning.

kidney scan—Used to detect kidney disease, trauma, and tumors, and to evaluate hypertension. Used to study patients with demonstrated or suspected sensitivity to iodinated radiographic contrast media.

liver scan—Used to detect primary and metastatic malignancy, biliary obstruction, abscesses, and cysts; sometimes used for the evaluation of hepatitis or cirrhosis, hepatomegaly, jaundice, and rupture.

spleen scan—Used to detect splenomegaly and splenic rupture.

thyroid scan—Used to detect hyperthyroidism and the localization of nodules. Preoperative and postoperative scans are done for patients with thyroid carcinoma.

cisternogram—Used to localize cerebrospinal fluid leaks, "normal pressure" hydrocephalus, and evaluation of the functional status of ventricular shunts. This procedure is done rarely.

lung perfusion—Used to detect a pulmonary embolus.

lung ventilation—Used to detect a pulmonary embolus. This procedure is usually done with a lung perfusion. Ventilation is done first and may be followed with the lung perfusion.

white blood cell scan—Used to determine the source of an infection in questionable cases. The image shows where many of the labeled white blood cells (WBC) go, i.e., to the site of the infection.

All scans can usually be done on an outpatient basis. The medical assistant should be aware of any special preparation that is required of the patient be-

fore having the scan and the approximate time each scan takes so that the patient can be briefed on what to expect. Tables 12-1 and 12-2 outline the most common scans and time required for each. Similar reference sheets should be available in the physician's office for the medical assistant to refer to when necessary. (The medical assistant's responsibilities relating to the diagnostic studies presented in this unit, and similar tables for x-ray examinations, are given on pp. 387–390.)

POSITION OF PATIENT FOR X-RAY STUDIES

Radiograms are made by directing beams of x-rays through the x-ray tube toward a specific body part. The body part to be radiographed must be positioned correctly between the film-containing cassette and the x-ray source. The body part to be filmed is positioned closest to the cassette.

When the physician orders x-ray film to be taken, and when radiologists interpret the film, they will use special terms to designate the position or direction of the x-ray beam and the patient's position. Before the x-ray film is taken, markers are placed on the film-containing cassette to indicate the position used, the patient's identification, and the date (Figs. 12-13 and 12-14).

Table 12-1. Common scans that *do not* require special patient preparation, and approximate time required for each

Scan	Procedure	Approximate time required
Brain scan	IV (intravenous) injection and scan immediately. Wait 2 hr and take delayed scan.	Initial injection and flow study—15 min Delayed scan—45 min
Bone scan	IV injection done and wait 3 hr, then scan.	1 hr plus 3-hr interval
Bone marrow scan	IV injection and begin scan in 15 min.	1 hr
Cisternogram	Injection into lumbar subarachnoid space via lumbar puncture.	Following injection, scans are done at 6, 24, 48, and 72 hr intervals
Kidney and/or spleen scan	IV injection and scan immediately. For some kidney scans, hydration of patient will be necessary.	45–60 min
Liver scan	IV injection and wait 15 min for scan.	45 min
Lung perfusion scan	Inject and scan immediately.	45 min
Lung ventilation scan	Patient inhales radioactive xenon gas. Serial films are taken for 30 min while patient breathes inert xenon gas.	40 min
Thyroid scan*	IV injection of Technitium 99m and scan; or patient is given Iodine-123 orally and scanned either immediately or 4 to 24 hr later, respectively.	45 min
White blood cell scan	Draw 50cc blood; label WBC with Indium III, then inject cells back into patient. Scan 24 hr later.	60 min

*X-ray intravenous iodionated dyes will interfere with the thyroid studies and must not have been done within 3 months of study. Vitamins with iodine interfere with thyroid studies and must be discontinued for at least 2 weeks before study. Synthyroid or other thyroid medications must be stopped for at least 2 weeks before thyroid studies.

Table 12-2. Scans that *do* require special patient preparation, and the approximate time required for each

Scan	Procedure	Approximate time required
Cardiac scans	If patient is going to have Thallium-201 heart scan, there should be NPO (nothing by mouth) for at least 3 hr before examination. Other cardiac scans need no special preparation.	
Thallium-201 heart scan	Injection IV and scan immediately. Scan is done with patient on a treadmill and at 85% stress. Delayed 6 and 24 hr films.	
Pyrophosphate heart scan	IV injection and scan immediately; then 1½ and 3 hr delayed films.	30–45 min
Cardiac wall motion scan	IV injection and scan immediately.	30–45 min
Gallium scan	For tumor localization and abscess. Patient is NPO for 6 hr before 24 hr examination. Does not have to be NPO for initial injection. Injection is given IV, and scans are taken at following times: 6 hr, 24 hr, 48 hr, 72 hr.	
Gallium scan of chest (only)	No preparation necessary; scan in 6 hr and 24 hr only.	
Gallium scan of abdomen (all orders should be obtained from physician)	NPO from midnight on evening of injection. Barium enema preparation evening of examination. Tap water enemas until clear on morning of 24 hr examination. Each day after 24 hr film, patient to have 30 ml milk of magnesia (light laxative) at hour of sleep to continue until examination is completed.	
Hepatobiliary scan	NPO 2 hr before. IV injection, then scan immediately.	60 min

Basic Positions for Proper Exposure of Body Part

anteroposterior (AP)—The x-ray beam is directed from front to back. The patient may be in a supine or standing position, having the back near the film and the front facing the x-ray tube (Fig. 12-14).

posteroanterior (PA)—The x-ray beam is directed from back to front. The patient is usually in an upright position, having the back facing the x-ray tube and the front near the film (Fig. 12-15).

lateral—The x-ray beam is directed from one side. In the RL (right lateral) view, the right side of the body is near the film, and the x-ray tube is pointed toward the left side (Fig. 12-16). For the LL (left lateral) view, the left side of the body is nearest the film.

oblique—The x-ray beam is directed at an angle. These views are often used to outline areas that would be hidden and superimposed in the AP and PA views.

Terms to Describe the Patient's Position

supine—The patient is lying on the back, with face up (Fig. 12-9).

prone—The patient is lying on the abdomen, face downward.

recumbent—The patient is lying down.

Other Terms to Describe Direction of X-Ray Beam

axillary—The beam is directed toward the axilla.

mediolateral—The x-ray beam is directed from the midline toward the side of the part being filmed.

supine mediolateral—The patient is in the supine position, and the x-ray beam is directed from the midline toward the side.

craniocaudal—The x-ray beam is directed from the superior to inferior levels (from head to toe).

RADIOLOGICAL DANGERS, HAZARDS, AND SAFETY PRECAUTIONS

Dangers

X-rays do constitute a potential danger both to patients and health personnel; therefore, proper precautions must be taken at all times.

Massive or excessive exposure to radiation can cause tissue damage and various ill side effects (see pp. 381 and 384). Tissue destruction to diseased areas is aimed for in radiotherapy, but in diagnostic radiology exposure to radiation should be kept within safe limits, because radiation has a cumulative effect over a period of time. That is, the radiation a person receives today adds to the dose one will receive tomorrow, and these add to the dose one received yes-

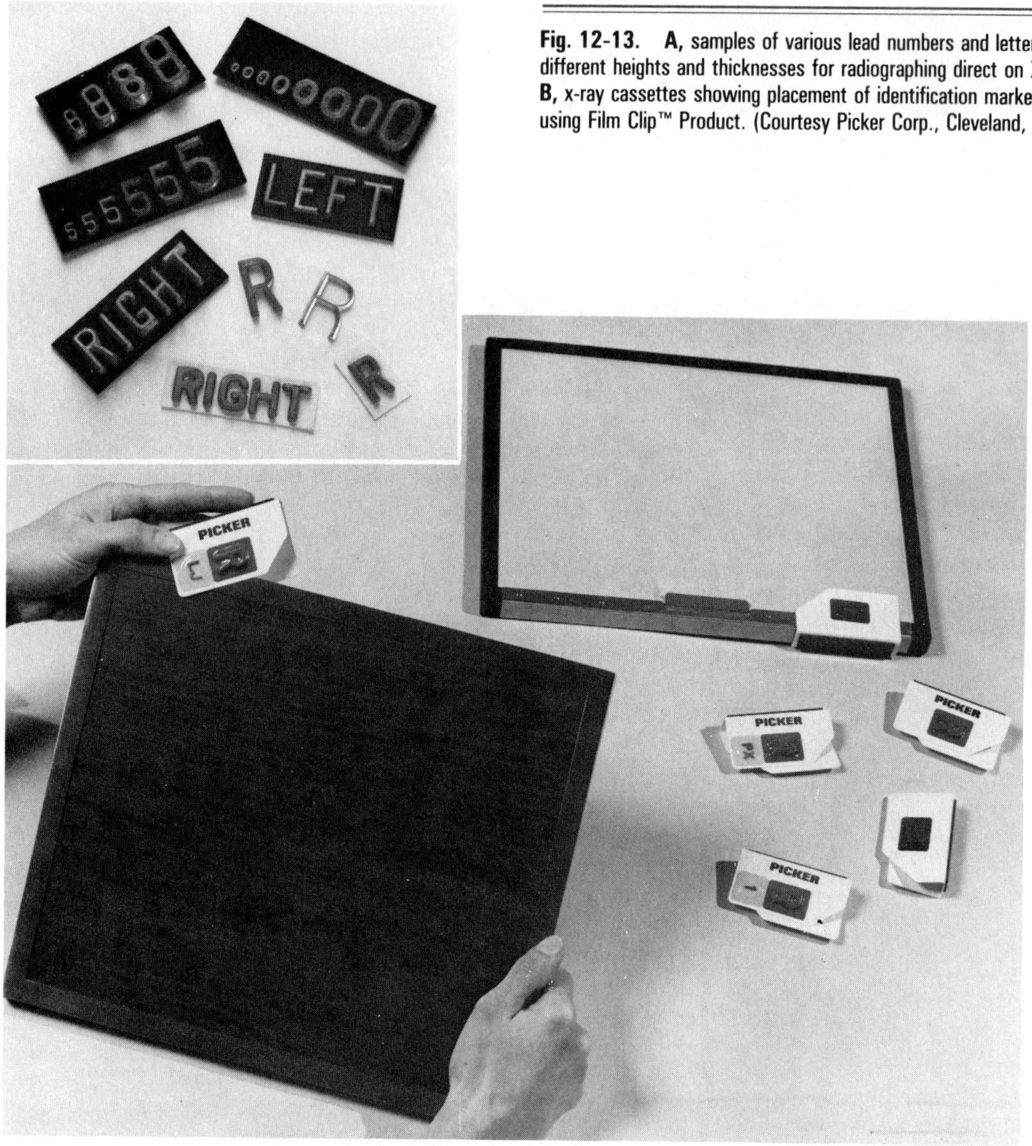

Fig. 12-13. **A,** samples of various lead numbers and letters in different heights and thicknesses for radiographing direct on X-ray film. **B,** x-ray cassettes showing placement of identification markers (lead) using Film Clip™ Product. (Courtesy Picker Corp., Cleveland, OH)

terday to accumulate a total radiation dosage. (Doses of radiation are measured in rads or rems or roentgens.) Thus everyone should avoid all unnecessary radiation exposure. On the other hand, patients must be helped to realize the importance of any radiological examination as an aid for the diagnosis and treatment of a disease process compared with the effects, if any, of the radiation dose that will be received. Newer machines and techniques currently used have significantly reduced the amounts of radiation exposure compared with the same examinations of 10 or more years ago.

When radiation goes beyond a safe limit, body tissues may begin to break down. Blood cells, skin, eyes, and reproductive cells are some of the tissues most sensitive to radiation. Overexposure to radiation can result in a lowered red blood cell and white blood cell count because of disturbances of bone marrow and other blood-forming organs; burns on the skin, and cancer; damage to the germinal cells in the ovaries and testes; and also damage to a fetus, especially in the first 3 months of pregnancy. Radiation also apparently predisposes individuals to the development of cataracts.

Studies have shown that massive and prolonged exposure to radiation can result in a higher incidence of cancer, especially of the lymph glands, and the various types of leukemia.

Hazards

Hazards of x-rays include the direct x-ray beam itself from the x-ray machine, which travels through an opening in the x-ray tube. Lead (which is able to stop x-rays from traveling) is in the x-ray tube housing to prevent the rays from escaping except through the opening.

Fig. 12-14.   Technologist placing cassette with patient in position to obtain an AP (anteroposterior) view. (Courtesy General Electric Co., Medical Systems Division, Milwaukee, WI)

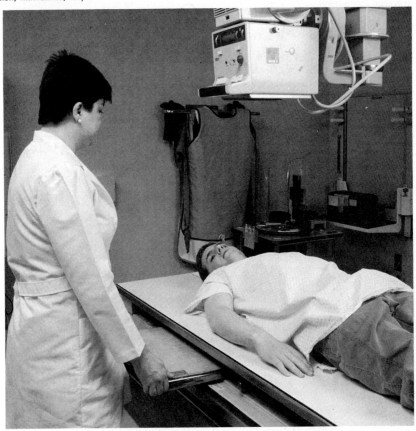

Fig. 12-15.   Patient in the PA (posteroanterior) position for chest x-ray film. (Courtesy General Electric Co., Medical Systems Division, Milwaukee, WI)

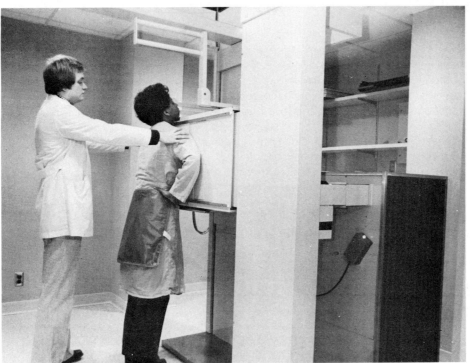

Fig. 12-16. Patient positioned for right lateral view of the chest (lung). (Courtesy Picker Corp., Cleveland, OH)

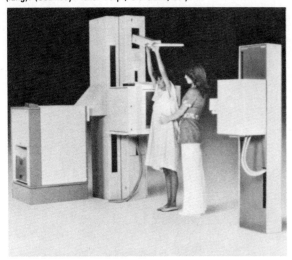

A second hazard is scattered radiation of two types: *Leakage radiation* is radiation that may escape (leak) from the head of x-ray machines, and this is dangerous to the operator. Therefore, frequent inspection of all x-ray equipment is to be performed by a licensed radiation physicist. Once the primary beam of radiation strikes and reacts on the patient or anything else in its path, it is then called *secondary radiation*, which can be emitted in all directions. Secondary radiation is radiation that has deviated from its original path, being strongest close to the patient. Therefore, distance is an important factor in radiation protection; that is, the further one is away from the patient, the better the protection one has from any form of radiation.

Lead screens or shields are used to separate x-ray personnel operating the controls of the machine from the patient receiving the radiation. These protect the personnel from secondary radiation. The walls of the x-ray room are also lined with lead, which absorbs secondary radiation when struck by it and thus prevents radiation from passing through the walls into adjacent areas, exposing others to the radiation. In most facilities, when x-ray machines are in use, a red light flashes on outside the room, indicating to others that radiation is being given and therefore they should not enter the room. In some facilities there are interlocking devices by which the door won't open when radiation is being used. Sometimes these devices interact with the x-ray equipment so that the machines won't work unless the door is locked.

Safety Precautions

X-ray personnel and medical assistants exposed to possible radiation can control the potential dangers by adhering to the following prescribed safety precautionary measures:

1. Have the equipment inspected frequently by a qualified person to assure that there is no leakage of radiation.
2. Stay behind the lead shield in a lead-lined room when the x-ray machine is being used.
3. Wear a lead apron and protective rubber-lead gloves if it is absolutely necessary to hold the patient or to remain in the room during any radiological procedure. On these occasions, always face the patient so that the lead apron is closest to the patient, or stay away from the patient. Never assume that you must hold or support the patient, and do not make this a routine. Certain techniques can be used to maintain the patient in the correct position.
4. Wear a film badge on outer clothing at the neck at all times when your job involves exposure to any type of radiation, including exposure to radionuclides. A film badge is a small device that contains x-ray film that is sensitive to radiation and thus records the level and intensity of radiation exposure, which is measured in rads, rems, or roentgens. These badges are to be submitted periodically (weekly in some facilities) to a film badge service for evaluation, thus providing a means for warning personnel when dangerous levels of radiation exposure are near.
5. Have a periodic blood count performed to determine if a blood dyscrasia is present. Blood counts do not measure the amount of radiation, but can indicate if there is any apparent radiation damage to blood cells.

To protect the patient from unnecessary radiation exposure, adhere to the following:

1. Before making arrangements for a patient to have x-ray examinations, routinely ask
   - If and when the patient has had other x-ray studies or therapy and the nature of these.
   - If the patient has been exposed to any radiation for other reasons, such as in employment or experimental situations.
   - If it is possible that a female patient is pregnant. These inquiries are important, as it may be that the patient has received excessive doses of radiation and further exposure at that time may be detrimental to the patient's health status. When it appears that the patient has been exposed to a large amount of radiation recently, and when a woman suspects that she is pregnant, inform the physician of this, without alarming the patient, and before making arrangements for the x-ray studies. Provided with this information, the physician may want to change the order for x-ray studies at that time. The physician will weigh the

facts: that is, how urgent is the need for the x-ray examination versus what is the risk to the patient or fetus, who will receive the additional radiation exposure.

2. Position the patient correctly for the x-ray film if licensed to do so (unlicensed personnel should not position patients for x-ray procedures) and when this is one of your assisting duties. Accuracy of the film requires that the patient assume and maintain the correct position without moving during the exposure time. If this is not attained, distortion on the film will result, thus requiring the patient to be exposed to additional radiation while a repeat film is taken.

3. Shield the patient's abdomen and reproductive organs with a lead apron when appropriate, especially patients who are pregnant, patients of childbearing age, and children.

MEDICAL ASSISTANT RESPONSIBILITIES

The medical assistant's responsibilities relating to radiological procedures used in the physician's office are to prepare the patient, provide reassurance when needed, and employ the safety measures relevant to x-ray equipment. When the physician employs a radiographer, the assistant may not do any of these functions.

When outside sources are used, the assistant is responsible for calling the radiologist's office or hospital x-ray department to schedule the examination and for furnishing the patient's name, the referring physician's name, and the type of examination.

One of the most important communications between the medical assistant and radiology department involves the scheduling of multiple x-ray procedures that are ordered at one time for the patient. Consultation will be needed to sequence the procedures so that they will not interfere with each other and to decide how many procedures can be done on the same day. The medical assistant should give all the information to the radiology department so that they can schedule the examinations in proper sequence. The general rule is that examinations *not* using a contrast medium are done *before* examinations that do use a contrast medium; for example, a chest x-ray would be done before a barium enema. The patient is to take the physician's written requisition(s) to the x-ray department on the day of the examination.

In either situation, before the scheduled date, patients should be informed of the approximate amount of time that the examination will take so they can schedule other activities accordingly and not get unduly upset or surprised if the examination takes an hour or so. Also, certain x-ray examinations require special patient preparation the day before or the

morning of the study, or both. To prepare the patient, the medical assistant must know and go over the instructions orally with the patient to ensure that these are understood, and provide written instructions to be taken home. Many physicians' offices have preprinted individual instructions to be followed before x-ray studies, or they may use product literature provided by pharmaceutical companies for patient use. Written instructions are essential, as oral instructions can easily be forgotten. Repeat examinations required because of poorly given or misunderstood instructions are unnecessary radiation exposures and expenses for the patient.

For the x-ray studies discussed in this unit, Tables 12-3 and 12-4 group those that do not require special patient preparation and then those studies that do require individual patient preparation (listed as individual, because the specific preparation may vary among different radiology departments). The approximate amount of time required for each examination is also listed. Samples of individual patient prepara-

Table 12-3. X-ray examinations that *do not* require special patient preparation

Examination	Time required
Barium swallow	½ to ¾ hr
Arthrogram	1½ hr
Diskogram, lumbar or cervical	1 hr
Hysterosalpingogram	1 hr
Lymphangiogram	6 hr
Mammogram	½ to ¾ hr
Xeroradiography	Depends on area being studied
Thermography	Depends on area being studied
Tomography	1 hr
Computed tomography	1 to 2 hr (no preparation if contrast medium *not* used)
Abdomen (flat plate)	20 min
Chest	20 min
KUB	10 min; 45 min when it includes intravenous urography
Skull series	20 to 30 min
Paranasal sinuses	20 to 30 min
Bone	15 min to 1 hr, depending on type and area being studied
Magnetic resonance imaging	1 hr (will vary with body part being examined)
Digital radiography	1 hr
Ultrasound of the gallbladder	1 hr

Table 12-4.   X-ray examinations *requiring* special individual patient preparation

Examination	Time required	Sample preparation
Barium enema	30 to 60 min	Take 2 oz (4 tbl) castor oil at 4:00 PM the day preceding x-ray examination (may be taken in grape juice or root beer). No solid foods on day preceding examination; just liquids such as fruit juice, clear soup, Jello, water, plain tea, or black coffee, but no milk products. NPO after midnight. No breakfast on day of examination. *or* Enemas till bowels are clear the evening before. NPO after midnight. Rectal suppository in the morning.
Barium meal (upper GI series)	30 to 60 min for stomach, but up to 90 min with small bowel examination. More films may be taken 6 hr or 24 hr later	Nothing to eat or drink after 10:00 PM the evening before examination. No breakfast, no fluids, and no cigarettes in the morning. Stomach must be empty. *or* Nothing to eat or drink after 8:00 PM. Do not eat breakfast. No water. Report to x-ray office.
Angiogram	1 to 3 hr	No breakfast when any of these examinations are done in the early morning; or no lunch if they are done in the afternoon.
Arteriogram	1 to 3 hr	
Angiocardiogram	2 hr	
Cerebral angiogram	2 to 3 hr	
Bronchogram	1 hr	NPO
Myelogram	1 hr	NPO
Computed tomography	1 to 2 hr	NPO for 4 hr before if a contrast medium is used.
Cholecystogram (gallbladder series)	1 to 2 hr	Evening before x-ray examination, eat a light supper, consisting of nonfatty foods such as lean meat (small portion) and fresh vegetables cooked without butter and no eggs, mayonnaise, French dressing, fried or fatty foods. After supper swallow gallbladder tablets with water, taking one at a time. Eat nothing after evening meal. Water, however, may be taken in moderate amounts until bedtime. Do not take a laxative. Do not eat breakfast. Report to x-ray department. *or* Low-fat evening meal. Telepaque tablets the evening before. NPO after midnight.
Intravenous cholangiogram	3 hr	NPO
Intravenous pyelogram (IVP)	1½ hr	Take 2 oz (4 tbl) of castor oil or 3 tablets Dulcolax at 4 PM the day before x-ray examination. Eat a light supper. Do not drink anything, even water, after midnight. Eat no breakfast, no fluids. *or* Laxatives or enemas night before examination. NPO for 8 hr before examination.
Retrograde pyelogram	1 to 1½ hr; usually done in operating room	NPO
Pneumoencephalogram	2 to 4 hr	NPO
Pneumoencephalomyelogram	2 to 4 hr	NPO
Ultrasonography		
Pelvic ultrasound	25 to 45 min up to 2 hr	Afternoon before the examination, take 3 Dulcolax tablets and 3 glasses of water to clear the bowel. On the day of examination, use a Dulcolax rectal suppository 3 hr before examination. Then take 3 to 4 glasses of water 45 min before the exam and do not urinate. *A full urinary bladder is essential for this examination.*

Table 12-4   (*continued*)

Examination	Time required	Sample preparation
		or
		A full urinary bladder is essential. Please do not empty your bladder for 1 to 2 hr before examination. Drink 4 to 6 glasses of any liquid 45 min before examination. Use one Dulcolax suppository 3 hr before examination.
Abdominal ultrasound		Take 1 Mylicon tablet 4 times daily for 2 days before examination. *Do not eat* solid food after 8:00 AM on day of examination. You may take fluids as desired.
		or
		Take 10 oz of citrate of magnesia and 3 glasses of water at noon the day before examination. Take 3 Dulcolax tablets at 6:00 PM with an additional 3 glasses of water. The evening meal should consist of clear fluids but no milk products. Have nothing other than liquids after midnight. Do not eat breakfast the day of examination.
Renal ultrasound		Drink 2 glasses of water 1 hr before examination.
Thyroid ultrasound		No preparation needed.
		Nothing in mouth 3 hr before examination.
Obstetrical ultrasound		A full urinary bladder is essential. Do not empty your bladder for at least 1 hr before exam. Drink 4 to 6 glasses of any liquid 45 min before examination.

tions are given for common examinations. Similar reference sheets should be made available for the medical assistant in the physician's office or clinic.

After the x-ray examination has been completed, the medical assistant must check to ensure that a written report is received and then filed in the patient's chart after being reviewed by the physician, and that the x-ray films, when sent to or when taken in the physician's office, are stored and handled correctly.

Preparation of Patient and Assisting with Radiographs in the Physician's Office

Procedure	Rationale
1. Identify the patient, check if the special preparation was followed (when applicable), and explain the following: • The value of the examination • How the machine operates • Whether it will hurt • What clothing and other articles must be removed • How to put on the patient gown, that is, with the opening in the front or back • What position will be required • The importance of remaining still during the examination	X-ray procedures performed in the office are used for diagnostic or screening purposes. If a required special preparation was not followed, the examination must be cancelled and rescheduled. The patient can be told that x-ray examinations are painless, with the exception of those requiring the instillation of a contrast medium. Then, on these occasions, an uncomfortable feeling can be expected, rather than pain. The patient is to remove clothes, watches, all metal, dentures, jewelry, and hairpins, which may interfere with the accuracy of the x-ray film. These objects will produce shadows on the film and may obscure details that should be observed.

Preparation of Patient and Assisting with Radiographs (*continued*)

Procedure	Rationale
	The patient gown is usually to be put on with the opening in the back. For films of the breast, all clothing from the waist up is removed. The physician will determine the position to be maintained by the patient; you will explain to the patient what it will be (refer to p. 383). Movement of the body during the examination will cause distortion on the film. It is then necessary to repeat the examination, which provides additional radiation exposure for the patient.
2. Drape the patient as necessary. Shield the abdominal regions with a lead apron, especially for patients who are pregnant, patients of childbearing age, or children.	Drapes may be used to provide warmth and to protect the patient's modesty, but are *not* to interfere with the body part being filmed.
3. Reassure the patient as required. Radiographs are taken on either very sick patients or those who come in for diagnostic purposes, but they all must be given support and attention.	Careful and complete explanations to the patient help provide reassurance and reduce fears and confusion. Offer assistance to the patient when getting on and off the x-ray table. Remain calm and quietly cheerful. Any reassurance to a nervous patient is helpful.
4. Be empathetic and courteous; remain calm.	The patient will be lying on or standing against a cold, hard plate. In an empathetic and courteous manner, emphasize the importance of remaining still in the proper position. Distortion on the film will occur unless the required position is maintained.
5. When the examination has been completed by the physician or x-ray technician or radiographer, ask the patient to wait in the dressing room while the films are developed.	The patient remains while films are developed to ensure that clear films have been obtained for study. This is much more convenient for everyone than to have the patient return later for retakes if the preliminary films are not clear.
6. If it is necessary to obtain another film, explain to the patient that the physician requires another film for study.	Careful communication is important, as you must avoid creating fears in the patient that unnecessary exposure to radiation will result or that the individual taking the x-ray was incompetent, thus necessitating another film.
7. Dismiss the patient after it has been determined that the films are satisfactory. If the x-ray film showed the presence of a fracture, make arrangements for immediate treatment.	The physician will read the films later, then the patient is to be notified; *or* schedule a future appointment for a time when the physician can review the results with the patient.
8. Record the procedure on the patient's chart.	Charting example: August 1, 19_____. PA and lateral chest x-rays taken by Dr. Mouer. Results—negative. Detailed report to follow. Film No. 8179 Cassandra Quinn, CMA

PROCESSING X-RAY FILM

One of two ways may be used to process x-ray film in a darkroom. Processing may be done either manually or mechanically by use of an automated film processor. It takes about 1 hour to complete the manual processing cycle, whereas if you use an automated processor, the processing cycle will produce a ready-to-read radiograph in as little as 90 seconds up to 10 minutes, depending on the processor used.

The conditions and steps involved in manually processing x-ray film are outlined in Figure 12-17.

Fig. 12-17.   Basic manual processing of x-ray film. (Reprinted courtesy of Eastman Kodak Company, Rochester, NY)

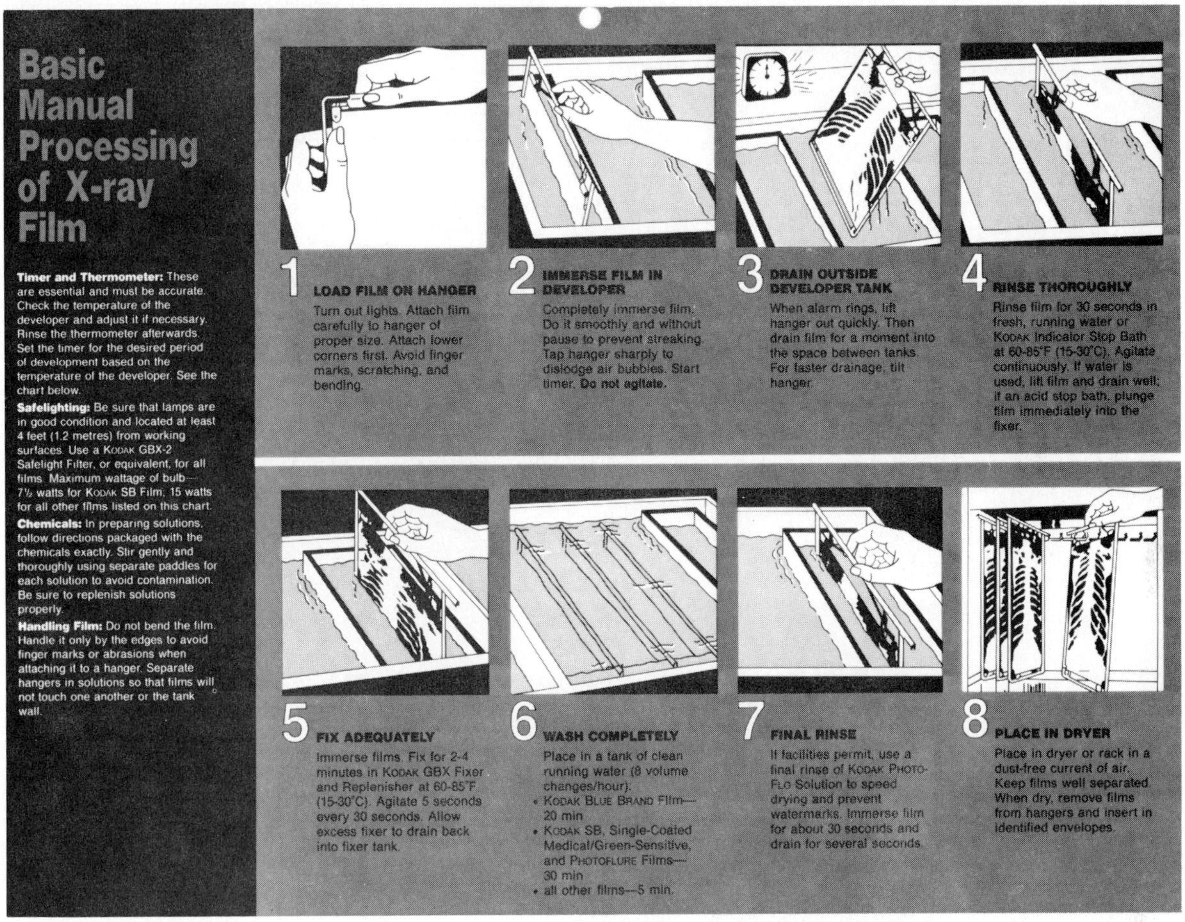

Basic Manual Processing of X-ray Film

Timer and Thermometer: These are essential and must be accurate. Check the temperature of the developer and adjust it if necessary. Rinse the thermometer afterwards. Set the timer for the desired period of development based on the temperature of the developer. See the chart below.

Safelighting: Be sure that lamps are in good condition and located at least 4 feet (1.2 metres) from working surfaces. Use a KODAK GBX-2 Safelight Filter, or equivalent, for all films. Maximum wattage of bulb 7½ watts for KODAK SB Film. 15 watts for all other films listed on this chart.

Chemicals: In preparing solutions, follow directions packaged with the chemicals exactly. Stir gently and thoroughly using separate paddles for each solution to avoid contamination. Be sure to replenish solutions properly.

Handling Film: Do not bend the film. Handle it only by the edges to avoid finger marks or abrasions when attaching it to a hanger. Separate hangers in solutions so that films will not touch one another or the tank wall.

1 LOAD FILM ON HANGER
Turn out lights. Attach film carefully to hanger of proper size. Attach lower corners first. Avoid finger marks, scratching, and bending.

2 IMMERSE FILM IN DEVELOPER
Completely immerse film. Do it smoothly and without pause to prevent streaking. Tap hanger sharply to dislodge air bubbles. Start timer. Do not agitate.

3 DRAIN OUTSIDE DEVELOPER TANK
When alarm rings, lift hanger out quickly. Then drain film for a moment into the space between tanks. For faster drainage, tilt hanger.

4 RINSE THOROUGHLY
Rinse film for 30 seconds in fresh, running water or KODAK Indicator Stop Bath at 60-85°F (15-30°C). Agitate continuously. If water is used, lift film and drain well; if an acid stop bath, plunge film immediately into the fixer.

5 FIX ADEQUATELY
Immerse films. Fix for 2-4 minutes in KODAK GBX Fixer and Replenisher at 60-85°F (15-30°C). Agitate 5 seconds every 30 seconds. Allow excess fixer to drain back into fixer tank.

6 WASH COMPLETELY
Place in a tank of clean running water (8 volume changes/hour).
• KODAK BLUE BRAND Film— 20 min
• KODAK SB, Single-Coated Medical/Green-Sensitive, and PHOTOFLURE Films— 30 min
• all other films—5 min.

7 FINAL RINSE
If facilities permit, use a final rinse of KODAK PHOTO-FLO Solution to speed drying and prevent watermarks. Immerse film for about 30 seconds and drain for several seconds.

8 PLACE IN DRYER
Place in dryer or rack in a dust-free current of air. Keep films well separated. When dry, remove films from hangers and insert in identified envelopes.

Always consult the manufacturer's recommendations for the procedures used for manual processing, as these can vary with different products.

Some films are designed only for automated processing. These films should not be processed manually except in emergency situations.

Three elements are required for proper automated processing. These include a processor, the correct film(s), and special chemicals. These components are designed to work together to produce a quality radiograph. Follow the manufacturer's recommendations for feeding the film into an automated processor. Usually you will feed the film squarely into the processor and feed multiple films simultaneously. The processor will transport, process, dry the film, and replenish and recirculate the processing solutions (Fig. 12-18).

After the manual or automated processing procedure has been completed, the radiograph is ready for viewing on an illuminated viewbox (see Fig. 12-10) or is to be placed in a special file envelope labeled with the patient's name, the date, and the x-ray number when used.

STORAGE AND MANAGEMENT IN OFFICE

X-Ray Materials

When x-ray materials are used in the office, they require special storage attention. These supplies must be protected from damage caused by exposure to moisture, heat, and light. Film must be kept in a dry, cool place, preferably in a lead-lined box. The lead-lined box protects the film from any x-rays that may escape during filming.

When unexposed film is to be placed into a cassette for use, the film packets are to be opened only in the darkroom with only the darkroom light on. Before development, the exposed film obtained after the radiological procedure is completed must also be stored in a lead-lined box to protect it from secondary radiation, which would spoil the radiograph recorded on the film.

X-ray developer solutions must also be stored in a moisture-free, cool location, because they are of extreme importance in the processing of quality radiographs.

Fig. 12-18. **A,** Roller transport system of an automated x-ray film processor. Diagram showing how the rollers transport films through the various sections of an automated processor. The arrangement and number of components in the various assemblies may differ from model to model but the basic plan is the same. (Reprinted courtesy of Eastman Kodak Company, Rochester, NY) **B,** Automatic x-ray film processor. **C,** Developing a radiograph using an automatic processor in the darkroom.

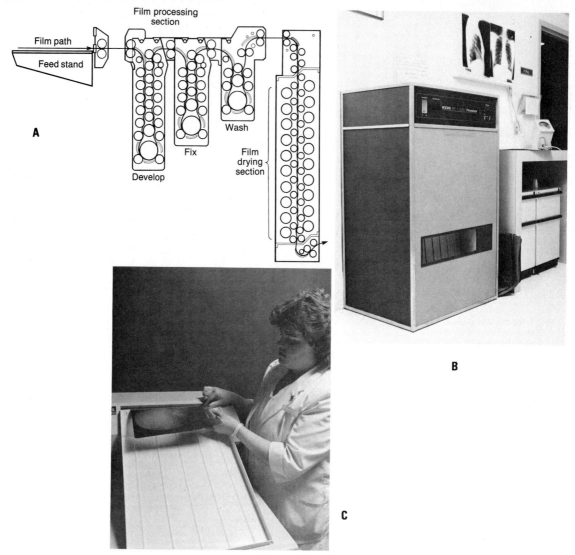

X-Ray Films, Reports, and Records

Frequently there is much controversy over the ownership of medical records, reports, and x-ray films. The important thing to remember is that this type of property legally belongs to the medical facility where it is made or recorded. It does not belong to the patient. All x-ray films obtained on a patient are the sole property of the physician's office or hospital that performed the radiological examination. Written x-ray reports from the radiologist are to be sent to the referring physician, but the actual films usually remain in the files of the office or hospital that did the filming. At times these films can be loaned out to the referring physician for further study, reference, or review as needed to confirm a diagnosis or to compare old films with current ones. At other times the radiologist's office routinely sends the films to the referring physician so that they may be kept as part of the patient's permanent medical record in the office, but they still remain as the legal property of the radiologist. Presently in a few states patients can request, pay for, and obtain copies of the original x-ray film.

Radiological films are permanent records for current or future reference (as opposed to fluoroscopy, which can be viewed only at the time of the examination unless the procedure was recorded on a videotape or 35 mm film). Special file envelopes are available to keep exposed film in. These envelopes must be labeled with the patient's name, the date, and the number, if and when used. (Some places file films by number rather than by the patient's name. In this case, the number *must* be recorded on the patient's medical record for a cross-reference.)

X-ray films placed in filing envelopes should be filed in a dry, cool storage area, preferably in a metal cabinet; ones no longer needed for current reference should be filed in a permanent storage file so that they are available for future reference.

CONCLUSION

This unit has given you an introduction to various diagnostic procedures used in the field of radiology. In addition, the medical assistant's responsibilities in these fields, though limited, have been discussed. Numerous additional studies may be performed in these specialty areas of medicine for the diagnosis and treatment of disease processes. It is not within the scope of this book to discuss all of them in detail. There are various sources to which you may refer to expand your knowledge on these procedures. Check with your instructor for additional enrichment assignments and references in areas of your own particular need and interest. A tour through the radiology and nuclear medicine departments of a modern hospital, especially a large teaching hospital, would make you aware of the dramatic progress that has been made in these fields of medicine.

When you feel that you know the information presented in this unit, arrange with your instructor to take a performance test.

REVIEW OF VOCABULARY

The following reports received in a physician's office pertain to some of the diagnostic examinations discussed in the preceding pages. Read these and be prepared to discuss the contents with your instructor. A dictionary or other reference books may be used to define the terms that you are not familiar with. In addition, it is suggested that you read more on these examinations elsewhere so that you may gain a more complete understanding of the procedures.

PATIENT NO. 1: Upper GI series

Preliminary film reveals no significant soft tissue or osseous abnormality.
There is a small lesser curvature antral ulcer measuring 7 mm at its neck and 4 mm deep. No mass is identified, and peristalsis passes through the area with ease. No abnormalities are seen of the distal esophagus, remaining stomach, duodenal bulb, duodenal loop, or proximal small bowel.
CONCLUSION: Small lesser curvature antral ulcer.

Follow up x-ray studies done by another physician

Comparison with previous study of 7-02-87 reveals near-complete clearing of the lesser curvature antral ulcer. A tiny barium collection measuring about 2 to 3 mm remains in the same location with some adjacent thickened folds.
Duodenal bulb, duodenal loop, and proximal small bowel show no abnormalities.
Distal esophagus appeared normal without evidence of hiatus hernia or reflux.
Incomplete fusion of the L-5 spinous process demonstrated.
CONCLUSION: Near-complete clearing of the lesser curvature antral ulcer. L-5 spina bifida occulta.

PATIENT NO. 2: Barium enema

Following a water cleansing preliminary enema, the colon was filled quite readily from rectum to cecum including terminal ileum.
The descending colon is displaced quite strikingly forward and toward the midline in the region of the previously described soft tissue mass closely related to the lower pole of the left kidney. There is no mucosal distortion, and the deformity is mainly that of extrinsic pressure rather than an intrinsic or invasive lesion.
The only other abnormality is a small area of kinking with slight narrowing of the lumen in the proximal transverse colon just distally to the hepatic flexure. That portion of the colon is quite redundant, and this is most likely a kink at the site of redundancy and not a true lesion; however, if surgery is contemplated, direct palpation of this area is suggested. The colon is otherwise normally outlined and so is the terminal ileum. It empties quite well.
CONCLUSION: Extrinsic pressure and displacement of the left colon by the previously described mass without evidence of any direct invasion. Small area of kinking and narrowing of the lumen at the proximal portion of the transverse colon, most likely normal and simply due to local redundancy.
Otherwise normal study of the colon.

PATIENT NO. 3: Barium enema

This is compared with similar study of 8/26/84. On the preliminary film there is some barium in the pelvis from previous study. Gas pattern is unremarkable. The large bowel is filled in retrograde manner with barium. Free reflux into the terminal ileum was seen, and the appendix fills. There are a few diverticula deep in the sigmoid, which account for the retention of the barium seen on the scout film. The left colon now distends completely with no evidence of ischemic colitis and no residual stricture noted. The remainder of the colon is unchanged.
IMPRESSION: Normal barium enema without residual from the previously described ischemic colitis. Diverticulosis of the sigmoid colon.

PATIENT NO. 4: Excretory urography with tomography

Preliminary examination demonstrates normal psoas and renal shadows.

There is an ovoid homogeneous increased density approximately 13 cm in maximum dimension in the left midabdomen.

Three calcified lymph nodes are in the right lower quadrant.

Opaque medium appears promptly and in good concentration demonstrating normal calyces, pelves, and ureters. The vesicle outline is normal with minimal retention after voiding.

The left midabdominal mass moves independently from the lower pole of the left kidney, particularly noted in the erect position, and is separate from it. The mass has well-delineated margins and appears to be of homogeneous density. Ultrasound would readily distinguish a cystic from a solid lesion separating such as a mesenteric cyst from a solid mesenchymal or epithelial tumor, or lymphoma. An ovarian tumor would be unusual in this location but possible.

CONCLUSION: Normal excretory urinary tract. Left midabdominal mass lesion, discussed above.

PATIENT NO. 5: Ultrasound consultation

CHIEF COMPLAINT: Right upper quadrant pain.

ULTRASOUND OF THE GALLBLADDER: The gallbladder is well seen. There is some slightly echogenic material in the dependent part of the gallbladder, but this is not definitely particulate, and there is no acoustic shadowing. Ducts are unremarkable.

IMPRESSION: The material in the gallbladder described above most likely represents sludge. This is not considered definitely abnormal.

PATIENT NO. 6: Chest x-ray report

In AP projection there is a mild dextroconvex curvature of the lower thoracic spine. The bony thorax is otherwise unremarkable.

The heart, vessels, and mediastinal structures are normal.

Clear lungs are well expanded with sharp costophrenic angles. There is no evidence of active disease.

PATIENT NO. 7: Facial bones x-ray report

The facial bones including the orbits are intact.

A smooth, 1 × 1.5 cm soft tissue opacity lies about the posterior aspect of the roof of the left maxillary sinus.

CONCLUSION: Facial bones negative for fracture. Soft-tissue mass about the roof of the left maxillary sinus. The possibility of a blow-out fracture of the orbit might be considered and should be clinically correlated.

REVIEW QUESTIONS

1. Mrs. G. B. Emerson, a 46-year-old, 164 pound woman has been scheduled for a barium enema and a cholecystogram. Mrs. Emerson does not understand why she must have these tests.

Explain the nature and purpose of these tests to her and the special directions that she must follow before having these tests performed.

2. The physician has ordered a PA and lateral chest x-ray film to be taken on Mr. T. Rankin. Explain how the patient will be positioned when these films are taken.

3. Mrs. C. A. Lunatto has had extensive radiotherapy and now is experiencing diarrhea and some loss of scalp hair. List four other side effects that she may experience with continued radiation therapy.

4. Mr. K. Cole is suspected of having kidney disease. List five diagnostic studies that the physician may order to help diagnose the problem.

5. Ms. B. Milius has discovered several lumps in her breast while doing a breast self-examination and has now come to the physician for a checkup. List three studies that the physician may order for this patient to help diagnose the condition.

6. Mrs. Gwen Boyd is scheduled for ultrasonography to determine if she is pregnant, because other tests have proved unsuccessful. She feels apprehensive about having this test done and is fearful of the pain she expects to have during this test. Explain the nature and purpose of this test, indicating if pain is to be expected.

7. Explain the nature and purpose of computed tomography (CT). State the advantages of this technique and equipment over other types of radiological examinations.

8. Explain the nature and purpose of magnetic resonance imaging. State the advantages of this technique over other types of radiological equipment.

9. List four advantages of digital radiography.

10. What is a film badge, and why is it used?

11. List three ways to protect the patient from unnecessary radiation exposure when having x-ray examinations.

12. Discuss the medical assistant's responsibilities relevant to x-ray procedures performed in the physician's office; at an outside facility.

13. Describe how an x-ray film should be stored in the office.

14. Mr. B. Wingate had a myelogram performed last month and now is in your office stating that he wants the x-ray films to take home. Define myelogram. Explain to Mr. Wingate why he cannot have the films to take home.

PERFORMANCE TEST

In a skills laboratory, a simulation of a joblike environment, the medical assistant student will demonstrate skill in performing the following activities without reference to source materials. Time limits for each of the following activities are to be assigned by the instructor (see also pp. 32 and 35).

1. Communicate proper preparation for x-ray procedures to the patient.
2. Prepare the patient for and assist the patient during an x-ray examination.
3. Position the patient for the AP, PA, LL, and RL x-ray exposure, if licensed to do so.
4. Care for and store an x-ray film in the office.
5. Demonstrate safety hazards and precautionary measures relevant to x-ray equipment.

The student is to perform the above with 100% accuracy.

PERFORMANCE CHECKLIST

The medical assistant students are to design their own performance checklists for the performance test.

Unit XIII

Diagnostic Allergy Tests and Intradermal Skin Tests

COGNITIVE OBJECTIVES

On completion of Unit XIII, the medical assistant student should be able to apply the following cognitive objectives.

1. Define and pronounce the terms listed in the vocabulary.
2. Discuss the nature, causes, signs, and symptoms of allergies.
3. List methods used for the diagnosis and treatment of allergies.
4. Describe and differentiate between the following tests:
   Patch test
   Scratch test
   Intradermal skin tests
   Mantoux test for tuberculosis
   Tine tuberculin test
5. Describe how to determine the results for each of the tests given in No. 4.

TERMINAL PERFORMANCE OBJECTIVES

On completion of Unit XIII, the medical assistant student should be able to do the following terminal performance objectives:

1. Select the correct equipment and supplies needed to perform diagnostic allergy and intradermal skin tests.
2. Correctly perform, and read and record the results of the following tests:
   Patch test
   Scratch test
   Intradermal skin tests
   Mantoux test for tuberculosis
   Tine tuberculin test
3. Prepare the patient and the equipment, and administer an intradermal injection in the correct body site.

The student is to perform the above activities with 100% accuracy.

Vocabulary

allergen (al'-er-jen)—Any substance that induces hypersensitivity.

allergy (al'er-jē)—An unusual and increased sensitivity (hypersensitivity) to specific substances that are ordinarily harmless.

anaphylaxis (an"ah-fi-lak'sis)—An unusual or hypersensitive reaction of the body to foreign protein and other substances; frequently caused by drugs, foreign serum (tetanus, and so on), and insect stings and bites.

atopy (at"o-pē)—A hypersensitive state that is subject to hereditary influences, such as hay fever, asthma, and eczema.

contact dermatitis—Dermatitis caused by an allergic reaction resulting from contact of the skin with various substances, such as poison ivy, or chemical, physical, and mechanical agents.

dermatitis (der"mah-tī'tis)—Inflammation of the skin.

induration (in"du-rā'shun)—An abnormally hard spot; a process of hardening.

vesicle (ves'ĭ-kl)—A circular, blisterlike elevation on the skin containing fluid.

wheal (hwēl)—A temporary, more or less round, elevation on the skin that is white in the center and often accompanied by itching.

ALLERGIES

The study and diagnosis of allergies are closely related to the field of immunity (review pp. 112–113). When a foreign agent (antigen) enters the body, antibodies are produced that attack and render the antigen harmless. This reaction is part of the body's natural defense mechanisms. However, in some instances, when the same antigen enters the body again, the antibodies, rather than protecting the body, set up an antigen-antibody reaction, producing harmful or uncomfortable results, such as the signs and symptoms of an allergy.

An allergy is the abnormal individual hypersensitivity to substances (allergens) that are usually harmless. Allergens, substances capable of inducing hypersensitivity, can be almost any substance in the environment. Examples of allergens to which patients have become sensitive are dust, animal hairs, plant and tree pollens, mold spores, soaps, detergents, cosmetics, dyes, food, feathers, plastics, and even some valuable medicines. When the allergen is in contact with or enters the body, it sets off a chain of events that brings about the allergic reaction. The allergen in itself is not directly responsible for the allergic reaction. An allergy does not develop on the first contact with the allergen, but can develop on the second contact or even years later after repeated contact with the allergen.

Signs and symptoms of allergies include sneezing, stuffed-up and running nose, watery eyes, itching, coughing, shortness of breath, wheezing, rashes, skin eruptions, slight local edema, and also mild to severe anaphylactic shock, which can be fatal unless treated.

Diagnosis and Treatment of Allergies

In order for the physician to correctly treat the patient's condition, the allergen responsible for the reaction must be identified. After obtaining a detailed case history from the patient, the physician may order one of three skin tests: (1) patch test, (2) scratch test, or (3) intradermal test. The medical assistant may do these tests or prepare the equipment and assist the physician with the procedure. The principle involved is that when a minute amount of various suspected allergens is applied to the skin in these tests, a mild allergic reaction occurs at the site of the offending allergen without causing any serious symptoms.

As many as 20 to 30 tests may be necessary before the offending allergen or allergens are identified. Control tests using the diluent without the active allergen are essential in each type of testing. Positive reactions at the other test sites can be compared with the appearance at the control site to verify that they are a true allergic reaction and not merely an irritating reaction to the diluent or trauma to the skin area.

Ready-made bottled preparations of allergen materials or diagnostic sets with vials containing up to 39 various allergens are available for testing.

Once the offending allergen has been identified, the first step in treatment is to avoid it. At times a special diet may have to be designed for the patient, or special antiallergic cosmetics and such may have to be used. When the allergen is animal hair, the patient will have to avoid the animal and may have to give away a household pet. Patients with hay fever or asthma often have to move to a different locale or plan a trip to a place free from the offending pollen during certain seasons of the year. Often patients can be cured of allergies by receiving a series of desensitization treatments. For these treatments patients are given the allergen(s) in gradually increasing amounts in order to reduce their sensitivity to those substances, or to build up their resistance to the point of immunity. Allergies that are resistant to cure may be controlled with certain medications such as antihistamines, epinephrine, aminophylline, and cortisone preparations.

Patch Test

Formerly used to detect tuberculosis, the patch test has been proved unreliable for that use. Today the patch test is most often used to diagnose skin allergies, especially contact dermatitis. This is the simplest type of skin test. To determine tissue hypersensitivity, gauze is impregnated with the substance to be tested and then applied and left in contact with an intact skin surface for 24 to 72 hours (usually 48 hours).

Equipment

Antiseptic and sponge to cleanse the skin or an alcohol sponge
Containers with the allergen(s) to be tested
Small gauze dressing(s) and squares of cellophane *or* commercially prepared protective covering patches
Adhesive or paper tape

Procedure	Rationale
1. Wash your hands.	
2. Assemble the supplies.	
3. Identify and prepare the patient.	Explanations help gain the patient's cooperation, help alleviate fear of the unknown, and help the patient relax.
• Explain the procedure.	
• Provide a patient gown if needed.	
• Position in a comfortable sitting position with the arm exposed and well supported, or the back exposed if the patch is to be applied there.	

Patch Test (*continued*)

Procedure	Rationale
4. Cleanse the skin site to be used, and allow it to dry.	The anterior forearm or the upper back are frequent test sites. The forearm is the preferred site for adults, and the back is the preferred site for children.
5. Place a drop or two of the specific allergen on the gauze dressing; cover this with a square of cellophane.	
6. Place the gauze on the skin site and attach with tape.	Commercially prepared covering patches come ready to be applied and do not need the cellophane covering.
7. Write the name of the test substance on the tape, or write a number on the tape and in the patient's record with the name of the allergen used.	When a positive reaction occurs, it is vital that the correct allergen be identified. Correct record keeping is a must. As many as 20 to 30 patches may be applied at one time on the back.
8. Instruct the patient.	The patch is to be kept in place for varying lengths of time, depending on the allergen used and the physician's order (minimum: 24 hours) up to 72 hours. Frequently it is left in place for 48 hours. Explain to the patient if intense itching occurs to remove the patch and contact the physician immediately for further instructions. Also the patient must be told to avoid wetting or scratching the test site until the patch is removed so that the allergen will not be spread over a large area.
9. Record the test on the patient's record.	Charting example: August 4, 19_____, 1 PM Patch tests done on forearm ×2.
10. Remove the patch at the specified time and read the results (observe the reaction). Discard the patch in a designated covered container.	The test result is negative when there is no reaction on the skin; the test result is positive when the skin is reddened (erythematous) or swollen, or when vesicles are present.
11. Instruct the patient when and if to return for another appointment.	
12. Leave the treatment room clean.	
13. Wash your hands.	

14. Record the reaction on the patient's record.	Charting example:
	August 6, 19_____, 1 PM
	   Skin patches removed.
	   Results of the test—negative.
	     Ari Sabir, CMA

Scratch Test

In the scratch test, one or more scratches are made in the skin, then a drop of the substance to be tested is placed in the scratch and left for 30 minutes. The scratch test is frequently used for detecting types of allergies. Kits to be used for this test come in various sizes with various numbers of allergens. Some physicians may keep multiple-dose bottles of allergens for common allergies rather than using the test kits. The history obtained from the patient will usually indicate the type and number of tests to be performed.

Equipment

Commercially prepared kit with needles for each test and the allergen solutions, either in a capillary tube or bottle. When the prepared kit is not used, you will need the bottles containing the allergens to be tested and 26 gauge needles (a dull sterile knife may also be used)

Two small towels

Washable ink pen

Toothpick or medicine dropper (to be used when the substance is provided in a bottle)

Patient gown

Procedure	Rationale
1. Wash your hands.	
2. Assemble the equipment.	
3. Identify and prepare the patient:	
• Explain the procedure.	Explanations help gain the patient's cooperation and help the patient relax.
• Ask the patient to disrobe to the waist and put the gown on with opening in back.	
• Position the patient in a prone position (face down) on the examining table with the back exposed, *or* sitting with the arm well supported and exposed.	
4. Wash the back (or arm) with soap and water; dry thoroughly.	The skin must be thoroughly cleansed and dried before the scratches are made.
5. Write test numbers 2 inches apart on sections of the skin to correspond with the allergen container numbers.	Use a pen with washable ink. Each allergen container is numbered. Incorrect readings are avoided because the allergen number corresponds with the numbered section on the skin.
6. Make a ⅛-inch scratch with the needle supplied in the kit *or* with a 26 gauge needle *or* with a dull sterile knife.	Do not penetrate the skin or cause bleeding. Only a superficial scratch is to be made on the skin.
7. Place a drop of the allergen on the scratch. For solutions supplied in a capillary tube: break the tube in two and allow the solution to drop onto the scratch. For solutions supplied in separate bottles: using a toothpick end or a medicine dropper, pick up a drop of the solution and drop it onto the scratch.	Use only a minute quantity of the allergen solution to avoid severe allergic reactions. When placed on the scratch, some of the solution will be absorbed into the deeper layers of tissue.
8. Make each additional scratch with a separate needle. Use a clean toothpick or medicine dropper for each solution to be tested.	
9. Allow the allergen solution to set for 30 minutes with the back or arm exposed to the air.	Make sure that the patient is not chilled; provide extra covering over areas of the body not used for testing.
10. Wipe the excess solution from each scratch separately.	Avoid spreading the solution in one scratch to another scratch.
11. Read the results (observe the skin reactions). NOTE: Test results may also be read 24 hours later to check for delayed reactions.	Test results are interpreted as: NEGATIVE: No reaction has occurred after 30 minutes. POSITIVE: The appearance of redness or swelling or a wheal at the test site. Positive results are designated as slight (1+), moderate (2+), or marked (3+).
12. Give the patient further instructions: • To dress and feel free to leave. • To return in 24 hours for a delayed reaction reading. • To schedule a future appointment for consultation.	
13. Remove used supplies from the treatment room; dispose of in designated covered containers; leave the treatment room clean and neat.	
14. Wash your hands.	
15. Record the test and results on the patient's chart.	Charting example: August 4, 19_____, 1 PM 20 scratch tests administered. Results— positive to dust, cat hair, and plant pollen. Negative to other substances. Mary Donovan, CMA

INTRADERMAL SKIN TESTS

In intradermal (intracutaneous) tests, a small amount of the substance under study is injected into the substance of the skin. These tests are used to determine allergies, to determine the patient's susceptibility to an infectious disease, and to diagnose infectious diseases such as tuberculosis (the Mantoux test) and diphtheria (the Schick test). For all these tests, the general rules for administering injections apply (refer to pp. 256–257, Intradermal Injections and Instructions for Administering Injections). Commercial trays of prepackaged sterile syringes are available for intradermal allergy tests (Fig. 13-1).

Administration of an Intradermal Injection

Equipment

Alcohol sponge or skin antiseptic and cotton ball
Tuberculin syringe, as fine calibrations are needed (0.5 or 1.0 ml)
Needle ⅜ or ½ inch, 26 or 27 gauge (see Fig. 7-7)
Solution to be injected

Procedure	Rationale
1. Wash your hands.	Steps 1 through 11 listed here correspond to steps 1 to 11 under intramuscular injection technique, pp. 257–259 in Unit VII.
2. Assemble the equipment.	
3. Prepare the syringe and needle for use.	
4. Compare the physician's order with the medication label.	
5. Check the medication label three times during preparation.	
6. Cleanse the vial rubber stopper, insert the needle, and withdraw the needed amount of solution into the syringe.	
7. Identify the patient, and explain the procedure.	
8. Select the injection site, and position the patient comfortably.	For intradermal injections, the dorsal surface of the forearm, about 4 inches below the elbow, is used. For patients over 60 years of age, loss of skin turgor in this area can contribute to bruising or to extravasation of the testing solution. To prevent these problems, inject the solution into the area over the trapezius muscle (on the back), just below the acromial process (Fig. 13-2).
9. Cleanse the injection site with the alcohol sponge and allow to dry.	
10. Remove the needle cover.	
11. Expel air bubbles from syringe.	
12. Stand in front of the patient. With your *nondominant hand,* grasp the middle of the patient's forearm on the posterior side, and pull the anterior skin taut.	
13. Hold the barrel of the syringe between your thumb and other fingers of your *dominant hand;* have the bevel of the needle facing upward.	
14. Insert the needle into the skin at a 10 to 15 degree angle (Fig. 13-2; see also Fig. 7-17).	The angle used to insert the needle is almost parallel to the skin. The point of the needle is inserted into the most superficial layers of the skin.
15. Inject the solution slowly. NOTE: This type of injection does not require aspiration before the solution is injected.	As the drug is injected, a small pale bump will rise over the point of the needle in the skin. If the injection is given subcutaneously (that is, no bump forms), or if a significant part of the solution leaks from the injection site, the test should be repeated immediately at another site that is at least 2 inches (5 cm) away.

Procedure	Rationale
16. Withdraw the needle, and wipe the injection site gently with the alcohol sponge.	*Do not* apply pressure or massage the skin. The medication is *not* to be dispersed into the underlying tissues.
17. Observe the patient for any unusual reaction, such as general febrile reaction, faint feeling, and shock.	
18. Position the patient for safety and comfort, and provide further instructions.	Have the patient lie down if feeling faint, or sit for a few minutes to ensure that no unusual reaction will occur.
19. Tell the patient when the test results will be read. Schedule a future appointment when necessary. The patient may be dismissed if the results are not to be read until a day or two later. If the test result is to be determined within the next half hour or so, let the patient rest comfortably and safely.	The skin reaction is read at various times, depending on the test done. Check with the physician or the literature that accompanies the drug used. Most allergy skin tests will be read within 20 to 30 minutes; the Mantoux test for tuberculosis will be read within 48 to 72 hours, and other tests at varying times within 48 hours.
20. Remove and dispose the used syringe and needle correctly.	A disposable needle shaft is to be broken at the hub; the tip of a disposable syringe should be bent or crushed so that it is rendered useless. Reusable syringes and needles should be flushed with water, then separated and placed in a designated cleaning solution until prepared for sterilization (see Unit IV).
21. Wash your hands.	
22. Record the procedure on the patient's chart.	When several skin tests are given, record the site of each injection with the name of the substance injected. This avoids confusion when the results are read.
23. Read the skin reaction.	Many tests are read as either positive or negative depending on the amount of redness (erythema) or hardening (induration). For some tests the areas of redness or induration must be measured in millimeters. Follow the directions provided with the test solution.

24. Record the reaction on the patient's chart.	Charting example:
	August 5, 19____, 4 PM
	   Reaction of Mantoux test given August 3, 19____, 4 PM is negative.
	   M. E. Burgdorf, CMA

Fig. 13-1. Prepackaged tray of sterile intradermal syringes for allergy testing. (Courtesy Becton-Dickinson, Division of Becton, Dickinson and Co., Rutherford, NJ)

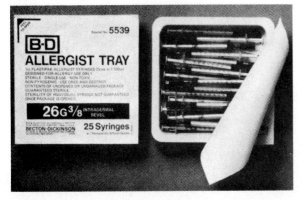

Mantoux Test for Tuberculosis

The standard test recommended by the American Lung Association to help detect infection with *Mycobacterium tuberculosis* is the Mantoux test. The Mantoux test is performed by injecting intradermally exactly 0.1 ml of tuberculin PPD (purified protein derivative). This dose contains 5 TU (tuberculin units) of tuberculin PPD. The reaction is read 48 to 72 hours later. Only induration is considered when interpreting the test results.

Fig. 13-2. **A,** administering an intradermal injection at 10 to 15 degree angle on dorsal surface of forearm, about 4 inches below elbow. **B,** administering intradermal skin test over the trapezius muscle just below the acromial process on elderly patients.

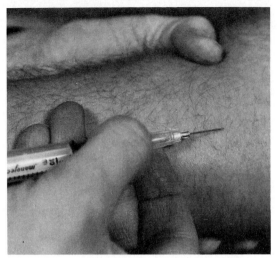
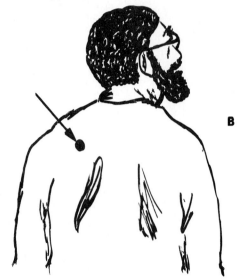

Equipment

Alcohol sponge
Tuberculin syringe (0.5 or 1.0 ml) with a ⅜ or ½ inch 26 or 27 gauge needle
Tuberculin PPD

Procedure

Follow the intradermal injection technique described above, measuring 0.1 ml of tuberculin PPD into the syringe for administration.

Reading Mantoux Skin Reactions

Read 48 to 72 hours after the injection.
Consider only induration (area of hardened tissue) when interpreting the results.
Measure the diameter of induration transversely (lying in crosswise direction) to the long axis of the forearm and record in millimeters.
Disregard erythema (redness) of less than 10 mm.
Disregard erythema greater than 10 mm if induration is absent, because the injection may have been made too deeply. Testing should be repeated in this case.

Interpreting Tuberculin Reaction

Positive reaction. Induration measuring 10 mm or more indicates hypersensitivity to the tuberculin PPD and is interpreted as positive for present or past infection with *Mycobacterium tuberculosis.* A positive reaction does not necessarily signify active disease. Further diagnostic procedures must be performed before a diagnosis of tuberculosis is made.

Doubtful reaction. Induration measuring 5 to 9 mm means that retesting may be indicated using a different test site.

Negative reaction. Induration of less than 5 mm indicates a lack of hypersensitivity to the tuberculin, and tuberculosis infection is highly unlikely.

Tine Tuberculin Test

The intradermal tine tuberculin test provides a convenient screening method for skin tuberculin reactivity in individuals and in large population groups. The reactivity of this test is comparable to, or more potent than, the intermediate strength Mantoux test (5 TU) administered intradermally. The disposable tine unit used for this test consists of a stainless steel disc, with four tines or prongs 2 mm long, attached to a plastic handle. The tines have been dipped in a solution of Old tuberculin containing stabilizers and then dried. The entire unit is sterile, and the protected portion will remain sterile as long as the plastic cap is not removed (Fig. 13-3, A).

Equipment

Alcohol sponge (acetone, ether, or soap and water can also be used)
Tine unit
Millimeter ruler (supplied with the Tine unit)

Fig. 13-3. **A,** tine unit for tuberculin testing. **B,** administering the tine tuberculin test.

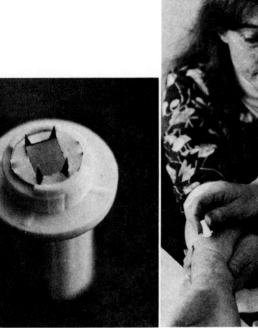

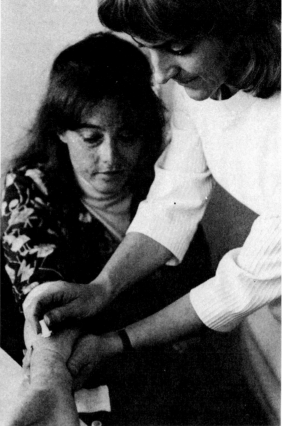

Procedure for Tine Tuberculin Test

Procedure	Rationale
1. Wash your hands.	
2. Assemble the equipment.	
3. Identify the patient, and explain the procedure.	Explain what is to occur and how it may feel. Explanations help gain the patient's cooperation and alleviate any apprehension.
4. Expose the patient's forearm, cleanse the skin with the alcohol sponge, and allow the skin to dry.	The preferred site for the administration of this test is the volar surface of the upper third of the forearm, over a muscle belly. Hairy areas and areas without adequate subcutaneous tissue, such as over a tendon or bone, should be avoided. The area must be clean and thoroughly dry before application of the tine test.
5. Remove the protective cap on the tine unit while holding the plastic handle.	The protective cap is removed to expose the four impregnated tines.
6. With your nondominant hand, grasp the upper third of the patient's forearm on the posterior side firmly and stretch the anterior skin tightly (Fig. 13-3).	A firm grasp of the patient's forearm is necessary, because the sharp momentary sting from the tine unit may cause the patient to jerk the arm and cause scratching.
7. With your dominant hand, apply the disc by puncturing the skin. Hold approximately 1 second before withdrawing.	Sufficient pressure must be exerted so that the four puncture sites and a circular depression of the skin from the plastic base are visible on the patient's skin.

Procedure for Tine Tuberculin Test (*continued*)

Procedure	Rationale
8. Discard the tine test unit in the appropriate container for waste materials.	The tine test unit must *never* be reused.
9. Instruct the patient when to return for the reading of the test results.	Tests should be read in 48 to 72 hours.
10. Wash your hands.	

11. Record the test on the patient's medical record.	Charting example:
	August 27, 19_____, 11 AM
	  Tine test administered in left forearm. Patient to return August 29, 19_____, 11 AM for reading of the reaction.
	    Sissy Block, CMA

12. Read the reaction in a good light with the patient's forearm slightly flexed.	Tests should be read in 48 to 72 hours. The extent of induration is the sole criterion; erythema without induration is insignificant. Determine the size of the induration in millimeters by inspecting the site and palpating with gentle finger stroking. The diameter of the largest single reaction around one of the puncture sites should be measured with a millimeter ruler (Fig. 13-4). Interpretation of tuberculin test reactions as recommended by the American Lung Association follow. • POSITIVE REACTION: Induration measuring 5 mm or more. The significance of this test and the management of the patient are the same as for one who reacts with 10 mm or more of induration to the standard Mantoux test. Further diagnostic procedures must be considered, such as a chest x-ray, laboratory examinations of sputum and other specimens, and confirmation using the Mantoux method. Chemotherapy should not be started solely on the basis of a single positive tine test. • DOUBTFUL REACTION: Induration of 2 to 4 mm. Patients in this group should have a Mantoux test done, and management should be based on the Mantoux reaction. • NEGATIVE REACTION: Induration of less than 2 mm. Patients in this group do not need to be retested unless they are in contact with a tuberculosis case or if there is suggestive clinical evidence of the disease.

13. Record the time and results on the patient's record.	Charting example:
	August 29, 19_____, 11 AM
	  Results of the tine test administered August 27, 19_____, at 11 AM are negative.
	    Sissy Block, CMA

REVIEW OF VOCABULARY

Read the following report and define the italicized terms.

Ms. Amy Fenster came to the office with an obvious case of *contact dermatitis*. Patient stated that she had been working in her garden when the signs and symptoms started and feels that poison ivy may be the *allergen*.

No other known *allergies;* patient has never experienced *anaphylaxis* nor any previous *dermatitis*.

Family history includes the presence of various *atopies* in both her mother and father.

Further studies will include a *scratch test,* in addition to a *Mantoux test* that is required by her present employment.

A. *Wheal*, MD

Fig. 13-4. Reading the reaction of a tine tuberculin test. **A,** palpate the area for presence of induration. **B,** using a millimeter ruler, measure the largest single reaction around one of the puncture sites.

A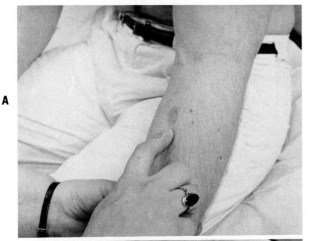

B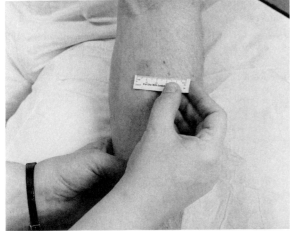

REVIEW QUESTIONS

1. Define the term *allergy,* and list six signs and symptoms of an allergy.
2. A patch test is left in place for a minimum of _____ hours up to a maximum of _____ hours.
3. List two body sites that are frequently used to apply a patch test. Which is the preferred site for adults? For children?
4. Describe how you would read and record the results of:

   Patch test   Mantoux test
   Scratch test   Tine tuberculin test
5. What body site would you use to administer an intradermal injection?
6. Why don't you massage the skin after administering an intradermal injection?
7. Where would you administer the tine tuberculin test? What is the purpose of this test?
8. Why are control tests essential in each type of allergy skin test?

PERFORMANCE TEST

In a skills laboratory, the medical assistant student will demonstrate skill in performing the following activities without reference to source materials. Time limits for the performance of each procedure are to be assigned by the instructor (see also pp. 32 and 35).

1. Select and prepare the supplies and equipment, then perform the following procedures:
   Patch test
   Scratch test
   Intradermal skin test (intradermal injection)
   Mantoux test
   Tine tuberculin test
2. Read and record the results of the above tests.

   The student is expected to perform these procedures with 100% accuracy.

PERFORMANCE CHECKLISTS

Patch Test

1. Wash your hands.
2. Assemble the equipment.
3. Identify and prepare the patient; explain the procedure; position the patient.
4. Cleanse the skin.
5. Prepare the dressing with the allergen.
6. Apply the impregnated dressing to the skin.
7. Label the test allergen with name or number.
8. Instruct the patient.
9. Record the test on the patient's record.
10. Remove the patch, and read the results.
11. Instruct the patient.
12. Leave the treatment room clean.
13. Wash your hands.
14. Record the results on the patient's record.

Scratch Test

1. Wash your hands.
2. Assemble the equipment.
3. Identify and prepare the patient, explain the procedure, and position the patient with the test site exposed and supported.
4. Wash the skin site.
5. Write test numbers 2 inches apart on skin.
6. Make a ⅛ inch scratch.
7. Place one drop of the allergen on the scratch.
8. Make additional scratches, and apply other allergens as needed.
9. Allow the allergen to set for 30 minutes.
10. Wipe off excess solution.
11. Read the results.
12. Instruct the patient.
13. Leave the treatment room clean.
14. Wash your hands.
15. Record the test results on the patient's record.

Intradermal Skin Test and Mantoux Test

1. Wash your hands.
2. Assemble equipment.
3. Prepare the syringe and needle for use.
4. Check the physician's order.
5. Identify the medication label three times.
6. Cleanse the stopper of the vial, insert the needle, and withdraw the required amount of solution.
7. Identify the patient, and explain the procedure.
8. Select the injection site, and position the patient.
9. Cleanse the injection site.
10. Remove the needle cover, and expel air bubbles from the syringe.
11. Facing the patient, grasp and support the forearm to be injected with your nondominant hand; pull the anterior skin taut.
12. Insert the needle at a 10 to 15 degree angle.
13. Inject the solution slowly.
14. Withdraw the needle; wipe the injection site gently. *Do not* massage the injection site.
15. Observe the patient for any unusual reaction; position the patient for safety and comfort.
16. Instruct the patient.
17. Remove and dispose of used needle and syringe correctly.
18. Wash your hands.
19. Record the procedure on the patient's record.
20. Read the results.
21. Record the results on the patient's record.

Tine Tuberculin Test

1. Wash your hands.
2. Assemble the supplies.
3. Identify and prepare the patient; explain the procedure; position the patient with a forearm exposed.
4. Cleanse the skin on the forearm.
5. Remove the protective cap on the tine unit.
6. Grasp the patient's forearm; with your dominant hand, puncture the skin with the tine unit; hold for 1 second before withdrawing.
7. Discard the tine unit in container for waste.
8. Instruct the patient.
9. Wash your hands.
10. Record the test on the patient's record.
11. Read the reaction in a good light; the patient's forearm should be slightly flexed.
12. Record the time and results on the patient's record.

Unit XIV

Physical Therapy

COGNITIVE OBJECTIVES

On completion of Unit XIV, the medical assistant student should be able to apply the following cognitive objectives:

1. Define and pronounce the terms listed in the vocabulary.
2. Differentiate between physical medicine and physical therapy; a physiatrist and a physical therapist.
3. List 11 modalities and/or techniques employed for treatments in physical therapy, indicating the nature and purpose or use of each.
4. Describe the differences between ultraviolet radiation, diathermy, ultrasound, and local applications of heat and cold.
5. State the physiological reactions that occur with applications of heat and with applications of cold.
6. Discuss the principles of preparation and patient care for applications of heat and cold.
7. List examples of dry and moist applications of heat and cold, and describe how to apply these to a patient.
8. Outline the types and uses of traction, massage, and exercises.
9. Differentiate between electrotherapy and electrodiagnostic techniques, explaining the nature and purpose of each.
10. Identify the medical assistant's responsibilities relevant to physical therapy procedures.
11. Outline the steps for performance checklists for the application of heat and cold treatments and other physical therapy modalities listed in this unit.
12. Define and discuss the principles of body mechanics.
13. Discuss the safety precautions and techniques to use when helping patients getting in and out of wheelchairs.

TERMINAL PERFORMANCE OBJECTIVES

On completion of Unit XIV, the medical assistant student should be able to do the following terminal performance objectives.

1. Assemble supplies and equipment necessary to correctly apply applications of heat and cold.
2. Apply the various hot and cold applications using safety precautions to avoid injury to the patient or yourself.
3. Demonstrate proficiency in communicating proper preparation of the patient for physical therapy treatments.
4. Discuss with the instructor the desired and undesired effects of applications of heat and cold.
5. Design a teaching-instruction program for the patient who will be using the following modalities at home:

   Heating pad   Moist cold compress
   Hot water bottle   Ice pack
   Hot moist compress   Alcohol sponge bath
   Ice bag
6. Design a performance checklist to be used for the application of the following:

   Dry heat applications   Dry cold applications
   Moist heat applications   Moist cold applications
7. Demonstrate correct standing, lifting, and bending techniques.
8. Demonstrate safe techniques when helping a patient to get in and out of a wheelchair.
9. Assist patients in learning how to walk with crutches and with a cane.

The student is to perform the above activities with 100% accuracy.*

Vocabulary

arthritis (ar-thrī′tis)—Inflammation of a joint.
bursitis (bur-sī′tis)—Inflammation of a bursa. The most commonly affected is the bursa of the shoulder.
conduction (kon-duk′shun)—The passage or conveyance of energy, as of electricity, heat, or sound.

*It is suggested that the student review Diagnostic and Therapeutic Procedures, and Organizing the Recordings of Diagnostic Procedures, in Unit IX, pp. 285–288 before proceeding with this unit.

debridement (da-brēd-ment')—The process of removing foreign material and devitalized tissue.

hypothermia (hī'pō-ther'mē-ah)—Low body temperature.

light therapy or phototherapy (fō'tō-ther'ah-pē)—The use of light rays in the treatment of disease processes. By custom, this includes the use of ultraviolet and infrared or heat rays (radiation).

modality (mō-dal'ĭ-tē)—Therapeutic agents used in physical medicine and physical therapy.

psoriasis (so-rī-'ah-sis)—A chronic inflammatory recurrent skin disease characterized by scaly red patches on the body surfaces. The lesions are seen most often on knees, elbows, scalp, and fingernails. Other areas frequently affected are the chest, abdomen, palms of the hands, soles of the feet, and backs of the arms and legs. The cause is unknown, although a hereditary factor is suggested.

sprain (sprān)—A joint injury in which some fibers of a supporting ligament are ruptured, but continuity of the ligament remains intact. There may also be damage to the associated muscles, tendons, nerves, and blood vessels.

strain (strān)—An overexertion or overstretching of some part of a muscle.

tendinitis (ten"dĭ-nī'tis)—Inflammation of a tendon; one of the most common causes of acute pain in the shoulder.

Physical medicine or physiatrics (fiz'ē-ah'triks) is the medical discipline that uses physical and mechanical agents in the diagnosis, treatment, and prevention of disease processes and bodily ailments. The therapeutic use of these agents in conjunction with patient education and rehabilitation programs (rather than by medicinal or surgical means) is called physical therapy (PT). Physicians who specialize in this field are **physiatrists** (fiz"e-ah'trist). Specially trained licensed individuals skilled in the techniques of physical therapy (physiotherapy) and qualified to administer treatments and tests prescribed by a physician are physical therapists (physiotherapists).

A great variety of modalities and techniques using the properties of heat, cold, electricity, water, light, mechanical maneuvers, and exercise is used in physical therapy. The *purpose* and *aim* of physical therapy is to relieve pain, increase circulation, restore and improve muscular function, build strength, and increase the range of motion or mobility of a joint. Aside from treating patients with neuromuscular conditions, physical therapy is involved with a significant number of physical conditioning programs, particularly for patients with cardiac and pulmonary conditions. Chest therapy is also given to patients with pulmonary conditions to help clear secretions and keep the air passageways open and clear. Patient education is a major area in physical therapy — that is, phys-

ical therapists teach and train patients how to perform essential activities that they can do themselves for their condition and how to avoid recurrences of certain problems.

Generally speaking, physical therapy treatments are given by physical therapists or the physician; therefore, the duties of the medical assistant may be limited. However, the medical assistant in the physician's office is often required to administer some types of physical therapy treatments under the direction and supervision of the physician. In addition, at the physician's request, the medical assistant should be able to explain the nature and purpose of the treatment or test to the patient, or provide adequate instructions to be followed by the patient at home. It is too often assumed that patients who are to use heat or cold applications at home know how to do so without assistance. The medical assistant will wish to ensure that these patients understand the dangers of using heat or cold to excess and the importance of using the correct solution at the proper temperature.

Some acquaintance with the various modalities used in physical therapy is therefore a requirement for the well-trained medical assistant. The following pages are devoted to briefing the medical assistant on various physical therapy modalities and techniques employed and their uses and purposes. Additional materials that may be studied or demonstrations for using the equipment are provided by the manufacturers of the modalities.

For any of the subsequent treatments that may fall within the scope of the medical assistant's duties on the job, the basic steps as stated in previous units for all procedures must be implemented. The medical assistant should now be able to organize the information that will be presented on various treatments into the following briefly stated procedural steps. These steps can also be used as a guideline for a performance test checklist.

1. Check the physician's order.
2. Wash your hands.
3. Assemble the equipment and supplies needed.
4. Identify the patient, and explain the nature and purpose of the treatment.
5. Prepare the patient: position correctly and comfortably, and drape as necessary.
6. Prepare supplies for use.
7. Proceed with the treatment, and time it accurately.
8. Observe the area to which the treatment has been applied frequently for desired or adverse reactions.
9. Remove the application used for the treatment.
10. Attend to the patient's safety and comfort; provide further instructions as indicated.
11. Properly care for the used equipment and supplies.
12. Wash your hands.

13. Record the treatment and the results obtained. Charting example:

September 9, 19_____, 9 AM

Hot moist compress applied to a wound on the inner aspect of the right forearm at 110° F for 1 hour. On completion of the treatment, the skin appeared pink, and the wound appeared clean; no evidence of suppuration present. Dry dressing was applied. Patient stated that most of the pain was relieved and that the compress provided much comfort.

Kim Worth, CMA

ULTRAVIOLET LIGHT

Ultraviolet rays are rays beyond the violet end of the visible spectrum. They are produced by the sun and by sun lamps. Although ultraviolet rays produce very little heat, they can cause tanning on the skin or a sunburn (redness, erythema) and are capable of killing bacteria and other microorganisms and activating the formation of vitamin D.

Ultraviolet rays (light) are used therapeutically in the treatment of acne, psoriasis, pressure sores, and wound infections. The purposes of this treatment are to stimulate growing epithelial cells and cause capillary hyperemia and to increase cellular metabolism and vascular engorgement, which increases the skin's defenses against bacterial infections.

Various forms of apparatus provide ultraviolet rays. Before receiving ultraviolet treatment, the patient's sensitivity must first be determined. This is done by exposing different areas of the patient's skin to different dosages of the rays for different time periods. The following day the patient returns so that the response can be determined. A little redness on the skin area is wanted, but not a real burn. For example, if 20 seconds of exposure gives the maximum coloration to the skin that is wanted without giving any more, the treatment is started with a 20 second exposure period to the ultraviolet light; then, depending on the light used, the exposure time is usually increased by 10 second intervals. The number of treatments to be given depends on how well the patient is responding.

When this treatment is given, the light must be placed at least 30 inches away from the patient and directed *only* on the area(s) to be treated.

Timing of the exposure period *must be exact*, as excessive exposure can cause severe sunburn up to second and third degree burns. Dark goggles should be worn by both the patient and the operator of the light to protect their eyes.

The patient *must never* be left unattended while being exposed to this light. If you are timing the exposure period and for some reason have to leave the room, you must disconnect the light and resume the treatment when you return. Some lights will turn off automatically, but it is still important for the operator to be present in the room when the patient is receiving this treatment to ensure that undesired burns do not result.

DIATHERMY

Diathermy is a heat-inducing wavelength that is part of the electromagnetic spectrum. It is the therapeutic use of a high frequency current, the purpose being to generate heat within a part of the body. Diathermy works by inducing an electrical field, a conduction field in the tissues, and thereby heats the tissues and increases the circulation.

Diathermy is used in the treatment of muscular problems and sometimes for the treatment of arthritis, bursitis, and tendinitis.

The term *diathermy* is also applied to the many different machines available for this purpose.

Depending on the machine used, the applicator is generally placed at least 1 inch away from the patient's skin. The heating element of some machines has a spacer built into it—that is, there is a space between the outside cover on the unit and the actual heating element. With these machines the element is placed directly against the skin, because it is the outside cover of the unit and not the actual heating element that is in contact with the skin. The built-in spacer of these machines provides the required distance between the skin and the heating element.

Other machines have pads on the applicators. When these machines are used, towels (1-inch thickness) are placed between the pad and the patient's skin.

When giving diathermy treatments, you must watch for desensitized skin areas, because patients have to be able to feel the heat; otherwise they can get burned without realizing that they are getting burned. Areas of skin breakdown and other reactive areas such as inflamed areas must be avoided.

The electrical field of diathermy is attracted by metal. Therefore patients who have metal implants, such as joint implants, cannot receive diathermy treatments. Also patients cannot be wearing any jewelry or other metal objects such as buckles and hairpins, and cannot be positioned on a metal table or chair, but must be on wooden furniture. If these practices are not followed, the patient may receive severe burns, because metal will become hot once the diathermy unit is turned on. Duration of the treatment is usually 15 to 20 minutes and should be timed carefully. It must be explained to the patient that a warm, comfortable feeling should be experienced, and if it becomes uncomfortable, to inform the operator of the unit. If the patient complains that the treatment is becoming too hot, it must be stopped to avoid burning the patient. To operate any of the diathermy units available, you must carefully follow the instructions for use supplied by the manufacturers of each unit. Currently, diathermy is no longer used very much in many facilities. It has been replaced by ultrasound.

ULTRASOUND

Ultrasound is also part of the electromagnetic spectrum. Therapeutic ultrasound is a very specific part of the sound spectrum that provides acoustic vibration with frequencies beyond human ear perception. This form of treatment utilizes high frequency sound waves to penetrate deep tissue layers. Sound waves transform into heat whey they reach deep tissues. (Ultrasound is also used for diagnostic purposes. Review p. 376 in Unit XII.)

Ultrasound vibrates on a molecular level. The two effects obtained from ultrasound are a mechanical effect and a heating effect. The mechanical effect, the vibration that causes the heating, is most noticeable on connective tissues, such as tendons and ligaments. A heating effect is produced on almost all tissues with the exception of bone, as bone reflects ultrasound; that is, ultrasound is reflected from bone.

Ultrasound is of value for the treatment of pain syndromes, to relax muscle spasm, and to provide deep penetration of heat and stimulate circulation in small areas, as when used to increase blood supply to tissues in patients with vascular disorders. It is also used in breaking up calcium deposits and in loosening scars.

Ultrasound is applied by means of an applicator with a sound head, approximately 2 inches in diameter, that extends off from the special machine. Since ultrasound is not conducted through the air, a conducting medium must be spread on the patient's skin over the area to be treated. Special gels are available for this; mineral oil can also be used, but it is not as effective. After the gel is applied to the skin, the operator of the machine holds the sound head and moves it in a steady up-and-down and rotary motion over the skin. The applicator must be in motion when used to prevent internal burns or tissue damage. Special care must also be taken when this treatment is used on patients with implants, such as joint implants, as ultrasound will tend to vibrate and loosen the implant. Also heat will build up in the metal (Fig. 14-1). Ultrasound can also be applied under water for treatment of the hands and feet. The water then acts as the conducting medium for the ultrasound. The length of any treatment will depend on the size of the area being treated, but is usually under 10 minutes. For example: ultrasound treatment to the lower back is applied for 6 to 7 minutes on one side. The minimal

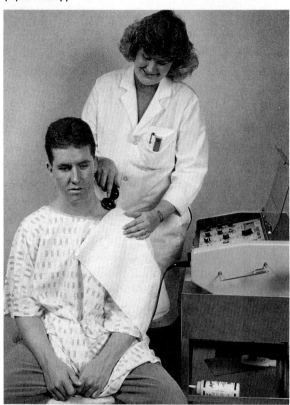

Fig. 14-1. Ultrasound therapy applied to patient's shoulder in physical therapy.

number of ultrasound treatments to be given to be effective varies from 5 to 12.

After use, the sound head should be cleansed with alcohol. Instructions for use of the ultrasound machines are supplied by the manufacturers and must be followed carefully.

LOCAL APPLICATIONS OF HEAT (THERMOTHERAPY) AND COLD (CRYOTHERAPY)

Dry and moist applications of heat and cold have been employed universally as an effective means of treatment by individuals in the home, and by physicians, nurses, medical assistants, and physical therapists, either in an office or hospital setting. Tolerance for the temperature changes that occur when heat or cold is applied to the body varies with the individual and also varies in different parts of the body. Generally, the more sensitive skin areas to these changes are those that are not usually exposed; the less sensitive areas are those that are exposed, usually having thicker and tougher layers of skin, such as areas on the soles of the feet or the palms of the hands.

Once heat or cold is applied to the skin, certain physiological reactions occur in the body, heat hav-

Table 14-1. Physiological reactions produced by heat and cold applications

Body Function	Heat	Cold
Blood vessels in area	Dilated (increasing circulation)	Constricted (decreasing circulation)
Heat production	Decreased	Increased (by shivering)
Blood pressure	Lowered	Elevated
Respiratory rate	Increased	Increased
Tissue metabolism	Increased	Decreased

ing the opposite effect to that of cold except for respiratory rate changes (Table 14-1).

Heat or cold modalities are to be placed on a bare body surface for only *short durations.* An important fact to remember is that the prolonged use of heat (more than 1 hour) produces reverse secondary effects; that is, blood vessels will then constrict, thus decreasing blood supply to the area. The prolonged use of cold (more than 1 hour) also has a reverse secondary effect; that is, blood vessels will dilate, thus increasing circulation and tissue metabolism. In other words, the immediate effect of heat applications is vasodilation, whereas the prolonged effect is vasoconstriction. Likewise, the immediate effect of cold applications is vasoconstriction, whereas the prolonged effect is vasodilation. Therefore, heat applications should not be left in place for long periods of time. Cold applications can be used for longer periods than heat, depending on the desired effects. The physician will usually indicate the temperature (that is, warm or hot, tepid, cool, cold, or very cold) and the time period to be used for the following applications of dry and moist hot and cold applications.

Principles for Preparation and Patient Care

Because applications of heat and cold are common treatments, the medical assistant should keep in mind the following principles regarding preparation and patient care:

1. Learn exactly where and for how long the application is to be placed on the patient's body.
2. Position the patient comfortably so that the treatment can be maintained for the designated time period.
3. Avoid accidents — be sure that the patient is positioned safely and will not fall. Place solutions in a convenient location and so that they will not spill.
4. Test the solution (with a bath thermometer) or the device you are using to be sure that it is at the exact temperature that the physician ordered or the recommended temperature for the method used.
5. Remove any dressings covering the area to be treated. (Review the procedure for a dressing

change, pp. 174–177). Apply a clean dressing, if ordered, when the treatment is completed.
6. Keep the application at the ordered temperature. Generally, compresses and packs cool off within 15 to 20 minutes and then will have to be reheated and reapplied. If the temperature of the device or the solution changes, it will not accomplish its purpose and may even harm the patient.
7. Keep the patient warm during the application of heat; drape sheets or blankets can be used to cover the patient. When blood vessels dilate (as with the application of heat), more blood comes to the surface of the body and the body is cooled by the surrounding air. Thus, the patient can easily become chilled unless protected with coverings.
8. Check the patient's skin frequently during the application to observe for any skin changes, as well as any signs of burns or frostbite. Report any signs of burns or frostbite *immediately.*
9. Provide further instructions to the patient, as indicated, on completion of the treatment.

Thermotherapy

Superficial heat treatments can be administered with dry or moist heat applications. These local heat applications are used to relieve pain, to promote muscle relaxation and reduce spasm, to increase circulation to an area to relieve congestion and swelling by dilating the blood vessels, and to speed up the inflammatory process to promote suppuration (pus formation) and drainage from an infected area. In addition, dry heat applications are used to dry and heal surgical incisions and sutures, perineal lacerations, and skin ulcers.

Dry Heat

Dry heat applications frequently used include the following:

• Infrared radiation (heat lamps)
• Electric light bulbs
• Electric heating pads
• Hot water bottles

Infrared radiation is dry heat application by means of a heat lamp. The term *infrared* usually refers to the heat lamp. Infrared rays from these lamps provide surface heat and penetrate the skin to a depth of about 5 to 10 mm. At times, a plain gooseneck lamp is used, because the *incandescent light bulb* is a source of infrared rays. Heat lamps must be kept at least 2 to 4 feet away from the skin, varying with the type and intensity of the lamp used. The skin must be clean and free of any ointment or medicinal substances. The duration of the treatment is *usually 15 to 20 minutes,* because prolonged or intense application can lead to burning and blistering of the skin.

Electric heating pads are to be placed in a protective covering, such as a towel or pillow case, and then applied to a dry area. They must never be used over moist or wet areas or dressings where moisture could come in contact with the electricity. Patients must be instructed not to lie on the pad because burns could result. The heat selector switch is usually set on the low or medium setting and left for an accurately timed period. (The amount of heat and period of time to be applied are to be designated by the physician.)

A *hot water bottle* is to be filled only about half full and have the air expelled before it is sealed. This allows the hot water bottle to be lighter and more pliable so that it can be molded to the area where it is to be applied. It is essential to test the temperature of the water accurately with a thermometer before it is poured into the hot water bottle. Water not exceed-

Fig. 14-2. **A,** testing temperature of hot water before placing it into hot water bottle. **B,** expel air from half-filled hot water bottle before using. **C,** cover the hot water bottle before applying to patient.

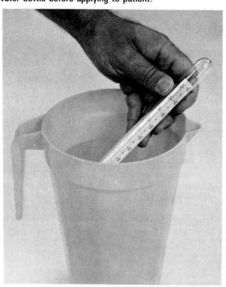
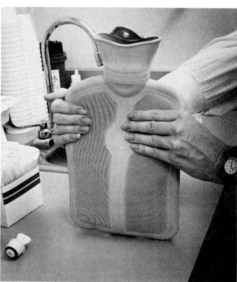
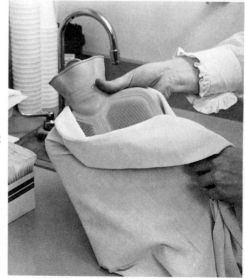

ing 125°F (32°C) is to be used. The accepted temperature ranges are from 115° to 125°F (46° to 52°C) for patients 2 years and older, and from 105° to 115°F (41° to 46°C) for children under 2 years and elderly patients. (The very young and the very old tend to be more sensitive to applications of heat and to cold.) Hot tap water is placed into a pitcher so that the temperature can be tested with a bath thermometer. The outside of the hot water bottle must be dry and then placed into a protective covering, such as a pillowcase or towel, before it is applied to the patient. This protective covering should remain dry unless the hot water bottle is placed over moist dressings to keep them warm (Fig. 14-2).

The patient should experience a feeling of warmth but not be uncomfortable; burns must be avoided. When the hot water bottle is left on for any length of time, it will need to be refilled with hot water so that the desired temperature is maintained. After use, the hot water bottle must be washed thoroughly with warm water and detergent, rinsed, and allowed to dry before being stored. The bottle should be stored with the stopper in place and air inside to prevent the sides from sticking.

Moist Heat Applications

Moist heat applications frequently used include the following:

- Hot soaks
- Hot compresses
- Hot packs

For a *hot soak,* the body part to be treated is immersed gradually (to allow the patient to become accustomed to the heat change) in tap water or a medicated solution of 105° to 110°F (41° to 44°C). *Unless otherwise ordered, the body part is kept immersed for 15 to 20 minutes.* This form of treatment can be used for heat application to the hands, arms, feet, or legs. The process of having the body from the neck down immersed in water in a special tank called the Hubbard tank, or the body or a limb immersed in a whirlpool tank, is more frequently referred to as *hydrotherapy* (see p. 416). Soaks applied to open wounds require the use of sterile (aseptic) technique, a sterile container, and a sterile solution. The water or solution temperature should be maintained as much as possible throughout the treatment. This can be accomplished by removing some of the solution every 5 minutes or so and adding more hot solution. Care to avoid burning the patient must be taken when the hot solution is added. The hot solution should be added to the container at the point farthest away from the patient's skin and stirred quickly into the cooler solution (Fig. 14-3).

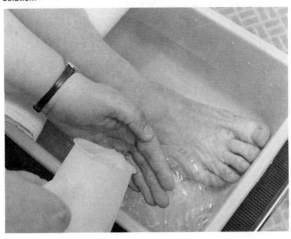

Fig. 14-3. During a hot soak add more hot solution to container at point farthest away from patient's skin and stir quickly into cooler solution.

The patient should be positioned comfortably to prevent strain or pressure on the area treated and also to prevent fatigue. The patient's skin is to be observed during the treatment for excessive redness, at which time the limb is to be removed from the solution until it has cooled. Remember that the observations made during the treatment must be recorded on the patient's record. On completion of the treatment, the limb should be dried with a towel by patting, *not* rubbing. For an open wound, only the surrounding area should be patted dry. The towel used should not touch the open wound. Observation of the area is necessary after the treatment, because this information is to be recorded on the patient's record. Soaks *differ* from compresses and packs in that soaks are used for shorter periods of time and usually at lower temperatures.

Hot moist compresses and packs. There are two basic differences between compresses and packs: (1) different materials are used for each, and (2) a pack is usually applied to a more extensive body area than a compress is.

A *compress* used for the application of moist heat is prepared by taking a soft square of gauze or similar absorbent material (a clean washcloth can also be used), soaking it in hot water, then wringing it out manually or with the use of forceps, to avoid excessive wetness. This material is then applied to a limited body area, such as the finger or a small area on the arm, for a designated period of time (Fig. 14-4). (*Dry compresses* are used to apply pressure or medications to specific restricted areas.)

A *pack* used for the application of moist heat is prepared in the same manner as a compress except that flannel or similar materials are used. Commercially prepared hot packs filled with a silica gel (for example, Hydrocollator packs) are also used. Packs are usually applied to a more extensive body area.

Fig. 14-4. **A,** wring out hot compress to avoid excessive wetness before it is applied. **B,** applying hot compress to body area.

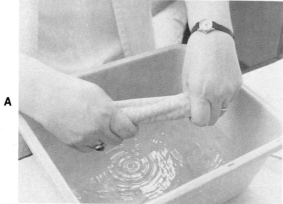

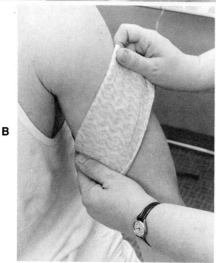

Both compresses and packs are to be applied to the skin area slowly so that the patient can gradually adjust to the heat. The recommended water temperature for soaking gauze, flannel, or similar materials is 105° to 110°F (41° to 44°C). Commercially prepared packs are kept in a hot water bath at 140° to 160°F (60° to 71°C) until used and then wrapped in towels before being applied to the patient's skin. Both compresses and packs should be as hot as the patient can comfortably tolerate. A plastic covering can be placed over or wrapped around the compress or pack to concentrate and hold the heat over the area treated for as long a time as possible.

During these treatments, the patient's skin should be checked frequently to ensure that the skin is not burning and to observe for signs of increased redness or swelling. All observations must be recorded on completion of the treatment. If the patient experiences pain or is uncomfortable, the plastic covering should be removed or unwrapped to release some of the confined heat. If the area remains painful, the pack or compress is to be removed and cooled somewhat before being reapplied. This is done to prevent burning the skin.

Additional compresses or packs should be made ready for use when the applied one cools. The length of these treatments will vary according to the physician's order. *Generally they will be prescribed for 15 to 20 minutes,* but at times may be applied for 1 hour. On completion of the treatment, the compress or pack is removed and the skin patted dry. When these treatments have been applied to an open wound, *only* the surrounding area is to be patted dry. The open wound is *not* to be touched. A clean sterile dressing is applied to an open wound when ordered by the physician. Used equipment and supplies are to be cared for properly. The treatment and all observations are to be recorded on the patient's record.

Cryotherapy

Cryotherapy, the therapeutic use of cold, is applied with dry or moist cold applications. Cold applications are used to

1. Prevent edema or swelling
2. Relieve pain or tenderness (cold produces a topical anesthetic effect)
3. Reduce inflammation and pus formation (cold inhibits microbial activity in the early stages of the infectious process)
4. Control bleeding (the peripheral vessels constrict with the application of cold, thus resulting in a decreased blood flow)
5. Reduce body temperature

Cold is commonly used following strains, sprains, and bruises, and also for muscle spasm and tenderness. Any type of acute injury responds fairly well to cold. During the acute phase of an injury when there may be bleeding in the area, you do not want to use heat. The old rule of thumb for treating such injuries was to apply cold for the first 24 hours, then apply heat. Currently, many health care practitioners frequently wait longer than 24 hours before using heat applications on patients, and often use cold continually when good results are being obtained.

The physician should indicate the temperature to be used for cold applications. The temperatures of the water are described as follows:

- Tepid: 80° to 93°F (26.7° to 33.9°C)
- Cool: 65° to 80°F (18.3° to 26.7°C)
- Cold: 55° to 65°F (12.3° to 18.3°C)
- Very cold: Below 55°F (below 12.5°C)

The selection of the temperature to use will depend on the

- Condition of the patient
- Sensitivity of the patient's skin

- Area to be covered
- Method to be used

The duration of the application depends on the temperature; for example, an ice massage will be given for a shorter time period (5 minutes) than a cold compress or pack (20 to 30 minutes). Colder temperatures can be tolerated best on small areas for short periods of time. It is usually considered dangerous to keep skin temperatures below 40°F (4.4°C) for long periods except when ice is used for anesthesia.

Dry Cold

Dry cold applications frequently used include the following:

- Ice bags
- Ice collars

An *ice bag* is filled one-half to two-thirds full with small pieces of ice; air is expelled from the bag by twisting the top and then capped (Fig. 14-5). At this time the bag should be checked for leaks. Small ice pieces reduce the amount of air spaces in the bag, which results in better conduction of cold and also allows the bag to mold better to the contour of the body part. Once sealed, the ice bag is dried and placed in a protective covering, which provides comfort for the patient and absorbs moisture that condenses on the outside. To be effective, the ice bag is placed on the skin for 30 to 60 minutes, as designated by the physician. If the treatment is to be continuous, the ice bag is applied for 30 to 60 minutes and then removed for 1 hour. By doing the procedure in this manner, the tissues are allowed to react to the immediate effects of the cold.

The patient's skin must be checked periodically for signs of decreased swelling or redness. Signs of excessive coldness, which include mottled and pale skin and excessive numbness in the body part, must be noted when present. When or if this occurs, the ice bag must be removed and the physician notified.

Ice collars are rubber or plastic modalities that are smaller than ice bags and look like a medium-sized rectangle. They are used on the neck, on small areas, or wrapped around a body part.

Moist Cold

Moist cold applications frequently used include the following:

- Cold compresses
- Cold packs
- Ice massage
- Alcohol sponge baths

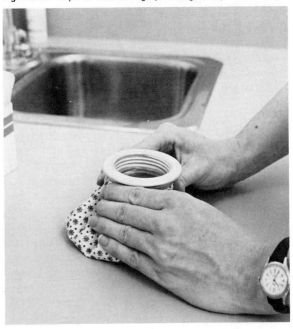

Fig. 14-5. Expel air from ice bag by twisting the top and then cap.

Moist cold compresses are generally applied to small areas, and *cold packs* are used on larger body areas, as are hot applications. Compresses may be used for treating a headache, a tooth extraction, or an eye injury. The area to which the compress is to be applied will determine the type of material used. For example, a clean washcloth can be used on the head or face; surgical gauze dressings with a small amount of cotton filling can be used for eye compresses. The material used for the compress is immersed in a clean basin containing ice chips or small pieces of ice and a small amount of cold water. To avoid dripping, the material is wrung out manually or with the use of forceps and then placed on the skin for the time period designated by the physician (*usually 20 to 30 minutes and then repeated every 2 hours*). Compresses should be changed frequently to maintain a cold application. Most patients will tell you when the compress no longer feels cold. Placing an ice bag over the compress helps keep the compress cold and reduces the number of times that it must be changed. The patient must be checked periodically during this treatment for any changes, such as a decrease or increase in swelling or redness on the area, or a decrease or increase of pain. On completion of the treatment, the skin should be patted dry if necessary. The treatment and observations made are to be recorded on the patient's record.

Cold packs (ice packs) may be applied to a small area but are generally used on larger areas, such as an arm or leg. At times they can be applied to the whole body to lower the temperature. In this case, hypothermia pads or blankets may be used, rather than ice packs. These are used in hospitals with the patient under close observation for temperature and skin changes. Manufacturers of hypothermia units provide complete instructions for use, which must be followed precisely.

To apply a cold or ice pack, first wrap the extremity in wet toweling and then pack ice chips around it; place an additional towel over the ice to reduce the melting rate. *Generally, these are applied for 20 to 30 minutes.* Commercial cold packs are also available. These are kept in a freezer until used. They do not freeze stiff, thus are pliable and can be molded to fit the contour of the body part.

Ice massage is simply massaging the area with ice. This can be as simple as freezing water in a paper cup and then rubbing it over the affected area for approximately 5 minutes (Fig. 14-6).

In the past *alcohol sponge baths* were recommended and used frequently, both in hospital and at home, for reducing a patient's elevated temperature. Presently they are more commonly done in a home situation, because they have been replaced in many hospitals or health care facilities by hypothermia pads or blankets. A mixture of half alcohol and half tepid water is used for an alcohol sponge bath. Because alcohol vaporizes more quickly than water, heat is removed from the skin surface rapidly when this mixture is applied to the body in contrast to using just a cold bath.

An alcohol sponge bath should *not* exceed 30 minutes. The patient should be draped with covers, and a hot water bottle may be applied to the feet to avoid excessive chilling and shivering. An ice bag may be applied to the head to promote comfort and relieve a headache, if present. Only the area being sponged is to be exposed. Two clean washcloths are needed—while one is being used, the other is to be cooling in the alcohol-water solution. Each extremity should be sponged for approximately 5 minutes, the back and buttocks for 5 to 10 minutes, the trunk and abdomen for 5 minutes. Moist cool cloths can be placed over large superficial blood vessels in the neck, axilla, and groin during the procedure as additional aids to lower the body temperature. The temperature should be recorded 30 minutes after the sponge to determine if the treatment has been effective.

Patients should be cautioned *not* to use alcohol sponge baths indiscriminately, because alcohol has a tendency to dry out the skin. In addition, if a fever does not break after the application of two or three alcohol sponge baths given in the home, the physician should be notified.

HYDROTHERAPY

Hydrotherapy is the use of water in the treatment of disease processes. Since these treatments are usually not performed in the physician's office, the patient will be referred to a physiotherapy department in a hospital or to a physical therapist's office. On other occasions the patient may be instructed to apply hot or cold soaks, compresses, or packs at home.

Modalities utilized for hydrotherapy include the Hubbard tank, the whirlpool, and a larger pool, all with varying temperatures of hot or cold water, as designated by the physician for each patient's care.

These three modalities are used primarily to promote relaxation, circulation, and early motion (by exercising) of the injured body part. Other uses include those discussed previously under Local Applications of Heat, p. 410. It is also used to cleanse and debride the skin, for example, in patients who have extensive burns. The Hubbard tank is a large tank in which the whole body can be immersed either in a sitting or lying position. It is basically a large whirlpool in which body exercises may also be done. The whirlpool is a tank of agitating water in which an arm, leg, or body can be immersed. The mechanical action of the water movement provides hydromassage, is very relaxing, and stimulates circulation. Body exercises cannot be done in the whirlpool tank because it is too small. The pool used in physical therapy is like a medium-sized swimming pool. Many types of exercises can be performed in the pool, because once in the pool, the effects of gravity can be reduced. For example, patients who are not strong enough to stand up alone

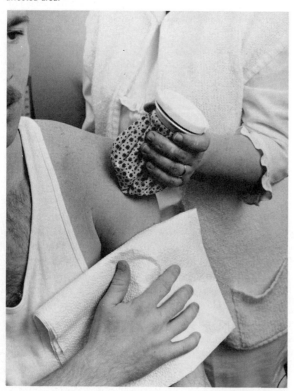

Fig. 14-6. Ice massage is one form of cryotherapy that can be used to decrease pain. Freeze water in paper cup and then rub it over affected area.

can stand up in the pool because they are supported by the water. The water also produces a heating or cooling effect, depending on the temperature used.

PARAFFIN WAX HAND BATH

Another form of heat application used for patients with rheumatoid arthritis is the hot paraffin wax hand bath. The purposes of this treatment are to relieve pain, increase circulation, and decrease the duration of morning stiffness of the fingers, hands, and wrists. An advantage of this treatment over moist heat applications is the longer-lasting (2 to 3 hours) circulatory changes that it can produce. This procedure can be performed at home, in the physician's office, or in a physical therapy department. Special containers are available for storing and heating the wax; or in a home situation, a double boiler may be used. Seven parts of canning grade paraffin wax are melted and heated to 126°F (52°C) and mixed with one part mineral oil. The *dry* hand and wrist are rapidly dipped in the warm paraffin and removed. This is done repeatedly until a fairly good coat of wax is covering the area. After each immersion, the wax is allowed to harden. The wax-covered area is then covered with a towel or aluminum foil or a newspaper, which acts as an insulator to help retain the heat. The wax (paraffin) is left in place for 15 to 20 minutes, then peeled off and replaced in the container for the next application. The fingers and wrist are then generally put through range-of-motion exercise, because the heat relieves pain and thus enables the patient to exercise the fingers and wrist with greater mobility. NOTE: One must be very careful that the hand and wrist are dry when placed in the warm paraffin wax. If there is moisture or water on the hand, it will conduct heat much more quickly and will burn the area. Burns are prevented when the area immersed is dry and dipped and removed rapidly.

TRACTION

Traction is the process of pulling or drawing, as applied to the musculoskeletal system for dislocated joints, fractured bones, or diseased peripheral joints (for example, arthritic joints). This therapy may be used in the physician's office, but more frequently is applied by physical therapists. Traction devices can also be set up for home use. Traction is used to

- Obtain and maintain proper position
- Correct or prevent a deformity
- Decrease or overcome muscle spasms
- Lessen or prevent contractures
- Facilitate healing
- Promote better movement of the area

- Lessen and prevent severe stiffening of peripheral joints
- Achieve vertebral distraction

Methods and Devices

Weight or Static Traction.   This method of traction is applied with weights of varied poundages that are connected to the end of a pulley mechanism. For example, the patient's head is placed in a head harness, which is attached to a rope with weights on the end. The rope is attached to a pole or door top so that it stretches up over the head and then is displaced downward where the weights are attached.

Elastic Traction.   Elastic traction is applied with elastic appliances that exert a pull on the affected limb.

Mechanical Traction.   Mechanical traction is applied by means of units that give an intermittent type of traction. They are set to pull and hold a set amount of tension for a set period of time and then to relax for a set period of time. They will continue to pull and relax as long as they are set.

Manual Traction.   Manual traction is applied by therapists using their hands to exert a pull on the affected part. In addition to other musculoskeletal problems, manual traction is frequently used to treat peripheral joint disease, such as arthritic joints, to distract the joint surface in order to obtain more movement and prevent severe stiffening.

Skin Traction.   Skin traction is applied by placing foam rubber pads, or some other material, with a weight attached to the end along the sides of the affected limb. For support, this application is wrapped with elastic bandages.

Skeletal Traction.   Skeletal traction is applied only in the hospital. Surgically installed pins and wires or tongs (for example, head tongs) are used to apply a pulling force directly on a bone.

MASSAGE

Massage was probably the first form of physical therapy. Individuals instinctively rub or massage an area after incurring an injury or bruise. After administering an injection, we rub the injection site, which is also a type of massage. Massage can be that simple, but it is also a highly skilled technique. Massage is a systematic and methodical pressure applied to bare skin by stroking, rubbing, kneading or rolling, tapping or pounding with the fingers or cupped hand, or by quick tappings with alternating fingertips. The type of massage used most frequently in the physician's office and clinics is stroking. Also tapotement, the pounding or cupping with a cupped hand, is used on patients with chest congestion, because this helps loosen the secretions and clear the congestion. Other purposes of massage are to

- Aid circulation by removing blood and waste products from injured tissues and by bringing fresh blood to the injured part, which helps the healing process
- Relax muscles and relieve spasms
- Reduce pain
- Help restore motion and function to the affected part
- Prevent swelling, as after the administration of an injection
- Reduce edema

To apply massage effectively, the therapist or assistant must be in a comfortable position to avoid straining, and the hands should be warm, to avoid discomfort to the patient. The patient must also be in a comfortable position so that beneficial results are more easily obtained.

EXERCISES

Therapeutic exercise is the performance of prescribed physical exertion to

- Improve one's general health status
- Improve one's general health status after being afflicted with disabilities affecting the neuromuscular, skeletal, cardiovascular, integumentary, respiratory, and urinary systems, in addition to treatment for congenital defects, prenatal and postnatal care, and psychiatric problems
- Correct a physical deformity
- Improve muscle tone and strengthen muscles
- Restore the strength of muscles that have atrophied or weakened because of disease processes
- Restore motion after a fracture, injury, or any form of immobilization
- Aid circulation
- Improve coordination

Exercises may be performed in the physician's office, in physical therapy departments, or the patient may be given instructions and taught the exercises to be performed at home. Patients who are to do exercises at home must be *taught* how to do them and not just *told* what to do. Reasons for the exercise program must also be explained to the patient. The medical assistant responsible for these duties should have the patient perform the exercises while in the office until the motions involved are fully understood to ensure that the patient is capable of performing the prescribed exercise program.

Classifications

Active Exercises.   All the motions involved in the exercise are performed totally by the patient and may involve the use of weights, pulleys, rubber balls, or similar appliances that the patient is to squeeze or manipulate.

Passive Exercises.   In these exercises, movement to the part is done by another person or outside force without any voluntary participation from the patient (Figs. 14-7, 14-8, and 14-9).

Aided Exercises.   In these exercises, the patient is helped to move muscles that are too weak to move on their own strength. Exercises that are performed in a pool are also considered aided exercises.

Active Resistance Exercises.   In these exercises the patient voluntarily applies pressure or movement of the part, and another individual applies resistance to the motion.

Range-of-Motion Exercises.   These exercises are designed to assist joint mobility and normal functioning, for example, bending the fingers, or twisting the wrist around in a normal motion, or rotation of the leg in a circumscribed fashion. They can be either active or passive exercises (Figs, 14-7, 14-8, and 14-9).

Joint Mobility Terminology

abduction—movement of a body part away from the midline of the body, as when moving the arm out to the side (see Fig. 14-7).
adduction—movement of a body part toward the midline of the body, as when bringing a raised arm down to the side of the body. The opposite of abduction.
extension—movement of a joint that opens it or that increases the angle between the bones (Figs. 14-7 and 14-8).
hyperextension—the extension of a limb or part beyond normal limits.
flexion—bending of a joint so that the angle between bones is reduced, as in bending the arm at the elbow or the leg at the knee or the toes. Opposite of extension (Fig. 14-8).
dorsiflexion—movement that bends a body part backward, as of the hand or foot.
eversion—movement that turns a body part outward; movement of the ankle that turns the foot outward.
inversion—movement that turns a body part in-

Fig. 14-7. Abduction of thumb and finger extension. **A,** with one hand hold the patient's fingers straight. Bend the patient's thumb towards the palm with your other hand. **B,** move the patient's thumb back, pointing away from the hand. Repeat this movement. **C,** rotate the thumb (in a circle). These exercises should be done on the good hand as well as on the weak hand.

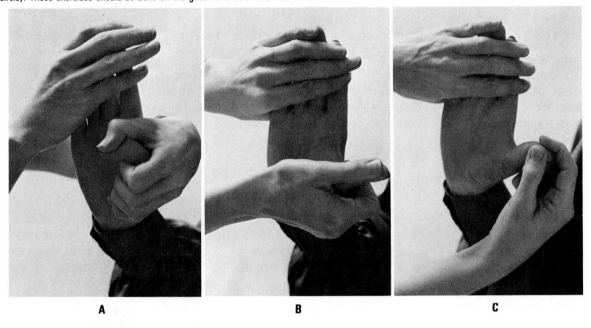

A   B   C

Fig. 14-8. Toe extension and flexion. **A,** support patient's foot and pull up on the toes. **B,** support patient's foot and push toes down.

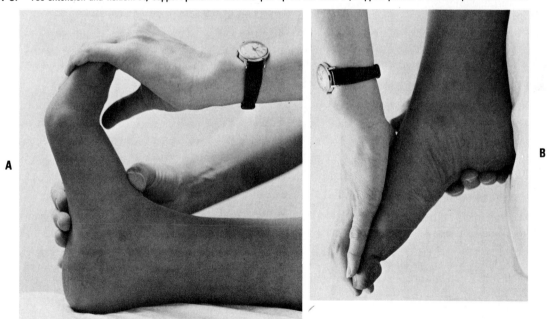

A   B

ward; movement of the ankle that turns the foot inward (Fig. 14-9).

pronation—movement of the arm to have the palm facing downward.

supination—movement of the arm to have the palm facing upward. Opposite of pronation.

rotation—the process of turning around an axis. The rotation of a bone on its central axis.

external rotation—outward rotation.

BODY MECHANICS

Body mechanics is the way you handle yourself safely and effectively, essentially how you hold yourself together in dynamic posture, when you are moving around, lifting, pulling, pushing, stooping, or carrying, or when performing any type of manual labor. It is also how you use your body when sitting, standing, or lying down. Safe body mechanics include the princi-

Fig. 14-9. Inversion of foot. **A,** support patient's foot and turn whole foot outward. **B,** support patient's foot and turn whole foot inward.

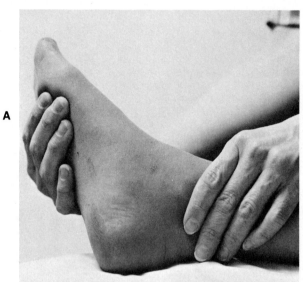

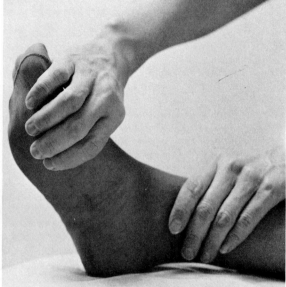

ples of proper body alignment, balance, and movement. When you apply these principles you can minimize the amount of energy you expend, and also improve your strength and flexibility when sitting, standing, and walking. An important aspect of using correct body mechanics is that you can prevent muscle and back fatigue, pain, strain, and injury.

Many individuals involved in the health care field often have to move and/or lift patients and equipment. Every time you lift, stand, sit, or even lie down, you are using your back. Therefore it is crucial that you know how to use safe and effective methods for moving and lifting for your own protection and also so that you are capable of teaching patients how to use these same methods for their own safety and protection. These same methods apply to all activities involving body movement and posture in everyday life. Safe and effective body mechanics keep the spine balanced when you stand, sit, or lie down. These proper movements are extremely important both on the job and at home. Good posture is necessary, as without this the overall spinal structure can be weakened and the back will be more susceptible to injury.

Correct standing, lifting, and bending habits must be developed, practiced, and maintained. The following is a general guide for proper use of the body.

Standing

Good posture and muscles help to keep your spine balanced when standing. Stand with your feet apart and one foot slightly in front of the other to provide a stable and wide base of support. When having to stand for a long period of time with little movement, place one foot on a low stool to help keep your spine

in balance. Don't twist or lean forward when standing and lifting; move your feet instead, and keep your upper body in line with your hips.

Sitting

For the least strain and injury to your back, keep the three normal curves of your spine in balanced alignment. Sit straight in a chair that supports your lower back or add a support to your lumbar curve by placing a pillow or a towel rolled up to 4 to 6 inches behind that area. When sitting on a stool, lean forward and rest your upper body lightly on your elbows and arms.

Lifting Techniques

1. Assess the load before beginning to lift. Get help when in doubt about lifting alone.
2. Clear the area where the lift will take place; for example, move chairs out of the way.
3. Explain the procedure to the patient (when the load you will be lifting is a patient and continue to communicate during the procedure so that the patient can work with you and not against you).
4. Keep the weight as close to your body as possible when lifting rather than reaching forward.
5. Attain and maintain a firm grip on the object or patient throughout the lift.
6. Keep your back straight and body weight over your feet (if possible). Don't bend the lower back at the lumbosacral area (Fig. 14-10).
7. Use your leg muscles during the lift. Bend your knees sufficiently (not your waist) so that your large leg muscles will be used.

Fig. 14-10. Good body mechanics. Keep your back straight and body weight over your feet when lifting.

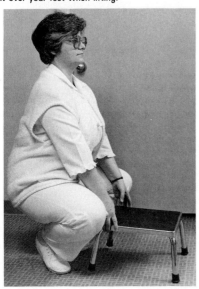

8. Establish a firm, stable foot position. Place your feet 10 to 12 inches apart and point them in the direction of the lift. One foot may be placed in front of the other for balance (Fig. 14-10).
9. Move your feet with the direction of the lift. *You must avoid twisting your back.*
10. Avoid jerking and jolting. Use even, smooth movements.
11. When two people are required to perform the lift, one person is to act as the leader. The leader should set and call the signals for beginning the lift and subsequent moves.
12. Bend your knees as much as possible when lowering the object or patient at the completion of the lift.
13. Use the appropriate type of lifting technique for the situation.
14. Use the "hip-bend" lift for loads that you cannot get close to, such as when helping or lifting a patient from the examining table, or when getting something from a place that is hard to reach. Once again get as close to the load as possible. Then put your buttocks out behind you, keeping your head and back in a straight line (this will help to balance and protect your spine). Then bend your knees (not your waist), and lift using your leg, buttock, and abdominal muscles (Fig. 14-11).

Remember that proper techniques are just as important when bending without lifting. Squat, don't bend (Fig. 14-12).

Use both sides of your body when lifting, pushing, pulling, or carrying so that the weight will not pull the body into a strained position.

Wear comfortable low-heeled shoes. Wearing high heels or clogs can throw your dynamic posture off and make you compensate when trying to maintain balance.

WHEELCHAIRS

Wheelchairs are mobile chairs of various shapes and sizes that are equipped with large wheels and brakes. Some are moved around manually and others are motorized. When a patient will be using a wheelchair for a long period of time or permanently, the physical therapist will work with a medical product store to obtain a wheelchair that will meet the patient's needs. The therapist will provide the store with all of the patient's information, such as size, disability, activities planned for the days ahead (for example, does the patient plan to go hiking in the wheelchair or use it just around the house), description of the patient's house and area where the chair will be used, and also what type of brakes are needed and if the chair should have right- or left-handed propulsion.

Many patients who will be using the wheelchair forever are taught how to maintain it. For example, young patients who have spinal cord injuries will be taught how to maintain the wheelchair just as they would be taught to maintain a bicycle, such as how to fix a broken wheel or broken brakes. All patients are taught safety techniques for using a wheelchair, such as how to lock and unlock the brakes, how to kick the

Fig. 14-11. The hip-bend lift for loads that you cannot get very close to.

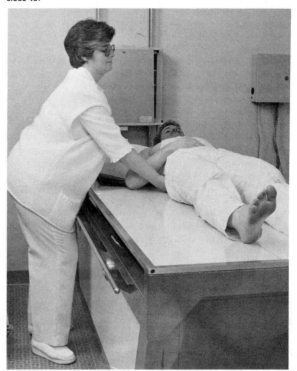

Fig. 14-12. Squat, don't bend. Correct (on the left side); wrong (on the right side).

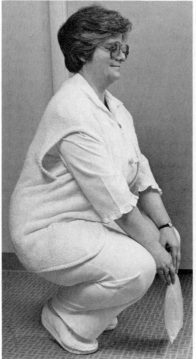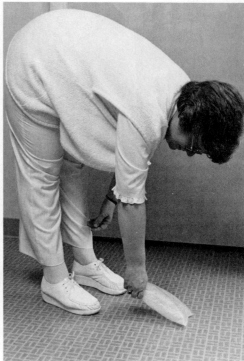

footrest out of the way, how to operate the different pieces of the wheelchair, and how to maneuver it in and out of different spaces. The patient will practice using the wheelchair in the hospital before going home to ensure safe functioning at home.

Wheelchair Transfers

Safety precautions and techniques to use when helping patients to get in and out of a wheelchair include the following:

* Obtain help from another person if you think that you will be unable to accomplish the transfer safely for yourself and the patient.
* Use the strong muscles in your legs and not the weaker muscles in your back when transferring a patient.
* Always move the patient toward the strong side if one side is stronger than the other.
* Support the patient's strong side when assisting with the move.
* Position the wheelchair parallel to the examining table to where the patient will be moving.
* Explain the procedure to the patient.
* Lock the wheels.
* Move the footrests out of the way.
* Position a step stool near the examining table.
* Stand facing the patient.

* Have the patient move forward in the chair. Stay directly in front of the patient. This is important so that you don't twist, as twisting will hurt your back.
* Bend down with your knees. *Do not* bend your back. Then put your arms under the patient's arms and your hands firmly over the patient's scapulae. Have the patient's hands rest on your shoulders (Fig. 14-13, *A*).
* Give a signal and lift upward so that the patient will rise to a standing position.
* Have the patient step up onto the stool and pivot with the back to the table (Fig. 14-13, *B*).
* Ease the patient to a sitting position.
* Place one arm on the patient's shoulder and the other arm under the patient's knees (Fig. 14-13, *C*).
* Using a *single* smooth move, raise the patient's legs onto the table and lower the head and trunk into the supine position.
* Attend to the patient's comfort and safety.

To Transfer a Patient from the Examining Table to a Wheelchair Use the Following Technique:

* Explain the procedure to the patient.
* Position the wheelchair parallel to the examining table.
* Lock the wheels and move the footrests out of the way.
* Place one arm under the patient's shoulders and your other arm under the knees.

Fig. 14-13. **A,** assisting patient out of wheelchair. **B,** assisting patient on to examining table. Have patient step up onto stool and pivot with back to table. **C,** assisting patient to lie down on examining table. Place one arm on patient's shoulder and the other arm under patient's knees.

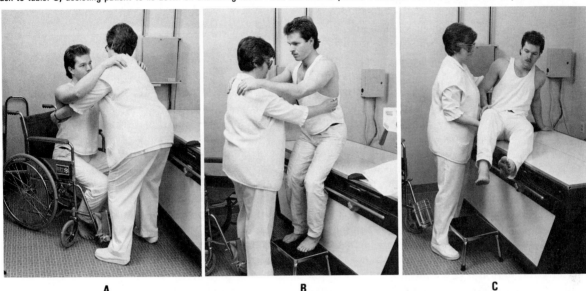

A   B   C

- Using a *single* smooth move, assist the patient to rise to a sitting position. Pivot a quarter of a turn at the same time so that the patient will be sitting on the edge of the examining table with the feet dangling over the side.
- Stand facing the patient.
- Put your arms under the patient's arms and your hands firmly over the patient's scapulae. Have the patient's hands rest on your shoulders.
- Give a signal, lift upward, and raise the patient to a standing position.
- Pivot a quarter of a turn so that the back of the patient's knees touch the edge of the wheelchair.
- Ease the patient into the wheelchair.
- Position the footrests and the patient's feet on them.
- Attend to the patient's safety and comfort.

CRUTCHES

Crutches are wooden or metal supports used to aid a person in walking. The most common types are the tall crutch, which reaches from the ground up to the axillae (axillary crutches), and the Lofstrand or Canadian crutch (forearm crutch), which is a shorter crutch. The Lofstrand or Canadian crutch is an aluminum tube with a hand bar on which the patient supports his/her weight and a metal cuff that fits around the forearm. The metal forearm cuff will support the patient when having to let go of the handbar as when grasping onto a handrail to climb stairs or when standing still. At the base of all crutches is a rubber tip that prevents slipping (Fig. 14-14). The type of crutch used will depend on the patient's disability. For example, if the patient has broken or sprained one

ankle, axillary crutches will be used. When the patient will be on crutches for a long time and/or has only limited mobility in the legs and/or is wearing leg braces, or is a paraplegic, forearm crutches may be used. Patients with severe arthritis who have poor use of their hands may use platform crutches. When using these crutches, patients use their forearms to lean on the crutches.

Fig. 14-14. Two types of crutches: axillary *(left)*, and Lofstrand or Canadian *(right)*. Note the rubber tip at the base of the crutch, which prevents slipping.

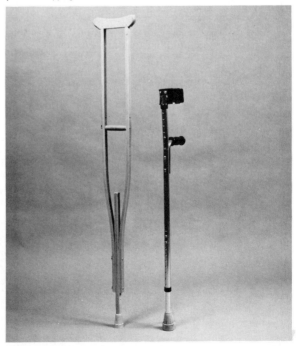

Axillary crutches should be measured for each patient so that they will not cause pressure on the axillae. Teaching the patient crutch-walking gaits may be the responsibility of the medical assistant if a physical therapist is not available. First you must instruct the patient in practicing correct standing posture, which is head and chest up, abdomen in, pelvis tilted inward, the feet straight, and a 5 degree angle bend in the knee joint. Tell the patient *not* to look down at the feet. Have the patient practice standing with the support of the crutches to get familiar with them and to bear weight on the palms of the hand and not on the axillae. You must teach the patient *not* to rest the body's weight on the axillary bars of the crutch for more than a few minutes at a time because pressure on the axillae will cause pressure on the brachial plexus. Excessive pressure on the brachial plexus can lead to severe and sometimes permanent paralysis in the arms. Teach the patient to bear weight on the palms of the hands (Fig. 14-15). Demonstrate the proper hand and arm position and gait before the patient tries to use the crutches. By doing this you will help the patient to understand how the crutches are to be used. Concentration on a normal rhythmic gait must be accomplished.

Gaits

In crutch-walking gaits, each foot and crutch is called a point. For example, in a two-point gait, two points of the total of four (two crutches and two legs) are in contact with the ground when taking one step. The type of gait to be used will depend upon the patient's condition. Crutch gaits include the following:

- **Two-point gait:**
  1. The first type of two-point gait is when you put both crutches ahead of you and hop forward with one foot (Fig. 14-15, *A*). This is a nonweight bearing gait.
  2. The second type of two-point gait is contralateral walking and a reciprocal walk. Put your left crutch and right foot forward; then put your right crutch and left foot forward, and repeat.
- **Three-point gait:**
  This may be used when one leg is stronger than the other. Put your crutches forward and then bring the weaker leg through the crutches. Next bring the stronger leg forward, and then repeat, crutches out, then one leg, then the other leg. This is a partial weight-bearing gait.
- **Four-point gait:**
  Put your right crutch forward, then the left foot, then the left crutch, and then the right foot, and repeat (Fig. 14-15, *B*).
- **Swing-to gait:**
  Put the crutches forward and then swing the legs up to the same point (Fig. 14-15, *C*).
- **Swing-through gait:**
  Put the crutches forward and then swing the legs past them (Fig. 14-15, *D*).

The last two gaits are commonly used by paraplegics who are using forearm crutches.

Instructions For Using A Single Crutch or Cane

Always hold a single crutch or cane on the *opposite* side of the injury. People normally walk contralaterally, that is, when your left arm swings out, your right

Fig. 14-15. Crutch walking gaits. **A,** two-point gait. **B,** four-point gait. **C,** swing-to gait. **D,** swing-through gait.

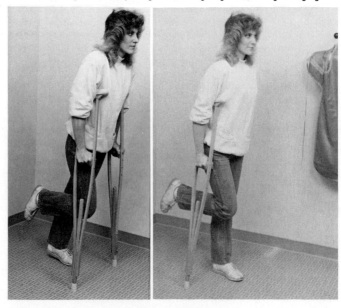

A

Fig. 14-15 *(continued)*

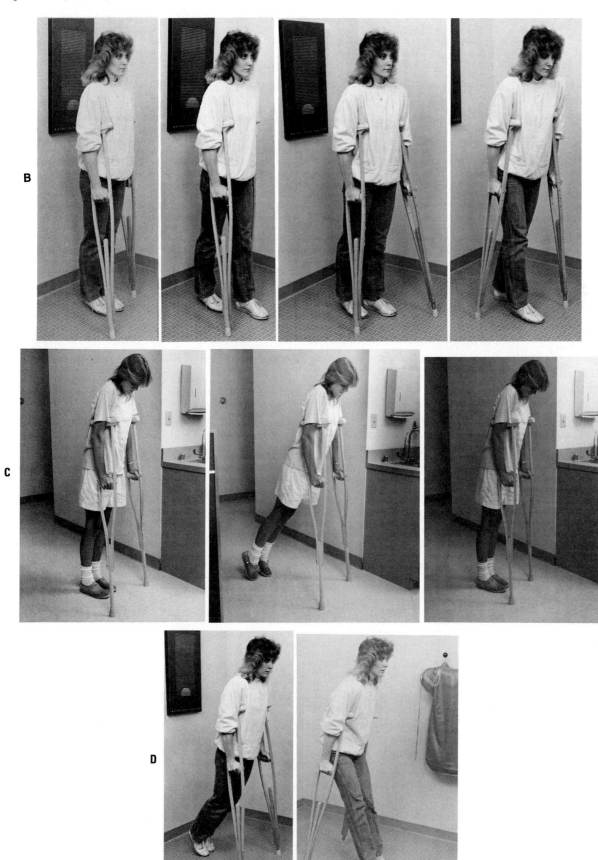

leg goes out. Think of a crutch or cane as an extension of your arm. As your arm swings out, your opposite leg will go out. With the crutch on the opposite side, it will support and take the weight off of the injured leg.

ELECTROTHERAPY UTILIZING GALVANIC AND FARADIC CURRENTS

Galvanic current is a steady direct current (DC); faradic current is alternating current (AC) produced by induction. Both are currents of low voltage that are used for many therapeutic purposes. The basic use for galvanic and faradic currents is for muscle stimulation, used to retrain patients when they have had nerve injuries. For example, as the injured nerve regenerates, the body may have forgotten how to contract a muscle, so frequently these treatments are given to somewhat remind them and get them functioning once again.

Galvanic stimulation (or faradic if it works) can be used just to maintain the contractility of the muscle while waiting for the nerve to regenerate. Once the nerve is cut or degenerates, or if the nerve itself does not conduct stimuli, galvanic current (direct current) is the only thing than can be used. Direct current will work directly on muscle tissue even when there is no intact nerve. Faradic current (alternating current) cannot be used, as it will not work on muscle tissue in this case. Galvanic current is also used for **iontophoresis** (ī-on"to-fo-rē'sis). Iontophoresis or ionotherapy is the introduction of ions into the body through the skin by means of an electric current for therapeutic purposes.

Faradic current is used mainly for the stimulation of weak muscles whose nerve supply is normal. This current causes contractions, which in turn increase blood supply to the muscle and thus help the muscle gain strength. Increased circulation will also help to decrease edema. Faradic current is also used to decrease pain as it helps to block pain sensations.

These treatments can be applied in various ways. To stimulate muscles, the current must be interrupted. This is accomplished by a hand interrupter or an interrupter that is built into the equipment. Basically, to apply these currents, two electrodes padded with cotton that has been soaked in salt water are placed over the area to be treated. The soaked pads prevent the occurrence of severe wounds. When small muscles are worked on, a very small applicator can be used. This has a push button on it so that specific jolts of current can be given. This apparatus can also be used when using what is called a surged current or a ramped current. These are currents that start out with nothing, then begin and increase up to a designated point and then decrease. With these a smooth contraction and then a smooth relaxation is obtained. In addition to muscle stimulation, these currents can also be used on muscle spasms and on areas around hematomas, bruises, and such. Electrostimulation therapy is also used with biofeedback for muscle reeducation. The biofeedback machine allows the patient to hear the muscle contract and relax. This is especially helpful postoperatively and for controlling chronic pain.

ELECTRODIAGNOSTIC EXAMINATIONS

Electrodiagnostic examinations used by physical therapy are performed by means of electrical stimulation applied to muscles and nerves. Various types of examinations are available, all having clinical value in the diagnosis and prognosis of some neuromuscular disorders. Two additional major electrodiagnostic examinations used for different clinical purposes are the electroencephalogram (EEG), which records the electrical impulses of the brain, and the electrocardiogram (EKG or ECG), which records the electrical action of the heart. The EKG is discussed in Unit XV.

Electromyographic examinations specifically measure the electrical activity in a muscle as a result of nerve conduction. A needle electrode is introduced into a muscle belly to study muscle action potentials. It will also measure just the general electrical excitability of the muscle cells. The recording obtained (the electromyogram) can be most specific diagnostically, as it not only tells you that something is wrong, but will point out exactly what is wrong. It helps distinguish any weakness from neuropathy from that of other causes.

Other examinations available test the reaction time of a muscle to a shot of electricity; the threshold is tested, that is, how much electricity it takes to get a reaction from the muscle. The results obtained are compared with normal levels. Any deviation or fluctuation from the established norm helps diagnose certain problems, such as damaged nerve and muscle tissues.

Nerve conduction studies are performed to test the speed with which the nerve is conducting; again, this helps the physician diagnose.

Special electrodiagnostic equipment is used for each of these tests, which are generally performed by a physical therapist or a physician. The medical assistant will not operate this equipment, but may be expected to keep it clean and ready for use. The medical assistant may also be expected to explain the nature and purpose of the examination to the patient.

DISABILITIES WITH MODALITIES USED

To provide the medical assistant with a broader insight to the various types of patient conditions that benefit from physical therapy, Table 14-2 lists common disabilities with the common physical therapy modalities used for each.

Table 14-2. Patient conditions that benefit from physical therapy

Disability	Common Modalities Used	Disability	Common Modalities Used
Amputations	Bed positioning Exercise Crutch training Prosthetic care and training	Fractures of upper and lower extremity	Biofeedback and electrical stimulation therapy Exercise Gait training
Arthritis and other rheumatic diseases	Heat Hot paraffin wax bath Exercise Pool Transfer techniques *Occupational therapy:* 　Splinting (Fig. 14-16), functional exercise, self-care instructions, such as dressing		Modalities to control pain and edema, e.g., heat and/or cold applications
		General surgery	Graduated exercise program
		Heart surgery and pulmonary congestion	Bronchial hygiene that includes postural drainage and chest tapotement
Burns	Hubbard tank Heat Exercise Whirlpool Massage Splinting		Breathing exercises Endurance exercises
		Infectious diseases	Graduated exercise program
Cardiovascular disease (Cardiac and Pulmonary Rehabilitation)	Bronchial hygiene e.g., postural drainage, chest tapotement Graduated exercise program *Occupational therapy:* 　Pacing activities: work simplification energy conservation	Low back pain	Constant pelvic traction (in bed and in clinic) Intermittent pelvic traction Heat Massage Pool Exercise Body mechanics instruction *Physical and occupational therapy:* 　Mobilization of soft tissues and joints— manual therapy 　Ergonomics— assessment and modification 　Industrial programs for employee evaluation, work capacity, and modification training
Cerebral palsy	Exercise; neurological facilitation exercises Functional training *Occupational therapy:* 　Self-care instruction, such as feeding and dressing		
Cerebrovascular accident (CVA)	Bed positioning Exercise—basic calisthenics → progress up to walking → running → riding bicycles Neurological facilitation exercises Transfer techniques Gait training *Occupational therapy:* 　Splinting, self-care instructions, such as dressing, training in one-handed activities	Lymphedema (after CVA, mastectomy, or sprain)	Jobst Intermittent Pressure Pump Exercise
		Muscle spasm	Heat Cold Massage Exercise
		Muscle disease	Pool Exercise
Congenital defects	Exercise Functional training	Multiple sclerosis	Ice baths for relief of spasticity Exercise Gait training Transfer activities Dressing training
Debility	Exercise Gait training		
Diabetes	Exercise		

(Table 14-2 continues)

Table 14-2 (*continued*)

Disability	Common Modalities Used	Disability	Common Modalities Used
Neck pain	Occupational therapy	Psychiatric problems (continued)	Pool
	Intermittent cervical traction or collars		Relaxation techniques
	Constant vertical traction		*Occupational therapy:* Therapeutic crafts and remedial games
	Heat		
	Massage	Pulmonary problems (emphysema, bronchitis, asthma)	Bronchial hygiene
	Exercise		Breathing exercises
	Ice		Endurance exercises
	Also see "Low back pain"		Outpatient pulmonary rehabilitation clinic
Osteoporosis	Bracing as indicated		Graduated rehabilitation with low flow oxygen
	Exercise		*Occupational therapy:* Pacing activities: work simplification energy conservation
	Graduated weight bearing		
	Modalities for pain control		
Parkinson's disease	Exercise		
	Gait training	Renal failure and transplants	Graduated exercises
Peripheral nerve injuries	Electrical stimulation		Maintenance exercises
	Exercise	Scoliosis and other postural defects	Bracing
	Splinting		Exercise
	Occupational therapy		Body mechanics instruction
Peripheral vascular diseases	Buerger's exercises		Posture instruction
	Gait training	Spinal cord injuries	Bracing
	General exercises		Exercise
Poliomyelitis	Bronchial hygiene		Gait training
	Exercise		Transfer activities
	Gait training with braces		Wheelchair mobility
	Heat		*Occupational therapy:* Self-care instruction, such as dressing and splinting
	Pool		
Pressure sores and wound infections	Ultraviolet light (bacteriocidal)		
	Bed positioning		
Prenatal and postnatal situations	Exercise	Sprains	Heat
	Breathing instruction		Cold and compression
Psoriasis	Ultraviolet light (bactericidal)		Exercise
			Gait training
Psychiatric problems	Exercise		
	Heat		

Fig. 14-16. Examples of splints as applied to patient's finger, wrist, and forearm.

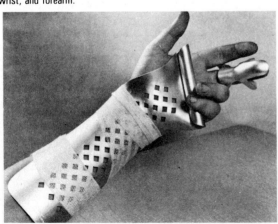

CONCLUSION

You have now completed the unit on physical therapy. After you have practiced the procedures and are ready to demonstrate your skills and knowledge attained, arrange with your instructor to take a performance test.

There are various types of patient conditions and disabilities that benefit from physical therapy. Numerous other procedures, tests, and modalities are used in a physical therapy department. It is not within the scope of this book to discuss all of them in detail. A clinical experience or a field trip to a physical therapy facility would be most valuable to you; here you could see firsthand the use of the various modalities and techniques.

REVIEW OF VOCABULARY

The following are statements taken from patient charts. Read these and be able to explain the nature of the types of treatment each patient has received.

PATIENT NO. 1

On January 14, the patient was working for the Webster Construction Company in custodial activity. He was using a mop, and after pulling the mop through the wringer, he experienced right paralumbar pain. The next morning the patient couldn't move because of severe pain. He had an appointment at the Crossroads Clinic, and medications were prescribed. Later the patient saw Dr. Treadmill who recognized the problem as one involving compensation. Furthermore, Dr. Treadmill obtained x-ray films and prescribed physical therapy. Physical therapy involved massages, infrared therapy, ultrasound therapy, and pelvic traction. Temporary relief came from these measures. About 8 or 9 days ago, however, because of persistence of the trouble, the patient was referred to me.
The patient stated that the pain in the right lower extremity prevents work. It is "static," by which the patient means it is not worsening or improving.
The patient in formative years had an occasional "kink" in the back, but was never off work and never had professional attention.

PATIENT NO. 2

Patient brought in a prescription to continue treatment for 3 more weeks. The physician felt that physiotherapy was helping and will see the patient at the end of 3 weeks. Patient states pain is gradually decreasing . Treatment: hot packs; ultrasound at 1.5 w/cm² for 7 minutes to left low back; exercise as before. Patient does exercises well and reports that she continues them at home.

Will Kerrigan, RPT

REVIEW QUESTIONS

1. Define, and state the purposes and time duration of application for each of the following:
   a. Ultraviolet light treatments
   b. Diathermy treatments
   c. Ultrasound treatments
   d. Application of moist and dry heat
   e. Application of moist and dry cold
2. How full should a hot water bottle be filled when applied to a patient? Why?
3. State the temperature of the water you would use when applying a hot water bottle to a 70-year-old man; to a 2-year-old child.
4. Define and discuss the principles of body mechanics.
5. Why should the patient's skin be checked frequently during any form of hot or cold application?
6. List five physiological reactions produced by heat applications, and five produced by cold applications.
7. List five situations in which cold applications may be used for treatment.
8. List five situations in which hot applications may be used for treatment.
9. List two modalities used in hydrotherapy. Explain each briefly. List two uses for each.
10. List five uses or purposes of exercises.
11. Differentiate between active and passive exercises.
12. State three purposes of traction, and three purposes of massage.
13. State two types of electrodiagnostic examinations, and explain each briefly.
14. Discuss the principles of electrotherapy utilizing galvanic and faradic currents.

PERFORMANCE TEST

In a skills laboratory, the medical assistant student will demonstrate skill and knowledge in performing the following activities without reference to source materials. The student will need a partner to play the role of the patient. Time limits for the performance of each procedure are to be assigned by the instructor (see also pp. 32 and 35).

1. To the outer aspect of the patient's right forearm, and to the inner aspect of the patient's left lower leg, prepare, apply, and remove the following:
   a. Hot water bottle
   b. Hot compress
   c. Ice bag
   d. Cold compress
2. Discuss the purpose and physiological effects of hot and cold treatments with your instructor.
3. Demonstrate with a partner:
   a. Active exercises of the right arm
   b. Passive exercises to the right arm
   c. Active-resistant exercises to the patient's right hand
4. Using the information provided in this unit, correctly write out the procedural steps and a performance checklist for the following applications of heat or cold:
   a. Heating pad
   b. Hot water bottle
   c. Hot moist compress
   d. Hot soak
   e. Ice bag
   f. Ice pack
   g. Moist cold compress
   h. Alcohol sponge bath

5. Using the information you outlined in No. 4, design a teaching-instruction sheet for the patient to use at home for each of the hot and cold applications listed.
6. Demonstrate safe and effective body mechanics when lifting a patient or heavy object.
7. Assist patients in learning how to walk with crutches, and with a cane.

8. Assist patients getting in and out of a wheelchair.

PERFORMANCE CHECKLIST

The medical assistant students are to design their own step-by-step procedures and performance checklists for the performance test.

Unit XV

Electrocardiography

COGNITIVE OBJECTIVES

On completion of Unit XV, the medical assistant student should be able to apply the following cognitive objectives:

1. Define and pronounce the terms in the vocabulary and text of this unit.
2. Explain the cardiac cycle and conduction system of the heart.
3. Explain how the heartbeat is controlled.
4. List eight components recorded on the electrocardiogram cycle, and relate these to the electrical activity of the heart.
5. State the normal time required for the cardiac cycle.
6. Describe electrocardiograph paper, and indicate the significance of each small block and each large block.
7. List four factors that are interpreted from an electrocardiogram.
8. Describe how to monitor an electrocardiogram for abnormal and erratic tracings.
9. List three types of common artifacts that may be seen on an EKG and the causes for each.
10. Describe electrodes and electrolytes, and state the purpose of each.
11. List the 12 leads recorded on a standard electrocardiogram; state the electrical activity that each is recording; and recognize each recorded lead by interpreting the identification code used.
12. Discuss the phrase, *standardizing the electrocardiograph,* indicating the importance of this. Illustrate and explain the universal standard of EKG measurement.
13. Discuss the concepts of the Phone-A-Gram, the computerized electrocardiograph.
14. Discuss the automatic electrocardiograph. State the advantages of this electrocardiograph.

TERMINAL PERFORMANCE OBJECTIVES

On completion of Unit XV, the medical assistant student should be able to do the following terminal performance objectives:

1. Demonstrate proficiency in communicating proper preparation of the patient for electrocardiography and in preparing the room and equipment.
2. Demonstrate the proper procedure for the application of the electrodes and lead wires to the patient.
3. Locate and mark the six positions used to record the chest leads.
4. Demonstrate the proper procedure for recording the electrocardiogram with a standard electrocardiograph and the Phone-A-Gram system, mounting the finished product, and caring for the equipment after use.

The student is to perform the above activities with 100% accuracy 90% of the time (9 out of 10 times).

Vocabulary

amplify (am'plĭ-fi)—To enlarge, to extend.

arrhythmia (ah-rith'mē-ah)—A variation from the normal or an irregular rhythm of the heartbeat.

atrium (ā'trē-um)—One of the upper chambers of the heart. The right atrium receives deoxygenated blood from the body, whereas the left atrium receives oxygenated blood from the lungs. (The plural is *atria.*)

cardiac (kar'dē-ak) **arrest**—Sudden and often unexpected cessation of the heartbeat. Permanent damage of vital organs and death are probable if treatment is not given immediately.

defibrillation (dē-fĭ"brĭ-lā'shun)—The application of electrical impulses to the heart to stop heart fibrillation.

electrocardiograph (ē-lek"trō-kar'dē-ō-graf")—The instrument used in electrocardiography.

fibrillation (fĭ"brĭ-lā'shun)—A cardiac arrhythmia characterized by rapid, irregular, and ineffective electrical activity in the heart. Ventricular fibrillation is a common cause of cardiac arrest.

myocardial infarction (MI) (mĭ"ō-kar'dē-al infark'shun)—The formation of ischemic necrosis in the heart muscle due to an interference of blood supply to the area.

myocardium (mĭ"ō-kar'dē-um)—The heart muscle.

Fig. 15-1. The treadmill stress test.

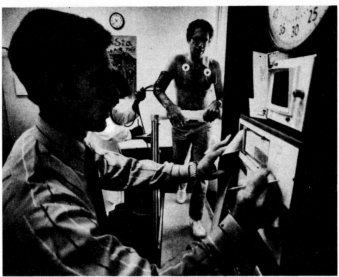

oscilloscope (ŏ-sil′o-skōp)—An instrument used to display the shape or wave form of the electrical activity of the heart and other body organs (comparable to a television screen).

pacemaker (pās′māk-er)—The pacemaker of the heart is the sinoatrial node located in the right atrium.

pericarditis (per″ĭ-kar-di′tis)—Inflammation of the pericardium, the fibroserous sac enveloping the heart.

rhythm strip—An EKG recording of a single lead that is used to determine the *rhythm* of the heartbeat, such as a fast, slow, regular, or irregular rhythm, and certain types of ventricular fibrillation. It is also used to determine if the patient is experiencing any type of heart block, such as third-degree heart block. The rhythm strip gives a one-dimensional picture of the beating of the heart to demonstrate the rhythm of the heartbeat *only,* in contrast to the 12 lead EKG, which can show damage to the heart and other conditions. Data from the rhythm strip can be a useful screening tool because frequent runs of arrhythmias can be more easily observed. The rhythm strip can also be used to confirm the basic assessment made on the 12-lead EKG. Current use of the rhythm strip is to record Lead V_1, and possibly Leads V_2 and V_s, although one could record any lead that is desired. Rhythm strips are frequently recorded from a continuous cardiac monitor in intensive care units in the hospital and by paramedics out in the field in emergency situations.

ventricle (ven′trĭ-kl)—One of the lower chambers of the heart. The right ventricle receives deoxygenated blood from the right atrium and pumps this blood through the pulmonary arteries to the lungs; the left ventricle receives oxygenated blood from the left atrium and pumps this blood out through the aorta to all body tissues.

Additional terms are defined in the text of this unit on electrocardiography.

The science and art of electrocardiography combine advanced electromedical technology with the science and art of medical practice. Present-day electrocardiographs present physicians with precise information by amplifying the minute electrical currents produced by the heart on a graphic record or tracing. This record or tracing is called an electrocardiogram, abbreviated EKG or ECG, defined simply as a graphic representation of the electrical activity (currents) produced by the heart during the processes of contraction and relaxation. More precisely, the EKG records the amount of electrical activity, the time required for this activity to travel through the heart during each complete heartbeat, and the rate and rhythm of the heartbeat. Many physicians now include an electrocardiogram as part of a complete physical examination especially for patients 40 years of age and older. It is also advisable to have an EKG or a treadmill stress EKG before any serious jogging or other exercise program is started.

The *treadmill stress test* is used for noninvasive cardiac evaluation to aid physicians in patient diagnosis and prognosis with electrocardiograms taken under controlled exercise stress conditions. During this test of increased stress and work, abnormal electrocardiographic tracings (that do not appear during an EKG taken when the patient is resting) may appear. The test is done in the presence of a physician, and the patient is constantly monitored. Systems used record and monitor the patient's EKG while it is being monitored by the physician (Fig. 15-1).

Fig. 15-2.   Your heart and how it works. (Courtesy and by permission of the American Heart Association, Inc.)

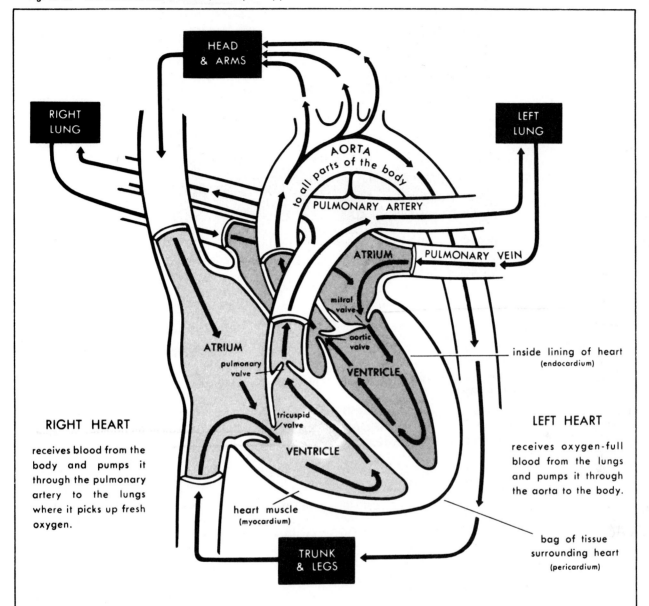

Your heart weighs well under a pound and is only a little larger than your fist, but it is a powerful, long working, hard working organ. Its job is to pump blood to the lungs and to all the body tissues.

The heart is a hollow organ. Its tough, muscular wall (myocardium) is surrounded by a fiberlike bag (pericardium) and is lined by a thin, strong membrane (endocardium). A wall (septum) divides the heart cavity down the middle into a "right heart" and a "left heart". Each side of the heart is divided again into an upper chamber (called an atrium or auricle) and a lower chamber (ventricle). Valves regulate the flow of blood through the heart and to the pulmonary artery and the aorta.

The heart is really a double pump. One pump (the right heart) receives blood which has just come from the body after delivering nutrients and oxygen to the body tissues. It pumps this dark, bluish red blood to the lungs where the blood gets rid of a waste gas (carbon dioxide) and picks up a fresh supply of oxygen which turns it a bright red again. The second pump (the left heart) receives this "reconditioned" blood from the lungs and pumps it out through the great trunk-artery (aorta) to be distributed by smaller arteries to all parts of the body.

Frequently physicians will have medical assistants take the electrocardiogram. To be valuable members of the health team, those who take EKGs must acquire related knowledge and develop skills; that is, they must know what they are doing, why and how to do it, and then do it well.

The following pages are designed to help medical assistants acquire this knowledge and skill by discussing the nature and purpose of the EKG, the equipment and materials needed, preparation of the patient and equipment, ways to monitor the record for abnormal and erratic tracings, procedure for taking the EKG, and mounting the record obtained.

Before going further, it is suggested that you review the anatomy of the heart to maximize your understanding of electrocardiography (Fig. 15-2).

THE CARDIAC CYCLE AND EKG CYCLE

The term *cardiac cycle* refers to one complete heartbeat, which consists of contraction (systole) and relaxation (diastole) of both atria and both ventricles. The many cells of the heart are arranged so they act together as one network or system. Throughout this network, two types of electrical processes, called depolarization and repolarization, are transmitted. When depolarization occurs, the cells are stimulated, and the myocardium (the heart muscle) contracts; as repolarization occurs, the myocardium relaxes. To understand the electrical activity of the heart, think of the heart as consisting of two separate cell networks, one being the atria and the other the ventricles. The two atria contract simultaneously; then as they relax, the two ventricles contract and relax, rather than the entire heart contracting as a unit. Any disturbance in the processes of the cardiac cycle will cause a change in the electrical forces needed to maintain normal, rhythmic heart beats and may produce an arrhythmia. Depending on the degree of the disturbance, it could be a minor disruption of rhythm or a major life-threatening arrhythmia.

Each of these cell networks (the atria and the ventricles) is considered separately on the electrocardiogram, the graphic recording of these electrical forces produced by the heart. That is, the waves or deflections recorded on the electrocardiograph paper represent the sequence of events that occur during the cardiac cycle. The normal EKG cycle consists of waves that have been arbitrarily labeled P, QRS, and T waves. Each wave corresponds to a particular part of the cardiac cycle (Fig. 15-3). The *P wave* reflects contraction (depolarization) of the atria. The *QRS wave* (QRS complex) reflects the contraction (depolarization) of the ventricles. This wave follows the P wave. The *T wave* reflects ventricular recovery (repolarization of the ventricles). A T wave reflecting the repolarization of the atria is not visible, because it is

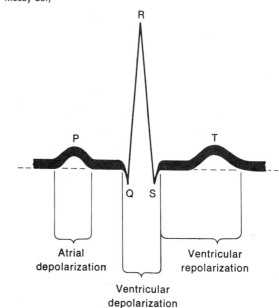

Fig. 15-3. Normal EKG deflections. (From Conover, M.B.: Understanding electrocardiography, ed. 3, St. Louis, 1980, The C. V. Mosby Co.)

obscured by the QRS wave. A T wave follows every QRS wave. Occasionally, another wave, the *U wave*, appears after the T wave. It is a small wave and usually shows up on EKGs of patients who have a low serum potassium level. In some animal laboratory studies, U waves have been produced during the repolarization stages of the Purkinje fibers.

Because the ventricles are much larger than the atria, the QRS and T waves are normally much larger than the P wave.

The *P-R interval* reflects the time it takes from the beginning of the atrial contraction to the beginning of ventricular contraction. The P-R interval is measured from the beginning of the P wave to the beginning of the QRS complex (Fig. 15-4).

The *ST segment* reflects the time interval from the end of the ventricular contraction (depolarization) to the beginning of ventricular recovery (repolarization). It is normally a flat (isoelectric) line that is measured from the end of the S wave (of the QRS complex) to the beginning of the T wave.

The *Q-T interval* reflects the time it takes from the beginning of ventricular depolarization to the end of ventricular repolarization. This interval gives a better picture of the total ventricular activity. It is measured from the beginning of the QRS complex to the end of the T wave.

The *baseline*, a flat horizontal line that separates the waves, may be seen to run the length of the EKG tracing. This is known as the isoelectric line. The waves of the EKG cycle will deflect either upward (positive deflection) or downward (negative deflection) from the baseline (isoelectric line). This line is present when there is no current flowing in the heart, that is, after depolarization or after repolarization of

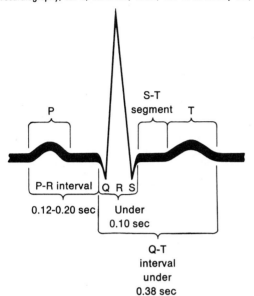

Fig. 15-4. EKG intervals. (From Conover, M.B.: Understanding electrocardiography, ed. 3, St. Louis, 1980, The C. V. Mosby Co.)

the heart. The baseline (isoelectric line) present after the T wave reflects the period when the entire heart is resting or in its polarized state.

Observing and measuring the configuration and location of each wave in relation to the other waves and baseline, the intervals and the segments in each cycle, and then between each EKG cycle allows the physician to interpret and analyze the rate, rhythm, and conduction of the heart. Abnormalities detected in the EKG cycles help diagnose cardiac problems, for example, myocardial infarction (MI), pericarditis, myocarditis, left ventricular hypertrophy, atrial and ventricular arrhythmias, nodal block, atrial and ventricular fibrillation, in addition to a variety of other conditions such as acid-base imbalance, effects of various drugs, metabolic diseases, autonomic hyperactivity, and hyperventilation.

Control of the Heartbeat: Conduction System of the Heart

To understand the interpretation of an electrocardiogram, one must know the mechanism by which the heartbeat originates. Stimulation of the heartbeat originates in the sympathetic (acting to increase the heart rate) and parasympathetic (the vagus nerve, acting to slow the heart rate) branches of the autonomic nervous system. Although the heart is under the control of the nervous system, the myocardium (heart muscle) itself is capable of contracting rhythmically independently of this outside control. Despite this property of automaticity, impulses from the autonomic nervous system are required to produce a rapid enough beat to maintain circulation and life effectively. Without the nerve connection, the heart rate may be less than 40 beats per minute instead of

the usual 70 to 90 per minute (average 80 beats per minute).

Specialized masses of tissue in the heart form the conduction system, regulating the sequence of events of the cardiac cycle. These include the sinoatrial node (SA node), the "pacemaker" of the heart, located in the upper right-hand corner of the right atrium adjacent to the opening of the superior vena cava; the atrioventricular node (AV node), located near the intraventricular septum in the inferior wall of the right atrium and near the tricuspid valve; the bundle of His (or atrioventricular bundle), located in the interventricular septum, which then divides into the left and right bundles; and the Purkinje fibers, which terminate in the ventricles.

The electrical impulse of the cardiac cycle travels first to the sinoatrial node, from which wavelike impulses are sent through the atria, stimulating first the right and then the left atrium, and eventually sweep over the heart. In a comparable manner, if one drops a pebble in water it will generate waves that travel outward from the point of origin.

When the atria have been stimulated, the impulse slows as it passes through the atrioventricular node. Slowing of the impulse at the AV node allows the resting ventricles (in diastole) to fill with blood from the atria. This wave of excitation (stimulation) then spreads down to the bundle of His, then to the right and left bundle branches, which then relay the impulse to the Purkinje fibers, an interlacing network terminating in the ventricle's musculature. The Purkinje fibers distribute the impulse in the right and left ventricles, causing them to contract. Stimulation of the muscle of the ventricle begins in the intraventricular septum and moves downward, causing ventricular depolarization and contraction. Mechanically, the ventricles empty blood into the pulmonary (or lesser) circulation by way of the pulmonary artery and the right and left pulmonary branches, and into the systemic (or greater) circulation by way of the aorta. This stimulation or impulse must spread through the muscle of both atria and both ventricles before mechanical contraction can occur. To complete the cardiac cycle, the entire heart now relaxes momentarily, and then a new impulse is initiated by the SA node to repeat the whole cycle.

The electrical wave front that originates in the SA node and spreads throughout the heart then spreads through the body. From the body surface it is possible to pick up these electrical impulses and record them on specialized paper (the electrocardiograph) or display them on an oscilloscope (comparable to a television screen).

Time Required for Cardiac Cycle

Each cardiac cycle takes approximately 0.8 second. With this time limit, there are 75 heart beats per min-

Fig. 15-5. EKG paper with section enlarged. **A,** number of large squares between recorded R waves indicate rate of heartbeat per minute. **B,** one large square enlarged.

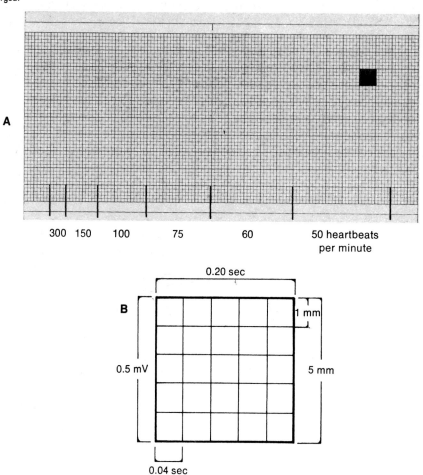

300   150   100   75   60   50 heartbeats
                                                          per minute

ute. When the heart beats more than 75 times per minute, the cycle requires less time. Conversely, when the heart beats fewer than 75 beats per minute, the cardiac cycle requires more than 0.8 second.

Heart Sounds During Cardiac Cycle

Typical sounds are elicited from the heart during each cardiac cycle. These sounds are described as *lubb dupp* as heard through a stethoscope. The first sound, *lubb* or systolic sound, is a longer and lower-pitched sound and is believed to be from the contraction of the ventricles and vibrations from the closing of the cuspid valves. The second sound, *dupp* (the diastolic sound), is shorter and sharper and occurs during the beginning of ventricular relaxation. It is thought to be due to the vibrations of the closure of the semilunar valves (pulmonic and aortic valves). Since these sounds provide information about the valves of the heart, they have clinical significance. Variations from normal in these sounds indicate imperfect functioning of the valves. Heart murmurs are one type of abnormal sound heard and may indicate stenosis or incomplete closing of the valves (valvular in-

sufficiency). It is important to remember that the electrocardiogram does not record these sounds. They can be heard when a stethoscope is put on the chest wall over the apex region of the heart.

ELECTROCARDIOGRAM

Electrocardiogram Paper

To understand the significance of each wave and interval of various heights and widths recorded by an electrocardiograph, the medical assistant needs to know the significance of the small and large blocks on the EKG paper (Fig. 15-5, *A*). On the horizontal line, one small block represents 0.04 seconds (Fig. 15-5, *B*). On the vertical axis, one small block represents 1 mm. Since a large block is five small blocks wide and five deep, each of them represents 0.2 second (horizontal) and 5 mm (vertical).

Notice all the lines. Every fifth line (horizontal and vertical) is usually printed darker than other lines, producing blocks (squares) that are 5 mm × 5 mm. Thus, two of the larger blocks equal 10 mm or 1 cm.

These measurements, accepted internationally, allow physicians to interpret cardiac time (rate) on the horizontal line and cardiac voltage on the vertical axis, and thus determine if the electrical activity of the heart is within normal limits.

Electrocardiograph paper is heat-sensitive and pressure-sensitive. When the machine is on and running, a heated stylus moves over the paper to record the cardiac cycles. Being pressure-sensitive, EKG paper must be handled carefully to avoid markings that would blemish the actual tracing.

Interpretation

When the physician interprets an EKG, the following factors are usually determined:

- *Rate.* How many beats per minute; determined are the atrial rate and the ventricular rate.
- *Rhythm.* Whether the heart rhythm is regular or irregular; determined are the atrial rhythm and the ventricular rhythm.
- *Conduction time.* How long it takes for the impulse originating at the SA node to stimulate ventricular contraction (review the conduction system, p. 435); determined are the P-R interval and the QRS duration.
- *Configuration and location.* Of each wave, the ST segment, the P-R interval, and sometimes the Q-T interval.

These findings are then recorded and reviewed by the physician to help establish a diagnosis or evaluate current treatment.

Because many physicians expect the medical assistant who takes a patient's EKG to monitor the graph for abnormal or erratic tracings, you should be aware of the following:

Heart Rate and Rhythm

In a normal EKG, all heartbeats consist of three major units, the P wave, the QRS complex, and the T wave, and appear as a similar pattern, equally spaced.

Briefly, the rate of a particular rhythm may be determined from the EKG simply by noting the distance between two R waves. As seen in Figure 15-5, *A*, two large squares between R waves means that the rate is 150 beats per minute; three large squares between R waves means that the rate is 100 beats per minute. Similarly, four large squares between R waves indicates a heart rate of 75 beats per minute. To get this rate per minute, divide the number of large squares between the R waves into 300. NOTE: If the rhythm is irregular, counting the squares in a single R-R interval will give an approximate rather than the precise rate that would be obtained with a perfectly regular rhythm.

To determine if heart rhythm is regular or irregular, the distance between each P wave and then between each R wave is measured. If the distance between all P waves is the same, atrial rhythm is regular; if the distance varies, rhythm is irregular. Similarly, if the distance between all R waves is the same, ventricular rhythm is regular, and if not, it is irregular.

Artifacts

Artifacts are defects (unwanted activity) on the electrocardiograph *not* caused by the electrical activity produced during the cardiac cycle. Since the EKG will pick up and record every kind of electrical activity it can find, artifacts may appear, making the recording difficult to interpret. To remedy this situation, the medical assistant should understand what causes artifacts, how they can be eliminated or greatly minimized, and use the correct recording technique.

There are several types of artifacts, the most common being somatic tremor (muscle movement), wandering baseline (baseline shift), and alternating current (AC) interference.

Somatic Tremor. These artifacts can be identified by the unnatural baseline deflections, ranging from irregular vibrations in amplitude and frequency (jagged peaks of irregular height and spacing) to large shifting of the baseline (Fig. 15-6, *A*). Muscle movement, either voluntary or involuntary, produces artifacts caused mainly when the patient

- Is tense and/or apprehensive
- Moves or talks
- Is in an uncomfortable position
- Suffers from a nervous disorder that causes constant tremors, such as Parkinson's disease

The best way to avoid these patient-produced artifacts is to prepare the patient well, both emotionally and physically, preferably in a pleasant and relaxing atmosphere. The following will aid in patient preparation:

- Gain the full cooperation of the patient.
- Explain the procedure and what you will be doing.
- Position the patient comfortably, with limbs well supported.
- Offer assistance and reassurance as needed.
- Have patients suffering from a nervous disorder put their hands, palms down, under their buttocks or take a deep breath. This will help reduce artifacts. (See also Preparation of Patient, p. 441.)

Wandering Baseline (Baseline Shift) (Fig. 15-6, *B*). Causes of this artifact include the following:

1. Electrodes that are applied too tightly or too loosely

Fig. 15-6. EKG artifacts. **A,** somatic tremor artifact. **B,** wandering baseline. **C,** alternating current artifact. (From Conover, M.B.: Understanding electrocardiography, ed. 3, St. Louis, 1980, The C. V. Mosby Co.)

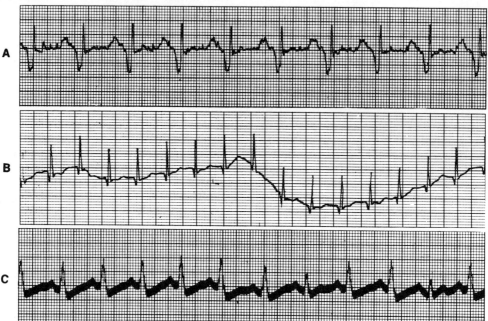

2. Tension on an electrode as a result of an unsupported lead wire that is pulling the electrode away from the patient's skin
3. Too little or poor quality electrolyte gel or paste on an electrode
4. Corroded or dirty electrodes
5. Skin creams or lotions present on the area where the electrode is applied

To prevent artifacts, correct and attentive technique when applying the electrodes with the electrolyte gel or paste is a must. Wash the electrodes after each use and occasionally with kitchen cleanser, but *never* use steel wool. Electrolyte gels or pastes that are left on the electrode can cause corrosion, which makes the electrode a poor conductor of cardiac electrical currents. The tips of the lead wires must also be kept clean.

Ensure that the patient's skin where the electrodes will be applied is clean; if necessary wash the area briskly with alcohol or the presaturated electrolyte pads before applying the electrode.

Alternating Current (AC) Interference. AC artifacts appear as a series of small regular peaks (or spiked lines) on the electrocardiogram (Fig. 15-6, C).

Alternating current is our standard source for electrical power. AC present in electrical equipment or wires can radiate or leak a small amount of energy into the immediate area. When a patient is present in this area, some of the AC may be picked up by the body, which in turn is detected by the electrocardiograph. Thus, an electrocardiogram with AC artifacts

results. Common causes of AC interference artifacts include the following:

1. Improper grounding of the electrocardiograph
2. Presence of other electrical equipment in the room
3. Electrical wiring in walls or ceilings
4. X-ray or other large electrical equipment being used in adjacent rooms
5. Lead wires crossed and not following the contour of the patient's body
6. Corroded or dirty electrodes
7. Faulty technique of the operator

To minimize or eliminate AC interference, correct technique is required. The EKG unit must be properly grounded. Check the instructions in the operator's manual supplied with each unit by the manufacturer. Newer units have three-prong plugs that are inserted into a properly grounded three-receptacle outlet. Older units may have a two-prong plug. In this case a ground wire from the unit is connected to a suitable ground, such as a cold water pipe.

Unplug other electrical equipment in the room. When x-ray equipment is being used in adjacent rooms, it may be necessary for you to wait until that procedure is completed or move to another room to record the EKG. Moving the patient table away from the wall may help minimize interference caused from electrical wiring. Lead wires must be straight and positioned to follow body contour; the line cord is to be away from the patient, and the unit should be near the patient's feet, not head. Electrodes must be cleaned after each use and occasionally should be scrubbed with a kitchen cleanser.

Additional Problems

When recording an EKG, one may encounter a few additional erratic tracings which may appear as follows:

- An indistinct tracing usually caused by (1) the stylus heat being too low, (2) a bent stylus, (3) incorrect stylus pressure, or (4) a broken stylus heating element, which results in no tracing
- A straight line but no tracing, caused by the patient cable not being plugged in correctly
- A break between complexes, caused by a loose or broken lead wire

When the medical assistant cannot correct the cause of an artifact, inform the physician and call the manufacturer's or other repair service, according to office policy.

EKG Electrodes and Electrolytes

Electrodes (also called sensors) are small metal plates placed on the patient to pick up the electrical activity of the heart and conduct it to the electrocardiograph. The standard 12-lead electrocardiograph has five electrodes: two to be attached to the fleshy part of the arms, two to be attached to the fleshy part of the legs, plus one floating electrode that will be placed in six different positions on the chest when recording the chest leads.

In the machine, this electrical current is changed into mechanical action, which is recorded on the EKG paper by a heated stylus. To help conduct this electric current, an electrolyte is applied to each electrode. Electrolytes are available in the form of gels, pastes, or flannel materials presaturated with an electrolyte solution.

Once the electrodes are correctly secured to the patient with rubber straps, lead wires are fastened to them. These lead wires extend off the patient cable, which is attached to the electrocardiograph machine.

EKG Leads

The standard 12-lead electrocardiograph system records electrical activity from the frontal and horizontal planes of the body by using 12 leads as follows:

Standard Limb or Bipolar Leads

The first three leads to be recorded on a standard EKG are known as Lead I, Lead II, and Lead III. These are called bipolar leads, because each of them uses two limb electrodes that record simultaneously the electrical forces of the heart from the frontal plane; that is, Lead I records electrical activity between the right arm (RA) and left arm (LA); Lead II records activity between the right arm and left leg; Lead III records activity between the left arm (LA) and left leg (LL) (Fig. 15-7, A).

The right arm is considered as a negative pole and the left leg as a positive pole. The left arm will either be negative or positive depending on the lead; in Lead I, it is positive; in Lead III it is negative.

Upright (positive) deflections on the EKG indicate current flowing toward a positive pole; inverted (negative) wave deflections indicate current flowing toward a negative pole. For example, in Lead I, the flow of current will be from a negative to a positive pole; thus the wave deflections on the recording will be upright.

Augmented Leads

The next three leads are the augmented leads, designated as aV_R, aV_L, and aV_F. The aV stands for augmented voltage; the R, L, and F stand for right, left, and foot (leg). Augmented leads are unipolar and also record frontal plane activity.

Lead aV_R records electrical activity from the mid-

Fig. 15-7. **A,** lead triangle showing position of standard limb leads. **B,** lead triangle showing position of augmented leads.

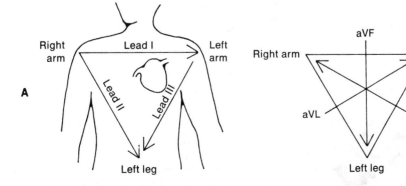

Fig. 15-8. Leads of routine electrocardiogram. (Courtesy The Burdick Corporation, Milton, WI)

Standard or bipolar limb leads	Electrodes connected	Marking code	Recommended positions for multiple chest leads (Line art illustration of chest positions)
Lead I	LA & RA	1 dot	
Lead II	LL & RA	2 dots	
Lead III	LL & LA	3 dots	
Augmented unipolar limb leads			
aVR	RA & (LA-LL)	1 dash	
aVL	LA & (RA-LL)	2 dashes	
aVF	LL & (RA-LA)	3 dashes	
Chest or precordial leads			
V	C & (LA-RA-LL)	(See data on right)	

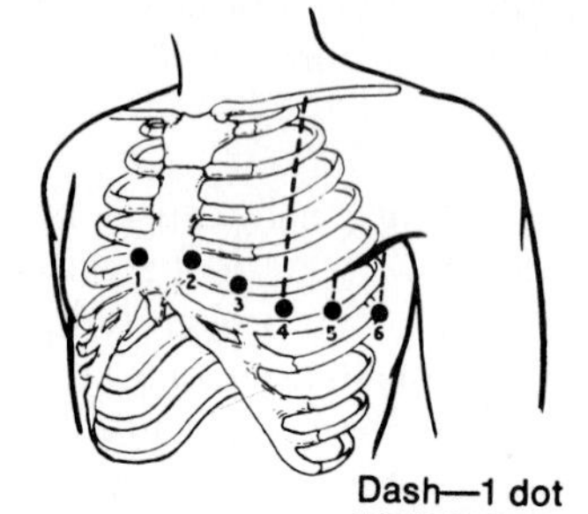

Dash—1 dot

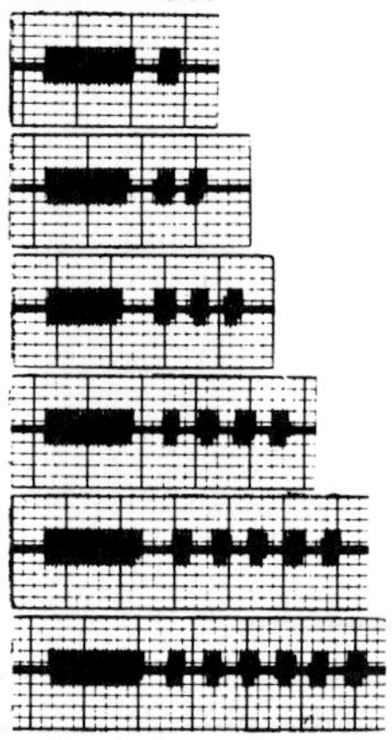

V_1 Fourth intercostal space at right margin of sternum
V_2 Fourth intercostal space at left margin of sternum
V_3 Midway between position 2 and position 4
V_4 Fifth intercostal space at junction of left midclavicular line
V_5 At horizontal level of position 4 at left anterior axillary line
V_6 At horizontal level of position 4 at left midaxillary line

point between the left arm and left leg to the right arm.

Lead aV_L records electrical activity from the midpoint between the right arm and left leg to the left arm.

Lead aV_F records electrical activity from the midpoint between the right arm and left arm to the left leg (Fig. 15-7, B).

Chest or Precordial Leads

The last six leads of the standard 12-lead EKG are the chest or precordial leads. These leads are also unipolar and are designated as V_1, V_2, V_3, V_4, V_5, and V_6.

This third set of leads records electrical activity between six points on the chest wall and a point within the heart. To obtain these recordings, the chest electrode is to be moved to six predesignated positions on the chest. Figure 15-8 shows the location of these positions. It is imperative that the correct position be used for each lead recording.

All 12 leads discussed can be interpreted separately or in combination. Each lead presents a picture of a different anatomical part of the heart, thus allowing the physician to determine areas of damage or problem areas.

When doing an EKG, the machine automatically connects the proper electrode potentials for Leads I, II, III, aV_R, and aV_F. To record the chest leads, the chest electrode must be moved manually to each of the assigned chest positions.

Suggested Codes for Marking Leads

Certain codes are used to identify each lead recorded. Without these codes it would be difficult to determine which lead one was interpreting and also would be impossible to mount the recording with proper lead identification. An example of codes used is seen in Figure 15-8. On older machines the leads are coded (marked) by depressing the lead marker button. New machines will automatically code for each lead as it is being recorded.

Standardizing the Electrocardiograph

The diagnostic value of an EKG depends on an accurate recording. Standard techniques have been adapted to provide a recording that can be interpreted anywhere in the world, assuming the EKG machine used has been calibrated according to universal measurements.

The universal standard of EKG measurement is the

following: 1 millivolt of cardiac electrical activity will deflect the stylus precisely 10 mm (1 cm) high. This is equal to 10 small blocks on the EKG paper (see also the section on EKG paper, pp. 436–437).

Before any EKG is recorded, the machine must be standardized; that is, it must be checked to determine if it is set to record according to the universal measurement.

To standardize the machine, turn the main power switch on. The stylus should be positioned to run along on one of the dark horizontal lines. Set the lead selector swith to STD and the record switch to RUN. Quickly depress and release the standardization button. The standardization mark should go 10 mm high and 2 mm wide. It will appear as an open-ended rectangle (the open end being along the baseline). A slight slant may be seen in the top right corner, which is normal, but any other deviation from this is not and must be corrected. To correct any deviation, turn the standardization adjustment knob and repeat the procedure until the correct standardization mark is obtained.

It is important to consult the instruction manual provided by the manufacturer of each EKG machine, as the above procedure may vary slightly among the various machines on the market.

The universal standard for recording an EKG is at a speed of 25 mm/second. This can be increased on the machine to run the paper at 50 mm/second when segments of the EKG are close together or when heart rate is rapid. A notation of this *must* be made to alert the physician of this change to allow an accurate interpretation of the record.

Preparation and Procedure for Obtaining Electrocardiograms

Equipment

Bed or examining table (preferably without any metal attachments)
Linen sheet or blanket
Electrocardiograph with patient cable lead wires
Electrolyte gel *or* paste *or* presaturated electrolyte pads
Electrodes and rubber straps
Gauze squares
Patient gown

Preparation of Electrocardiograph Room

1. The room should be as far away as possible from all x-ray and other electrical equipment that may cause artifacts on the electrocardiogram.
2. The room should be comfortably warm, quiet, pleasant, and not crowded with medical instruments, which may make the patient apprehensive.
3. The electrocardiograph (and patient) should be

positioned away from wires, cords, and any other source of AC interference.
4. The bed or examining table must be wide enough so that the patient may rest comfortably with the extremities well supported; otherwise muscle tension or tremors may cause artifacts.

Preparation of Patient

The quality of the record obtained is influenced by scrupulous attention to fundamental rules regarding the preparation of the patient. The medical assistant who is confident, but empathetic, will make it easier for the patient to relax, both mentally and physically.

1. Explain the nature and purpose of the electrocardiograph to the patient. Tactfully help the patient realize that full cooperation (that is, relaxing and not talking, moving, or chewing gum) will help produce a recording that will help the physician diagnose and treat the patient's condition (when applicable).
2. Assure the patient that no shock or other sensation will be felt.
3. Have the patient remove any jewelry that would interfere with the electrode placement or come in contact with the electrolyte.
4. Have the patient remove shoes and clothing from the waist up; women are to remove nylons. A patient gown should be put on with the opening in the front.
5. Help the patient assume a recumbent position on the table with arms at the sides and legs not touching. The extremities must be well supported on the table.
6. Place a cover over the patient with arms and lower legs exposed. Protecting the patient from cold or any other discomfort is very important. A small pillow can be placed under the head.
7. Locate and mark the six chest locations on the patient. (You can use a felt tip pen or such and wash the markings off after with an alcohol sponge.) The patient gown over a woman's chest can be adjusted so as not to expose the breasts and cause possible embarrassment and apprehension and still allow you to adequately locate and record the chest lead positions.
8. Inquire if the patient has any questions before you begin the recording.

Application of Electrodes and Connection of Lead Wires

1. Expose the patient's arms and legs.
2. Attach one end of each rubber strap to each electrode (Fig. 15-9, *A*).
3. Place a small amount of electrolyte gel or paste, about the size of a pea, on the electrode (Fig. 15-9, *B*).

Fig. 15-9. **A,** attaching rubber strap to electrode. **B,** place small amount of electrolyte gel on electrode. **C,** presaturated electrolyte pad and electrode applied to arm. **D,** electrolyte pad, electrode, and rubber strap applied to arm. (Courtesy The Burdick Corp., Milton, WI)

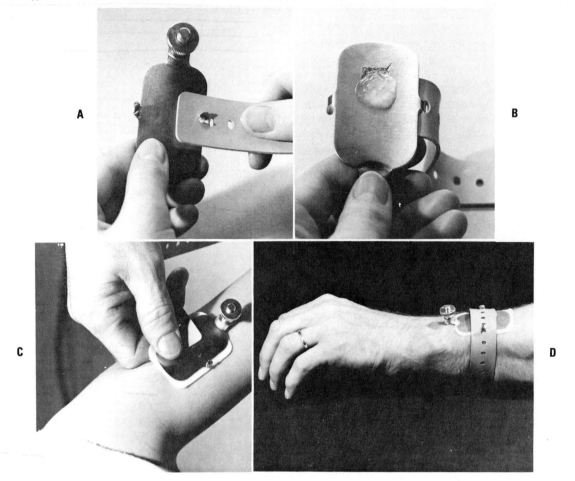

4. Using the side of the electrode, rub the electrolyte into the skin on the fleshy part of the right arm. The area rubbed should not be much larger than the size of the electrode and should be slightly reddened by the rubbing. (If there is lotion or cream on the skin, it must be removed with an alcohol sponge before the electrolyte and electrode are applied.)

5. Place the electrode on this skin area, pull the rubber strap around, and fasten it to the electrode. The electrode must not be pressing against the table or other body parts. The electrode must not be fastened too loosely or too tightly. Try to move the electrode about once secured in place. If it slips or slides on the limb, it is too loose and must be tightened; if the skin is pinched on either side of the electrode, the strap is too tight and must be loosened.

6. Using a gauze square, wipe any excess gel or paste from around the electrode.

7. Follow this same procedure to apply the electrodes to the left arm and to the right and left legs over the fleshy part of the lower leg, not over the bone. By applying the electrodes to the fleshy areas on the limbs, the chance of undesirable muscle artifacts is minimized. Also use equal amounts of gel or paste on each electrode.

8. When using presaturated electrolyte pads rather than a gel or paste, rub the skin with the pad, then place it on the skin. The electrode is to be placed directly on top of the pad (Fig. 15-9, *C* and *D*).

9. *If taking an EKG on a patient who has a cast, amputation, or prosthesis, place the electrode above the affected area. The electrode for the other extremity must then be placed in the same location opposite the first. For example, if the patient has a cast extending from the knee to the ankle on the right leg, place the electrode on the inside of the upper right leg. The electrode for the left leg must then be placed on the inside of the upper left leg. If the electrodes are not placed in this manner, that is, if one electrode is placed on the upper part of the right limb above the cast and the other electrode is placed on the fleshy part of the lower left leg, the electric vector would be changed, and abnormal results would occur on the electrocardiogram.*

10. Leave the chest electrode unattached but not touching a direct surface, *or* position it on the first chest position using the electrolyte of choice.

11. Firmly connect the patient cable lead wires to the proper electrodes so that the lead wire connector faces the patient's feet. Each wire is alphabetically coded: RA — right arm, LA — left arm, RL — right leg, LL — left leg, and C — chest. In addition, each lead wire is color coded to provide additional identification for the operator. It is very important that the lead wires are connected and arranged to follow the contour of the body without any strain placed on the electrodes so that the possibility of AC artifacts is minimized (Fig. 15-10).
12. Plug the patient cable into the patient cable jack on the machine. Make sure that it is pushed all the way in.
13. Before beginning the recording, routinely check that all connections are secure, that the patient cable is supported on the table or over the patient's abdomen to prevent pulling of the cable, and to see if the patient has any questions.

Recording the Electrocardiogram (Fig. 15-11)

Limb leads

1. Set the lead switch to STD (standard).
2. Turn recorder switch to ON. (Some machines will require a warm-up period before recording. Check the instruction manual to determine if this is the case for the equipment that you are using.)
3. Turn recorder switch to RUN.
4. Center the baseline by turning the centering dial or position control knob.
5. Check the standardization; quickly depress and release the standardization button several times

Fig. 15-10. Application of electrodes and connection to unit in correct positions. (Courtesy The Burdick Corp., Milton, WI)

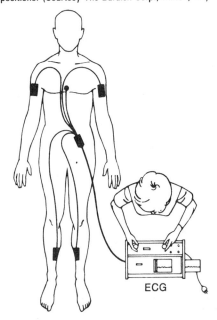

ECG

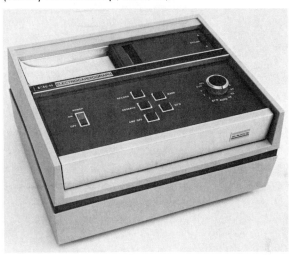

Fig. 15-11. Single-channel electrocardiograph. Can be used in the manual mode or in the automatic mode. When used in automatic mode, the EK-8 records a complete 12-lead EKG in just 38 seconds. (Courtesy The Burdick Corp., Milton, WI)

while the lead selector is on STD and the recorder switch is on RUN. The height of the standardization measurement should be 10 mm or two large squares from the baseline.
6. Turn the lead selector switch to Lead I.
7. Mark the identification code for the lead immediately after it is selected, unless the machine does this automatically.
8. Run for a few heartbeats; depress the standardization button quickly if the physician requires proof of standardization for each lead. This standardization mark should be inserted between the T wave (or U wave when present) of one complex and the P wave of the next complex.
9. Record at least 8 to 10 inches. This provides ample tracing of the lead.
10. Turn lead selector to Lead II.
11. Repeat steps 7, 8, and 9.
12. Turn the lead selector to Lead III and repeat steps 7, 8, and 9.

Augmented leads — aV_R, aV_L, aV_F

13. Turn the lead selector to lead aV_R, mark the identification code, insert a standardization mark if required, and record 5 to 6 inches (see steps 7 and 8).
14. Turn the lead selector to lead aV_L, and repeat step 13.
15. Turn the lead selector to lead aV_F, and repeat step 13.
16. Turn the machine off.

Chest leads

17. Leave the limb electrodes and patient cable wires in place.

18. Position the chest electrode over the first chest position, V_1, applying the electrode with gel *or* paste *or* presaturated electrolyte pad in the same manner used on the limbs.

19. Turn the lead selector to STD, the recorder switch to RUN, and depress the standardization button.

20. Turn the recorder switch to OFF to prevent excessive movement of the stylus.

21. Turn the lead selector switch to V.

22. Turn the recorder switch to ON.

23. Mark the identification code for the lead, and insert standardization marks as described in step 8, when required.

24. Record 5 to 6 inches.

25. Turn the recorder switch to OFF.

26. Move the chest electrode to the next position. Start again with step 21; repeat until all the chest leads have been recorded, that is, lead V_1 through lead V_6.

27. When all the leads have been recorded satisfactorily, turn the lead selector to STD, the recorder switch to OFF, and unplug the power cord.

28. Disconnect the lead wires, unfasten the rubber straps, and remove the electrodes from the patient.

29. Wipe any electrolyte from the patient's skin.

30. Assist the patient as needed. Provide further instructions as indicated.

31. Label the recording with patient's name, date, and your initials.

32. Clean all equipment, and return it to the proper storage area.

33. Wash your hands.

34. Record the procedure.

35. Mount the recording, using the preferred mount as indicated by the physician; record the required information on the mount. Sign your name to the mounted electrocardiogram.

36. Give the mounted electrocardiogram to the physician for review and interpretation.

Throughout the recording of the EKG, make sure that the stylus stays on the same baseline (Fig. 15-12). Use the position control knob if any adjustment is necessary. Constantly watch for the appearance of any artifact. If they do occur, determine the cause, and correct the problem (refer to pp. 437–439).

Mounting an Electrocardiogram

Mounting the electrocardiogram is important so that the recording can be protected, easily seen by the physician, and inserted into the patient's medical record after the physician has reviewed and interpreted it. There are a variety of commercially prepared mounts available for use, or the recording can be mounted on a plain piece of paper. Regardless of the method chosen to mount the EKG, each lead must be correctly identified. In addition, the patient's name, address, age, sex, and the date of the recording must be documented. Other information may be included varying with the physician's request, such as drugs the patient is taking, especially cardiac drugs such as digitalis and quinidine, height, weight, blood pressure, and occupation. See Figure 15-13 for sample mounts and specific directions for mounting the electrocardiogram.

PHONE-A-GRAM: THE COMPUTERIZED EKG

For over 2000 years, physicians from Hippocrates to Laënnec and Einthoven and many others have sought to improve diagnostic accuracy. Phone-A-Gram joined this distinguished group in 1971 by providing a

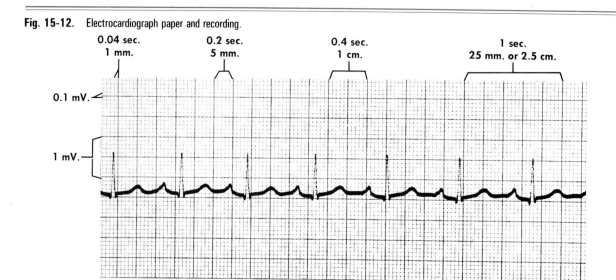

Fig. 15-12. Electrocardiograph paper and recording.

Fig. 15-13. **A,** sample EKG mount for mounting three-channel electrocardiogram strip. Directions are given on mount. **B,** sample EKG mount with instructions for use with single-strip electrocardiograms. **C,** information to be recorded on back of single-strip EKG mount. (Courtesy Hewlett-Packard, Palo Alto, CA)

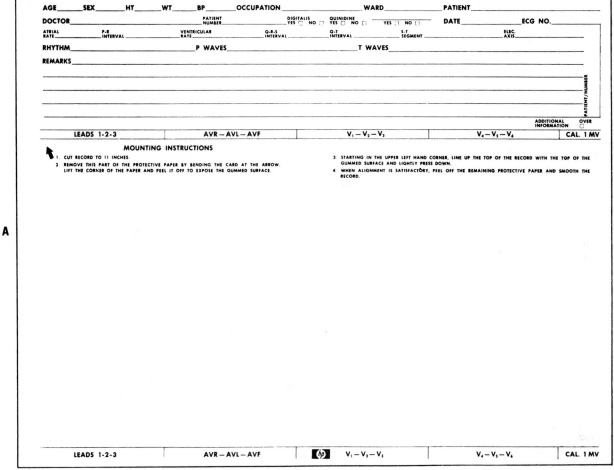

A

(Fig. 15-13 continues)

computerized EKG system to help physicians diagnose heart disease. In the late 1950s the U.S. Public Health Service started investigating the use of computers in the analysis of EKGs. By 1969, following the expenditure of millions of dollars, the Health Care Technology Division, National Center for Health Service Research and Development, had approved a computer-assisted EKG analysis program. In 1971 Phone-A-Gram System received the Public Health Service certificate, ensuring faithful reproduction of an EKG analysis program.

Today Phone-A-Gram provides a complete EKG *service* and all the necessary equipment to over 2400 physicians, hospitals, and clinics throughout the United States. The unmatched speed and accuracy of the computer now provide physicians everywhere with a second opinion for the diagnosis of a patient's condition and save much time and money.

Phone-A-Gram's EKG system includes a portable automatic EKG transmitter (a standard model, a scout model, or the stripchart recorder model), all the auxiliary equipment, and a personal hookup into the na-

tional network (Data Center), which receives, converts, processes, analyzes, and prints out all EKG information for ready reference.

All EKG transmitting units are single-channel units with the features of automatic lead switching and standardization across all 12 leads. The units are compact, portable, and extremely reliable. The *standard model unit* is the simplest to operate and *does not* produce a stripchart. This eliminates the need for and cost of graph paper. It is battery powered and can be easily transported from one location to another. The *scout model* is the same as the standard unit but can be used in conjunction with a conventional electrocardiograph to produce an on-site tracing as the EKG is being transmitted. When using this model to get an on-site tracing, an audiocable is attached to the standard electrocardiograph. The *stripchart recorder* (Fig. 15-14) is a compact, single-channel, automatic lead-switching electrocardiograph with a built-in transmitter. It can run a preview tracing and then produce single-channel tracings simultaneously as the EKG is transmitted.

Fig. 15-13 *(continued)*

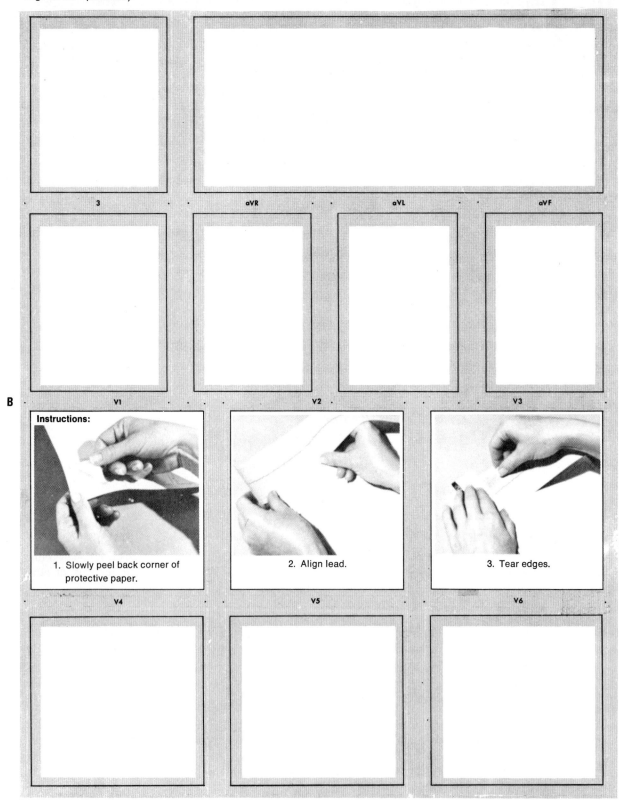

Fig. 15-13 *(continued)*

NAME_____DATE_____CODE_____

ADDRESS_____

TEL. NO._____ OCCUPATION_____

AGE_____SEX_____HT._____WT._____B.P._____

PHYSICIAN_____

HISTORY_____

DIGITALIS_____QUINIDINE_____OTHER_____PAT. POS._____

AURIC. RATE_____   P WAVES_____   Q-T INT._____

VENT. RATE_____   P-R INT._____   S-T SEG._____

RHYTHM_____   Q-R-S INT._____   T WAVES_____

FINDINGS:_____

C

REMARKS:_____

PATIENT

Fig. 15-14. Phone-A-Gram stripchart model. (Courtesy Phone-A-Gram System, San Francisco, CA)

1. Start/reset switch: Used to start the instrument. Instrument will automatically stop at the end of test. If the instrument stops in the middle of a test, this is because an electrode has either fallen off or is not making proper contact with the patient's skin.

2. Recorder chart switch: This three-position switch allows the user the option of either producing or not producing a tracing at the time the ECG is being transmitted to Phone-A-Gram system. When a tracing is not desired the switch should be set on STOP position. When a tracing is desired it should be set on AUTO position. The FEED position is only used at the end of a test to feed the tracing out of the recorder so it can be torn off.

3. Gain switch: This switch is normally left in the *1* position. If the patient's heart waves are large enough to go off the graph the switch should be moved to the ½ position. If the patient's heart waves are too small to measure the switch should be moved to the *2* position.

4. Strip chart recorder: Produces a 12-lead tracing automatically. Use only ECG paper provided by Phone-A-Gram system. Other types may damage recorder. When your supply of paper is low you may reorder by calling our customer service department.

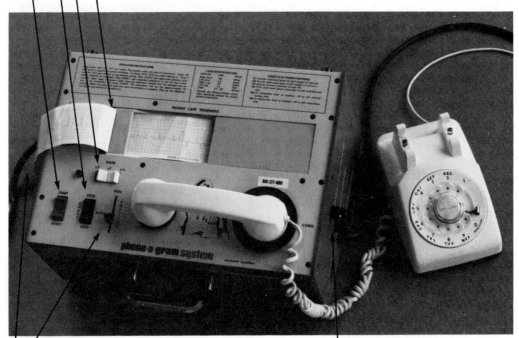

5. Stylus/pen position knob: Allows user to center the baseline in the middle of the tracing before the test begins.

6. Patient cable socket: Patient cable plugs in here.

7. Fuse access: If fuse blows replace with your spare ½ amp slo-blow type fuse only.

The patient is prepared for the EKG by attaching the electrodes to the chest, arms, and legs in the usual manner, although when using the Phone-A-Gram system, all six chest lead electrodes are applied to the patient's chest before you begin to record the EKG.

A standard telephone is used to dial the Data Center (Fig. 15-15). The telephone handset is placed on the Phone-A-Gram unit, and the EKG is transmitted at the push of a button (Fig. 15-14). The unit picks up signals from the patient and transmits them over the telephone to the Data Center.

Phone-A-Gram Data Centers are staffed 24 hours a day, 7 days a week, by technicians fully trained to receive and process computer-interpreted EKGs. They monitor transmissions, evaluate the quality of EKG tracings, and identify and solve common technical problems. Phone-A-Gram's computer prints out the 12 lead measurements and interpretations. The complete printout, stripchart, and analysis are mailed to the physician the same day (Fig. 15-16). In an emergency or upon request, the technician calls the reports back to the physician within minutes. Phone-

Fig. 15-15. Phone-A-Gram Data Center, equipped with most technically advanced telephone system. Phone-A-Gram unit picks up signals from patient and transmits these signals over telephone to Data Center, where EKG is processed. (Courtesy Phone-A-Gram System, San Francisco, CA)

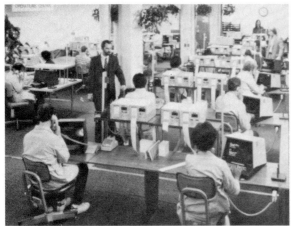

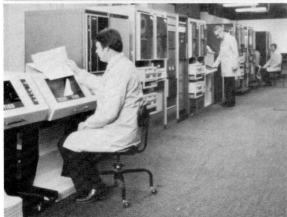

A-Gram's staff cardiologists will automatically review EKGs when necessary and will also provide special optional services as required, such as telephone consultations. In addition, other special services such as serial comparison of EKGs and pediatric EKG interpretations can be obtained on request.

The accuracy of a computer-analyzed EKG, like the manually read EKG, depends on the current state of the art and science of electrocardiography. The criteria for diagnosis incorporated into the Phone-A-Gram computer software analysis program represent the most recent in the state of the science. Phone-A-Gram EKG interpretations are a combination of computers and cardiologists. Expert cardiologists agree that this method represents the optimum in EKG analysis and provides the most clinically relevant and accurate interpretations available.

The physician receiving a Phone-A-Gram computer or cardiologist's report should relate the interpretative statements to the clinical circumstances, symptomatological findings, and other diagnostic test results in determining the appropriate plan of treatment for the patient.

Procedure for Using the Phone-a-Gram System for EKGs*

1. Prepare the electrocardiograph room.
2. Obtain the pertinent patient data: name, sex, age, height, weight, blood pressure, medication, and the clinical reason for the EKG. This information is needed when you call the Data Center before transmitting the EKG recording. It is recommended that you convert the last three items to the appropriate codes listed in Table 15-1 on p. 451 to expedite the telephone procedure.
3. Prepare the patient (see p. 441).
4. Insert the patient cable into the side of the instrument. Push it straight in all the way. *Do not* attempt to screw it in or twist it in any way, because this could cause damage to the unit and/or cable.
5. Attach the 10 suction cup electrodes to patient cable tips and check to see that each electrode fits snugly onto the tip of each lead wire. If any are loose, gently expand the metal tip of the lead wire with a small screw driver until a secure fit is achieved. The tips of the lead wires are color-coded and lettered for ease of identification (Fig. 15-17).
6. When all electrodes are attached to the patient cable, anchor the cable under one of the patient's legs or right arm and rest the cable on the patient's lap while you apply the electrode gel to the skin.
7. Rub the skin area for each electrode position vigorously with gauze saturated in alcohol (particularly during cold, dry weather) to remove dead skin and oils from the body surface. Next apply a drop of electrode gel to the appropriate areas and work it into the skin in a circular pattern about the size of a nickel, being careful that gel from one electrode position does not overlap onto that for another position. Since the gel forms a seal around the rim of the suction cup, a sufficient amount should always be used to ensure good contact. If the patient has an extremely hairy chest, use additional gel, spread the hair, and if necessary shave the area before attaching the electrodes. Figure 15-17 illustrates the correct positions for the V_1 through V_6 electrodes to obtain accurate results. It is important that actual counting and feeling for rib (intercostal) spaces is done routinely, since patient anatomies may differ. NOTE: *Spacing should appear equidistant from one electrode to the next with no crowding or gaps.*
8. Properly applying the six chest electrodes and two arm electrodes is a quick and easy procedure. To achieve maximum suction and contact,

*Modified from Phone-A-Gram System Operating Handbook, San Francisco, Phone-A-Gram System.

Fig. 15-16. Latest, most technologically advanced computer system in combination with revolutionary device called Printer Plotter produce unique Phone-A-Gram report format. Printer Plotter format *eliminates hand mounting* of tracing, because it is produced on one sheet of paper. *File storage convenience* is afforded, because report can be folded to an 8½ × 11 inch size before being placed on the patient's chart. (Courtesy Phone-A-Gram System, San Francisco, CA)

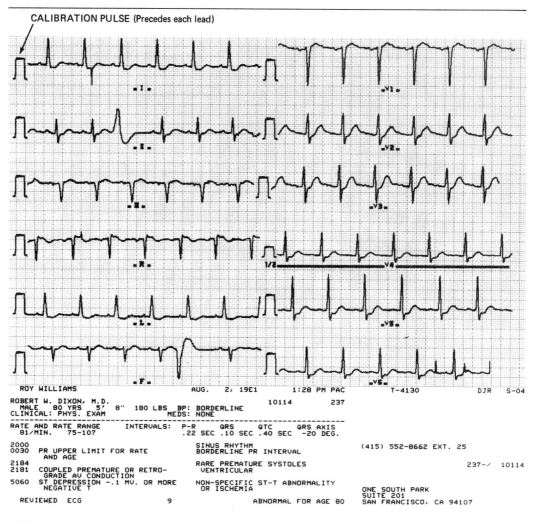

CALIBRATION PULSE (Precedes each lead)

```
ROY WILLIAMS                          AUG.   2, 19E1      1:28 PM PAC       T-4130          DJR     S-04
ROBERT W. DIXON, M.D.                                10114        237
   MALE   80 YRS   5'  8"   180 LBS   BP: BORDERLINE
CLINICAL: PHYS. EXAM               MEDS: NONE
--------------------------------------------------------------------
RATE AND RATE RANGE      INTERVALS:  P-R     QRS       QTC      QRS AXIS
  81/MIN.    75-107                 .22 SEC .10 SEC .40 SEC  -20 DEG.

2000
0030   PR UPPER LIMIT FOR RATE          SINUS RHYTHM                (415) 552-8662 EXT. 25
       AND AGE                          BORDERLINE PR INTERVAL
2184                                    RARE PREMATURE SYSTOLES
2181   COUPLED PREMATURE OR RETRO-      VENTRICULAR                        237-/  10114
       GRADE AV CONDUCTION
5060   ST DEPRESSION -.1 MV. OR MORE    NON-SPECIFIC ST-T ABNORMALITY
       NEGATIVE T                       OR ISCHEMIA                 ONE SOUTH PARK
                                                                   SUITE 201
       REVIEWED  ECG            9             ABNORMAL FOR AGE 80   SAN FRANCISCO, CA 94107
```

grasp the electrodes in a syringe-type manner, depress the rubber bulb with your thumb, and push down firmly on the patient's skin before releasing.

9. Attach the leg electrode to a meaty area of the calf. Arrange excess lead wires on the patient's lap so that there is no strain or pull on any of the electrodes. If strain exists or any electrode is leaning to one side, hold the electrode in place by the rubber bulb and swivel the lead wire (where it is labeled, for example, LA) clockwise or counter-clockwise so that the electrode cup ultimately lies flat on the patient's skin.

10. *Standard model only* — After all electrodes are attached to the patient, press the START button and allow the unit to run for at least 15 seconds to test that all connections are properly made. If the red light comes on, this indicates that one or more of the electrodes is not making proper contact, a lead has actually fallen off, or the patient cable is not inserted properly into the unit. Recheck the patient and test the instrument again. When the red light stays out, press the RESET button to stop the unit (see Fig. 15-14 for operation if you have the stripchart model equipment). Instruct the patient to lie still, relax, and breathe normally without expanding the chest excessively and not to talk or move. *Do not* touch the patient, the cable, or the Phone-A-Gram instrument during transmission.

11. Now you are ready to make the telephone call to the Data Center, using the Data Center number that is affixed to the transmitting unit.

12. Telephone procedure — Proceed as follows when the Data Center operator takes your call:
    • This is account number #_____

Table 15-1. Phone-A-Gram codes for blood pressure, medication, and clinical reason information

The listed *Blood Pressure, Medication Class,* and *Clinical Reason* codes are the ones the Phone-A-Gram computer program takes into account in producing the analysis. You should use the appropriate codes whenever possible, particularly for medications, since Phone-A-Gram is not familiar with all brand name drugs.

Code   Blood pressure

BO	Normotension—Systolic pressure 100 to 139 mm and diastolic pressure 89 mm or below
B1	Borderline hypertension—Systolic pressure 140-159 mm or diastolic pressure 90-94 mm
B2	Hypertension—Systolic pressure 160 or above or diastolic pressure 95 mm or above
B3	Hypotension—Systolic pressure 99 mm or below
B4	Unknown

Code and medication class

DO	None	D8	Antihypertensive
D1	Digitalis	D9	Alpha-adrenergic
D2	Quinidine/procaine/lidocaine	D10	Beta-adrenergic
D3	Antiarrhythmic	D11	Parasympathomimetic
D4	Diuretic	D12	Phenothiazine
D5	Potassium	D13	Tranquilizer
D6	Nitroglycerin	D14	Thyroid
D7	Beta-blocking	D15	Unknown/other

Code and clinical reason

R0	None given	R8	Arrhythmia
R1	Physical exam	R9	Pacer, demand rate
R2	Pre-op	R10	Pacer, fixed rate
R3	Chest pain	R11	Lung disease
R4	Acute myocardial infarct	R12	Cardiac surgery
R5	Prior myocardial infarct	R13	Rheumatic heart disease
R6	Congestive heart disease	R14	Congenital heart disease
R7	High blood pressure	R15	Pericarditis

Courtesy and with permission of Phone-A-Gram System, San Francisco, CA.

- Dr. _____ office (or _____ Hospital)
- The patient's name is _____
- Sex _____
- Age _____
- Height _____
- Weight _____
- Blood pressure* _____
- Medication* _____
- Clinical reason* _____

If you desire any special service(s), such as an immediate callback report, it should be requested at this time.

13. The Phone-A-Gram operator will then advise you when to start the transmission process. The patient should again be reminded to lie still, breathe normally, and not talk.

14. To transmit, simply place the mouthpiece of the telephone snugly in the black cup and then press the START button. The instrument will then auto-

*It is recommended that a code be used to expedite the telephone procedure. Please see the list of codes in Table 15-1.

matically calibrate itself, switch from one lead to the next, and shut itself off at the end of the test. It takes a total of 75 seconds to transmit the EKG (Fig. 15-18).

15. When the white light goes off and the tone stops, pick up the telephone and the Data Center operator will inform you within seconds if the EKG was of good quality. If the tracing was of poor quality, the Data Center operator will ask you to rerun the test after the problem is corrected. If for any reason you get cut off before getting confirmation on the quality of the tracing from the operator, call the Data Center back immediately before disconnecting the patient and inform the operator that you were cut off.

16. The tracing and complete computer printout will be mailed to you on the same day. If you requested an immediate callback on the EKG, the results will be called back before being mailed. Approximately 5 seconds of heartbeat is automatically recorded at the Phone-A-Gram Data Center for each of the 12 leads (Figure 15-16).

Fig. 15-17. Phone-A-Gram System's lead wire color codes, alphabetical codes, and six chest electrode positions. (Courtesy Phone-A-Gram System, San Francisco, CA)

LEAD WIRE COLOR CODES AND ALPHABETICAL CODES

Electrode location	Alphabetical code	Color code
Right arm	RA	White
Left arm	LA	Black
Right leg	RL	Green
Left leg	LL	Red
Chest	V1-V2-V3-V4-V5-V6	Brown

SIX CHEST ELECTRODE (PRECORDIAL) POSITIONS

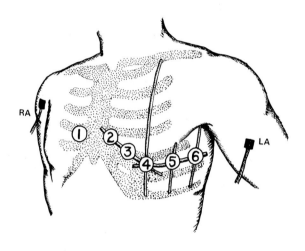

V1   Fourth intercostal space, right margin of sternum
V2   Fourth intercostal space, left margin of sternum
V3   Midway between position V2 and V4
V4   Fifth intercostal space at junction of left mid-clavicular line
V5   Fifth intercostal space at anterior axillary line
V6   Fifth intercostal space at left midaxillary line

ELECTRODE POSITIONS

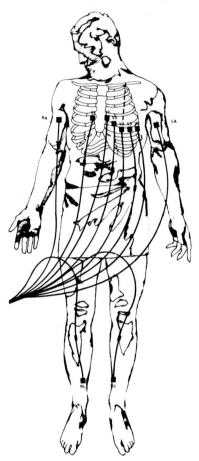

The four limb electrodes should be adhered to the following areas shown

Left arm/Right arm/
Left leg/Right leg

Fig. 15-18. Phone-A-Gram EKG being recorded on site and transmitted to Data Center. (Courtesy Phone-A-Gram System, San Francisco, CA)

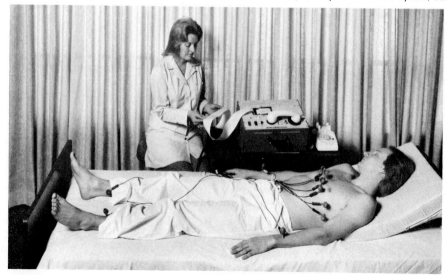

17. Disconnect the patient cable tips from the electrodes and remove the electrodes from the patient.
18. Wipe any electrode gel from the patient's skin.
19. Assist the patient as needed. Provide further instructions as indicated.
20. Clean all equipment and return it to the proper storage area.
21. Wash your hands.
22. Record the procedure on the patient's chart.

CLEANING ELECTRODES

All 10 of the suction cup-type electrodes must be wiped clean immediately after each EKG is completed to prevent residual buildup and subsequent contact problems. Use only alcohol or soap and water to clean electrode surfaces, since polishes, commercial cleaners and other such items if used can cause artifacts in the EKG tracing. Also, never use a scrub brush to clean the electrode surfaces, because the metal plating is very thin and can be scraped away, thus rendering the electrodes useless.

THE ROLE OF THE COMPUTER IN EKG ANALYSIS

The computer is used to obtain a large number of precise measurements from the EKG waveforms. These measurements coupled with the pertinent patient data — sex, age, height, weight, blood pressure, medications, and clinical reason for the EKG — are then compared against range criteria for normal and abnormal cardiac conditions. The results of these comparisons are printed out along with the patient and account data and a set of routinely used EKG interval measurements (P-R, QRS, QTC, QRS axis) in an easy-to-read, understandable report. The computer-generated report represents, in the majority of cases, what would be reported by a cardiologist reading the same EKG.

THE EFFECT OF COMBINING COMPUTER ANALYSIS AND CARDIOLOGIST REVIEW

Inherent to the computer analysis program are two automatic flagging systems. One identifies possible and actual acute conditions (for example, acute myocardial infarction), which are automatically reviewed by a cardiologist. An immediate callback report is then given to the physician. The other flagging system represents an array of preselected cardiac conditions (for example, complex arrhythmias) that are routinely reviewed by a staff cardiologist before being sent back to the physician.

Reports that have been reviewed by a staff cardiologist will contain the statement *Phone-A-Gram reviewed EKG* at the bottom of the left-hand corner of the printout, in addition to the signature of the reviewing cardiologist.

OPTIMAL USE OF THE PHONE-A-GRAM EKG REPORT

The unique Phone-A-Gram EKG report format includes the *interpretive statements* (descriptive) on the right-hand column and the *diagnostic criteria statements* (objective EKG findings) on the left-hand column. Simply stated, the criteria reflect the objective EKG data that were used to arrive at each interpretation. This criteria-interpretive statement format allows the physician to apply the diagnostic criteria to the actual tracing to verify the reported interpretation(s). Directly above this data is the rate and rate range, interval measurements, and pertinent patient information that was used in arriving at the interpretation(s). In the lower right-hand corner is an overall severity classification of the EKG, which summarizes the interpretative statements and suggests clinical significance (for example, *within normal limits for age* or *abnormal for age*) (Fig. 15-16).

NEWEST TECHNOLOGY: AUTOMATIC ELECTROCARDIOGRAPHS

The newer electrocardiographs have fewer operating controls and are much easier to use. With these new machines you *don't* have to adjust controls such as position, sensitivity, heat, paper speed, run, and lead markers. You just set one switch to select the format that you want to record. Different *positions* on the electrocardiograph set it at different speeds and sensitivities. On Hewlett-Packard's 4700 models many different formats can be selected. The 10 preset EKG format selections are on a pull-out card under the machine. Directions for use are on top of the electrocardiograph. Thus there is no need to memorize the format selections available (Fig. 15-19, *A*).

There are different operating modes of the electrocardiograph that will produce three different EKG reports. These modes include the following:

- Auto Mode: By pushing this button and selecting a format position by turning the format switch, you instruct the electrocardiograph to automatically record the routine diagnostic 3-channel 12-lead EKG. Multiple leads are recorded simultaneously. If you wish, you can also add a rhythm strip recording. The final single-page report will have 10 seconds of continuous 12-lead information plus the rhythm strip.

Fig. 15-19. **A,** the new HP 4760 series PageWriter cardiographs can provide analysis reports, measurements and/or interpretation at the office in under 90 seconds. **B,** all new HP 4760 PageWriter cardiographs have a complete alphanumeric keyboard. A wide range of patient data can be entered through this keyboard onto the EKG record. (Courtesy-Hewlett Packard, Palo Alto, CA)

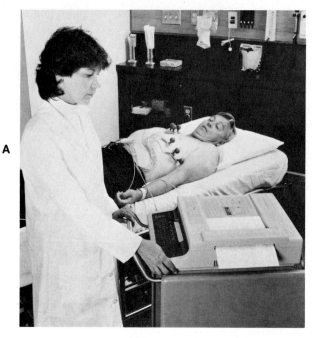

A

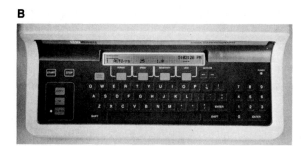

B

- Manual Mode: By pushing this button and selecting a format position by turning the format switch, you instruct the electrocardiograph to record 3 leads for detailed waveform examinations. You can choose which leads you will record from one of the preset formats.
- Rhythm Mode: By pushing this button and selecting a format position by turning the format switch, you instruct the electrocardiograph to record a single-lead rhythm strip. Format selection determines which and for how long the rhythm strip will be recorded.

These electrocardiographs allow you to make an exact copy of the EKG that you just took simply by pushing the *copy* button. Lead identification marks, lead switching marks, and frequency changes are printed on every record. A one-page EKG on standard 8½ by 11 inch heavy-weight paper is produced. The page is easy to read, handle, store, and interpret, and does not require mounting.

Some electrocardiographs have a complete alphanumeric keyboard through which you can enter a wide range of patient data including the patient's name, the requesting physician, name of the facility, and the operator's initials on the EKG record (Fig. 15-19, *B*). Other 3-channel electrocardiographs can be operated manually or automatically by the push of a touch pad. The EKG record is produced on standard size paper that can be mounted on card or folder-format mounts (Fig. 15-20). When operating these new electrocardiographs, which is relatively easy, you must first attach all 10 electrodes (one on each arm, one on each leg, and six on the chest) to the patient and then select the type of report that you wish to record.

There are also single-channel electrocardiographs that can be operated manually or automatically (Fig. 15-11).

Another new machine, the *portable interpretive* electrocardiograph, is also available (Fig. 15-21). Using a clinically proven computerized program, the Burdick E500 analyzes 10 seconds of data from all 12 leads simultaneously in just 3 seconds and also provides you with the reason for its interpretation. Up to 60 EKGs can be stored in memory for review and printout at a later time. Wherever there is a phone line, the E500 can transmit data from the patient's location to other units for overread so that the physician can take it along if visiting the patient at home or in a care facility. The unique LCD display shows actual waveforms for each lead, permitting continuous monitoring while the EKG is being taken. The display also indicates if leads are improperly connected, thereby eliminating paper waste caused by false

Fig. 15-20. The high-volume, easy-to-operate, three-channel EKG that makes its own copies. Can be operated manually or automatically. (Courtesy The Burdick Corp., Milton, WI)

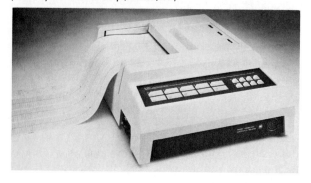

Fig. 15-21. Portable Burdick E500 interpretive electrocardiograph. (Courtesy The Burdick Corp., Milton, WI)

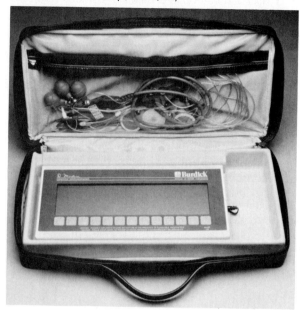

starts. A comprehensive report of all pertinent information is provided on one compact 8½ by 11 inch, easy-to-file sheet. Demographic information on the patient in addition to medications that the patient may be taking, heart rate interval measurements, date and time are included on every printout.

CONCLUSION

Having completed the unit on electrocardiography, you should have acquired a basic understanding of the technique for taking EKGs and the importance of this vital diagnostic procedure.

After you have practiced the procedures and are ready to demonstrate your skills and knowledge attained, arrange with your instructor to take a performance test.

REVIEW OF VOCABULARY

The following are EKG reports received in the physician's office from a consulting cardiologist's office. These are presented to expose the medical assistant to ways in which the interpretation reports of the patient's EKG may be written. Normal and abnormal EKG findings are given.

PATIENT NO. 1
EKG of 12-12-87 showed frequent PVCs (premature ventricular contractions). Rhythmic strip showed numerous PVCs.

PATIENT NO. 2
The patient's EKG showed normal sinus tachycardia of 145, with right axis; P pulmonale was noted inferior laterally; there were ST-T wave changes consistent with ischemia; no significant change since the reading on 9-30-87.

Gary Greaves, MD

PATIENT NO. 3
INTERPRETATION:
  Rate: 75
  Rhythm: sinus
  P waves: normal
  P-R interval: normal
  Position: Intermediate heart
  QRS waves: deep SV_{1-5}
  T waves: normal
CONCLUSION: Intermediate heart within normal limits.

J. Dobbins, MD

PATIENT NO. 4
INTERPRETATION:
  Rate: 60
  Rhythm: sinus
  P waves: normal
  P-R interval: 0.16
  Position: horizontal heart
  QRS waves: deep SV_{1-4}
  T waves: normal
CONCLUSION: Horizontal heart within normal limits.

Sally Eton, MD

PATIENT NO. 5
INTERPRETATION:
  Rate: 108
  Rhythm: sinus tachycardia
  P waves: normal
  P-R interval: 0.18
  Position: normal axis
  QRS waves: deep SV_{1-4}
  T waves: normal
CONCLUSION: Within normal limits except for mild sinus tachycardia.

Carol Overkamp, MD

PATIENT NO. 6
INTERPRETATION:
  Rate: 52
  Rhythm: sinus bradycardia
  P waves: notched
  P-R interval: 0.16
  Position: left axis deviation
  QRS waves: Deep Q_1, aV_L, V_{5-6} with
  T waves: low T waves
CONCLUSION: Sinus bradycardia, left atrial enlargement, and left ventricular hypertrophy.

Erik Evans, MD

PATIENT NO. 7
INTERPRETATION:
  Rate: 60
  Rhythm: sinus
  P waves: notched

P-R interval: 0.18
Position: horizontal heart
QRS waves: slurred ST_1, aV_L, V_{5-6} with
T waves: low T waves
CONCLUSION: Horizontal heart with left atrial
enlargement, left anterior hemiblock, and old
anterolateral myocardial damage.

John Dunn, MD

REVIEW QUESTIONS

1. Draw and label the waves, intervals, and segments of an electrocardiogram. Explain what each component signifies.
2. Explain what is happening in the heart during the processes of depolarization and repolarization.
3. List eight abnormalities that may be detected on the electrocardiogram.
4. Mr. Perry Bloom is having an EKG done and wants to know if the record will pick up his heart sounds and what each of the little squares on the EKG paper mean. State and explain the answer that you give to this patient.
5. The physician expects you to monitor the recording of Mr. Bloom's EKG. List three items that you will look for.
6. During the recording of Max Sugar's EKG, he continually coughs and moves his hand to cover his mouth. What type of artifact would you expect to see on the record?
7. When recording Ms. Lillian Bell's EKG, the stylus continually wanders off the baseline. Describe the actions you would take to try to remedy this situation.
8. Explain to Ms. Maurine McArthur how and why the physician in your office can read her EKG taken on another machine by a different physician in another city.
9. Mrs. D. Bernstrom wants to know why you have to put that "gooey paste" on her body when you are applying the electrodes. State your reply to this patient.
10. Mrs. Sara Pace wants to know how you can tell if your EKG machine is working properly and what all those "funny little" waves on the EKG paper mean. What would you tell her?
11. State what the following items on the electrocardiograph are used for.
    • The STD button
    • The position control knob
    • The lead selector knob
    • The recorder switch
12. In the process of recording Mr. Dan Orlando's EKG, you suddenly notice that there is no tracing on the paper. What could the cause of this be, and how would you remedy the situation?
13. Mrs. Colette Kelly's EKG tracing is very light and hard to distinguish. What could be the cause of this, and how would you remedy the situation?
14. Illustrate identification codes for each of the 12 leads on a standard EKG.

PERFORMANCE TEST

In a skills laboratory, the medical assistant student will demonstrate skills in performing the following activities without reference to resource materials. For these activities the student will need five different individuals to play the role of the patient. Time limits for the performance of the following are to be assigned by the instructor (see also pp. 32 and 35).

1. Prepare the patient for an electrocardiogram.
2. Locate the six chest lead positions on at least five different individuals; then apply the electrodes and lead wires, and record the electrocardiograms of these individuals.
3. Mount the recordings obtained in No 2.
4. Correctly care for the equipment after use.

The student is to perform the above activities with 100% accuracy 90% of the time (9 out of 10 times).

PERFORMANCE CHECKLIST

Obtaining an Electrocardiogram

1. Assemble supplies; prepare the room and equipment for use.
2. Prepare the patient.
   a. Explain the nature and purpose of the EKG.
   b. Have the patient disrobe and put the patient gown on with the opening in the front; jewelry that will interfere with the electrodes is to be removed.
   c. Position and drape the patient.
   d. Locate and mark the six chest positions.
   e. Explain that the patient must remain still and not talk during the recording.
   f. Give reassurance as needed.
   g. Ask if the patient has any questions before you begin the recording.
3. Apply electrodes with electrolyte to the four limbs.
4. Attach the patient cable lead wires to the electrodes.
5. Plug the patient cable into the patient cable jack on the machine.
6. Check once more to ensure that all electrodes and lead wires are correctly and securely attached.
7. Set the lead selector to STD and the recorder switch to ON. (Some machines require a warm-up period.)
8. Turn the recorder switch to RUN.
9. Center the baseline by turning the position control knob.
10. Check the standardization.
11. Turn the lead selector to Lead I.
12. Mark the identification code and record 8 to 10 inches of Lead I.
13. Insert standardization mark between the T wave of one complex (or the U wave if present) and the

P wave of the next complex when this is required by the physician.

14. Continue recording Leads II, III, aV$_R$, aV$_L$, and aV$_F$ in the same manner, but turn the lead selector to the appropriate position, and mark the identification code for each lead. Record only 5 to 6 inches of the augmented leads.
15. Turn the machine off.
16. Position the chest electrode for the first chest lead.
17. Turn the lead selector to STD, the recorder switch to RUN, and depress the standardization button.
18. Turn the recorder switch to OFF.
19. Turn the lead selector switch to V.
20. Turn the recorder switch to ON.
21. Mark the identification code for the chest lead, and insert standardization marks if required (see step 13).
22. Record 5 to 6 inches.
23. Turn the recorder switch off.
24. Move the chest lead to the next position. Start again with step 19; repeat until all the chest leads have been recorded.
25. Turn the lead selector to STD, the recorder switch to OFF, and unplug the power cord.
26. Disconnect the lead wires, unfasten the rubber straps, and remove the electrodes from the patient.
27. Wipe any electrolyte off the patient's skin; assist the patient as needed, and provide further instructions.
28. Label the recording.
29. Clean the equipment, and return it to the storage area.
30. Wash your hands.
31. Record the procedure.
32. Mount the recording and label it.
33. Give the mounted recording to the physician.

Unit XVI

Common Emergencies and First Aid

COGNITIVE OBJECTIVES

On completion of Unit XVI, the medical assistant student should be able to apply the following cognitive objectives:

1. Define first aid and the related terminology presented in this unit.
2. State what factors constitute a medical emergency.
3. List four fundamental rules and general procedures to follow in a medical emergency.
4. Explain how to administer cardiopulmonary resuscitation.
5. Explain how to give first aid treatment for a victim who is choking.
6. List six common warning signals of a heart attack.
7. Discuss the 911 emergency telephone system.
8. State the purpose of a poison control center.
9. Define and list eight signs and symptoms of a cerebral vascular accident (CVA).
10. List five types of shock and the usual causes of each.
11. List at least 10 signs and symptoms of shock.
12. Differentiate between arterial, venous, and capillary bleeding.
13. List four methods used to control severe bleeding.
14. Explain what is meant by the *pressure point method,* and list the seven pressure points used to control severe bleeding.
15. Differentiate between a first, second, and third degree burn.
16. Explain what is meant by the *rule of nine* in reference to burns.
17. Differentiate between insulin reaction and diabetic coma by stating the signs, symptoms, and causes of each.
18. Explain when you should and should not induce vomiting when the victim has ingested a poisonous substance.
19. State and describe the first aid treatment for all the emergency situations discussed in this unit.
20. List at least 15 items that should be included in a first aid kit.

TERMINAL PERFORMANCE OBJECTIVES

On completion of Unit XVI, the medical assistant student should be able to do the following terminal performance objectives.

1. Demonstrate the proper first aid care to be used for all the medical emergencies presented in this unit.
2. Demonstrate the proper application of a tourniquet.
3. Locate the seven pressure points, and demonstrate how to use them to control severe bleeding.

Vocabulary

antidote (an'tĭ-dōt)—An agent used to counteract a poison.

biological death—The condition that results when the brain has been deprived of oxygenated blood for a period of 6 minutes or more, and irreversible damage has probably occurred.

clinical death—The state that results when breathing and circulation have stopped.

concussion (kon-kush'un)—The injury that results from a violent blow or shock.

  concussion of the brain—A violent disturbance of the brain caused by a blow or fall.

contusion (kon-too'zhun)—A bruise, indicating injury to tissues without breakage in the skin. Discoloration appears because of blood seepage under the surface of the skin.

epinephrine (ep"ĭ-nef'rin)—A hormone produced by the adrenal glands. Epinephrine can be administered parenterally, topically, or by inhalation. It is used as an emergency heart stimulant, to relieve symptoms in allergic conditions, and to counteract the lethal effects of anaphylactic shock.

tourniquet (toor'nĭ-ket)—A constricting device used to compress an artery or vein to stop excessive bleeding or to prevent the spread of snake venom.

Additional terms will be defined under their respective topics in this unit.

When someone is injured or suddenly becomes ill, there is a critical period — before medical help is obtained — that is of the utmost importance to the victim. What you do, or what you don't do, in that interval of time can mean the difference between life and death. For serious conditions, the victim *must* receive medical attention, as first aid is not meant to resolve serious problems.

First aid is defined as the immediate and temporary care given the victim of an accident or sudden illness until the services of a physician can be obtained. It is the help that *you* can provide in emergencies until trained medical emergency personnel or a physician take over. You owe it to yourself, the patients under the care of your physician-employer, your family, and the general public to know and understand the simple procedures that can be rendered quickly and intelligently in an emergency.

First aid is more than a dressing or a cold compress. The victim suddenly has new problems and needs. Both emotional and physical needs of the victim must be cared for. Your contributions include offering well-chosen words of encouragement, a willingness to help, the uplifting effect of your evident capabilities and calmness, and the performance of temporary physical care to alleviate pain or a life-threatening situation.

It is frequently a responsibility of the medical assistant to deal with an emergency before the physician or other emergency teams arrive. The medical assistant who can exercise good judgment, remain calm, avoid panicking others, and be familiar with the procedures for emergency care, can administer care in an orderly manner and thereby renders great service to the patient and the physician. Whether in the physician's office, at home, or on the street, *prompt action must be taken.*

Each year more than 1 million Americans die from sudden death. In many cases of sudden death, especially death from heart attacks, the victim could have been saved if the early warning signs of heart attack were known, if someone close by could have performed cardiopulmonary resuscitation, or if the victim had been transported quickly to a hospital, or received first aid or medical attention at the scene of sudden illness or injury. *Time* is of essence in any medical emergency in which breathing and heartbeat have ceased. Within 4 to 6 minutes after the heart stops, brain damage begins. Thus, the importance of the medical assistant knowing what to do and acting quickly in a medical emergency cannot be overemphasized. *Know what constitutes an emergency, whom to call for help, and what to do.* An emergency exists when life is threatened, when situations develop that endanger a person's physical and/or psychological well-being, or when pain and suffering occur.

When an emergency occurs in the physician's office, the medical assistant should notify the physician. If the physician is not in the office and is not expected momentarily, the assistant should call for a nearby physician; if none can be reached for immediate help, call the local emergency medical service system, or an ambulance, or the fire and rescue squad, or the police department. The medical assistant is *not* to assume the responsibility for making a diagnosis and providing medical treatment, but *is* expected to make a reasonable judgment (that may require medical knowledge) of the situation and to provide immediate first aid care.

Medical assistants should perform *only* those procedures that they have been trained to do, and when in the office or health care agency, only with the prior consent of the physician. An office policy should be established between the physician and assistant as to what should be done in the case of office emergencies, and in the case of emergency telephone calls received from patients.

The fundamental rules and general procedures to follow in an emergency are few but very important.

1. Remain calm, reassure the patient, be empathetic, and do not panic. Act in an orderly organized manner. Have a reason for what you do; avoid injury to yourself; know the limits of your capabilities; and avoid further injury to the patient.
2. Survey the situation to determine the nature of the emergency. A primary survey includes the ABCs for all emergencies; that is, check the patient for an open airway, for *breathing*, and for *circulation*. A secondary survey is to examine the total body to determine what is wrong.
3. Take immediate steps to remedy the situation. Your responsibilities for the type of care to provide will vary in each situation and depend on the nearness of medical help, the seriousness of the injury or illness, and the immediate environment.
4. Seek medical help if needed and be able to describe the nature of the patient's condition. Think of yourself as a reporter who must obtain concise and relevant information to act on and then report. Seek answers to questions that begin with who, what, when, where, why, and how.

Provided in this unit is important information in concise and convenient form on common emergencies and the first aid treatment to be administered. Cardiopulmonary resuscitation (CPR) and care for choking victims, and then care for patients in shock are presented first. Other common emergencies are then discussed in alphabetical order. Read and study the contents of this unit carefully, and keep this or other first aid references in a convenient place where they will be on hand for quick reference when needed.

The purpose of this unit is to provide a review and

reference source for first aid treatment to use for common emergencies. It is not intended to be used as a substitute for a certified first aid program of study. Currently it is a requirement of all accredited medical assistant programs of study for the students to complete a recognized certified first aid and CPR course. Medical assistants who completed their training and studies before this requirement was made should enroll in a certified first aid and CPR course if they have not already done so. Courses are offered by the American Red Cross and at many community colleges. Cardiopulmonary resuscitation courses for basic life support are also provided by the American Heart Association in numerous communities. All medical assistants should then take a refresher course in first aid every few years and in CPR every year.

CARDIOPULMONARY RESUSCITATION IN BASIC LIFE SUPPORT FOR CARDIAC ARREST

Cardiopulmonary resuscitation, commonly known as CPR, is a combination of artificial respiration and artificial circulation. CPR should be started immediately by individuals properly trained to do so in emergency situations in which cardiac arrest occurs. To repeat, CPR must be performed by those properly trained in the skill. The performance of CPR is *not recommended unless one has had proper training and practice in the procedure,* because serious adverse consequences may result because of faulty technique. Therefore, the following information is to serve as a review and reference source *after* you have completed a training course and before you take your next refresher course.

The *goal* of CPR is life support. When trained in CPR techniques, you must start life support techniques as quickly as possible and continue them until one of the following has occurred:

1. An effective respiration and pulse are restored to the victim
2. You are completely exhausted and cannot continue CPR
3. Care of the victim is turned over to medical or other properly trained personnel
4. The victim is pronounced dead

Basic and Advanced Life Support

Life support is divided into two systems: basic and advanced life support. Basic life support can be carried out by trained lay and medical persons and includes the following:

Basic ABC steps
    A — airway opened

    B — breathing restored
    C — circulation restored

Supplementary techniques
    Proper positioning of the victim, that is, in the supine position.
    Jaw thrust maneuver — may be required when the head-tilt alone is unsuccessful for opening the airway. This technique *without* the head-tilt is the safest to use on a victim who possibly has a neck injury.
    Opening the mouth — at times it may be necessary to force the mouth open for ventilation or to remove foreign bodies or to allow drainage of vomitus or blood.
    Mouth-to-stoma resuscitation — when the victim has had a laryngectomy, a stoma will be present in the neck through which the person breathes; in this case, mouth-to-stoma resuscitation must be performed.
    Adjunctive equipment — to be used only by those trained in its use.

Advanced life support is to be performed *only* by trained medical personnel and includes the following (Fig. 16-1):

Fig. 16-1. Advanced life support being administered to a patient by medical personnel in hospital emergency room.

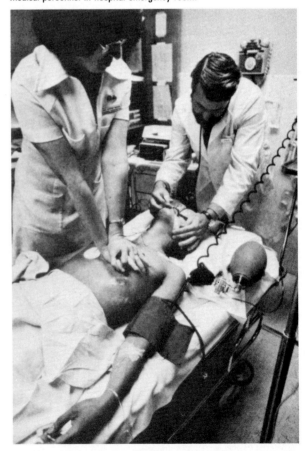

- Definitive therapy
  - Diagnosis
  - Drugs
  - Defibrillation
- Cardiac monitoring and stabilization
- Transportation
- Communication

HEART ATTACK: SIGNALS AND ACTIONS FOR SURVIVAL*

There are many causes of sudden death: poisoning, drowning, suffocation, choking, electrocution, and smoke inhalation. But the most common cause is heart attack. Everyone should know the usual early signals of heart attack and have an emergency plan of action.

The most *common signal* of a heart attack is:

- Uncomfortable pressure, squeezing, fullness or pain in the center of the chest behind the breastbone, which may spread to the shoulder, neck, jaw, or arms (the pain may not be severe)

Other signals may be:

- Sweating
- Nausea, and maybe vomiting
- Shortness of breath *or*
- A feeling of weakness
- Apprehension

Sometimes these signals subside and return.

Action:
1. Recognize the ''signals''
2. Stop activity and sit or lie down
3. *Act at once if pain lasts for 2 minutes or more* — call the emergency rescue service or go to the nearest hospital emergency room with 24-hour service.

CARDIOPULMONARY RESUSCITATION (CPR)

Basic CPR is a simple procedure, as simple as A-B-C, Airway, Breathing, and Circulation. *The following brief review is based on the 1986 standards for CPR. This is to be used only for review purposes. It is not to be used for learning the procedure for performing CPR.*

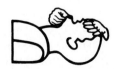

*Reprinted by permission of the American Heart Association, Inc.

Airway

If you find a collapsed person, determine if the victim is conscious by shaking the shoulder and shouting ''Are you all right?'' If no response, shout for help. Then open the airway. If the victim is not lying flat on the back, roll the victim over, moving the entire body at one time as a total unit.

To open the victim's airway use the head-tilt/chin-lift maneuver. Lift up the chin gently with one hand while pushing down on the forehead with the other to tilt head back. Once the airway is open, place your ear close to the victim's mouth:

- Look — at the chest and stomach for movement.
- Listen — for sounds of breathing.
- Feel — for breath on your cheek.

If none of these signs are present, the victim is not breathing.

If opening the airway does not cause the victim to begin to breathe spontaneously, you must provide rescue breathing.

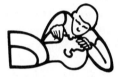

Breathing

The best way to provide rescue breathing is by using the mouth-to-mouth technique. Take your hand that is on the victim's forehead and turn it so that you can pinch the victim's nose shut while keeping the heel of the hand in place to maintain head tilt. Your index and middle fingers of your other hand should remain under the victim's chin, lifting up.

Immediately give two full breaths (1 to 1.5 seconds per breath) using the mouth-to-mouth method.

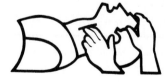

Check Pulse

After giving the two breaths, locate the victim's carotid pulse to see if the heart is beating. To find the carotid artery, take your hand that you are using on the victim's chin and locate the voice box. Slide the tips of your index and middle fingers into the groove beside the voice box. Feel for the carotid pulse. Cardiac arrest can be recognized by absent breathing and an absent pulse in the carotid artery in the neck.

If you cannot find the pulse, you must provide artificial circulation in addition to rescue breathing.

Activate the Emergency Medical Services System (EMSS). Send someone to call 911 or your local emergency number if this has not already been done. If you are alone, perform CPR for 1 minute, then call the EMSS if possible. If it is not feasible to summon the EMSS, continue with CPR.

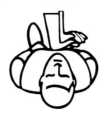

Cardiac Compression

Artificial circulation is provided by external cardiac compression. In effect, when you apply rhythmic pressure on the lower half of the victim's breastbone, you are forcing the heart to pump blood. To perform external cardiac compression properly, kneel at the victim's side near the chest at the level of the victim's shoulders. Locate the notch at the lowest portion of the sternum with your hand that was on the victim's chin. Put your middle finger on this notch and your index finger next to it. Using your hand that was on the victim's forehead, place the heel of this hand on the lower half of the sternum, close to the index finger of your other hand. Place your other hand on top and parallel to the one that is in position. Be sure to keep your fingers off the chest wall. You may find it easier to do this if you interlock your fingers.

Bring your shoulders directly over the victim's sternum as you compress downward, keeping your arms straight. Depress the sternum about 1½ to 2 inches for an adult victim. Then relax pressure on the sternum completely. However, *do not* remove your hands from the victim's sternum, but *do* allow the chest to return to its normal position between compressions. Relaxation and compression should be of equal duration.

If you are the only rescuer, you must provide both rescue breathing and cardiac compression. The proper ratio is 15 chest compressions to 2 full, slow breaths. You must compress at the rate of 80 to 100 times per minute when you are working alone since you will stop compressions when you take time to breathe.

When there is another rescuer to help you, position yourselves on opposite sides of the victim if possible. One of you should be responsible for interposing a breath (1 to 1.5 seconds) after each fifth compression, maintaining an open airway, and monitoring the carotid pulse for adequate chest compressions. The other rescuer, who compresses the chest, should use a rate of 80 to 100 compressions per minute.

Rescuers	Ratio of Compressions to Breaths	Rate of Compressions
1	15 : 2	80 to 100 times/min
2	5 : 1	80 to 100 times/min

CPR FOR INFANTS AND SMALL CHILDREN

Basic life support for infants and small children is similar to that for adults. A few important differences to remember are given below.

Airway

Be careful when handling an infant that you do not exaggerate the backward position of the head tilt. An infant's neck is so pliable that forceful backward tilting might *block* breathing passages instead of opening them.

Breathing

Don't try to pinch off the nose. Cover both the mouth and nose of an infant or *small* child who is not breathing. Use small breaths with less volume to inflate the lungs. Give one small breath every 3 seconds for an infant (0 to 1 year) and one small breath every 4 seconds for a child (1 to 8 years). (For a child, a mouth-to-mouth seal should be made with the nose pinched tightly, as is done for adults.)

Check Pulse

The absence of a pulse may be more easily determined by feeling for the brachial pulse for infants (0 to 1 years). (Locate the carotid pulse for children 1 to 8 years, as you would for an adult.)

Circulation

The technique for cardiac compression is different for infants and small children. In both cases, only one hand is used for compression. The other hand may be slipped under the child to provide a firm support for the back.

For infants, use only the *tips* of two or three fingers to compress the chest. Place the index finger of the hand nearest the infant's legs just under an imaginary line between the nipples where it intersects with the sternum. Compress the chest one fingerbreadth below this intersection, at the location of the middle and ring fingers. Depress the sternum between ½ to 1 inch at a fast rate of 100 times a minute.

For children 1 to 8 years, use only the *heel* of one hand to compress the chest. Depress the sternum between 1 and 1½ inches, depending upon the size of the child. The rate should be 80 to 100 times per minute.

In the case of both infants and small children, breaths should be administered during the relaxation after every fifth chest compression.

	Part of Hand	Depress Sternum	Rate of Compression
Infants	Tips of 2 or 3 fingers	½ to 1 inch	100 per minute
Children	Heel of hand	1 to 1½ inches	80 to 100 per minute

Neck Injury

If you suspect the victim has suffered a neck injury, you must not open the airway in the usual manner. If the victim is injured in a diving or automobile accident, you should consider the possibility of such a neck injury. In these cases, the airway should be opened by using a jaw thrust, keeping the victim's head in a fixed, neutral position.

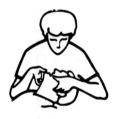

CHOKING

The urgency of choking cannot be overemphasized. Immediate recognition and proper action are essential. If the victim has good air exchange, or only partial obstruction, and is still able to speak or cough effectively, *do not interfere with his or her attempts to expel a foreign body.* The distress signal for choking is the gesture of clutching the neck between the thumb and index finger. *Prompt action is urgent in every case of choking.*

When you recognize complete airway obstruction by observing the conscious victim's inability to speak, breathe, or cough, the following sequence should be performed quickly on the victim in the sitting, standing, or lying position:

1. Manual thrusts (abdominal or chest) until effective, or the person becomes unconscious.
2. Finger sweep if the victim is unconscious.
3. If the victim becomes unconscious, shout for help. Place the victim on the back, face up. Open the airway and attempt to ventilate. If unsuccessful, deliver 6 to 10 manual thrusts, probe the mouth with the finger, and attempt to ventilate. It may be necessary to repeat these steps. *Be persistent.*

MANAGEMENT OF THE OBSTRUCTED AIRWAY

Heimlich Maneuver

The Heimlich maneuver (subdiaphragmatic abdominal thrusts or abdominal thrusts) is the technique recommended for relieving foreign-body airway obstruction. It may be necessary to repeat the thrust 6 to 10 times to clear the victim's airway. Never have your hands on the victim's xiphoid process of the sternum or on the lower margins of the victim's rib cage when performing this maneuver (Fig. 16-2).

Manual thrusts are a rapid series of thrusts to the upper abdomen or chest that force air from the lungs.

Heimlich Maneuver (Abdominal Thrusts) with Victim Sitting or Standing:

1. Stand behind the victim; wrap your arms around the waist.
2. Place the thumb side of your fist against the victim's abdomen in the midline slightly below the rib cage well below the tip of the xiphoid process and slightly above the umbilicus.
3. Grasp your fist with your other hand and press it into the victim's abdomen with a *quick upward thrust.*
4. Repeat if necessary.

Heimlich Maneuver (Abdominal Thrust) with Victim Lying:

1. Place the victim in a supine position; kneel astride the victim's hips/thighs.
2. Place the heel of your hand in the middle of the abdomen, slightly below the rib cage well below the tip of the xiphoid process and slightly above the umbilicus. Place your other hand on top of your bottom hand.

Fig. 16-2. Heimlich maneuver. (Courtesy Edumed, Inc., Cincinnati, OH)

A person choking on food will die in 4 minutes – you can save a life using the HEIMLICH MANEUVER*

Food-choking is caused by a piece of food lodging in the throat creating a blockage of the airway, making it impossible for the victim to breathe or speak. The victim will die of strangulation in four minutes if you do not act to save him.

Using the Heimlich Maneuver* (described in the accompanying diagrams), you exert pressure that forces the diaphragm upward, compresses the air in the lungs, and expels the object blocking the breathing passage.

The victim should see a physician immediately after the rescue. Performing the Maneuver* could result in injury to the victim. However, he will survive only if his airway is quickly cleared.

If no help is at hand, victims should attempt to perform the Heimlich Maneuver* on themselves by pressing their own fist upward into the abdomen as described.

WHAT TO LOOK FOR

The victim of food-choking:

1. Can Not Speak or Breathe.

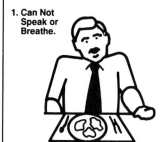

2. Turns Blue.

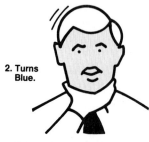

Heimlich Sign: Hand to neck signals: "I am choking!"

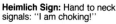

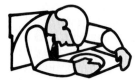

3. Collapses.

HEIMLICH MANEUVER*

RESCUER STANDING
Victim standing or sitting

☐ Stand behind the victim and wrap your arms around his waist.

☐ Place your thumb side against the victim's abdomen, slightly above the navel and below the rib cage.

☐ Grasp your fist with your other hand and press into the victim's abdomen with a **quick upward thrust.**

☐ Repeat several times if necessary.

When the victim is sitting, the rescuer stands behind the victim's chair and performs the maneuver in the same manner.

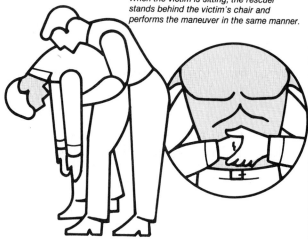

OR

RESCUER KNEELING
Victim lying face up

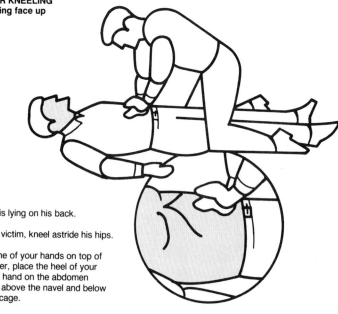

☐ Victim is lying on his back.

☐ Facing victim, kneel astride his hips.

☐ With one of your hands on top of the other, place the heel of your bottom hand on the abdomen slightly above the navel and below the rib cage.

☐ Press into the victim's abdomen with a **quick upward thrust.**

☐ Repeat several times if necessary

3. Rock forward, having your shoulders directly over the victim's abdomen and press into the abdomen and toward the diaphragm with a *quick upward thrust. Do not* press to either side.
4. Repeat if necessary.

Chest Thrusts

Chest thrusts are to be used *only* when the victim is markedly obese or in the later stages of pregnancy. The downward thrusts will generate effective airway pressures.

The Chest Thrust with the Victim Standing or Sitting:

1. Standing behind the victim, place your arms under the victim's armpits, and encircle the victim's chest.
2. Place the thumb side of your fist on the victim's sternum (breastbone), but not on the xiphoid process.
3. Grasp this fist with your other hand, and press on the victim's sternum with a quick backward thrust.

The Chest Thrust with the Victim in a Lying Position:

1. Place your hands in the same position used for closed chest compression.
2. Exert quick downward thrusts.

Infants and Children

For infants up to 1 year of age, the combination of back blows and chest thrusts continues to be recommended. *Back blows* are a rapid series of sharp whacks delivered with the hand over the spine and between the shoulder blades. The blows should be applied quickly, forcefully, and in rapid succession. For a child 1 to 8 years of age, the Heimlich maneuver is recommended.

Other Causes of Airway Obstruction

An adequate open airway must be maintained at all times in all unconscious patients.

Other conditions that may cause unconsciousness and airway obstruction include stroke, epilepsy, head injury, alcoholic intoxication, drug overdose, and diabetes.

Remember:
1. Is the victim unconscious?
2. If so, shout for help, open the airway, and check for breathing

3. If no breathing, give two breaths
4. Check carotid pulse
5. Activate the EMSS: Send someone to call 911 or your local emergency number
6. If no pulse, begin external cardiac compression by depressing the lower half of the sternum 1½ to 2 inches (for adults)
7. Continue uninterrupted CPR until advanced life support is available

> *CPR for one rescuer:*
>   15 : 2 compressions to breaths at a rate of 80 to 100 compressions a minute (four cycles per minute)
> *CPR for two rescuers:*
>   5 : 1 compressions to breaths at a rate of 80 to 100 compressions a minute

Periodic practice in CPR is essential to ensure a satisfactory level of proficiency. A life may depend on how well you have remembered the proper steps of CPR and how to apply them. You should be sure to have both your skill and knowledge of CPR tested at least once a year. It could mean someone's life. *See also Unit IV for AIDS Infection Precautions And CPR.*

EMERGENCY MEDICAL SERVICES SYSTEM (EMSS)

Any victim on whom you begin resuscitation must be considered to need advanced life support. He or she will have the best chance of surviving if your community has a total emergency medical services system. This includes an efficient communications alert system, such as 911, with public awareness of how or where to call; well-trained rescue personnel who can respond rapidly; vehicles that are properly equipped; an emergency facility that is open 24 hours a day to provide advanced life support; and an intensive care section in the hospital for the victims. You should work with all interested agencies to achieve such a system.

911: Emergency Telephone System

Many communities participate in the nationwide 911 emergency telephone system. To find out if it is in effect in your community, call information in your area.

The 911 telephone system *must be used only in emergency situations when you need help quickly.* Dial 911 only when you or someone nearby needs emergency medical help or an ambulance, when you see a fire or a crime in progress, and even when you suspect that a stranger may be in your home or you see him/her trying to enter or leave. Since 911 is a local service in each area, it is not necessary to dial any special access codes before the number. You only need to use three telephone digits — 911. You can dial 911 from any type of telephone, including coin-operated public telephones, without any charge (you don't have to put coins into a coin-operated telephone to dial 911). If you are calling for help for someone who does not live in your area, you should call the "O" operator instead of 911. This is because 911 is a *local* service and cannot be used to obtain help outside of your immediate area.

When you dial 911 you will reach a specially trained emergency operator. This operator will ask you a few important questions so that the type of help you need will be obtained without delay. Information that you will be asked includes the following:

- What is the emergency?
- Where is the emergency? (Include cross-reference streets when applicable.)
- What is your name and address?

Even if you can't talk, stay on the line. In many communities, the special nature of the 911 system allows the emergency operator to know exactly where you are so that help can come quickly. The emergency operator immediately assesses the problem and by pressing a button, notifies the appropriate public emergency agency. The operator stays on the line to be sure that your problem is handled properly to get the fastest emergency service and to see if other emergency services are necessary. The emergency operator also serves to keep the caller calm while waiting for help to arrive. Callers who are disconnected after dialing 911 can be called right back and in even greater emergencies, the operator can trace the location of the phone.

Remember to stay calm and don't hang up. The emergency operator should hang up before you do. Often people panic in an emergency situation. They may give the operator information in a hurried fashion and hang up to go back to the emergency scene before the operator has obtained adequate and correct information. When this happens, the proper help may not be able to reach you in an adequate time to meet the needs of the situation. In some communities your line can be left open until the proper type of emergency help arrives. This would allow special instructions to be given for the emergency while you wait for help to arrive, and if necessary, to determine your address if you are unable to give it.

Remember, 911 must be used only to report "real" emergencies. It must not be used for every call that you may have to make to the police department, the fire department, or an ambulance service.

SHOCK

Shock, a state of collapse or a depressed condition of the circulatory system, occurs when the vital organs of the body are deprived of circulating blood flow necessary to sustain their normal cellular activity. It is a physiological reaction of the body to severe injury or insult. Circulatory collapse may occur following hemorrhage, severe trauma, dehydration, massive infection, severe burns, surgery, increased peripheral resistance, decreased cardiac output, drug toxicity, pain, fear, or emotional distress.

Shock may be immediate or delayed, slight or severe, even fatal. Every injury is accompanied by some degree of shock and so should be treated promptly.

Types of Shock

Shock may be divided into five basic types, as the exact cause of shock is not always the same for every patient.

- **Traumatic shock.** Traumatic shock is the direct result of extracellular fluid loss as in extensive contusions or loss of plasma from large burned areas.
- **Hemorrhagic or hypovolemic shock.** Hemorrhagic or hypovolemic shock is produced by a decrease in the circulating blood volume. The blood loss may be external or internal (into a body cavity where it is no longer accessible to the circulatory system).
- **Cardiogenic shock.** Cardiogenic shock is the result of conditions that interfere with the heart's function as a pump. This may be a result of cardiac failure, secondary to myocardial infarction, coronary thrombosis, or certain disorders of the rate and rhythm of the heart.
- **Septic shock.** Septic shock results from bacterial infection. It may occur when there is massive infection of traumatized tissue or when toxic tissue products are absorbed. Gram-negative shock is a form of septic shock due to infection with the gram-negative bacteria (see Unit VI).
- **Neurogenic shock.** Neurogenic shock is the result of loss of peripheral vascular tone with subsequent dilation of the blood vessels, decreased heart rate, and a drop in the blood pressure to the point at which the supply of oxygen carried to the brain by the blood is insufficient. The patient then faints; thus this type of shock is frequently called fainting.

Signs and Symptoms of Shock

Five "Ps" denote the outstanding signs and symptoms of shock.

1. Prostration
2. Pallor
3. Perspiration
4. Pulselessness
5. Pulmonary deficiency

These will vary in intensity depending on the patient's condition and the injury or cause.

The most outstanding signs and symptoms of severe shock or the later stages of shock include the following:

1. The pulse is weak, rapid, and irregular.
2. Respirations increase in rate and are shallow.
3. Blood pressure is lowered — less than 90 mm Hg systolic.
4. The skin is markedly pale and may feel cold to the touch and moist with perspiration.
5. The lips, nailbeds, tips of the fingers, and lobes of the ears may be bluish (cyanosis).
6. The face may appear pinched and without expression.
7. There may be a staring of the eyes, which often lose their characteristic luster.
8. The pupils may be dilated, especially in the late stages.
9. Occasionally, the patient may be unusually anxious, restless, or excited.
10. When conscious, the patient appears quite disinterested in the surroundings and complains little of pain, although he or she may be groaning.
11. Later the patient may become apathetic and unresponsive. Eyes are sunken with a vacant expression.
12. If untreated, the patient will eventually lose consciousness, vital signs drop, and death may occur.

First Aid Care

In any emergency situation a routine procedure is to evaluate the situation for the possibility of shock and take measures to prevent it. The following objectives for preventing or treating shock should be met:

1. Improve circulation of blood; control bleeding when necessary.
2. Ensure an open airway and an adequate supply of oxygen.
3. Maintain normal body temperature, and keep the patient at rest.
4. Obtain medical assistance as and when required.

When treating a patient in shock:

1. Do a quick primary survey of the situation. Ensure the ABCs of all emergencies; that is, maintain an open airway, and check for breathing and circulation. Be prepared to give cardiopulmonary resuscitation if necessary.
2. Control severe bleeding if present.
3. Position the patient in a supine (lying) position with the lower extremities elevated 8 to 12 inches, *except* when there is a head injury, or if breathing difficulty is thereby increased, or if the patient complains of pain when this is attempted, or if the patient is vomiting. A patient with a head injury should be kept flat, or the head and shoulders may be propped up slightly.
4. Keep the patient warm, but do not overheat.
5. Loosen tight clothing.
6. Do not move the patient unnecessarily.
7. Avoid disturbing the patient with noise and questions.
8. Fluids may be given *only* when there are no contraindications and when medical help cannot be obtained for an hour or more. Fluids are not given to patients who are unconscious, have head injuries, are vomiting, are convulsing, have abdominal injuries, or are likely to require surgery. The recommended fluid to give is water, preferably water with 1 teaspoon of salt and ½ teaspoon of baking soda to each quart of water. Give this at 15 minute intervals as follows:

   • 4 ounces for adults
   • 2 ounces for children ages 1 to 12 years
   • 1 ounce for infants under 1 year of age

9. When necessary, administer oxygen, but only with the consent and directions of the physician.
10. Provide constant, kindly, tactful encouragement and extreme gentleness when caring for the patient.
11. Call the physician or hospital promptly when the patient is going into or is in the state of shock.
12. Arrange for ambulance transport as indicated. Do not attempt to move the patient alone without explicit instructions from the physician unless the immediate surroundings would cause further harm to the patient.

ABDOMINAL PAIN

All abdominal pain should be investigated, especially unusual pain that occurs rather suddenly and is accompanied by fever. Treatment varies with the cause of pain. For pain caused by trauma, keep the patient lying flat if possible, in case of internal bleeding. For pain caused from metabolic or pathological causes, keep the patient in a comfortable position until medical help arrives or the patient is transported to the hospital. For any abdominal pain:

• Keep the patient quiet and warm. Keep activity to a minimum.
• Do not apply heat.
• Do not give food, liquids, or laxatives.
• Place an emesis basin nearby in case the patient vomits.
• Check the patient frequently.
• Be empathetic.

Pathological processes causing acute abdominal emergencies are inflammation, hemorrhage, perforation, obstruction, and ischemia (lack of adequate blood supply). These medical emergencies require immediate care by a physician, because most often they require surgical intervention, although at times some may be treated medically.

ALLERGIC REACTION TO DRUGS (ANAPHYLACTIC REACTION)

Usually in an anaphylactic reaction or in any type of drug overdose reaction, the airway, breathing, and circulation will become impaired because of the effects of drugs on the central nervous system. Thus, a primary survey (the ABCs) must be done.

A = *airway*
 Ensure that the airway is open.
B = *breathing*
 After you ensure that the airway is open, make sure that the breathing is spontaneous; in other words, make sure that the patient is breathing on his or her own.
C = *circulation*
 Check for a pulse beat. The best place to check the pulse rate is at the carotid artery.

When any of these areas requires stabilization, do nothing else except stabilize the ABCs and call or send for medical help. A secondary survey should also be made to ensure that additional injury is not done to the patient. This is a quick head-to-toe check to observe for any obvious bleeding or injury that may require immediate attention. Oxygen and epinephrine should be available for administration on the physician's order. Usually 4 to 8 liters of oxygen is administered by mask or nasal cannula, and 1 to 3 ml epinephrine 1:1000 IU is administered subcutaneously. It is necessary to stay with the patient until medical help arrives to ensure the ABCs.

Constantly monitor the level of consciousness and vital signs, and maintain an adequate airway and ventilation.

Positioning the patient is also very important. Frequently when a patient goes into anaphylaxis, a lying position cannot be tolerated. Usually the patient must be in a sitting or a semi-Fowler position in order to expand the lungs and breathe more easily. Monitor the vital signs carefully, approximately every 2 or 3 minutes, note the skin color, and again monitor the airway. An oropharyngeal airway may be used at times to allow more air to get into the air passageways. When there is not a reversal within a reasonable time, rapid transport to the hospital is necessary.

You should encourage patients with known allergies to wear a Medic-Alert bracelet or necklace.

ASPHYXIA

Asphyxia may occur whenever there is an interference with the normal exchange of oxygen and carbon dioxide between the lungs and outside air. Common causes include obstruction of the airway caused by foreign bodies or the tongue, or by edema of the tissues, as seen in burns or inflammatory processes of the air passages. Drowning, electric shock, inhalation of smoke and poisonous gases, trauma to or disease of the lungs, bronchi, and trachea, or allergic reactions can all cause asphyxia. Basically the patient is apneic (not breathing). Treatment must be an immediate remedy of the situation. Follow the ABCs — check for an open airway, breathing, and circulation. Open the airway if necessary, and give artificial ventilation. Remove the underlying cause whenever possible. When there is absence of both breathing and heartbeat, cardiopulmonary resuscitation must be given immediately. Have oxygen available; it may be given when the patient is having difficulty breathing, and also is frequently administered after breathing resumes to treat the resultant hypoxia. Send for medical help or call the physician.

HUMAN, ANIMAL, SNAKE, AND INSECT BITES AND STINGS

Bites

Injuries caused from animal or human bites may cause punctures, lacerations, or even avulsions, as the person attempts to pull away from the animal or human. Human bites have a high potential for infection because of the high bacterial count in the human mouth. The danger of animal bites is rabies. Bites on the face, neck, or head are considered most serious and require immediate medical attention.

Human and Animal Bites

The first aid care for human and animal bites is a thorough washing with soap and water for 5 minutes and copious rinsing under running water. Benzalkonium chloride (Zephiran) may be applied to the wound and then covered with a sterile or clean dressing. Keep the patient quiet, and avoid movement of the affected part until attended by the physician. Report animal bites to the police or health department, because the animal should be kept for observation for rabies. Collect information from the patient for the possibility of rabies. If the animal is not found and it is believed that the animal was rabid, treatment for rabies will be administered. Also treatment against tetanus will be given.

Common Insect Bites

Bites from ants, mosquitoes, and chiggers can be cared for by washing the affected parts with soap and water, applying a paste made from baking soda and a little water, or applying calamine lotion. When swelling is present, cover the area with a cloth saturated with ice water.

Tick Bites

Don't try to tear an embedded tick loose. Cover it with heavy oil (mineral or salad) or petroleum jelly to close the tick's breathing pores. Frequently this will disengage the tick at once; if not, allow the oil or jelly to remain in place for 30 minutes. If the tick does not disengage after this time, remove it with tweezers, working slowly and gently so that all parts are removed. Wash the area with soap and water for 5 minutes. Do not touch the tick with your hands, because ticks can transmit several diseases. If the skin area becomes inflamed and swollen, or if the patient develops a fever, the physician must be notified.

Severe Reactions to Bites from Spider, Jellyfish, or Insect or Marine Animal of Unknown Origin

Try to remove the stinger with a sterilized needle or knife if it can be seen. Maintain an open airway; give cardiopulmonary resuscitation, and treat for shock when necessary.

Apply a constricting band 2 inches above and below the wound site. This band must not be applied so tightly that it will cut off arterial circulation. To ensure proper application, take the pulse below the band or insert a finger under the band. You should obtain a pulse rate and be able to slip your finger under the band. Remove the band after ½ hour if medical attention has not been obtained within that time.

Keep the affected part immobile and below the individual's heart level. The victim should lie quietly and be covered with a blanket to maintain warmth. Apply ice wrapped in a towel or plastic bag or cold compresses to prevent spread of the poison and to prevent and reduce swelling. Summon the physician, or have the victim taken to a hospital emergency room at once.

Snake Bites

Keep the part immobile and below the victim's heart level. Apply a constricting band 2 inches above and below the bite site when on the arm or leg. The band must be tied tightly enough to retard the blood flow in surface vessels, but not so tightly that it will ob-

struct blood flow in deep-lying vessels. There should be some oozing from the wound, and you should be able to slip your finger under the band and obtain a pulse beat if the constricting band is properly applied.

When the bite is from a poisonous snake and no physician is available, take a sterile knife or a razor blade (sterilize by putting over a flame for a few minutes if sterile instruments are not available) and make a ⅛- to ¼-inch longitudinal incision, no deeper than the skin, at each fang mark and over the suspected venom deposit point. Suck on the wound with your mouth or the suction cup from a snakebite kit for 1 hour or more. Rinse your mouth well after stopping the suction. Although snake venom is *not* a stomach poison, it is best not to swallow it.

Wash the wound with soap and water, blot dry, and apply a sterile dressing and bandage.

Apply ice wrapped in cloth or a plastic bag, or cold applications to the wound to slow absorption of the venom and retard swelling.

Treat for shock or give artificial respiration if necessary.

If the individual must walk, rapid movement must be avoided. Get medical attention as soon as possible. Call the nearest physician or hospital to notify them to prepare antivenin serum.

Stings of Bees, Wasps, Hornets

Try to remove the stinger with a sterilized needle or knife. Run cold water over and around the sting, or apply ice in a towel or plastic bag around it to relieve pain and slow the absorption of the venom. Calamine lotion may be applied to relieve any itching. A victim of massive stings should be soaked in a cool bath of baking soda solution (1 tablespoon per quart of water). If an allergic reaction develops, the victim must be immediately seen by the physician.

SEVERE BLEEDING (HEMORRHAGE)

Three types of bleeding can be observed from open wounds. Spurting of bright red blood from a wound indicates arterial bleeding; continuous flow of dark red blood indicates venous bleeding; and oozing of blood indicates capillary bleeding. Arterial bleeding is the most serious, requiring immediate control and medical intervention after the initial control to prevent severe shock or death. Generally, venous bleeding is easier to control than arterial bleeding, because there is less pressure on the blood flow in the veins than in the arteries. However, venous bleeding may also be life-threatening especially if several large veins are involved. Capillary bleeding is easily controlled by first aid measures and the body's own clotting mechanisms.

Immediate action is imperative for any wound accompanied by severe bleeding, because shock, loss of consciousness, and even death may occur from a rapid loss of blood in a short time.

Objectives of Wound Care

- To control the bleeding immediately
- To protect the wound from contamination and infection (as is feasible; in emergency situations where sterile dressings are not available, you must use materials on hand, even if not sterile. It is more important to save the person's life by controlling the bleeding than it is to worry about preventing infection)
- To treat for shock
- To obtain medical attention

Methods to Control Severe Bleeding (In Order of Preference)

Direct Pressure

Place a sterile dressing (or the cleanest cloth item on hand) over the wound site and apply hard, firm, direct pressure. This will usually be effective in controlling severe bleeding. In the absence of dressing or cloth materials, apply direct pressure with the hand or fingers, but only until a compress is obtained. If a dressing becomes saturated with blood, do not remove it, but place additional dressings directly over the saturated one and continue firm, direct pressure.

Maintain direct pressure by applying a pressure bandage over the dressings on the wound site until medical help is obtained. If bleeding resumes once pressure is released, reapply it, and get the person to the physician immediately.

Elevation

Elevate a limb above the person's heart level in conjunction with direct pressure, unless there is evidence of a fracture. Elevation helps reduce blood pressure within the limb, thus slowing down blood loss from the wound.

Pressure Points

When severe bleeding is not controlled with direct pressure and elevation of an affected limb, the pressure point method can be applied in conjunction with the first two methods. The pressure point method compresses the blood vessel supplying blood to the wound against an underlying bone or muscle tissue in an effort to close it off and reduce the amount of blood flowing through the vessel to the wound site. This method will control bleeding in all but a few circumstances. The exact position of the pressure point must be known and located quickly; otherwise significant blood loss will result. The seven pressure points follow (really fourteen, because there is one on the right and one on the left) (Fig. 16-3).

Temporal Artery.   Compression on the temporal artery may be used to control superficial wounds of the forehead or the frontal part of the scalp.

Facial Artery.   Upward and outward compression of the facial artery against the jawbone with two or more fingers may be used to control bleeding in the facial region.

Carotid Artery.   Compression of the carotid artery in the neck against underlying muscle tissue may be used to control *only* serious hemorrhaging in the head. When this pressure point is used, extreme care must be taken to avoid obstructing the person's airway. *Do not* apply pressure dressings around the neck.

Subclavian Artery.   Downward compression with the fingers on the subclavian artery just behind the collar bone (the clavicle) may be used to control bleeding in the arm and upper shoulder regions.

Brachial Artery.   Compression of the brachial artery against the bone with the fingers applied midway between the shoulder and elbow on the inside of the arm may be used to control bleeding from the arm, hand, and fingers.

Femoral Artery.   Compression of the femoral artery (in the center of the groin area) against the pelvic bone with the heel of the hand may be used to control bleeding from the leg.

Radial Artery.   Compression of the radial artery on the anterior side of the wrist on the thumb side may be used to control severe bleeding from the hand or fingers.

Compression of the ulnar artery (on the little finger, anterior side of the wrist) should be used in conjunction with compression of the radial artery when there is profuse hemorrhaging from the hand. If bleeding does not stop with compression on the radial and ulnar arteries, apply pressure to the brachial artery to control the bleeding.

Tourniquet

The use of a tourniquet is dangerous and should be used *only as a last resort* to control severe, life-threatening hemorrhage when direct pressure, elevation,

Fig. 16-3. Location of pressure points. (From Parcel, G.S.: First aid in emergency care, St. Louis, 1977, The C. V. Mosby Co.)

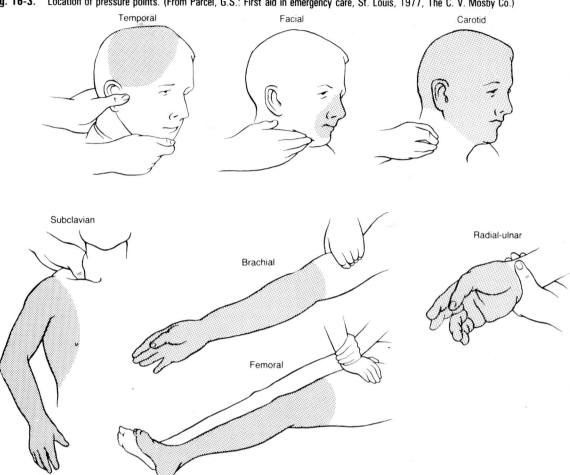

and pressure point methods fail to control the bleeding. The dangers of nerve damage, blood vessel damage, and tissue damage exist when a tourniquet is applied; thus, a tourniquet must be avoided unless a life could be lost. In essence, the decision to apply a tourniquet is a decision to risk the loss of the person's limb to save life. After the application of a tourniquet, it is imperative that the person be attended to by a physician. The following directions *must* be observed when a tourniquet is applied (Fig. 16-4).

1. Use appropriate materials at least 2 inches wide, such as a stocking, a cloth, a folded triangular bandage, or a blood pressure cuff, if available.
2. Apply the tourniquet just above the wound, or just above a joint when the wound is in or below a joint area.
3. Wrap the tourniquet material around the limb twice, and secure it with a knot.
4. Insert a strong stick or similar object between the two loops and twist this object to tighten the tourniquet until bleeding stops. Tourniquets must be applied tightly enough to stop the bleeding; if applied too loosely, bleeding will increase.

Fig. 16-4. Procedure for application of tourniquet. (From Parcel, G. S.: First aid in emergency care, St. Louis, 1977, The C. V. Mosby Co.)

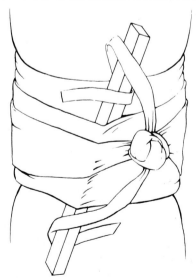

5. Wrap the ends of the tourniquet material around the stick or similar object, and tie it in place.
6. Make a written note of the time of application and the location of the tourniquet, and attach this to the person's clothing, or mark this information on the person. Frequently people will mark a large TK (for tourniquet) on the injured person's forehead with lipstick when at the scene of the accident.
7. *Never* release a tourniquet once it has been applied. A tourniquet must be removed only by a physician, who can provide supportive treatment for shock.
8. Elevate the limb slightly if this will not cause further injury.
9. Treat for shock, and give first aid for other injuries as required.
10. Transport the person immediately to receive medical attention.

Amputation

In cases of amputation, the amputated part should be kept cool and moist if possible, and taken with the victim to the physician. With the advent of microsurgery, amputated limbs can frequently be reattached successfully, providing there is minimal tissue damage to the surrounding tissues.

Further Wound Care

For capillary bleeding, direct pressure and the application of ice wrapped in a towel or plastic bag are useful. Remember that ice is not effective in controlling *severe* bleeding.

In all cases when caring for bleeding wounds, provide reassurance and emotional support to the victim, and remain calm. If possible, estimate how much blood was lost, because this will help the physician treat the person and determine if fluid replacement is necessary. However, remember that even an ounce of blood can discolor large numbers of dressings; and a cup of blood poured on the floor or ground covers a fairly large area, because when blood first comes from the vessels it is thin, and a small amount looks like a lot. Also observe the actual bleeding—is it a minimal, moderate, or heavy flow? This information will aid the physician, in addition to guiding your decision for the use of a tourniquet.

When bleeding stops, bandage the dressings firmly in place. Do not remove the initial dressings, because blood clots may be disturbed and bleeding resumed. Leave the cleaning and treatment of the wound to the physician.

Prevention of Contamination and Infection

To prevent infection, avoid, if possible, touching the wound with an unsterilized dressing or your unscrubbed hands. Do not disturb or remove the initial dressing placed over the wound.

BURNS

Burns are wounds caused by body contact with fire (dry heat), steam and scalding water (moist heat), electricity, chemicals, radiation (sun or nuclear rays), or lightning. Each year thousands of burns occur, many of which could have been prevented, and many of which are fatal in both the young and old. Burns involving over one third to one half of the body are often fatal, especially in children. Theories on the treatment for burns have undergone many changes over the years; many remedies were advocated and later rejected. Current thought on the matter can best be summed up by following the three Bs and the three Cs.

B = *burn*
  Stop the burning
B = *breathing*
  Check the breathing
B = *body examination*
  Examine where and how extensively the body has been burned, and assess any associated injuries

C = *cool*
  Cool the burn
C = *cover*
  Cover the burn
C = *carry*
  Carry the burn patient to the nearest medical treatment facility

In addition, current treatment practices *condemn* the application of greasy substances, ointments, powders, or antiseptics to a burned area.

Classification of Burns

Burns are classified as first, second, and third degree, depending on the depth of the wound; they are also classified according to the percentage of body surface involved (Figs. 16-5 and 16-6).

Depth of Wound

First degree burns involve only the outer layers of the skin. The skin is reddened without blister formation

Fig. 16-5. **A,** Cross-section showing structures of skin. **B,** Classification of burns by degree. (From Parcel, G.S.: First aid in emergency care, St. Louis, 1977, The C. V. Mosby Co.)

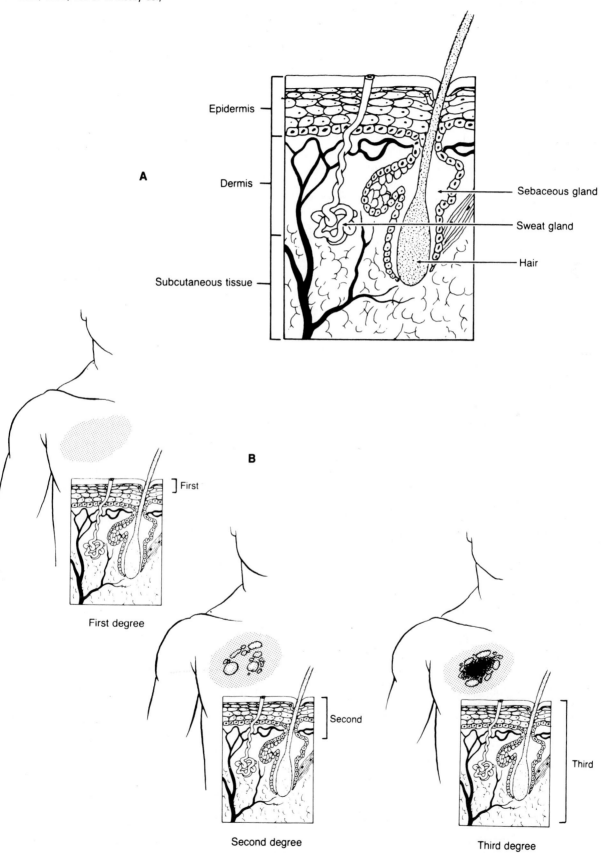

Fig. 16-6. Classification of burns by body surface area. (From Parcel, G.S.: First aid in emergency care, St. Louis, 1977, The C. V. Mosby Co.)

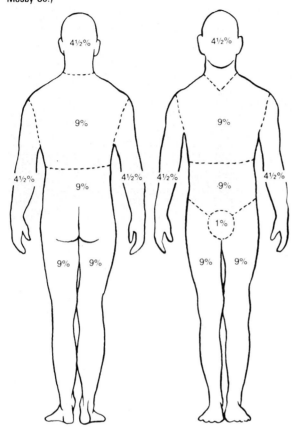

and is painful. The best example is a sunburn. *Second degree burns* involve deeper layers of the epidermis, are painful, and usually form blisters. *Third degree burns* are the most serious, destroying all layers of the skin including the hair follicles, and the sebaceous and sweat glands. Nerves are destroyed, thus the wound is painless. Muscles, blood supply, and bones may also be destroyed in third degree burns.

Body Surface

The percentage of total body surface involved usually determines the severity of the burn. The body surface is divided into areas by the rule of nine. Each arm is 9 percent, each leg is 18 percent, the front or back of the trunk is 18 percent, and the head and neck are 9 percent of the total body surface.

A first degree burn involving more than 20 percent of total body surface, or involving the face and airway, or impairing the person when walking or wearing clothes should receive medical attention. Any second or third degree burn involving more than 20% of the total body surface, or the feet, hands, or genitalia is considered a serious burn in need of medical attention. When more than 40% of total body surface is burned, it is considered a *severe burn*.

First Aid Treatment for Burns

Objectives For Care of First Degree Burns:

- To relieve pain
- To prevent the formation of blisters

Treatment

1. Immediately submerge the burned part in ice water, or place cold compresses directly on the burn.
2. Continue this treatment until pain has subsided when the cold is discontinued.
3. Apply a dry sterile dressing if the burn is in an area that will be irritated by clothing.
4. When running water is available, it is best to place the burned part under cold running water for 20 minutes. The reason is that, even though the top layers of the skin are cooled within a few minutes, the underlying tissue is still very heated, and the burn continues to cause tissue damage up to periods of 20 minutes after the initial burn.

Objectives for Treating Second and Third Degree Burns:

- Treat the person for shock
- Prevent infection
- Relieve pain

Second Degree Burn Care:

1. Immediately submerge the burned part in cold water for 1 to 2 hours, *or* place under running water for 20 minutes.
2. *Do not* break blisters or remove tissue.
3. Cover with a dressing or clean cloth that has been wrung out in ice water.
4. Apply a dry dressing as a protective bandage.

Third Degree Burn Care

1. Stop the burning; check for breathing; remove the burning agent. Remove any smoldering clothing; certain synthetics retain heat. Remove any jewelry on the burned area. Clothing and jewelry retain heat and also can become constricting as edema develops. Do a quick body assessment to determine the extent and severity of the burn.
2. Keep the person lying down with the head a little lower than the legs and hips, unless there is a chest or head injury, or if the person has difficulty breathing in this position.
3. Cool and cover the wound. Cover the burned areas with sterile dressings if available, or a cloth or sheet. Pour copious amounts of cool water, or saline, if available, onto the material covering the

wound. Continue pouring cool water onto the material every so often, as the burn continues to heat the water up to the material. If clean material is not available, water may be poured directly onto the wound. When the wound is cooled, wrap the person for transport to a medical facility. *Never open any blisters.* Covering the wound prevents moving air from reaching the wound, lessens pain, and reduces contamination.

4. If adjoining surfaces of skin are burned, separate them with gauze or cloth to keep them from sticking together (such as between the toes or fingers, ears and head, arms and chest).

5. *If* the victim is conscious, is not nauseated or vomiting, and medical help cannot be obtained for an hour or more, make a solution of ½ teaspoon baking soda and 1 teaspoon salt in a quart of water. Allow the adult patient to sip a half glass every 15 minutes to replace lost body fluids; a child 1 to 12 years, 2 ounces, and an infant about 1 ounce. Discontinue fluid if vomiting occurs.

6. For **chemical burns,** wash immediately with *copious* amounts of cool running water for at least 5 minutes (Fig. 16-7). Remove any clothing that was in contact with the chemical. If the chemical got on the face or eyes, flush the face and eyes with a gentle flow of cool water for at least 15 minutes (Fig. 16-8). Remove contact lenses if the victim is wearing them. Try to find out what chemical caused the burn so that you can tell the personnel at the emergency department where the victim will be taken. Also see the above steps. NOTE: *Never* flush a phosphorus burn with any type of solution, including water, as this could cause tissue sloughing. Instead, *soak* the affected area in water.

Fig. 16-7. For chemical burns, wash immediately with copious amounts of cool running water for at least 5 minutes.

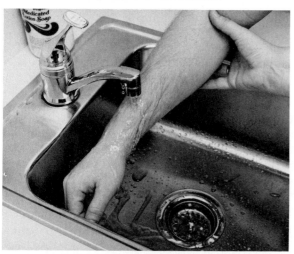

Fig. 16-8. If chemical gets on face, flush face and eyes with a gentle flow of cool water.

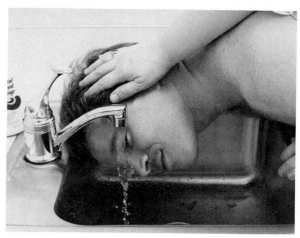

7. If possible while awaiting transport for the person, take the pulse, respiration, and blood pressure to assess impending shock.

8. Keep the patient warm and resting quietly. Chilling must be avoided to prevent additional discomfort and loss of energy.

9. Constantly provide emotional support for the patient.

10. Inform the patient before transfer is undertaken.

What *Not* to Do About Burns

- *Don't* pull clothing over the burned area—cut it away if necessary.
- *Don't* try to remove any pieces of cloth or bits of debris or dirt that are stuck to the burn.
- *Don't* try to clean the burn; *don't* use iodine or other antiseptics on it; and *don't* open any blisters that may form on the burn.
- *Don't* use grease, butter, ointment, salve, petroleum jelly, or any type of medication on *any* burn.
- *Don't* breathe on a burn, and *don't* touch it with anything except a sterile or clean dressing.
- *Don't* change the dressings that were initially applied to the burn until directed to do so by a physician.

CEREBRAL VASCULAR ACCIDENT (STROKE)

A cerebral vascular accident (CVA), also called a stroke, is a disorder of the blood vessels of the brain. It results in a lack of blood supply to parts of the brain. Main causes of a CVA include a cerebral thrombus or a cerebral embolus, cerebral hemorrhage, compression of cerebral arteries (as from edema or tumors), and arterial spasms. The symptoms and effects of a

CVA vary greatly. They can be slight or severe, temporary or permanent, depending on the cause, location, and extent of the damage in the brain. Signs and symptoms of a CVA may include the following:

- dizziness, mental confusion, headache, and poor coordination
- difficulty in speaking or loss of speech
- loss of bladder and bowel control
- paralysis or weakness on one or both sides of the body
- loss of vision, especially in one eye
- difficulty in breathing and in swallowing
- unequal size of the pupils
- loss of consciousness

First Aid Measures for a Cerebral Vascular Accident Include the Following:

1. Loosen all constricting clothing especially around the neck. This may help to improve breathing and circulation to the head.
2. Maintain an open airway.
3. Position the victim on the affected side so that secretions will drain from the mouth and thus prevent aspiration of saliva and mucus.
4. Keep the victim calm and provide reassurance that care is being provided.
5. If conscious, the victim may sit up or have the head elevated. This will help to lessen blood pressure in the head.
6. Do not give fluids unless the victim is able to swallow and is fully conscious. Discontinue all fluids if the victim vomits.
7. Seek medical attention as soon as possible. The victim will usually need to be hospitalized.
8. Be prepared to administer cardiopulmonary resuscitation if required.

CHEST PAIN

Chest pain can be associated with heart disease, lung disease, pain in the muscle fibers of the chest wall, and a few other conditions. It can be serious. It is advisable to treat all patients with chest pain as if they are heart patients. First aid measures include the following:

1. Observe the symptoms.
2. Keep the patient quiet and warm. Allow the patient to rest. Frequently the patient will find it easier to breathe when in a semisitting or upright position. Do not have the patient walk any distance.
3. Loosen all tight clothing.
4. Administer 4 to 6 liters of oxygen (if you are in the office and have prior directions and permission from the physician).

5. Contact the physician. When the physician cannot be reached, call the emergency medical system in your community, or an ambulance, or the fire department.
6. Stay with the patient until medical help arrives.
7. If the patient is conscious, inquire if she or he has any medication with her or him that is used for attacks of chest pain. The medication will usually be nitroglycerin tablets, which are taken sublingually. You may give them to the patient with the patient's consent.
8. When feasible obtain pertinent information from the patient. Use the PQRST method:
   P = provoking
   What provoked the pain? Was the patient doing any physical activity, experiencing emotional upset or excitement, or was the patient just sitting quietly reading or such?
   Q = quality of pain
   Is it a sharp pain, prolonged oppressive pain, or unusual discomfort?
   R = radiation of pain
   Where, if at all, does the pain radiate to? Is it in the center of the chest? Is it in the chest wall? Does it radiate to the abdomen or to the neck or to the left arm?
   S = severity
   How severe is the pain—mild, moderate, or severe?
   T = time
   When did the pain start? How long does it last? How frequently does it recur?
9. Keep an emesis basin handy in case the patient vomits.
10. At times it may be necessary to start artificial respiration or cardiopulmonary resuscitation if breathing and heartbeat have ceased.
11. If in the physician's office, you may connect the patient to the electrocardiograph and record a few tracings for the physician to interpret. Lead II and Lead V_1 are considered the monitoring leads.
12. Remain calm; offer emotional support and reassurance to the patient, because most patients will be anxious and frightened.

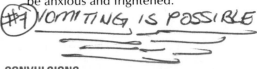
#9 VOMITING IS POSSIBLE

CONVULSIONS

Convulsions are the involuntary spasms or contractions of muscles caused by an abnormal stimulus to the brain, or by changes in the chemical balance in the body. The primary effort in first aid for convulsions is to protect the patient from causing harm to the body during the convulsion.

1. Move items near the patient that may cause harm. Ask curious onlookers to remove themselves from the immediate area.

2. Loosen clothing around the neck and in any other area where it is constricting.

3. Place a padded bite block between the teeth to protect against biting of the tongue. *Do not* insert a bite block when force is required to get it in place. If an appropriate bite block is not available, one can be made by wrapping and taping a couple of pieces of gauze around two tongue blades.

4. Do not restrain the patient's movements except to prevent injury. Protect the head at all times.

5. When movement has ceased, keep the patient lying down and allow to rest.

6. Ensure an open airway.

7. If bleeding from a bitten tongue, or excessive saliva, or vomit is present, turn the patient's head to one side to prevent aspiration of these excretions.

8. After all seizure activity has ceased, allow the patient to rest or sleep in a quiet, comfortable place until sufficiently oriented to time and place, and capable of moving without weakness.

Anyone who has experienced a seizure (convulsion) should be seen by a physician, although the occurrence of one seizure is not considered an emergency. If convulsive activity is repeated or occurs frequently, medical attention must be sought.

If reporting the convulsion to the physician, it is very important that you describe the convulsive activity; that is, whether the convulsion was generalized or localized, how and where it started, how many convulsions there were, and how long they lasted.

EPISTAXIS (NOSEBLEED)

Most nosebleeds are not serious and can be easily controlled. However, excessive bleeding requires medical attention and may require electrocauterization of the ruptured vessels causing the bleeding.

First aid for nosebleeds is relatively simple. Have the patient in a sitting position, and pinch the lower portion of the nose between the thumb and index finger for 5 to 10 minutes. When this does not control the bleeding, apply ice packs to the nasal and facial areas. Place a moistened gauze pad gently into the bleeding nostril, leaving one end of the gauze outside so that it can be removed easily, then pinch the nose between the thumb and index finger for 10 minutes. If this does not control the bleeding, medical attention should be obtained.

FAINTING (SYNCOPE)

Fainting is a partial or complete loss of consciousness of limited duration caused by a decreased amount of blood to the brain. A person may feel weak and dizzy, cold, nauseated, appear pale, perspire, and have numbness or tingling in the hands and feet before fainting; or one may faint suddenly. First aid management for patients who faint follows:

1. Lay the person flat with the head lowered slightly.

2. Ensure an open airway.

3. Loosen tight clothing.

4. Apply cold cloths to the face. These are beneficial because of their stimulating effect.

5. Pass aromatic spirits of ammonia back and forth in front of the person's nose to allow inhalation. Avoid holding them too close to the person's nose.

6. Observe the person carefully, looking for anything unusual.

7. Observe for local weakness of the arms and legs, and locate and count the pulse. These observations may be of great importance if the condition turns out to be something other than a fainting episode.

8. Keep the person resting quietly for at least 10 minutes after full consciousness has been regained.

9. Lower the head between the legs when the person is in a sitting position and begins to feel faint. Stay with the person, and protect against falling should fainting occur.

10. When fainting lasts more than a minute or two, keep the person warm and resting quietly, and summon the physician or transport to the hospital, for the condition may not be a simple episode of fainting. It may, in fact, be a symptom of diabetes, heart disease, epilepsy, stroke, or any one of many diseases.

FOREIGN BODIES IN THE EAR, EYE, AND NOSE

Ear

Foreign bodies lodged in the ear canal are frequently seen in children. *Do not* attempt to remove them. They must be removed by the physician, because of the possibility of injury to the eardrum (tympanic membrane) and ear canal tissue.

If the foreign body in the ear is a live bug or insect, instill a few drops of sterile oil into the ear canal. This will asphyxiate and stop the movement of the intruder.

Eye

Foreign bodies in the eye are irritating and can be harmful because of the possibility of their scratching the eye surface or becoming embedded in the eye tissue.

Instruct the patient not to rub the affected eye. Wash your hands, and examine the eye by pulling the lower lid down and turning the upper lid back. If the object is on either lid, take a moistened corner of a clean cloth and touch it lightly to try to remove it. Avoid applying any pressure on the eye. If the object is on the eye itself, do not attempt to remove it this way. At times when the object is located under the upper eyelid or on the eye, it may be dislodged by pulling the upper eyelid forward and down over the lower lid; tears may dislodge the object. The eye then may be flushed with clean water. (See also *Eye Irrigation* in Unit VIII.)

When the previous methods do not remove the object, it may be embedded. Cover the closed eye with a dressing, and summon the physician.

Nose

When the object cannot be removed easily, a physician must be consulted. Instruct the patient to avoid violent nose blowing and probing the nose, because these acts may only push the object deeper or injure the tissues of the nose.

FRACTURES

A fracture is a break in the continuity of a bone. Broad classifications of fractures are *open fracture* — one in which the bone penetrates the skin producing an open wound, and *closed fracture* — one in which there is no break in the skin. Closed fractures are much more common than open fractures. Not all fractures prevent the patient from moving the injured part; therefore, never ask the patient to move to determine the presence of broken bones. Movement of a fractured area may cause additional harm, and at times, permanent damage. Different types of fractures are illustrated in Figure 16-9.

First Aid for Fractures

1. Treat for shock and give artificial respiration when necessary; keep the patient warm and quiet.
2. Prevent movement of the injured part and adjacent joints, and *do not* move the injured part.
3. Elevate affected extremities when possible without disturbing the suspected fracture. This will help reduce hemorrhage, when present, and swelling.
4. Apply an ice bag to the painful area.
5. Never attempt to reduce (set) a fracture. This is the physician's responsibility.
6. Never attempt to push a protruding bone back into place.
7. For an open fracture, in addition to the above:
   - Control any serious bleeding.
   - Do not attempt to clean the wound.
   - Avoid contaminating the wound; do not touch the wound.
   - Do not replace bone fragments.
   - Cover the wound with a sterile dressing or clean cloth material, and secure in place with a bandage.
8. To prevent additional trauma when the patient has to be moved or transported, the injured part must be immobilized by applying splints or slings, and bandages. Splints must be long enough to reach beyond the joint above and below the break on both sides. Pad improvised splints to prevent additional pressure or injury, and tie them in place with bandages or strips of material. Make sure that the bandages or splints are not too tight. Normal circulation must not be hindered. Refer to a first aid textbook for additional information on the application of various types of splints.

Fractured Neck or Back

When there is a suspected neck, back, pelvis, or skull fracture, *do not* attempt to move the patient. Trained medical or ambulance personnel are required. When the patient experiences a numbness or tingling around the shoulders and cannot move the fingers readily, a neck fracture should be suspected.

When there is numbness or tingling in the legs, or pain when trying to move the back or neck, or when the feet or toes cannot be moved, a back fracture is suspected.

In either of the above cases, loosen the patient's clothing around the neck and waist. Do not move the patient, and do not let the patient attempt to move, as injury to the spinal cord may occur. Keep the patient warm and quiet, and treat for shock, as indicated. Call for medical help immediately. The patient will need to be transported by ambulance to the nearest hospital.

Fractured Jaw

When a fractured jaw is suspected, tie a bandage around the chin and over the head to stop movement. Do not manipulate the jaw. Medical attention is required for treatment.

HEAD INJURIES

The severity of head injuries can vary greatly. The patient may appear normal, experience a headache, have a momentary loss of consciousness or lack of memory, be dazed, or be unconscious. Bleeding from the mouth, nose, ears, or scalp may be present; pulse may be rapid and weak; pupils of the eyes may

Fig. 16-9. Types of fractures. (From Ingalls, A.J., and Salerno, M.C.: Maternal and Child Health Nursing, St. Louis, 1983, 5th Edition, The C. V. Mosby Co.)

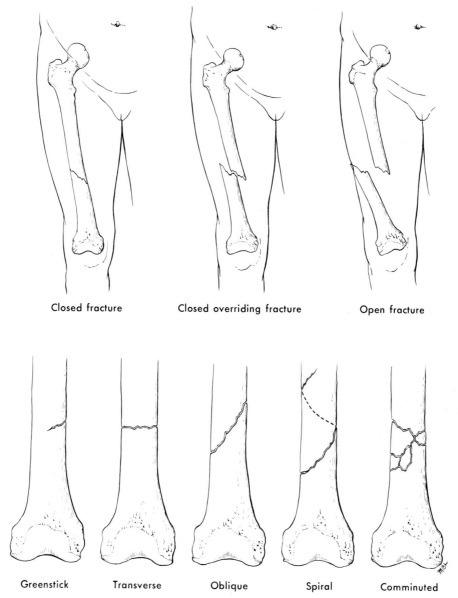

Closed fracture   Closed overriding fracture   Open fracture

Greenstick   Transverse   Oblique   Spiral   Comminuted

be unequal in size; and pallor, vomiting, or double vision may be present. *In all cases medical attention is imperative.* When the initial symptoms are minor, it must be remembered that even after a period of time, hours or days, the injured person may become drowsy or confused or unconscious as a result of a head injury. A prompt recovery from a state of minor signs and symptoms may not be an indication of the seriousness of the injury. The following steps and precautions should be taken:

1. Assess the patient's physical and mental status. For physical assessment, check for signs as stated above, and take the blood pressure if equipment is available. For mental assessment, when the patient is conscious, check for orientation as to time, place, name, and alertness, and ask the patient to repeat a simple phrase. Talking with the patient is a good way to check the level of consciousness and alertness.

2. Keep the patient at rest in a supine position if the face is ashen and gray, or raise the head and shoulders (together) if the face is flushed. *Never position the patient with the head lower than the rest of the body.*

3. Always ensure an open airway. Be prepared to give artificial respiration when necessary.

4. Control hemorrhage if present.

HO·70 Normal BS

120 ↑BS

5. Do not give fluids by mouth.
6. Apply a dressing to a scalp wound, and bandage it in place with a head bandage.
7. Take note of any period of unconsciousness, and record it.
8. Observe and record any changes in the pupils of the eyes.
9. Take and record the blood pressure and the time of any changes (if the equipment is available). When the blood pressure begins to rise and if the pupils begin to dilate, or the state of consciousness begins to decrease, this usually indicates an elevation of intracranial pressure.
10. If the patient is unconscious, gently turn the head to one side to prevent aspiration of any blood or mucus that may be present.
11. Keep the patient resting quietly until medical help arrives or the patient is transported to the hospital.

HYPERVENTILATION

Hyperventilation is a common complication of emotional upsets or hysterical situations. It usually affects persons who are anxious, high-strung, and have a history of job or home stress, anxiety from lack of sleep, sudden stoppage of prescribed drugs such as diazepam (Valium), or a history of drug usage that increases sensitivity of the respiratory centers, such as high concentrations of salicylate. These individuals usually unknowingly breathe too rapidly, which in turn disturbs the normal balance of carbon dioxide in the blood.

At the outset, individuals may feel a tightness in the chest and have a feeling of air hunger; they feel that they cannot fill the lungs because they can't get enough air. Frequently these individuals will become apprehensive, which only leads to increased hyperventilation and at times to syncope (fainting). Palpitation of the heart, abdominal pain, and a feeling of fullness in the throat may also occur.

Immediate first aid treatment is to have the individual breathe into a paper bag held tightly over the mouth and nose for 10 minutes or more to replace the carbon dioxide that has been given off during hyperventilation. Removing the victim from the surroundings is helpful, because frequently people who are trying to help the victim become excited and anxious, and unknowingly only promote the victim's anxiety and subsequent hyperventilation. In all cases, the first aider or medical assistant should be the calming influence and provide reassurance to the victim.

When frequent attacks of hyperventilation occur, it is recommended that the victim seek medical attention for treatment of the underlying cause(s).

INSULIN REACTION AND DIABETIC COMA

Diabetes mellitus is a disorder of carbohydrate metabolism in which the ability to oxidize and utilize carbohydrates is lost, and a subsequent derangement of protein and fat metabolism occurs. This results from disturbances in the normal insulin mechanism, a hormone secreted by the islands of Langerhans in the pancreas.

Adverse conditions can occur when a diabetic is undiagnosed or does not follow the therapy prescribed or when there is a disturbance in the normal functions of the body. All persons with diabetes, their immediate families, and persons in the health care professions should know the signs and symptoms and the treatment or immediate first aid for an insulin reaction (too much insulin or presence of insulin without food) and diabetic coma (a condition that may develop when there is lack of insulin in the diabetic patient's system) (Table 16-1). Diabetics should carry a card stating the fact that they are diabetic, their daily insulin or oral hypoglycemic drug dosage, their address, and the name and address of their physician. Many diabetics wear Medic-Alert bracelets or necklaces, which indicate their condition in case of emergency situations requiring treatment.

First Aid

Insulin reaction

1. If the patient is conscious, give some form of simple sugar, such as hard candy, sugar, or sweetened orange juice.
2. Seek medical attention if the patient does not respond readily to the above.
3. If the patient is unconscious, do not force fluids or food. Call the physician, or get the patient to the hospital immediately.

Diabetic coma. There is *no adequate first aid* treatment for hyperglycemia or diabetic coma. *Immediate medical treatment is necessary.*

OPEN WOUNDS

Types of wounds include abrasions, avulsions, incisions, lacerations, and puncture wounds. See pp. 170–171 and Fig. 5-27.

First Aid Care for Minor Wounds

1. Wash your hands thoroughly before treating any wound to minimize the possibility of infection.

Table 16-1. Signs and symptoms of insulin reaction and diabetic coma

	Insulin Reaction	Diabetic Coma
Onset	Gradual	Sudden
Skin	Perspiration, pallor, cold and damp skin	Flushed and dry skin, dry tongue
Behavior	Tremors, restlessness, fatigue, faint feeling, headache, confusion or strange behavior	Weakness, drowsiness, lethargy
Gastrointestinal tract	Extreme hunger, nausea	Thirst, nausea, and vomiting
Vision	Double vision	Eyeball tension low
Respiration	Shallow	Difficulty in breathing or air hunger
Pulse	Rapid or normal	Rapid, weak
Speech	Slurred	
Breath	No acetone smell	Sweet or fruity odor; smell of acetone
Level of consciousness	May have loss of consciousness	Coma if unattended
Blood glucose	Low (40–70 mg/100 ml)	High (over 200 mg/100 ml)
Urine test	Sugar—absent, or a trace at most Acetone—negative	Sugar—positive in high amounts Acetone—positive

2. Observe the wound to check for foreign objects, such as pieces of glass, wood, and dirt.
3. Control bleeding (see pp. 470–472).
4. Gently wash the skin around the wound with soap and water. Wash away from the wound, not toward it.
5. For minor cuts, scratches, and abrasions, wash the wound well with soap and water to remove foreign matter.
   • Lacerations and incisions may be irrigated with large amounts of water or normal saline. Do not apply an antiseptic unless instructed to do so by the physician.
   • For puncture wounds, gently squeeze the wound to encourage a small amount of bleeding to help wash out microorganisms. Then wash the wound with soap and water.
   • Wounds with severe bleeding should not be cleansed.
6. Cover the wound with a sterile dressing, and bandage it in place. Use the cleanest material on hand when sterile dressings are not available.
7. Refer the person to the physician for follow-up care. Tetanus immunization may be required. Lacerations, incisions, and avulsions will require medical attention, because they may have to be sutured.
8. Advise the person to be alert for signs of infection, and if present, to seek medical attention. Signs to watch for are
   • Swelling
   • Excessive redness
   • Heat and increasing tenderness
   • Drainage
   • Red streaks away from the wound
   • Fever
   • Excessive pain

POISONING

The symptoms of poisoning vary greatly and depend on the type and amount of substance taken. All types of poisonings are considered emergencies that require immediate attention. Points that should be considered when poisoning is suspected follow:

1. Look for any physical changes, such as an abrupt onset of pain or illness; burns or stains around the mouth or on the face, which would indicate poisoning with a caustic substance; breath odor, which may indicate the type of poison ingested; or depressed consciousness and irregular heartbeat.
2. Observe the surroundings for empty containers, spilled fluids, or containers of substances that would be poisonous if ingested.
3. Obtain information from the person or an observer when possible.

Objectives of First Aid Measures

1. To dilute or neutralize the poison.
2. To induce vomiting, *except* when the person has swallowed corrosive or petroleum products, when the person is unconscious, or when the person is convulsing.

3. To prevent absorption of the poison.
4. To maintain an open airway, breathing, and vital functions.
5. To obtain medical attention without delay.

First Aid

Speed is essential to stop absorption of a poison. First aid for poisoning depends on the type of poison ingested. It is not possible for the first aider or medical assistant to know exactly what to do for all cases, but general guidelines must be followed.

1. In all cases, monitor the person's vital signs, maintain an open airway, and be prepared to administer cardiopulmonary resuscitation if necessary.
2. Make every effort to determine what, when, and how much was ingested.
3. Obtain specific information to follow when this is possible. Call the physician, or the poison control center that is in the nearest city, or the hospital emergency physician. Antidote labels may be on the product ingested, but *caution* must be taken, because the label may be out-of-date and incorrect. Poison control centers are open 24 hours a day and maintain antidote information on several thousand available commercial products. Most states have a poison control center in the major cities. Keep this number on hand with other important telephone numbers.
4. Carry out the specific first aid instructions obtained.
5. When specific directions cannot be obtained, the following may be performed.
   • If the person is awake and able to swallow, milk or water may be given to dilute the poison.
   • *Do not induce vomiting* if the person (1) is unconscious or in a coma; (2) is having a convulsion; (3) has ingested a petroleum product, such as kerosene, lighter fluid, gasoline; (4) has ingested a corrosive substance, for example, strong acids or alkalis. In these situations, if the person can swallow, give the following:
      (a) For acids: milk, water, or milk of magnesia (1 tablespoon to 1 cup of water).
      (b) For alkalis: milk, water, any fruit juice, or vinegar; for persons 1 to 5 years old — 1 to 2 cups, for persons 5 years and older — up to 1 quart.
   • If the person has ingested a *noncorrosive* substance and is *not* unconscious or convulsing:
      (a) Give 1 tablespoon of syrup of ipecac, followed by 1 cup of water. Keep children active. Repeat the same dose in 15 minutes if vomiting has not occurred. *Repeat only once.*

   (b) If ipecac is not available, attempt to induce vomiting by giving milk or water and then placing the blunt end of a spoon or your finger at the back of the person's throat. Mild soapy water may also induce vomiting if ipecac is not available.
   (c) When retching and vomiting begin, place the person's head down with the head lower than the hips. This prevents vomitus from entering the lungs, causing further injury.
   (d) When the poison is unknown, save the vomitus, and take it to the physician or hospital for analysis.
   NOTE: The universal antidote of 2 parts burned toast, 1 part milk of magnesia, and 1 part strong tea that was formerly recommended is now believed to be *useless.* Therefore, *do not* waste time preparing this mixture for administration.
6. Arrange for transportation of the person to the physician or the hospital. *All cases of poisoning must receive medical attention.*
7. Remain calm at all times. Stay with the person, and provide reassurance.

Many poisoning cases are related to drug abuse. In order to determine the proper first aid care that should be given in these cases you should be aware of the characteristics of intoxication for drugs that are commonly abused. See Table 16-2 on pp. 484–485 for selected effects of commonly abused drugs.

POISON CONTROL CENTERS

Poison control centers have been established in many cities across the nation to provide quick and reliable information on possible poisonings or drug-related problems. They provide information on the appropriate first aid and clinical management to use for cases of suspected or known poisoning. Some centers also offer specialized poisoning treatment and consultant services, professional training, and poisoning prevention education for consumers. Many centers are staffed by clinical pharmacists 24 hours a day, every day of the year.

Not all states have poison control centers; some rely on centers in nearby cities. Some states have state designated centers that are located in 2 or 3 major cities in that state. Other states have poison control centers that are regional centers established by a particular city. These centers are usually financed locally. The centers are usually located at major hospitals or major medical universities. You should post the telephone number of the nearest poison control center near your telephone both at work and at home so that you are able to obtain information as quickly as possible when the need arises.

For a list of poison control centers in the United States write to:

Publication Office of Veterinary
   and Human Toxicology
Comparative Toxicology Laboratories
Kansas State University
Manhattan, Kansas 66506
Telephone: (916) 532-5679

FIRST AID KIT

Now is the time to check the first aid kit kept in the office, home, and family automobile. A properly equipped kit, with fresh supplies that are kept replenished after use, is a practical aid in relieving many minor injuries and ailments. It may even be lifesaving before medical help arrives. But, the best time to provide the office, home, or automobile first aid kit is *before* it is needed. The following first aid supplies are suggested:

1. Sterile gauze pads
2. Sterile gauze roller bandages
3. Adhesive tape
4. Adhesive dressings
5. Absorbent cotton — sterile
6. Triangular bandage
7. Elastic bandage
8. A mild antiseptic
9. Syrup of ipecac
10. Analgesic, such as aspirin and/or acetaminophen
11. Petroleum jelly
12. Calamine lotion
13. Aromatic spirits of ammonia
14. Tweezers
15. A scissors with rounded ends
16. Clinical thermometer
17. Flashlight
18. Safety pins
19. Sugar for diabetics
20. First aid book

For automobiles, the American National Red Cross suggests a specially designed compact unit with standardized first aid materials fitted into a case, like blocks. The packet is readily stored, and the supplies do not become easily disarranged. Each packet is clearly labeled, and instructions for use are included. These kits can be obtained at auto supply stores and department stores with contents selected to meet the purchaser's particular needs. Ask your physician about other medications for such things as car sickness, upset stomach, and allergies. Take some road flares for car safety.

Regardless of how well equipped the first aid kit is, its effective use depends on individuals knowing how to give aid properly. A course in first aid, as well as training in cardiopulmonary resuscitation (CPR), can be an invaluable investment. For additional drugs and supplies that may be kept in the physician's office or clinic for emergency situations, see "Emergency Tray" in Unit VII.

CONCLUSION

In the event of a sudden illness or an accident that causes trauma to a person, the trained, competent medical assistant should be prepared to properly administer the appropriate first aid treatment and obtain medical assistance as needed. In time of emergencies, prompt action must be taken. It is important that the medical assistant remain calm in all cases and provide care in a competent, orderly, and organized manner. Do not perform procedures that you have not been trained to do. To maintain your skills and knowledge in first aid and cardiopulmonary resuscitation, it is suggested that you enroll in a refresher course every few years.

REVIEW OF VOCABULARY

The following is a hospital discharge summary received in the office on one of the physician's patients who had been in an accident. After reading this, you should be able to discuss the contents with your instructor. Be prepared to define and explain any medical terms that are used. A medical dictionary, other reference books, and information given in preceding units of this book may be used as references for obtaining definitions or explanations of the contents of this report.

Discharge summary

PATIENT: Will Nelson
ADMITTED: January 10, 19_____
DISCHARGED: February 10, 19_____

DISCHARGE DIAGNOSES

1. Multiple facial fractures including fracture of the maxilla, mandible, nose, and right orbit.
2. Comminuted fracture, left patella.

HISTORY
This 22-year-old man was injured in a head-on motorcycle accident with another motorcycle at about 4:30 PM on January 10. The patient was brought to the emergency room of this hospital by ambulance.

(*Continues on p. 486*)

Table 16-2 Comparison of selected effects of commonly abused drugs

Drug category	Physical dependence	Characteristics of intoxication
Opiates	Marked	Analgesia with or without depressed sensorium; pinpoint pupils (tolerance does not develop to this action); patient may be alert and appear normal; respiratory depression with overdose
Barbiturates	Marked	Patient may appear normal with usual dose, but narrow margin between doses needed to prevent withdrawal symptoms and toxic dose is often exceeded and patient appears "drunk," with drowsiness, ataxia, slurred speech, and nystagmus on lateral gaze; pupil size and reaction normal; respiratory depression with overdose
Nonbarbiturate sedatives: glutethimide (Doriden)	Marked	Pupils dilated and reactive to light; coma and respiratory depression prolonged; sudden apnea and laryngeal spasm common
Antianxiety agents ("minor tranquilizers")	Marked	Progressive depression of sensorium as with barbiturates; pupil size and reaction normal; respiratory depression with overdose
Ethanol	Marked	Depressed sensorium, acute or chronic brain syndrome, odor on breath, pupil size and reaction normal
Amphetamines	Mild to absent	Agitation, with paranoid thought disturbance in high doses; acute organic brain syndrome after prolonged use; pupils dilated and reactive; tachycardia, elevated blood pressure, with possibility of hypertensive crisis and CVA; possibility of convulsive seizures
Cocaine	Absent	Paranoid thought disturbance in high doses, with dangerous delusions of persecution and omnipotence; tachycardia; respiratory depression with overdose
Marijuana	Absent	Milder preparations: drowsy, euphoric state with frequent inappropriate laughter and disturbance in perception of time or space (occasional acute psychotic reaction reported); stronger preparations such as hashish: frequent hallucinations or psychotic reaction; pupils normal, conjunctivas injected (marijuana preparations frequently adulterated with LSD, tryptamines, or heroin)
Psychotomimetics: LSD, STP, tryptamines, mescaline, morning glory seeds	Absent	Unpredictable disturbance in ego function, manifest by extreme lability of affect and chaotic disruption of thought, with danger of uncontrolled behavioral disturbance; pupils dilated and reactive to light
Phencyclidine	Unknown	Disinhibition, agitation, confusion, chaotic thought disturbance, unpredictable behavior, hypertension, meiosis, respiratory collapse, cardiovascular collapse, death
Anticholinergic agents	Absent	Nonpsychotropic effects such as tachycardia, decreased salivary secretion, urinary retention, and dilated, nonreactive pupils plus depressed sensorium, confusion, disorientation, hallucinations, and delusional thinking
Inhalants*	Unknown	Depressed sensorium, hallucinations, acute brain syndrome; odor on breath; often glassy-eyed appearance

*The term inhalant is used to designate a variety of gases and highly volatile organic liquids, including the aromatic glues, paint thinners, gasoline, some anesthetic agents and amylnitrite. The term excludes liquids sprayed into the nasopharynx (droplet transport required) and substances that must be ignited before administration (such as marijuana).

(Courtesy C. V. Mosby)

Characteristics of withdrawal	"Flashback" symptoms	Masking of symptoms of illness or injury during intoxication
Rhinorrhea, lacrimation, and dilated, reactive pupils, followed by gastrointestinal disturbances, low back pain, and waves of gooseflesh; convulsions not a feature unless heroin samples were adulterated with barbiturates	Not reported	An important feature of opiate intoxication, due to analgesic action, with or without depressed sensorium
Agitation, tremulousness, insomnia, gastrointestinal disturbances, hyperpyrexia, blepharoclonus (clonic blink reflex), acute brain syndrome, major convulsive seizures	Not reported	Only in presence of depressed sensorium or after onset of acute brain syndrome
Similar to barbiturate withdrawal syndrome, with agitation, gastrointestinal disturbances, hyperpyrexia, and major convulsive seizures	Not reported	Same as in barbiturate intoxication
Similar to barbiturate withdrawal syndrome, with danger of major convulsive seizures	Not reported	Same as in barbiturate intoxication
Similar to barbiturate withdrawal syndrome, but with less likelihood of convulsive seizures	Not reported	Same as in barbiturate intoxication
Lethargy, somnolence, dysphoria, and possibility of suicidal depression; brain syndrome may persist for many weeks	Infrequently reported	Drug-induced euphoria of acute brain syndrome may interfere with awareness of symptoms of illness or may remove incentive to report symptoms of illness
Similar to amphetamine withdrawal	Not reported	Same as in amphetamine intoxication
No specific withdrawal symptoms	Infrequently reported	Uncommon with milder preparations; stronger preparations may interfere in same manner as psychotomimetic agents
No specific withdrawal symptoms; symptoms may persist for indefinite period after discontinuation of drug	Commonly reported as late as 1 year after last dose	Affective response or psychotic thought disturbance may remove awareness of, or incentive to report, symptoms of illness
No specific withdrawal symptoms	Occasionally reported	Same as in LSD intoxication
No specific withdrawal symptoms; mydriasis may persist for several days	Not reported	Pain may not be reported as a result of depression of sensorium, acute brain syndrome, or acute psychotic reaction
No specific withdrawal symptoms	Infrequently reported	Same as in anticholinergic intoxication

Discharge summary (*continued*)

PHYSICAL EXAMINATION

At the time of admission, the patient was conscious. He was alert and oriented and aware of his surroundings. Physical examination revealed gross bleeding from mouth and nose. There were multiple contusions and abrasions over the face area. Blood pressure was 118/60, pulse was 74, respirations 16.

HEENT

The ears were clear. The eyes had marked ecchymotic areas present periorbitally, with diffuse edema in the periorbital area. The fundus on the left was clear. The fundus on the right was not seen. The nose was filled with blood clots, and there was some active bleeding in the nasal area. At the time of admission, this was not delineated clearly. There was a marked amount of blood in the right side of the mouth. The patient was unable to open his mouth because of deviation of the jaw. Neck was supple.

CARDIORESPIRATORY

Chest was clear to auscultation. There was a regular sinus rhythm with no murmurs.

GI

The abdomen was soft, without masses or organs palpable. Bowel sounds were active.

EXTREMITIES

There was ecchymosis and edema over the left knee.

NEUROLOGICAL

The patient was conscious. The deep tendon reflexes were within normal limits, and there were no pathological toe signs elicited.

DIAGNOSTIC DATA

X-ray studies at the time of admission revealed a fracture of the right patella, comminuted; and maxillary and mandibular fractures of the face. CBC at the time of admission revealed a hemoglobin of 12.6 gm with a hematocrit of 38%. The hemoglobin on January 26 was down to 10.5 gm with a hematocrit of 32% and WBC of 8300 with a normal differential. On February 2, hemoglobin was 11.7 gm with hematocrit of 34%. Urinalysis on January 27 was normal. Serum electrolytes were normal on January 13. The chloride was 101 mEq/L. PCO_2 content 30 mEq/L. Potassium 3.5 mEq/L. Sodium 135 mEq/L. Serum osmolality ran from 276 to 282. On January 13, hemoglobin had dropped to 8.6 and 8.7 gm, with a packed cell volume of 25% and mean proportional hemoglobin concentration of 34% and 35%. The patient was transfused with two units of blood at that time, and hemoglobin rose, on January 14, to 11.2 gm, with a packed cell volume of 32%. X-ray examinations on January 10, at the time of admission, of skull, facial bones, left ribs, and left knee revealed multiple fractures of the facial bones, including the nasal bones and the mandible. There was a fracture of the left patella and, postoperatively, on January 12, a PA view of the chest (portable) revealed a hazy infiltration in the right upper lung field, resembling pneumonitis. A film of the right hand, on January 12, revealed a very small chip fracture of the palm as described. A portable chest x-ray film, on January 16, revealed the small patch of hazy infiltration in the upper right field, which was probably due to lung contusion. The chest otherwise was unremarkable. On January 14, stereo views of the pelvis revealed a gas pattern, heavy in the visible part of the abdomen. Bony structures were intact. There were no signs of dislocation of the hips. X-ray film of the left arm revealed the elbow and wrist to be intact. Cervical spine was negative except for a fracture in the mandible as described. Lumbosacral spine showed anterior displacement of L-5 on S-1, and L-1 was wedged very slightly anteriorly. It was not believed that this was a fracture. Water's view of the sinuses revealed multiple facial bone fractures, evident with generalized haziness in the central part. On January 18, AP x-ray films of the facial bones revealed superior fractures of the nasal and maxillary bones, as well as the previously described fractured mandible. There were no specific changes.

HOSPITAL COURSE

On the night of admission, January 10, the patient was taken to the operating room where, under general anesthesia, the patient first had a tracheostomy by Dr. U. R. Belson. The patient then had a reduction of fracture of the mandible and maxilla with repair of facial lacerations and mucous membrane of the mouth and packing of the right antrum, reduction of nasal bones, and fixation of nasal packing. This was done by Drs. U. R. Belson, B. Beal, and I. B. Tucker. A simultaneous patellectomy was done on the left knee by Dr. P. Adamson. The patient did relatively well in the intensive care unit, postoperatively, maintained on antibiotics and tracheostomy care. On January 18, the patient was returned to the operating room where, under general anesthesia, Drs. U. R. Belson and I. B. Tucker performed open reduction of the fracture of the facial bones. The patient has continued to do well since that time on a general basis, requiring constant observation and very close and meticulous care of his tracheostomy site. He has been gradually ambulated from the bed to a wheelchair and ambulation in the room. The cast has been removed from the left leg. Sutures have been removed from his face. The patient was seen in consultation by Dr. I. B. Tucker, concerning the eyes, and he was found to have Berlin's edema from the fractures of the floor and rim of the right orbit. On January 11, the patient also was seen in consultation by Dr. P. Brown concerning advice for maintenance and following of his tracheostomy site and antibiotic therapy. The patient is being discharged today to his home, where he will be under observation by his father, Dr. W. F. Nelson, and will be followed by the physicians, as required, at General Hospital.

Andrew Berger, MD

REVIEW QUESTIONS

1. List three factors that determine if a situation is an emergency.
2. As a medical assistant you are responsible for rendering first aid when the need arises. Define first aid, and state the contributions you can make for the physical and psychological care of the victim in an emergency situation.
3. List four fundamental rules and procedures to follow in a medical emergency.
4. Mr. Bill Bailey has been experiencing uncomfortable pressure and pain in the center of the chest, shortness of breath, and slight nausea for the past 3 minutes. What medical condition would you suspect him to have? What type of action should be taken for this condition?
5. While having lunch with a friend, she suddenly clutches her neck between her thumb and index finger. What should this indicate to you?
6. Define shock. List and explain the five types of shock. List eight outstanding symptoms of shock.
7. Dave Rubin has just had minor surgery in the physician's office. As you are assisting him after the procedure, you observe that he is very pale and his skin quite cold to the touch. You immediately take his vital signs and find that the pulse is weak and rapid, the blood pressure 92/70, and respirations 34 and shallow. What condition would you suspect that he is experiencing? What must be your immediate actions?
8. Anna Westover is having a severe reaction to penicillin. Describe the first aid treatment that you could provide.
9. Ray Wood is cleaning the windows in your office. By accident, he breaks a window. He comes running to you at the desk. You observe that he is clutching his wrist and that there is bright red blood spurting from his wrist as well as from his hand and fingers. State the type of bleeding this would indicate, the vessel that may be cut, and the first aid treatment that you would administer.
10. List and locate the seven pressure points used to control severe bleeding.
11. State the difference between a first, second, and third degree burn.

12. After having blood drawn, Joanne Newman faints. State the first aid treatment that you would provide for this patient.
13. Ann O'Brien, a diabetic patient, is displaying the signs and symptoms of an insulin reaction. List six signs and symptoms of insulin reaction. State the immediate care that you could provide for Ann.
14. List six signs and symptoms of diabetic coma.
15. In the case of ingested poisoning, when should you *not* have the victim vomit?
16. When is the use of a tourniquet advisable?
17. List at least 15 items that you would include when compiling supplies for a first aid kit.

PERFORMANCE TEST

In a skills laboratory, with simulations of emergency situations, the medical assistant student is to demonstrate skill in performing the following procedures without reference to source materials. Time limits for the performance of each procedure are to be assigned by the instructor. The student will need a person to play the role of the patient.

1. Demonstrate the proper first aid treatment to be administered to patients who have experienced all the emergency situations given in this unit.
2. Demonstrate how to locate the seven pressure points to be used when controlling severe bleeding.
3. Demonstrate the proper method of applying a tourniquet to a patient's left arm, right leg.
4. Demonstrate on the manikin (if available) the correct method of administering cardiopulmonary resuscitation to an unconscious patient.

The student is to perform the above activities with 100% accuracy before passing this unit.

PERFORMANCE CHECKLIST

The medical assistant students are to design their own step-by-step procedures and performance checklists for the performance test.

Appendix A   Special Vocabulary

PART 1—VOCABULARY USED WHEN RECORDING INFORMATION OBTAINED FROM THE REVIEW OF SYSTEMS

The following vocabulary lists *some* of the terms that an examiner may use when recording the *subjective* findings of the review of systems (ROS) of a patient. Terms are presented in the order in which they appear in the patient's ROS and under the body part or system for which they are used in describing ROS findings (see also Unit II).

Eyes

photophobia (fo"to-fo'be-ah)—An abnormal visual intolerance to light.

Ears

tinnitus (tĭ-nī'tus)—A ringing or buzzing noise in the ears.

Nose

coryza (ko-rī'zah)—A head cold; an acute inflammation of the nasal mucous membrane with a profuse discharge.

epistaxis (ep"ĭ-stak'sis)—A nosebleed; hemorrhage from the nose. Many episodes of epistaxis are caused by the rupture of the small vessels over the anterior part of the cartilaginous nasal septum.

Respiratory

asthma (az'mah)—Recurrent attacks of difficulty in breathing (dyspnea) with wheezing that is caused by spasms in the bronchial tubes.

expectoration (ek-spek"to-ra'shun)—The coughing up, expulsion, or spitting out of material (mucus, sputum, or phlegm) from the throat, trachea, bronchi, or lungs.

hemoptysis (he-mop'tĭ-sis)—The spitting and/or coughing up of blood from the respiratory tract caused by bleeding in any part of the respiratory tract. In true hemoptysis sputum is frothy with air bubbles and bright red. (Hemoptysis must not be confused with *hematemesis*, in which a dark red- or black-colored substance is ejected from the gastrointestinal tract.)

hyperventilation (hi"per-ven"tĭ-lā'shun)—Abnormal deep and prolonged breathing; increase in the inspirations and expirations of air resulting from an increase in the depth or rate of respirations or both. This results especially with depletion of carbon dioxide. This condition is often associated with emotional tension or acute anxiety situations.

Cardiovascular (CV)

palpitation (pal"pi-ta'shun)—An unusually strong, rapid, or irregular heartbeat, usually over 120 beats per minute (normal heart rate varies between 60 to 100 beats per minute). Palpitation is often the result of strong exertion, nervousness, excitement, or the taking of certain medications. Palpitations may also result from a variety of heart disorders.

peripheral edema
(pĕ-rif'er-al)—Pertaining to the periphery, which means the surface or outward structures.
(e-de'mah)—An abnormal accumulation of fluid in the intercellular spaces of the body.

varicosity (var"i-kos'ĭ-te)—Pertaining to a varicose condition; distended, swollen veins.

Gastrointestinal

anorexia (an"o-rek'se-ah)—Loss of appetite. Anorexia can be caused by illness, emotional upsets, or unattractive food.

colic (kol'ik)—Pertaining to the colon; abdominal pain caused by spasmodic contractions of the intestinal tract.

constipation (kon"stĭ-pa-shun)—Difficult elimination of fecal material from the intestinal tract; often the infrequent passage of waste material that is hard to eliminate easily results in the passage of unduly dry and hard fecal material.

diarrhea (di"ah-re'ah)—The rapid movement of fecal material through the intestine, the feces having more or less fluid consistency; primarily a result of increased peristalsis in the intestinal tract.

distention (dis-ten'shun)—The state of being stretched out, or distended.

dysphagia (dis-fā'jē-ah)—Difficulty in swallowing.

flatus (fla'tus)—Air or gas in the gastrointestinal tract.

hemorrhoid (hem'ŏ-roid); also called **piles**—A dilated blood vessel in the anus that may bleed, cause discomfort or pain, and itch.

jaundice (jawn'dis); also called **icterus** (ik'ter-us)—A symptom of different disorders of the gallbladder, liver, and blood characterized by yellowness of the skin, mucous membranes, and whites of the eyes caused by excessive bilirubin in the blood and deposition of bile pigments.

melena (mĕ-lē′nah)—Black fecal material; blood pigments darken the feces.

Genitourinary (GU)

enuresis (en″u-re′sis)—The involuntary excretion of urine, especially at night during sleep; bedwetting; most commonly seen in children with physical or emotional problems.

frequency—(fre′kwen-se)—The need to urinate frequently.

hesitancy—Dysuria caused by nervous inhibition or obstruction in the vesical outlet.

incontinence (in-kon′ti-nens)—The inability to refrain from the urge to urinate. This may occur in times of stress, anxiety, or anger; after surgery; or because of obstructions that prevent the normal emptying of the urinary bladder, spasms of the bladder, irritation caused by injury or inflammation of the urinary tract, damage to the spinal cord or brain, or the development of a fistula (an abnormal tubelike passage) between the bladder and the vagina or urethra. The word also may refer to fecal incontinence caused by nervous disorders or weakening of the anal sphincter.

nocturia (nok-tu′re-ah)—Excessive urination at night.

potency (po′ten-se)—The ability of a male to have sexual intercourse.

renal colic (re′nal kol′ik)—Spasms accompanied by pain that radiates from the kidney region around to the abdomen and into the groin. Renal colic is experienced during movement of a stone in the ureter.

retention (rĕ-ten′shun)—The process of urine accumulating in the bladder because of the individual's inability to urinate.

urgency—The immediate need to urinate.

urination (u″rĭ-na′shun); also called **micturition** (mik″tu-rish′un)—Voiding; the act of passing urine from the body.

venereal (vĕ-ne′re-al) **disease**—A disease that is transmitted by sexual contact and intercourse. Veneral disease is now more commonly referred to as a *sexually transmitted disease.* Abbreviations used are VD and STD.

Female Reproductive

abortion (ah-bor′shun)—The termination of a pregnancy before the fetus is capable of surviving outside of the uterus. In lay terminology, **abortion** refers to a deliberate interruption of pregnancy by various methods, and **miscarriage** refers to the natural loss of the fetus (**spontaneous abortion**).

dyspareunia (dis″pah-ru′ne-ah)—Difficult or painful genital sexual intercourse in women.

gravida (grav′i-dah)—A pregnant woman. During the first pregnancy the woman would be referred to as Gravida I (**primigravida**), and so on with each succeeding pregnancy.

leukorrhea (loo″ko-re′ah)—An abnormal yellow or white mucus discharge from the cervix or vaginal canal. Leukorrhea may be a symptom of pathological changes in the vagina and endocervix.

menarche (mĕ-nar′ke)—The beginning of the menstrual functions in a woman.

menopause (men′o-pawz)—The period in a woman's life at which the menstrual cycles decrease and gradually stop; the period when menstruation and the ability to have a child cease because the ovaries stop functioning. Menopause is often referred to as **the change of life** and also called the **climacteric.**

parous (pa′rus)—Having borne at least one child. For example, if a woman has one live child and is now pregnant for the second time, she would be referred to as Gravida II, Para I (see **gravida**).

Endocrine

goiter (goi′ter)—An enlargement of the thyroid gland.

Skin

allergy (al′er-je)—An abnormal condition of individual hypersensitivity to substances (**allergens**) that are usually harmless. Allergens, substances capable of inducing hypersensitivity, can be almost any substance in the environment. Examples of allergens to which people become sensitive include dust, animal hairs, plant and tree pollens, mold spores, soaps, detergents, cosmetics, dyes, foods, feathers, plastics, and even some valuable medicines. When the allergen is in contact with or enters the body, it sets off a chain of events that brings about the allergic reaction. The allergen itself is not directly responsible for the allergic reaction. An allergy does not develop on the first contact with the allergen, but can develop on the second contact or even years later, after repeated contact with the allergen. Signs and symptoms of the allergies include sneezing, stuffed up and running nose, watery eyes, itching, coughing, shortness of breath, wheezing, rashes, skin eruptions, slight local edema, and mild to severe anaphylactic shock, which can be fatal unless treated.

mole (mōl)—A discolored blemish or growth on the skin; also called a **nevus.**

ulcer (ul′ser)—An open sore or lesion on the surface of the skin or mucous membranes of the body, produced by the sloughing of dead inflammatory tissues.

Musculoskeletal

atrophy (at'ro-fe)—A wasting away and decrease in size of a normal tissue or organ.

dislocation (dis"lo-ka'shun)—The displacement of a bone from its normal position in a joint.

fracture (frak'chur)—A break in the continuity of a bone. Broad classifications of fractures are **open fracture**, in which the bone penetrates the skin, producing an open wound; and **closed fracture**, in which there is no break in the skin.

spasm (spazm)—An involuntary sudden movement or contraction of a muscle or group of muscles, commonly accompanied by pain, and varying from mild twitches to severe convulsions. Spasms may be **clonic**, in which muscles alternate between contracting and relaxing; or **tonic**, in which the contraction of the muscle is sustained. Tonic spasms are the more severe type, because they are caused by diseases that affect the brain or central nervous system, such as rabies or tetanus.

tetany (tet'ah-ne)—A continuous tonic spasm of a muscle without distinct twitching. The spasms are usually sudden, periodic, or recurrent, and they involve the extremities.

Neurological

convulsion (kun-vul'shun)—Involuntary spasms or contractions of muscles caused by an abnormal stimulus to the brain or by changes in the chemical balance of the body.

paralysis (pah-ral'ĭ-sis)—A state caused by damage to parts of the nervous system resulting in impairment or loss of motor function in a part or parts of the body.

paresthesia (par"es-the'ze-ah)—An abnormal sensation experienced without an objective cause. Examples include a burning, tingling, or numb feeling.

tremor (trem'or)—An involuntary quivering or trembling movement of the body or limbs caused by alternate contractions of opposing muscles. Tremors may have a psychological or a physical cause or both.

vertigo (ver'ti-go)—A sensation of dizziness, rotation of oneself or of external objects in one's surroundings.

PART 2—VOCABULARY USED IN RECORDING PHYSICAL FINDINGS

The following vocabulary lists *some* of the terms that an examiner may use in recording the *objective* findings of the physical examination of a patient. Each term is presented under the body part or system for which it is used when describing the findings of the physical examination. The order in which the body part or system is presented follows the usual sequence that examiners follow in performing a physical examination.

Skin

abrasion (ah-bra'zhun)—A scrape on the surface of the skin or on a mucous membrane, for example, a skinned knee.

avulsion (a-vul'shun)—A piece of soft tissue that is torn loose or left hanging as a flap.

contusion (kon-too'zhun)—A bruise; an injury to the tissues without skin breakage. In a contusion blood seeps into the surrounding tissues from the injured and broken blood vessels, causing pain, tenderness, swelling, and discoloration of the surface skin.

cyanosis (si"ah-no'sis)—A bluish discoloration of mucous membranes and skin.

ecchymosis (ek"i-mo'sis)—A round or irregular nonelevated hemorrhagic spot on mucous membranes or skin. The appearance is that of a blue-black or purplish patch changing to yellow or greenish brown. An ecchymosis is *larger* than a petechia.

erythema (er"i-the'mah)—A redness of the skin caused by capillary congestion in the lower layers of the skin. Erythema will be present in any inflammatory process, infection, or injury of the skin.

jaundice (jawn'dis)—See in ROS vocabulary.

laceration (las"ĕ-rā'shun)—A tear or jagged-edged wound of body tissue.

petechia (pe-te'ke-ah)—A tiny, round, nonraised, purplish red spot caused by submucous or intradermal hemorrhage. Later a petechia will turn blue or yellow. Small red patches.

purpura (per'pu-rah)—Purpura is a hemorrhagic disease of obscure cause. It is characterized by the escape or discharge of blood from vessels into tissues under the skin and through mucous membranes, producing small red patches and bruises on the skin.

turgor (tur'gor)—The condition of normal tension or fullness in a cell.

ulcer (ul'ser)—See under ROS vocabulary.

urticaria (ur"tĭ-ka're-ah)—Also called **hives**. An inflammatory reaction of the skin characterized by the appearance of slightly elevated red or pale patches that are often itchy.

Eyes

acuity (ah-ku'ĭ-te)—Clearness, sharpness, or acuteness of vision.

adnexa (ad-nek′sah)—Accessory organs of the eye.

arcus senilis (ar′kus seni′lis)—An opaque white ring partially surrounding the margin of the cornea, usually seen in people 50 years old or older. This condition often occurs bilaterally and is a result of fat granules depositing in the cornea or lipoid degeneration.

fundus (fun′dus) (of the eye)—The back portion of the interior of the eye. The physician can observe this part of the eye by looking into or through the pupil of the eye with an ophthalmoscope.

nystagmus (nĭs-tag′mus)—The constant, involuntary, rhythmic movement of the eyeball in any direction.

papilledema (pap″il-ĕ-de′mah)—Edema and inflammation of the optic nerve, usually caused by intracranial pressure as a result of a brain tumor pressing on the optic nerve.

ptosis (to′sis)—A drooping of the upper eyelids caused by paralysis.

Ears

cerumen (sĕ-roo′men)—Earwax.

tympanic (tim-pan′ik) **membrane;** also called **eardrum**—A thin membrane that separates the middle ear from the outer ear.

Nose

nares (na′rēz)—The external openings into the nasal cavity; the nostrils.

nasal septal defect—A deviation of the bone and cartilage that divides the nasal cavity so that one part of the nasal cavity is larger than the other. On occasion this may produce difficulty in normal breathing, prevent normal drainage from infected sinuses, and interfere with the normal flow of mucus from the sinuses when one has a cold.

Neck

supple (sup′l)—Easily movable.

Respiratory System

fremitus (frem′ĭ-tus)—A vibration or tremor felt through the chest wall, usually during palpation.

    tactile fremitus—A vibration felt when a person speaks.

    tussive fremitus—A vibration felt when a person coughs.

    vocal fremitus—A vibration heard during auscultation of the chest wall when a person speaks.

friction rub; also called **rub**—A sound heard during auscultation that is produced when two serous membrane surfaces rub together.

rale (rahl)—An abnormal respiratory sound heard when the physician auscultates the chest. A rale indicates a pathological condition. There are many types of rales. Examples include a **dry rale**, which is a whistling or squeaky sound as heard in a person who has bronchitis or asthma; a **moist rale**, which is produced by fluid in the bronchial tubes; and a **crepitant rale**, which is a dry, crackling sound heard in the early stages of pneumonia when the person completes an inspiration.

resonance (rez′o-nans)—The quality of sound heard when the physician is examining the chest wall by percussion.

rhonchus (rong′kus) (pl. **rhonchi**)—A dry rale in the bronchus or a rattling in the throat.

rub—See under friction rub, above.

sputum (spu′tum)—The mucous secretion that comes from the lungs, bronchi, and trachea and that is ejected from the mouth. *Saliva* is not the same as sputum; saliva is secreted from the salivary glands in the mouth.

stridor (stri′dor)—A harsh shrill respiratory sound heard during inspirations in individuals who have laryngeal obstruction.

Cardiovascular System (CVS)

bruit (brū′ē)—A blowing sound heard over an aneurysm during auscultation of the cardiovascular system.

congestion (kon-jes′chun)—An abnormal accumulation of blood in a body part.

ecchymosis—See under Skin, p. 490.

engorgement (en-gorj′ment)—A distention of a body part with blood.

erythema—See under Skin, p. 490.

gallop (gal′op)—A disordered rhythm of the heart heard during auscultation. In a gallop rhythm three or four extra sounds are heard during the diastolic phase; the sounds are related to atrial contraction.

infarction (in-fark′shun)—A localized area of deficiency of blood in a part causing death to the cells. This is caused by blockage of arterial blood supply to the area. With reference to the heart, the term **myocardial infarction** is used. This pertains to the death of the cells in the myocardial layer of the heart caused by the lack of blood supply to the area.

ischemia (is-ke′me-ah)—The deficiency of blood in a body part. Ischemia may be caused by an obstruction in a blood vessel, such as from a clot or cholesterol deposits, or by a functional constriction.

murmur (mer′mer)—A sound heard during auscultation that is cardiac or vascular in origin, especially a periodic sound of short duration. This sound may be heard over the aortic valve, over the apex of the heart, or over an artery; all of these indicate possible disease in the particular area.

petechia—See under Skin.

purpura—See under Skin.

resuscitation (rĕ-sus"ĭ-ta'shun)—The act of restoring life or consciousness to a person whose respirations have stopped and who is thought to be dead.

rub; also called **friction rub**—See under Respiratory System.

> **pericardial rub** — A rub associated with inflammation of the pericardium. When this condition is present during auscultation the physician will hear a grating or scraping sound with the heartbeat.

thrill (thril)—A vibration that is felt by the physician when palpating the area over the heart, either during diastole or systole.

Abdomen

ascites (ah-si'tēz)—An abnormal excessive accumulation of serous fluid in the peritoneal cavity that may cause abdominal distention. Ascites can be caused by a variety of conditions, some of which are tumors, kidney and heart disease, inflammation of the abdominal cavity, and cirrhosis of the liver.

contour (kon'toor)—The outline or shape, as of the abdomen.

distention—See under ROS vocabulary.

flaccid—See under Musculoskeletal System.

hernia (her'ne-ah)—An abnormal projection or protrusion of an organ or tissue or part of an organ through the wall of the cavity in which it is normally contained.

protuberant (pro-tu'ber-ant)—With reference to the abdomen, an area that projects out or is prominent beyond the usual surface abdominal area.

scaphoid (skaf'oid)—In reference to the abdomen, appearing as having a hollowed anterior wall; boat-shaped.

rigidity—See under Musculoskeletal System.

Gastrointestinal System

caries (ka're-ēz, kăr'ēz)—The decay of teeth or bone.

distention (dis-ten'shun)—See under ROS vocabulary.

fissure (fish'er)—A slit or cracklike sore. For example, an anal fissure is a lineal ulcer at the border of the anus.

fistula (fis'tu-lah)—An abnormal tubelike passage from a tube, organ, or cavity to another cavity or organ or from an internal organ to a free body surface.

hemorrhoid (hem'o-roid)—A varicose (enlarged) vein in the mucous membrane just outside (external hemorrhoid) or inside (internal hemorrhoid) the rectum. Also called piles, these enlarged veins may be painful and itchy and may bleed.

peristalsis (per"ĭ-stal'sis)—A wavelike movement by which tubular organs and the alimentary canal propel their contents. Peristalsis is an involuntary movement seen in tubes that have both circular and longitudinal layers of smooth muscle fibers.

Reproductive System

adnexa (ad-nek'sah)—Accessory organs of the uterus (ovaries, uterine tubes, and ligaments).

atrophy (at'ro-fe)—A decrease in size of organs or tissues after having reached full functional development. Atrophy is seen in the female reproductive organs after menopause.

gravida—See under ROS vocabulary.

introitus (in-tro'ĭtus)—The opening into a body cavity or canal, as the opening into the vagina.

involution (in"vol-lu'shun)—The retrogressive change in the size and the vital processes of organs and tissues after they have fulfilled their functions, such as is seen after menopause or in the reduction in size of the uterus after birth.

parous—See under ROS vocabulary.

Musculoskeletal System (MS)

crepitation (krep"ĭ-tā'shun)—A crackling, grating sound produced by movement of the ends of a fractured bone.

exostosis (ek"sos-to'sis)—A new bony growth arising and projecting from the surface of a bone, characteristically capped by cartilage.

flaccid (flak'sid)—Relaxed, soft, weak, flabby; applied especially to muscles that lack muscular tone.

gait (gāt)—The style or manner in which a person walks.

kyphosis (ki-fo'sis); also called **hunchback**—When viewing a person from the side, the examiner sees an abnormal convexity in the curvature of the thoracic spine.

lordosis (lor-do'dis)—An abnormal forward curvature of the lumbar spine.

protuberance (pro-tu'ber-ans)—A part that projects or is prominent beyond the usual surface area.

rigidity (rĭ-jid'ĭ-te)—A state of being stiff or inflexible.

scoliosis (sko"le-o'sis)—A lateral curvature of the vertebral column that usually consists of two curves, one in the opposite direction from the first.

supple (sup'l)—Flexible, limber, or easily bent.

Extremities

claudication (klaw"dĭ-kā'shun)—Limping, lameness.

intermittent claudication—A severe pain, tension, and weakness in the calf muscles that occurs after walking is begun and that subsides when walking stops and the limb has been resting. This condition is seen in patients with occlusive arterial disease in the limbs.

clubbing (klub'ing)—A process or result of rapid reproduction of the soft tissue on the ends of the fingers and toes, as seen in adults with long-standing pulmonary disease.

edema (ĕ-de'mah)—An abnormal accumulation of fluid in the body's intercellular spaces. It can be local or general.

passive congestion (kon-jes'chun)—An abnormal accumulation of blood in an area on the body.

ulcer (ul'ser)—See under ROS vocabulary.

varicosity (var'ĭ-kos'ĭ-te) (pl. **varicosities**)—The condition of being varicose; a swollen, distended, enlarged, and twisted vein.

General

cachexia (kah-kek'se-ah)—A general state of ill health, wasting away, and malnutrition, as seen in many chronic diseases.

dehydration (de"hi-dra'shun)—The condition that results when water output exceeds water intake; the excessive loss of water from the tissues or body.

diaphoresis (di"ah-fo-re'sis)—Perspiration.

emaciation (e-ma"se-a'shun)—A condition in which the body is extremely thin and wasting away. Emaciation is generally caused by extreme malnutrition or diseases of the gastrointestinal tract.

fingerbreadth (fin'ger-bredth)—The width of the finger from side to side, used when measuring the width of something, such as a lesion, or when measuring the distance between two areas, for example, "two fingerbreadths from the umbilicus."

lethargic (leth'ar'gic)—The state of being indifferent, drowsy, or sluggish.

patulous (pat'u-lus)—The state of being open, spread apart widely, or distended.

tenderness (ten'der-nes)—A sensitivity to touch or pressure.

Appendix B   Summary of Studies Used for Diagnosing Conditions Affecting Body Organs and Systems

A history and physical examination are the preliminary steps, then individual or combined studies as outlined may be requested.

1. **Heart**
   a. Chest X-ray studies
   b. Electrocardiogram
   c. Serum enzyme levels
   d. Cardiac catheterization
   e. Angiogram
   f. Echocardiography (ultrasonography)
   g. Radioisotope and radionuclide techniques
   h. Cardiac scan
   i. Treadmill stress test (see Fig. 15-1)
   j. Magnetic Resonance Imaging (MRI)

2. **Vascular system**
   a. Angiography
   b. Venous pressure measurement
   c. Funduscopic examination
   d. Arteriography
   e. Cerebral angiogram
   f. Ultrasound techniques
   g. Splenoportography
   h. Bone marrow studies
   i. Lymph node biopsy
   j. Aortography
   k. Radionuclide studies (bone marrow scan)
   l. Arterial catheterization
   m. Digital radiography
   n. Positron Emission Tomography (PET)

3. **Respiratory system and chest**
   a. Pulmonary function tests
   b. Spirometry
   c. X-ray studies
   d. Bronchoscopy
   e. Bronchogram
   f. Tomography
   g. CT scan (computed tomography)
   h. Magnetic Resonance Imaging (MRI)
   i. Lung perfusion
   j. Lung ventilation

4. **Gastrointestinal (GI) system**
   a. Upper GI series
   b. Barium enema
   c. Sigmoidoscopy
   d. Fecal occult blood test
   e. Gastric analysis
   f. Gastroscopy
   g. Esophagoscopy
   h. CT scan
   i. Magnetic Resonance Imaging (MRI)
   j. Colonoscopy

5. **Liver, gallbladder, and pancreas**
   a. Laboratory tests, such as bilirubin blood levels, bromosulphalein (BSP), serum amylase and lipase for pancreatic disease, and tests for chronic malabsorption
   b. Biopsy of the liver
   c. Liver scan
   d. Abdominal x-ray films
   e. Cholecystogram
   f. Cholangiogram
   g. CT scan
   h. Magnetic Resonance Imaging (MRI)
   i. Hepatobiliary scan

6. **Kidney and genitourinary system**
   a. Cultures
   b. Urinalysis
   c. Blood urea nitrogen and creatinine blood tests
   d. Renal biopsies
   e. Cystogram
   f. Retrograde cystourethrogram
   g. Intravenous pyelogram (IVP)
   h. KUB (kidney, ureter, bladder) x-ray film
   i. Catheterization
   j. Cystoscopy
   k. Seminal fluid examination
   l. Aortogram
   m. Excretion urogram
   n. Vasogram
   o. Ultrasonography
   p. Kidney scan
   q. Magnetic Resonance Imaging (MRI)

7. **Female genital organs**
   a. Pelvic examination
   b. Pap smear
   c. Cultures
   d. Pregnancy test
   e. Dilatation and currettage (D & C) for endometrial biopsy (surgery)
   f. Laparoscopy (surgery)
   g. Hematocrit blood test
   h. Biopsy of the cervix
   i. X-ray studies, such as abdomen for fetus, hysterosalpingogram

j. Ultrasonography

k. CT scan

l. Magnetic Resonance Imaging (MRI)

8. Breast

a. Mammography

b. Thermography

c. Xeroradiography

d. Biopsy

e. Physical examination (palpation and inspection)

f. Self-examination for lumps, pain, or discharge from the nipple

9. Skin

a. Physical examination for rash, lesion, pain, itching, and appearance

b. Incisional biopsies

c. Excisional biopsies

d. Laboratory tests — culturing purulent lesions, smears, blood tests

e. Diagnostic skin tests for allergies and tuberculosis

10. Eye

a. Visual field defects (focal areas of blindness)

b. Physical examination and history to determine presence of

(1) Pain

(2) Blurring of vision

(3) Papilledema as seen through the ophthalmoscope

(4) Photophobia (uncomfortable sensitivity to light)

(5) Infections

(6) Nystagmus (flickering eye movements) — may be caused by a variety of central nervous system lesions

c. Clinical tests

(1) Eye charts or machines for testing visual acuity

(2) Visual field tests

(3) Funduscopic examination with the ophthalmoscope

(4) Tonometry

(5) Tests for refractive errors (myopia or hyperopia)

11. Bones and joints

a. Observation of pain, decreased mobility, deformity, and fractures

b. Physical examination

c. X-ray films, for example, of fractures, tumors, joints, skull, sinus cavities, teeth

d. Blood serum tests — calcium, phosphorus, alkaline phosphatase, sedimentation rate, rheumatoid factor (latex fixation titer), and uric acid levels

e. Whole blood test — red blood cell count

f. Cultures — for diagnoses of acute arthritis and osteomyelitis

g. Biopsy — to diagnose bone tumors

h. Arthrography

i. Diskography

j. Myelography

k. Pelvimetry

l. Bone scan

m. Magnetic Resonance Imaging (MRI)

12. Skeletal muscle

a. Physical examination, to observe atrophy, weakness

b. Laboratory tests, such as for the enzymes aldolase and creatine phosphokinase (CPK)

c. Electromyography

d. Muscle biopsy

e. Ultrasonography

13. Central nervous system

a. Physical examination — neurological examination of the motor and sensory systems

b. Lumbar puncture to examine the cerebrospinal fluid and the pressure of the fluid; chemical, serological, and culture tests may be performed

c. Angiogram

d. Skull x-ray films

e. Electroencephalogram (EEG)

f. Pneumoencephalogram

g. CT scan

h. Brain scan

i. Cerebral angiogram

j. Echoencephalogram (ultrasonography)

k. Myelogram

l. Positron Emission Tomography

m. Magnetic Resonance Imaging (MRI)

14. Mental illness

a. Physical examination

b. Screening laboratory tests

c. X-ray studies of the chest and skull

d. Electroencephalogram

e. Psychological assessment, such as personality inventory and intelligence testing

15. Endocrine system

a. Measurement of hormones — either hypersecretion or hyposecretion.

b. Laboratory measurements — presence of glucose in blood or urine, glucose tolerance test, measurements of the presence of hormones in blood or urine, and measurement of calcium and phosphorus levels (for the status of the parathyroid glands) in the blood and urine

c. Radionuclide studies — thyroid scan

d. CT scan

e. Magnetic Resonance Imaging (MRI)

16. Infectious diseases

a. Physical examination and history — often physical examination of lesions is sufficient for diagnosis, for example, rash of measles or chickenpox, swelling of parotid glands in mumps, pus draining from an abscess

b. Laboratory studies
   (1) Culture and sensitivity tests on throat, urine, sputum, purulent lesions, blood, and cerebrospinal fluid specimens
   (2) Smears — for determining gonorrhea and meningitis
   (3) White blood count and differential
   (4) Urinalysis
   (5) Gram stain
c. Immunological tests
   (1) Serology tests, tests for antibodies in the patient's blood serum, such as for syphilis and viral infections
   (2) Skin tests, such as the purified protein derivative (PPD) or the Tine test for tuberculosis
d. Radiologic tests
e. Gallium scans
f. White blood cell nuclear medicine scan
g. Ultrasound examinations
h. CT scan

17. **Immunological diseases**
   a. Skin tests — used for diagnosing allergies, such as the patch and scratch tests
   b. Laboratory tests — varied blood tests often specific for the type of disease and the body organ or system that is affected, such as the tests used in diagnosing rheumatoid arthritis and systemic lupus erythematosus (SLE)

Appendix C   Common Medical Terminology Combining Word Parts

In this appendix the basic elements of medical word-making are presented. A scientific vocabulary that conveys complex ideas and descriptions is needed. Our medical traditions and word sources have been commonly taken from Greek and Latin writings.

Learning a medical vocabulary becomes a matter of memorizing a few score Greek and Latin prefixes, suffixes, and word roots and combining them systematically to make thousands of precise terms.

When studying, the student should have at hand a good medical dictionary. Spelling, pronunciation, word structure, and usage need to be verified constantly if one is to build a medical vocabulary.

The base word we call the *root;* the combining modifier (or affix) we call the *prefix* when it is placed *before* the root, or the *suffix* when we place it *after* the root. Thus in the foregoing sentence, *pre-* and *suf-* are prefixes to *-fix.* Ophthalmo- (eye) and *-scope* (instrument for viewing) become *ophthalmoscope,* an instrument for examining the eye. *Oto-* (ear) and *-scope* become *otoscope,* an instrument for examining the ear. Combining the suffix *-itis,* meaning inflammation, with the base words *tonsilla, peritoneum, otos,* and *osteon,* we get *tonsillitis, peritonitis, otitis,* and *osteitis.*

Prefixes and suffixes give special meaning to the ideas the roots express. In English we have, for example, *before*hand, hand*iness* and hand*icraft.* Memorize the following commonly used prefixes, word elements, and suffixes. Get the feel of their usage in medical-word construction.

Prefixes and Word Elements	Common Usage	Examples*
a-, an-	without, absent	aplasia
ab-	away from	abduct
ad-	to, at	adhesive
aden/o	gland	adenosis
albo/o	white	albicans
album-	white, albumin	albuminuria
alveolo-	alveoli	alveolotomy
ana-,/an-	up, too much, backward	anaphylaxis
angi/o	blood vessel	angiogram
ankyl/osis	bent, crooked, adhesion	ankylosis
ante-	before	antefebrile
antero-	in front of, before	anterograde
anti-	against, opposed to	antibiotic, antibody
aort/o	aorta	aortitis
appendic/o	appendix	appendicitis
arteri/o	artery	arteriosclerosis
arthr/o	joint	arthropathy
audi/o	hearing	audiogram
auto-	self	autograft
bacteri/o	bacteria	bacteriuria
bi-	two	bilateral
blast-	germ cell	blastoma
blenno-: see muco-		
blephar/o	eyelid	blepharoplasty
brady-	slow	bradycardia
bronch/o	bronchus	bronchitis
bucc/o	cheek	buccal
burs/o	bursa	bursitis
cardi/o	heart	electrocardiogram
cephal/o	head	cephalogram
cerebr/o	cerebrum	cerebropathy
cervic/o	neck, cervix	cervical; cervicitis
cheil/o	lip	cheiloplasty

Prefixes and Word Elements	Common Usage	Examples*
cholecyst-	gallbladder	*cholecyst*ectomy
chondr/o	cartilage	*chondr*itis
coccus	coccus (bacterium)	strepto*coccus*
col/o	colon	*col*ostomy
colp/o	vagina	*colp*ostenosis
cost/o	rib	*cost*overtebral
crani/o	cranium	*crani*otomy
cyan/o	blue	*cyan*osis
cyst/o	bladder	*cyst*ocele
cyto-	cell	*cyto*plasm
dacry/o	tears	*dacry*agogic
dacryocyst/o	lacrimal sac	*dacryocyst*itis
dent/o	tooth	*dent*algia
derm-	skin	*derm*al
dermat/o	skin	*dermat*ology
dextr/o	to the right side	*dextr*ocardia
dia-	through	*dia*phragm
diplo-	double	*diplo*pia
dis-	to separate	*dis*articulate
doch/o	duct	chole*doch*ectomy
duoden/o	duodenum	*duoden*oscopy
dys-	difficult, painful	*dys*pnea
ec-, ex-	out of, away from	*ec*topy, *ex*crete
ecto-	outside	*ecto*pic
electro-	electric in nature	*electro*cardiogram
emesis	vomit	hemat*emesis*
encephal/o	brain, or enclosed within the head	*encephal*ogram
endo-	within, inside of	*endo*cardium
enter/o	intestine	*enter*ocolitis
epi-	on, over	*epi*dermis, *epi*dural
erythr/o	red	*erythr*ocyte
esophag/o	esophagus	*esophag*itis
esthesia	sensation	an*esthesia*
eti-	causation	*eti*ology
ex/o	outside	*exo*cardia
extra-	outside of	*extra*dural, *extra*peritoneal
gastro-	stomach	*gastro*enteritis
gen/o	producing	*gen*esis
gingiv/o	gums	*gingiv*itis
gloss/o	tongue	*gloss*itis
glyc/o	sugar	*glyc*ogen
gyne-, gyneco-	women	*gyneco*logy
hemat/o	blood	*hemat*emesis
hemi-	one half	*hemi*plegia
hem/o	blood	*hem*atoma
hepat/o	liver	*hepat*itis
hidr/o	sweat	*hidr*osis
hist/o	tissue	*hist*ology
hydr/o	water	*hydr*otherapy
hyper-	over, excessive, increased	*hyper*alimentation, *hyper*esthesia, *hyper*trophy
hyp/o	under, below, less	*hypo*tension, *hypo*dermic, *hypo*gastric
hyster/o	uterus	*hyster*ectomy
iatro	physician, medicine	*iatro*genic
im- (replaces *in-* before *b, m,* or *p*)	negative prefix, not	*im*balance
in-	negative prefix, not	*in*operable
in-	in, into	*in*clusion

Prefixes and Word Elements	Common Usage	Examples*
infra-	below	*infra*patellar
inter- (contrast *intra-*)	between, among	*inter*costal
intra-	within, inside of (separate the double *a* with a hyphen)	*intra*-articular, *intra*muscular, *intra*venous
intro-	into, within	*intro*spection
intus-	in, into	*intus*susception
ipsi-	self, the same	*ipsi*lateral
ir-	not	*ir*regular, *ir*reversible
ir-	in, into	*ir*radiate
ir/o, irid/o	iris	*irid*ocele
isch- (pronounced *isk*)	to suppress	*isch*emia
ischi/o (pronounced *iskee* [*o*])	ischium	*ischi*ectomy, *ischi*odynia
iso-	equal, alike	*iso*tonic
juxta-	near	*juxta*-articular, *juxta*position
kal-, kali-	potassium (K⁺)	*kal*emia
karyo-	nucleus	*karyo*cyte
kerat/o	horny tissue, cornea	*kerat*osis, *kerat*itis
keto-	carbonyl group (through German from Latin *acetum*, vinegar)	*keto*genic, *keto*sis
kilo-	one thousand	*kilo*gram, *kilo*meter, *kilo*volt
kine-, kinesi/o	movement	*kinesi*ology
labio-	lip (compare *labium*, lip, and *labrum*, edge or lip)	*labio*plasty
lacrima, lacrimo-	tears	*lacri*matory
lact/o	milk	*lact*igenous
lalo-	speech; babbling	*lalo*gnosis, *lalo*plegia, *lalo*rrhea
lamell/a	thin leaf or plate (a little lamina)	*lamell*iform
lamin/a	thin plate or layer	*lamin*ectomy
lapar/o	abdomen	*laparo*tomy
laryng/o	larynx	*laryng*itis
lepto-	delicate, slender, thin	*lepto*cyte, *lepto*meninges
leuko-, leuco-	white (*leuko-* is preferred)	*leuko*cyte, *leuk*emia (o omitted before another vowel)
levo-	to the left side	*levo*cardia, *levo*rotation
lip/o	fat, lipid	*lip*ase, *lipo*tropic
litho-	stone, calculus	*litho*nephritis
lob/o	lobe	*lob*ectomy
lymphaden/o	lymph gland	*lymphaden*opathy
lympho-	lymph	*lympho*blast, *lympho*sarcoma
macro-	large, abnormally long	*macro*scopic, *macro*cyte
malacia	softening	cerebro*malacia*
mamm/o	breast	*mamm*ogram
mast/o	breast	*mast*ectomy
melan/o	black	*melan*oma
mening/o	meninges	*mening*eal
meso-	middle, intermediate, mesentery	*meso*derm, *meso*appendix
metr/o	uterus	*metr*optosis
micro-	small (in Greek originally *short*)	*micro*scopic, *micro*cyte
mito-	thread, threadlike, mitosis	*mito*chondria, *mito*genesis
mon/o	one, single	*mono*blast, *mono*cular
mortem	death	post*mortem*
muco- (Latin); *myxo-* and *blenno-* (Greek)	mucus	*muco*sa, *muco*purulent, *myx*oma, *myx*orrhea or *blenn*orrhea
multi-	many, much	*multi*factorial, *multi*form
my-; see *myo-*		
mycet-, myc/o	fungus	*myc*ology, *myco*bacterial
myelo-	marrow, often specifically spinal cord	*myelo*blastoma, *myelo*cele, *myelo*cyte

Prefixes and Word Elements	Common Usage	Examples*
my/o	muscle	*my*atrophy or *myo*atrophy, *myo*cardial, *myo*tonia
myring/o	eardrum	*myring*oplasty
nas/o	nose	*nas*opharyngitis
natal	birth	*natal*ity
natr/i	sodium (Na⁺)	*natr*emia
necr/o	death	*necr*osis
neo-	new	*neo*natal, *neo*plastic
nephr/o	kidney	*nephr*itis, *nephr*ostomy
neur/o	nerve or nervous system	*neur*ectomy, *neur*odermatitis, *neur*ofibroma
non-	without; not	*non*union
normo-	normal, usual	*normo*blast, *normo*calcemia
nos/o	disease	*nos*ocomial, *nos*ology
oculo-	eye	*oculo*facial, *oculo*motor
odont/o	teeth	*odont*algia, *odonto*blast
olig/o	few, scanty	*olig*uria
onc/o	mass, bulk, tumor	*onc*ology
onych/o	nails	*onych*odystrophy, *onycho*gryphosis, *onycho*mycosis
oo- (Greek); *ov/i, ov/o* (Latin)	egg, ovum	*oo*genesis, *ovi*parous, *ovo*id
oophor/o	ovary	*oophor*ectomy
ophthalm/o	eye	*ophthalm*oscope
orchi/o	testes	*orchi*oplasty
orchid/o	testes	*orchid*ectomy
orth/o	straight, normal, correct	*orth*opedic
ost-, osteo-	bone	*ost*ectomy, *osteo*malacia
ot/o	ear	*ot*oscope
ox/o, oxy	oxygen	*oxy*genation
pan-	all	*pan*carditis, *pan*hysterosalpingo-oophorectomy
para-	beyond, beside, apart, accessory to	*para*-appendicitis, *para*colitis
partum	birth	post*partum*
ped-	child; foot	*ped*iatrics; *ped*al
peri-	around	*peri*anal, *peri*osteum
phagia	swallowing	dys*phagia*
pharyng/o	pharynx	*pharyng*itis
phasia	speech	dys*phasia*
phleb/o	vein	*phleb*itis
phobia	fear	acro*phobia*
phon/o	sound	*phono*cardiogram, *phono*myogram
phot/o	light (the radiation)	*phot*ometer
phren-, phrenic-	diaphragm, mind, of the phrenic nerve	*phren*ectomy or *phrenic*ectomy
phys-, physio-	nature, physiology, or physical things	*phys*iatry, *physio*therapy
pilo-	hair	*pilo*nidal
plegia	paralysis	para*plegia*
pneumato-, pneumo-, pneumon-	lungs, air in lungs, breath	*pneumo*encephalogram, *pneumon*ia
post-	after	*post*partum
pre-	before	*pre*natal
proct/o	rectum	*proct*oscope
prostat/o	prostate gland	*prostat*ectomy
pseud/o	false	*pseudo*ankylosis
pulm/o	lung; air or gas	*pulm*onary
py/o	pus	*pyo*cyst
pyel/o	kidney pelvis	*pyel*ogram
quadri-, quadru-	four	*quadri*ceps, *quadri*plegia

Prefixes and Word Elements	Common Usage	Examples*
radi/o	x radiation, radius bone, shortwave radiation	radioactive, radiocarpal, radiothermy
recto-	rectum	rectocele, rectosigmoid
ren/o	kidney	renal
retin/o	retina	retinitis
retro-	backward, behind	retrocecal, retrobulbar
rhin/o	nose, noselike	rhinitis
sacr/o	sacrum	sacrococcygeal, sacroiliac
salping/o	tube (uterine or auditory)	salpingectomy, salpingopharyngeal
sangui-	blood	sanguineous
sarc/o	flesh	sarcoidosis, sarcoma
scler/o	hard	scleredema, scleroderma
semi-	half, partly	semicoma, semiflexion
sinistr/o	left side; left	sinistraural, sinistromanual
spleno- (lien/o)	spleen	splenomegaly, lienectomy
spondyl/o	vertebra, vertebrae, spinal column	spondylitis, spondylolysis
staped/o	stapes	stapedectomy
staphyl/o	resembling a bunch of grapes	staphylococcus
sten/o	narrow, contracting	stenosis
stere/o	solid, three dimensional	stereognosis, stereogram
stomat/o	mouth	stomatitis
sub-	under, near, almost	subacute, subclinical, subungual
supra-	above	suprarenal
sym-, syn-, sys-, sy-	together; union or association	symphysis, synapse, syndrome
synov/io	synovial	synovitis
tachy-	swift, rapid	tachycardia
teno- (less used: tendo-, tendino-, tenonto-)	tendon	tenoplasty (tendinoplasty, tendoplasty), tenodesis, tenotomy
tetra-	four	tetrabasic, tetralogy
therm/o	heat	thermal, thermometer
thorac/o, thoracico-	chest	thoracalgia, thoracocentesis
thromb/o	clot, thrombus	thrombectomy, thromboembolism
thyr/o	thyroid	thyrotomy
tomo-	a cutting, a section	tomography
trache/o	trachea	tracheostomy
trans-	through, across	transfusion
tri-	three	triceps
tympan/o	typanic membrane or eardrum	tympanitis
ungu/o	nail	unguinal
uni	one	unilateral
ureter/o	ureter	ureteritis
urethr/o	urethra	urethritis
urin/o, ur/o	urine	urinalysis, urinometer
vas/o	vessel, a duct	vasoconstriction, vasectomy
ven/o	vein	venogram
xanth/o	yellow	xanthelasma, xanthochromia
xer/o	dry; dryness	xeroderma, xerography
xiph-, xiphi, xipho-	xiphoid process (swordlike)	xiphisternal, xiphocostal
zoo- (pronounced zō-ō, not zū)	animal	zoonosis
zyg/o	yoked, joined	zygapophysis, zygote

Suffixes	Common Usage	Examples*
-ac	pertaining to	cardiac
-al	pertaining to	oral
-algia	pain	arthralgia
-ase	an enzyme	amylase
-centesis	puncture and aspiration of	paracentesis, amniocentesis, anthrocentesis
-cele	hernia, cavity, tumor	hydrocele, rectocele
-clasis	breaking	osteoclasis
-clysis	to wash out	hypodermoclysis
-desis	binding	arthrodesis
-dynia	pain	cephalodynia
-ectasis	dilatation, distention	colpectasis
-ectomy	excision of an organ or part	appendectomy, gastrectomy
-emia	blood condition	hypervolemia, septicemia
-gnosis	knowledge	diagnosis
-gram	recorded; written	electrocardiogram
-graphy	making a graphic tracing or recording	electrocardiography
-ia	state; condition; disease	cardia
-iac	pertaining to	cardiac
-iasis	condition of; process or its result	cholelithiasis
-itis	inflammation	gingivitis, glossitis
-logy	word, reason, science, study of	pathology, etiology, embryology
-lysis	dissolution, releasing, freeing	hemolysis
-megaly	enlarged	hepatomegaly
-meter	measure	sphygmomanometer
-odynia	pain condition	ophthalmodynia (same as ophthalmalgia)
-oid	resembling, like	lipoid
-ologist	specialist; expert in the study of	cardiologist
-ology	study of science	cardiology
-oma	tumor	adenoma
-opia, opsia	vision	diplopia, hemianopsia
-ose	carbohydrate (sugars, starches, and celluloses)	glucose, cellulose
-osis	process, disease, abnormal increase	hepatosis
-para	bring forth (woman who has born viable young)	multipara, nullipara, primipara
-pathy	disease	neuropathy, myopathy, osteopathy
-penia	abnormal reduction in number	erythropenia, leukopenia, neutropenia
-pexy, -pexia	surgical fixation of an organ, suspension	nephropexy
-plasty	shaping or surgical formation of	arthroplasty, mammaplasty or mammoplasty, rhinoplasty
-pnea	breathing	dyspnea
-ptosis	drooping; sagging	nephroptosis
-ptysis	cough up	hemoptysis
-rrhage, -rrhagia	a bursting forth, excessive flow	hemorrhage, menorrhagia, metrorrhagia
-rrhaphy	surgical repair by suture	herniorrhaphy, tenorrhaphy
-rrhea	flow, discharge	dysmenorrhea
-scope	instrument for observing	otoscope, ophthalmoscope, bronchoscope, arthroscope, sigmoidoscope, laryngoscope
-scopy	examination of	gastroscopy
-sect	act of cutting, sectioning	dissect

Suffixes	Common Usage	Examples*
-stomy	(mouth) surgical creation of an opening of a viscus for drainage or for communication from one viscus to another	colo*stomy*, tracheo*stomy*, gastrojejuno*stomy*
-tome	instrument for cutting	myringo*tome*, osteo*tome*
-tomy	act of cutting, incising	tracheo*tomy*, gastro*tomy*
-trophy	nutrition, as it has to do with vitality and growth	a*trophy*, hyper*trophy*
-uria	urine condition	dys*uria*, an*uria*, olig*uria*

*As you study, find these words in the medical dictionary and include them in your vocabulary. Also note that the terminal vowel of some prefixes, usually *o* but often *i* or even *a*, is dropped when the word root begins with a vowel, such as *hyp*esthesia, *kal*emia, and *lamin*ectomy.

Appendix D The Patient's Bill of Rights

1. The patient has the right to considerate and respectful care.
2. The patient has the right to obtain from his physician complete current information concerning his diagnosis, treatment and prognosis in terms the patient can be reasonably expected to understand.
3. The patient has the right to receive from his physician information necessary to give informed consent prior to the start of any procedure and/or treatment. . . . Where medically significant alternatives for care or treatment exist, or when the patient requests information concerning medical alternatives, the patient has the right to such information [and] to know the name of the person responsible for the procedures and/or treatment.
4. The patient has the right to refuse treatment to the extent permitted by law, and to be informed of the medical consequences of his action.
5. The patient has the right to every consideration of his privacy concerning his own medical care program.
6. The patient has the right to expect that all communications and records pertaining to his care should be treated as confidential.
7. The patient has the right to expect that within its capacity a hospital must make reasonable response to the request of a patient for services.
8. The patient has the right to obtain information as to any relationship of his hospital to other health care and educational institutions insofar as his care is concerned [and] any professional relationships among individuals, by name, who are treating him.
9. The patient has the right to be advised if the hospital proposes to engage in or perform human experimentation affecting his care or treatment [and] has the right to refuse to participate.
10. The patient has the right to expect reasonable continuity of care.
11. The patient has the right to examine and receive an explanation of his bill regardless of source of payment.
12. The patient has the right to know what hospital rules and regulations apply to his conduct as a patient.

Adapted from American Hospital Association: Nurs. Outlook **24**:29, 1976.

Appendix E Universal Blood and Body Precautions

The following information should be taught when the seciton on Medical Asepsis and Hand Washing (p. 118) are discussed.

The following is in accordance with recommendations from the U.S. Public Health Service, Centers for Disease Control (CDC).

VOCABULARY

Aerosol Dispersion of fine particles into the air.

Body Substance Any fluid or substance produced by the body that can carry infectious agents, for example, blood, urine, sputum, and stool.

Body Substance Precautions (BSP) A system focusing on the cautious handling of potentially infectious body substances by using barrier precautions (gloves, masks, etc.).

Detergents Chemicals used for cleaning purposes, sometimes used in combination with germicides, for example, LpH and Staphene.

Universal Precautions (Same as Body Substance Precautions) Use of uniform infection control procedures with all patients and in all work situations, based upon the degree of exposure risk to body substances, but not based on diagnosis.

Waste Infectious waste is:

1. Laboratory wastes, including cultures of etiologic agents, that pose a substantial threat to health because of volume and virulence.

2. Pathologic specimens, including human tissue, blood elements, excrement, and secretions that contain etiologic agents, and attendant disposable fomites.

3. Surgical specimens, including human parts and tissue removed surgically or at autopsy, which in the opinion of the attending physician contain etiologic agents and attendant disposable fomites.

4. Sharps (needles, sharp disposable instruments, and glass slides.)

Contaminated waste is all moist waste, including products that have been in contact with the patient's bodily fluids or wastes that might attract vermin, (for example: tongue blades, diapers, urine cups, moist blood-stained dressings, nonsharp disposable instruments, and food wastes).

Other wastes are paper material and other office materials.

Infection control systems are designed to prevent health care workers from transferring infections to patients and health care workers from acquiring infections themselves. Infection precautions previously used were based on diagnosis. Body Substance Precautions (BSP) improve on the traditional systems because they protect workers during the period before a patient's diagnosis is known. Sometimes it is not possible to tell by looking if patients are infectious; and it is not practical to test all patients for all possible infections, nor is it timely because exposure would occur before test results are obtained. Pathologic agents may be present in body substances, even if they are not known to be present, and they may be transmitted from ostensibly clinically healthy individuals.

Body Substance Precautions (BSP) are designed for use with all patients, not just those who are identified as infected. BSP are based on the knowledge of how diseases are transmitted and how disease transmission is prevented. Body Substance Precautions (BSP) are based on degree of exposure risk to blood and other body substances, not on diagnosis, and precautions should be based on the degree of risk.

BSP with all patients should include routine use of appropriate barrier precautions to prevent skin and mucous membrane exposure when contact with the patient's blood or other body substances is anticipated. Because all patients and laboratory specimens are considered possibly infected, BSP provides protection from not only known infected cases but also from unrecognized cases, therefore protecting patients and health care workers alike.

Health care workers who have weeping dermatitis or exudative lesions should not take part in direct patient care and should not handle patient-care equipment until the condition is resolved.

BARRIER PRECAUTIONS

The following barrier precautions should be used.

Handwashing

Body substances that may contain disease microorganisms easily contaminate health care givers' hands. If these microorganisms enter an opening in the body, the mouth for example, infection can occur. Handwashing is one of the most effective means of infection control.

Handwashing should occur:

- before eating or preparing food, drinking, and smoking.
- before performing clean or sterile invasive procedures.
- before and after performing a clinical procedure.
- before and after assisting a physician with a clinical procedure.
- before and after touching wounds or other drainage.
- after coming in contact with blood or body fluids, mucous membranes, secretions, or excretions, such as saliva, urine, and feces.
- after handling soiled linen or waste.
- after handling devices or equipment soiled with body substances, for example, urine collection containers.
- after removing gloves.
- after using the toilet.
- after blowing your nose or coughing into your hands.
- between each patient contact.

The most important function of handwashing is to remove infectious organisms. No handwashing product on the market kills all disease-causing organisms. Physical removal, washing soil and organisms down the drain, is the most effective practice. If properly used, any approved handwashing product, whether antibacterial or not, will achieve this goal. Soap-impregnated towelettes should be used only in the field where handwashing facilities are not available; towelettes should not be substituted for soap and water in the office or clinic except during an internal disaster. Other chemicals, such as alcohol or bleach, should not be used for handwashing; they may damage skin and cause open or chapped areas, which are more easily infected.

Skin can become dry and chapped with frequent handwashing. Lotion used after handwashing will help replace the oils removed during handwashing. Hands must always be washed before using lotion. Using a lotion bottle while hands are dirty is likely to contaminate the lotion container and, thereafter, each user's hands. Claims that medicated lotions control this problem have proven less than satisfactory in test data. Each health care giver should use his or her own bottle of lotion, which can be left in a locker or other location convenient to the sole user, and the user should be aware if the lotion becomes contaminated. Community lotion bottles should not be left in staff bathrooms. (See the procedure for handwashing on page 118.)

Gloves

Gloves give the health care provider additional protection beyond that of intact skin and handwashing. Gloves provide additional safety, and they should be worn whenever contact with blood or other body fluids or tissue is expected. Both vinyl and latex gloves are suitable for patient care activities, and each has a 95% effectiveness rate. All gloves tear with heavy or prolonged use. This fact needs to be considered, and torn gloves should be replaced as soon as patient safety permits.

Gloves should be worn for the following procedures:

- when touching blood and body fluids, mucous membranes, or nonintact skin of all patients.
- when handling items or surfaces moist with blood or body fluids and substances.
- when performing venipuncture or other vascular access procedures.
- when working with blood, specimens containing blood, body fluids, excretions, and secretions.
- when cleansing reusable instruments and equipment. Wear heavy rubber gloves over disposable gloves, a plastic apron or gown, and safety glasses, goggles, or personal glasses when involved in decontamination activities of instruments and equipment.
- when decontaminating areas contaminated with body substances.
- when cleaning up blood spills and other contaminated areas. Small spills should be wiped up with disposable absorbent towels. Any broken glass should be scooped up with several paper towels and disposed of in a red sharps container. Finally, the area should be mopped with a disinfectant. Large blood spills also should be mopped up with a disinfectant.

Sterile gloves should be worn for all sterile procedures to protect both the patient and the care provider. *Nonsterile gloves* can be worn for nonsterile patient care procedures where worker protection is needed.

Finger cots or *gloves* should be worn while working to cover cuts, abrasions, rashes, or minor infections on the hands.

If a glove is torn or punctured by a needlestick or other accident, the damaged glove should be removed, hands rewashed, and a new glove put on as promptly as patient safety permits.

If gloves are contaminated, the care provider should not touch telephone receivers, other uncontaminated surfaces, or other areas of the same patient's body that may be uncontaminated.

Care providers must change gloves between patients and wash hands immediately after glove removal.

Gloves always should be removed when answering the telephone, opening a door or drawer, handling a record book or worksheet, and when performing other clean procedures.

Handwashing remains the most effective infection control procedure. Glove use, as described, is used to augment the barrier provided by intact skin against infectious agents. Gloves can transport infectious agents from one person to another or to the mouth as easily as ungloved hands; therefore, these policies are not to be interpreted as replacing the need for handwashing.

Masks and Protective Eyewear

Masks and protective eyewear should be worn to prevent exposure of the care provider's mucous membranes of the mouth, nose, and eyes during procedures that are likely to generate aerosol droplets or splashes of blood or other body fluids, and when cleaning equipment that may have disease-producing microorganisms on it. Masks should cover both the nose and the mouth, and fit close to the face so that air can be breathed only through the mask. Care providers should not loosen the mask. Over time, a mask will become impregnated with moisture from the breath, and it will be harder to breathe through the mask. When this occurs, the mask should be changed—not loosened. Masks should be discarded after each use or when they become damp. They are treated as regular, not infectious, waste.

Protective eyewear, such as personal glasses, goggles, safety glasses, or face shields, should be worn to protect the face from any splashes. Procedures in which eyewear might be needed include certain diagnostic procedures such as endoscopies or any invasive surgical procedure, and when cleaning and decontaminating reusable instruments and equipment. Face shields are best suited for nonpatient care activities such as sorting laundry. After use undamaged eyewear must be washed with soap and water and then dried before it is used again.

Gowns and Aprons

A gown or apron should be worn to protect the arms and clothes during all procedures that are likely to generate splashes or soiling from blood or body fluids. The care provider should wear a gown when cleaning noncontaminated equipment, when cleaning and decontaminating reusable instruments and equipment, and when performing procedures involving contact with large amounts of patient substances. When performing laboratory procedures, the care provider should wear either a long-sleeved gown with a closed front or a long-sleeved laboratory coat buttoned shut. The gown or laboratory coat should be removed when leaving the laboratory area. Care providers should change a gown or laboratory coat immediately if it becomes contaminated with blood or body fluids, and at appropriate periods to ensure cleanliness. Contaminated gowns and laboratory coats should be placed in a biohazard bag for sending to the appropriate laundry as arranged by the facility. If laboratory gowns or coats are contaminated with a microbiological agent because of a laboratory accident, the gown or coat should be sterilized in the steam sterilizer before it is sent to the laundry.

Disposable plastic aprons should be worn if there is a significant probability that blood or body fluids may be splashed. After the task is completed, the disposable apron, if contaminated, should be discarded in a biohazard container or sterilized in the steam sterilizer before it is discarded as ordinary waste. Used laboratory wear should never be stored with street clothes.

Sharps

Needles, scalpel blades, and any other sharps that can easily puncture the skin must be handled with extreme caution to prevent infection with HIV and hepatitis. Most needle sticks happen when used needles are not handled properly. Broken skin or mucous membrane contact and a needle stick or other blood-to-blood accident can transmit infection. The following procedures must be adhered to to prevent any undue infection.

1. Place used disposable needles and syringes, scalpel blades, and other sharp items in a rigid puncture-resistant disposable container with a lid (needle container) that is easily recognized (for example, a red container) and clearly marked as a biohazard. Preferably, the container should be made of rigid plastic. Do not use cardboard or paper containers. *Never* put needles or sharps in the trash or linen. This is dangerous to others.

2. Locate puncture-resistant containers as close as practical to the area where needles and other sharps will be used. The sharps containers should be located in each treatment room, at each laboratory table, and at any other area where syringes, needles, and slides will be used in the office or clinic.

3. Keep needle containers at a level where the top opening can be seen. Needles should not project from the top of the container.

4. *Never* try to take anything out of a needle box. If a needle will not go in easily and the box is not full, use a large syringe to disloge it. Do not push or force items with your hands. If the box is full, arrange to have it replaced.

5. Place the cover to close and seal the sharps containers when they are three-fourths full, and dispose of the container as infectious waste. No additional protective garb is necessary for handling these containers. One method of disposing of full sharps containers is to place the full container in a brown cardboard box labeled "infectious waste" and lined with plastic sheeting. The disposal box should be located in a centralized authorized area. A contract scavenger company should then pick up the sealed boxes and deliver them to an incineration company on a weekly basis.

6. Pick up improperly discarded needles with extreme caution and dispose of them in the nearest sharps container. Do not attempt to cap the needle. Wash your hands after you dispose of the needle. Use tongs or forceps to pick up sharps.

7. *Never* purposely bend or break by hand a used needle. *Never* recap a used needle unless absolutely necessary or in approved special circumstances. An example of a special circumstance when a needle should be recapped is in drawing blood for blood gases. To recap vacutainer needles, put the cap on the table, and slide the needle into it without holding the cap. Then tighten the cap at the needle hub.

8. *Never* remove a used needle from a used disposable syringe. Discard the syringe with the needle in place.

9. *Never* put a used needle into your pocket.

10. Wear gloves when doing laboratory work where a needle needs to be removed from a syringe. Discard the gloves immediately if they become contaminated with blood. It is preferable to use a needle disposal container that has an integral device for removing needles without necessitating touching the needles with your hands.

11. Discard vacutainer sleeves in the sharps container at the end of each day or when they are soiled with blood.

12. Place *reusable sharps* in a suitable puncture-resistant container after use and take them to the decontamination area where they will be cleaned and disinfected or sterilized. Wear protective garb, such as gowns, aprons, gloves, and face protection, while cleaning up.

Ventilation Devices

Mouthpieces, resuscitation bags, or other ventilation devices should be available to use in areas where the need for resuscitation is predictable. Use these devices on all patients instead of mouth-to-mouth resuscitation.

Laboratory Specimens

To control the spread of infection and to protect the health of employees, patients, and the public, all laboratory specimens should be handled and transported according to the following procedures:

1. Laboratory specimens should be contained for transport. Special secure, stiff, and impermeable containers, such as the igloo-type containers, should be used by messenger service personnel when transporting blood and other body fluids from the office or clinic to a laboratory. Specimen containers may be placed in test tube racks, then in the secure transport container. Some facilities also require that the specimen be placed in a Ziploc or other hand-sealed plastic bag and sealed shut before being placed in the secure transport container for delivery to the laboratory. If the specimen container is too large to fit in a sealable plastic bag, tape can be used to secure the cap and then enclose the entire item in a plastic bag with a twist tie. The laboratory work slip should be attached by rubber band or tape to the outside of the bag.

Specimen mailers must have a metal inner container and a rigid outer container to comply with CDC regulations. (See Figures 6-1 and 6-2 on page 192.)

Centrifuge all blood or body fluid specimens in carriers with safety domes. Decontaminate the carrier and dome according to the manufacturer's directions. Human tissue, blood, body secretions and excretions, or other specimens and cultures should be autoclaved before they are disposed of in a sanitary landfill.

2. Gloves should be used for handling laboratory specimens when contamination of the hands is anticipated. Care must be taken when collecting specimens to avoid contamination of the outside of the container or the laboratory slip. Put on disposable gloves and dispose of urine specimens in a toilet or utility sink and feces into toilets that empty into a sewer system. Sinks should then be rinsed thoroughly and toilets flushed. (To avoid cross-contamination, this sink should *not* be used for other activities such as preparation of clean supplies or supply of drinking water. Other sinks should be used for routine handwashing.) Dispose of specimen containers and gloves in a closed waste container lined with a strong plastic or vinyl bag.

3. Wash your hands after handling all specimens and after removing gloves. Hands and other skin surfaces contaminated with blood or other body fluids must be washed immediately and thoroughly. Decontaminate laboratory work surfaces with a disinfectant, such as a 1:10 dilution of sodium hypochlorite (household bleach) or Staphene germicide solution, when the procedures have been completed or if a specimen is spilled.

4. All potentially contaminated materials used in laboratory tests should be decontaminated, preferably by steam sterilization, before disposal or reprocessing. All infectious laboratory waste should be treated by steam sterilization, incineration, or disinfection before disposal to render the waste harmless. Promptly contact your supervisor when you have had an exposure to blood or other body fluids.

HANDLING OF EQUIPMENT, SUPPLIES, AND WASTE FROM PATIENT CARE AREAS AND THE LABORATORY, AND CARE OF ENVIRONMENTAL SURFACES

Waste equipment and supplies should be handled as follows:

Reusable Equipment

All used reusable equipment not classified as sharps should be placed as soon as possible, if appropriate, in an Environmental Protection Agency approved detergent such as Hemosol or Coleo, and transported to the decontamination area. Items that require sterilization or high-level disinfection first must be thoroughly cleaned and decontaminated. Cleaning and decontamination should be done by personnel wearing gloves, gown, and face protection. Each facility must develop cleaning and decontamination procedures appropriate to its needs.

Blood pressure equipment, scales, and other reusable room equipment should be decontaminated with a disinfectant solution at the end of each day. Stethoscope earpieces must be cleaned after each use with an alcohol swab. Tonometers must be disinfected with alcohol swabs, rinsed thoroughly in clean water, and then left to air dry or be dried with a clean non-lint material after *each* use. When visibly soiled, or at least weekly, centrifuges should be cleaned with 70% alcohol swabs or disposable cloths soaked in 70% alcohol or LpH solution mixed according to the product's directions. Tourniquets can be soaked in a 1:10 of 5% sodium hypochlorite solution for 15 minutes. Discard bloodstained tourniquets. After each use, goggles and heavy rubber gloves used during decontamination procedures must be decontaminated with alcohol. After each use brushes and buckets or basins used for decontamination procedures must be decontaminated with a detergent solution, rinsed, and then placed in a specifically designated area for such supplies. This equipment should be sterilized weekly.

Sharps

Sharps containers must be closed after they are filled and then disposed of as infectious waste. No additional protective garb is necessary when handling these containers.

Reusable sharps should be placed in containers suitable for transportation to the decontamination area where they will be cleaned, disinfected and sterilized. Employees who do this cleaning must wear protective garb (aprons, gloves, and face protection). (See also SHARPs on page 4.)

Tissues, Body Fluids, and Cultures

- Patient specimens and the containers that hold them should be collected and treated as infectious waste.
- Cultures and the containers that hold them should be collected and treated as infectious waste.
- Human tissues or body parts should be treated as infectious waste.

- Large volumes of blood or drainage, such as that from suction machines, should be flushed down the sewer or disposed of in collection containers and treated as infectious waste.
- Used disposable dialysis equipment should be treated as infectious waste.
- Large volumes of urine, stool, or dialysate should be flushed down the sewer with appropriate precautions to guard against spillage.

While awaiting transport for disposal, infectious waste must be held in covered or bagged leakproof waste containers. Infectious waste must be collected in identifiable containers or bags for transportation to a separate disposal site. If disposal cans without working lids are used, moist trash must be bagged before it is placed in an open can. All trash containers must have a liner thick enough to withstand necessary handling, and they must be tied closed when disposed of. Waste containers should be cleaned weekly with a disinfectant solution.

Other Waste

All other waste, such as paper towels and packaging materials, should be placed in regular waste containers lined with plastic or vinyl liners strong or thick enough to withstand necessary handling. For convenience, small items such as contaminated cotton balls may be disposed of in the sharps containers. Other disposable, moist waste generated by clinics or offices should be collected in *covered* foot-operated cans that are lined with moisture-impervious bags. When removed, the bags should be closed, not emptied, and disposed of as ordinary waste.

Each waste container liner must be removed as a single unit and tied shut without turning the container upside down to consolidate waste. Waste containers must be strong enough to resist tears and leaks under normal handling. Final disposal of waste is by approval of the local health officers and includes incineration, autoclaving, sewer system, or sanitary landfill.

Surfaces

- When body fluids are spilled, the visible material should be removed from surfaces followed by decontamination processes with an approved disinfectant, such as a 1:10 dilution of sodium hypochlorite (household bleach) or Bytech solution. Gloves must be worn for this process.
- Laboratory work surfaces should be decontaminated with a disinfectant, such as a 1:10 dilution of sodium hypochlorite or Staphene germicide solution at the completion of work activities or in the event of a specimen spill.

- Regular cleaning of diapering areas is recommended because of the potential for fecal-orally transmitted agents.
- Environmental surfaces in patient care areas should be cleaned with an approved disinfectant weekly, and as needed.
- Periodic cleaning of the clinic or office environment is good housekeeping rather than an infection control concern.
- Materials used for cleanup should be disposed of in the moist infectious waste covered container.
- Covers on examination tables and Mayo stands must be changed after each patient.
- At the end of the day, examination tables, counters, Mayo stands, and other equipment should be decontaminated with a disinfectant solution (for example, LpH solution).
- Supply closets should be dusted and cleaned at least monthly using a rag saturated with 70% alcohol to wipe the shelves, then allowing the shelves to air dry. The door to the room should be left open while this procedure is in progress to avoid any side effects from fumes.
- Janitorial staff must be taught how to handle and dispose of ordinary, contaminated, and infectious waste.

Uniforms and Clothing

Uniforms and clothing that are soiled with body secretions should be cleaned with soap and *cool* water, then washed following normal laundering procedures. Clothing with large amounts of contaminates should be changed as soon as possible.

Glossary

abdominal pulse—Abdominal aorta pulse.

abdominal respirations—The inspiration and expiration of air by the lungs accomplished primarily by the abdominal muscles and diaphragm.

accelerated respirations—More than 25 respirations per minute, after 15 years of age.

acetonuria (as"ĕ-tō-nu'rē-ah) or **ketonuria** (kē"tō-nu'rē-ah)—The presence of acetone or ketone in the urine.

acrotism (ak'ro-tizm)—Apparent absence of pulse.

addiction (ah-dik'shun)—An acquired physiologic and/or psychologic dependence on a drug with tendencies to increase its use.

agglutination (ah-gloo"tĭn-nā' shun)—A clumping together of cells, as of blood cells or bacteria. An example is when red blood cells (RBC) clump together as a result of an incompatible blood transfusion.

agranulocyte (a-gran'ū-lō-sīt")—A white blood cell (WBC) with a clear or nongranular cytoplasm. There are two types, monocytes and lymphocytes.

albuminuria (al-bū"mi-nu'rē-ah) —The presence of serum albumin in urine.

allergen (al-er-jen)—Any substance that induces hypersensitivity.

allergy (al'er-jē)—An unusual and increased sensitivity (hypersensitivity) to specific substances that are ordinarily harmless.

alternating pulse—Alternating weak and strong pulsations.

AMA—American Medical Association

amplify (am'plĭ-fī)—To enlarge, to extend.

anaerobic Culturette culture collection system—This system offers the same basic properties of the Culturette, plus a standardized and dependable anaerobic environment for transport of anaerobic bacteria. The transport medium once released maintains an anaerobic environment for up to 48 hours. Many laboratories request that the anaerobic culture system be used when taking a wound culture. (See also Culturette.)

anaphylactic (an"ah-fi-lak'tik) **shock**—An intense state of shock brought on by hypersensitivity to a drug, foreign toxin, or protein. Early symptoms resemble an allergic reaction, then increase in severity rapidly to dyspnea, cyanosis, and shock. This can be fatal if emergency measures are not taken immediately (see also Unit XVI, First Aid for Allergic Reactions to Drugs).

anaphylaxis (an"ah-fi-lak'sis)—An unusual or hypersensitive reaction of the body to foreign protein and other substances; frequently caused by drugs, foreign serum (tetanus, and so on), and insect stings and bites.

anemia (ah-nē'mē-ah)—There is a variety of forms of anemia, but broadly speaking it is a lack of red blood cells in the circulating blood or a reduction of hemoglobin or both. Anemia is thought of as a symptom of a disease or disorder; it is not a disease.

anesthesia (an"es-the'ze-ah)—The loss of sensation or feeling.

anisocytosis (an-i"-sō-sī-tō'sis)—A state of abnormal variations in the size of red blood cells in the blood.

anoscope (an'no-skōp)—A speculum or endoscope inserted into the anal canal for direct visual examination.

antidote (an'tĭ-dōt)—An agent used to counteract a poison.

antiseptic (an'tĭ-sep'tik)—A substance capable of inhibiting the growth or action of microorganisms, without necessarily killing them; generally safe for use on body tissues.

anuria (ah-nu're-ah)—The absence of urine.

apnea (ap-ne'ah)—Cessation or absence of breathing.

applicator—A slender rod of glass or wood with a pledget of cotton on one end used to apply medicine or to take a culture from the body.

arrhythmia (ăh-rith'mē-ah)—A variation from the normal or an irregular rhythm of the heartbeat.

arthritis (ar-thri'tis)—Inflammation of a joint.

artificial respiration—Artificial methods to restore respiration in cases of suspended breathing.

asepsis (ā-sep'sis)—The absence of all microorganisms causing disease; absence of contaminated matter.

aspiration/needle biopsy—Removal of material from internal organ by means of hollow needle inserted through the body wall and into affected tissue.

atopy (at"o-pē)—A hypersensitive state that is subject to hereditary influences, such as hay fever, asthma, and eczema.

atrium (ā'trē-um)—One of the upper chambers of the heart. The right atrium receives deoxygenated blood from the body, whereas the left atrium receives oxygenated blood from the lungs. (The plural is **atria.**)

auricle (aw'rĭ-kl)—The outer projection of the ear; also known as the **pinna** (pin'nah).

bactericide (bak-tēr'ĭ-sīd)—A substance capable of destroying bacteria but not spores.

bacteriology (bak-te"-re-ol'o-je) —The study of bacteria.

bacteriolysis (bak-te"re-ol'ĭ-sis)—The destruction of bacteria.

bacteriostatic (bak-te"re-o-stat'ik) —A substance that inhibits the growth of bacteria.

511

bacteriuria (bak-te"rē-u'rē-ah)—The presence of bacteria in urine.

band-form granulocyte—A granular WBC in a stage of development.

benign (be-nīn) **hypertension**—Hypertension of slow onset that is usually without symptoms.

bigeminal (bī-jĕm'ĭn-al) **pulse**—Two regular beats followed by a longer pause. It has the same significance as an irregular pulse.

bimanual (bi-man'u-al)—With both hands, as bimanual palpation.

biochemistry (bi"o-kem'is-tre)—The study of chemical changes occurring in living organisms.

biological death—The condition that results when the brain has been deprived of oxygenated blood for a period of 6 minutes or more, and irreversible damage has probably occurred.

biopsy (bi'op-se)—Removal of tissue from the body for examination.

biopsy (bi'op-se) **forceps**—Two-pronged instruments of varying sizes and shapes used to remove tissue from the body for examination.

Biot respiration—Irregularly alternating periods of apnea and hyperpnea; occurs in meningitis and disorders of the brain.

blood culture—Used in the diagnosis of specific infectious diseases. Blood is withdrawn from a vein and placed in or upon suitable culture media; then it is determined whether or not pathogens grow in the media. If organisms do grow, they are identified by bacteriological methods.

blood dyscrasia (dis-krā'zē-ah)—An abnormal or diseased condition of the blood.

BNDD—Bureau of Narcotics and Dangerous Drugs (a federal government agency of the DEA).

bowel movement—The elimination/excretion of fecal material from the intestinal tract.

bradycardia (brad-ĭ-kar'dĭ-ă)—Slow heart action; extremely slow pulse, generally below 60 beats per minute.

bronchoscope (brong'ko-skōp)—An endoscope designed specifically for passage through the trachea to allow visual examination of the interior of the tracheobronchial tree.

bronchoscopy (bron-kos'kō-pī)—Internal inspection of the tracheobronchial tree with the use of a bronchoscope; used for diagnostic or treatment purposes. For diagnosis, the physician will inspect the interior of the bronchi and may obtain a sample of secretions or a biopsy of tissue; for treatment, foreign bodies or mucus plugs that may be causing an obstruction to the air passages can be located and removed.

bursitis (bur-sī'tis)—Inflammation of a bursa. The most commonly affected is the bursa of the shoulder.

canthus (kan'thus)—The inner canthus is the angle of the eyelids near the nose; the outer canthus is the angle of the eyelids at the outside corner of the eyes.

cardiac (kar'dē-ak) **arrest**—Sudden and often unexpected cessation of the heartbeat. Permanent damage of vital organs and death are probable if treatment is not given immediately.

cassette (kah-set')—A light-proof aluminum or bakelite container with front and back intensifying screens, between which x-ray film is placed when used for x-ray examinations.

cautery (kaw'ter-ē)—A hot instrument used to cut or destroy tissue, causing hemostasis at the time.

cerumen (sĕ-roo'men)—Ear wax secreted by the glands of the external auditory meatus.

chemotherapy (kē"mo-ther'ah-pē)—The use of drugs (chemicals) to treat disease; a type of therapy used for cancer patients in which powerful drugs are used to interfere with the reproduction of the fast-multiplying cancer cells.

Cheyne-Stokes (chān-stōks) **respiration**—Respirations gradually increasing in rapidity and volume, until they reach a climax, then gradually subsiding and ceasing entirely for from 5 to 50 seconds, when they begin again. These are often a sign of impending death. Cheyne-Stokes respirations *may* be observed in normal persons (especially the aged) during sleep or during visits to higher altitudes.

clinical death—The state that results when breathing and circulation have stopped.

colicky—Acute intermittent abdominal pain usually caused by spasmodic contractions.

concussion (kon-kush'un)—The injury that results from a violent blow or shock.

concussion of the brain—A violent disturbance of the brain caused by a blow or fall.

conduction (kon-duk'shun)—The passage or conveyance of energy, as of electricity, heat or sound.

conjunctiva (kon"junk-tī'vah)—The delicate membrane lining the eyelids and reflected onto the front of the eyeball.

constant fever—High fever with a variation not exceeding 1 or 2 degrees F (.06° or 1.2° C) between morning and evening temperatures.

constipation (kŏn-stī-pā'shun)—A condition in which the waste material in the intestine is too hard to pass easily, or in which bowel movements are so infrequent that discomfort results.

contact dermatitis—Dermatitis caused by an allergic reaction resulting from contact of the skin with various substances, such as poison ivy, or chemical, physical, and mechanical agents.

contaminated, contamination (kon-tam"ĭ-nā'shun)—The act of making unclean, soiling, or staining, especially the introduction of disease germs or infectious material into or on normally sterile objects.

contraindication (kon"tra-in"dĭ-kā'shun)—Condition in which the use of certain drugs or treatments should be withheld or limited.

contusion (kon-too'zhun)—A bruise, indicating injury to tissues without breakage in the skin. Discoloration appears because of blood seepage under the surface of the skin.

cross-tolerance—Cross-tolerance can develop when tolerance to one drug increases the body's tolerance to drugs in the same category. For example, a tolerance to one depressant drug leads to a tolerance of other depressant drugs.

crude drug—An unrefined drug.

culture (kul'tūr)—The reproduction or growth of microorganisms or of living tissue cells in special laboratory media (the material on which the organisms grow) conducive to their growth. Various types of cultures follow.

culture medium—A commercial preparation used for the growth of microorganisms or other cells. (Types of culture media are described in Unit VI.)

Culturette—A commercially prepared bacterial culture collection/transport system, consisting of a sterile plastic tube with applicator. Modified Stuart's transport medium is held in a glass ampule at the bottom end, to assure stability of medium at the time of use. Transport medium is released only after the sample is taken, by crushing the ampule. A moist environment (not immersion) is maintained up to 72 hours to preserve the specimen.

Culturette II culture collection system—This is identical to the Culturette, with the exception that the plastic tube contains two applicators and the ampule contains twice the medium (1 ml).

cumulative action of a drug—A drug accumulates in the body;

it is eliminated more slowly than it is absorbed.

cystoscope (sist'o-skōp)—A hollow metal tube instrument (endoscope) designed specifically for passing through the urethra into the urinary bladder to permit internal inspection. The bladder interior is illuminated by an electric bulb at the end of the cystoscope. Special lenses and mirrors allow the bladder mucosa to be examined for calculi (stones), inflammation, or tumors.

cystoscopy (sis-tos'kop-ĭ)—Internal examination of the bladder with a cystoscope. Samples of urine for diagnostic purposes can be obtained by passing a catheter through the cystoscope into the bladder or beyond, up into the ureters and kidneys. Also, radiopaque dyes may be injected through the cystoscope into the bladder or up into the ureters when taking x-ray films of the urinary tract.

cytology (sī-tol'ō-jē)—The study of the structure and function of cells.

DEA—Drug Enforcement Administration. This is the federal law enforcement agency charged with the responsibility of combating drug diversion.

debridement (da-brēd-ment')—The process of removing foreign material and devitalized tissue.

defibrillation (de-fi"brĭ-la'shun)—The application of electrical impulses to the heart to stop heart fibrillation.

density—The quality of being dense or impenetrable.

dermatitis (der"mah-ti'tis)—Inflammation of the skin.

detail—The sharpness of the radiograph image.

diaphragmatic respiration—Performed mainly by the diaphragm.

diarrhea (di-a-re'a)—Rapid movement of fecal material through the intestine, resulting in poor absorption, producing frequent, watery stools.

digital (dij'it-al)—The use of a finger to insert into a body cavity, such as the rectum, for palpating the tissue.

dilute—To weaken the strength of a substance by adding something else.

disinfectant (dis"in-fek'tant)—A substance capable of destroying pathogens, but usually not spores; generally not intended for use on body tissue, because it is too strong.

diuresis (di"u-re-'sis)—An abnormal, increased secretion of urine as seen in diabetes mellitus, diabetes insipidus, or when drinking large amounts of fluid; this can be artificially produced by drugs with diuretic properties.

don—To put an article on, such as gloves or a gown.

drug idiosyncrasy (id"ē-o-sing'krah-sē)—An unusual or abnormal response or susceptibility to a drug that is peculiar to the individual.

drug tolerance—The decreased susceptibility to the effects of a drug after continued use. In this case an increased dosage would be required to produce the desired effects, as the initial dose would be ineffective.

dysplasia (dis-pla'ze-ah)—An abnormal development of tissue.

dyspnea (disp-ne'ah)—Labored or difficult breathing.

dysuria (dis-u're-ah)—Painful or difficult urination.

electrocardiograph (e-lek"tro-kar'de-o-graf")—The instrument used in electrocardiography.

electrolyte (e-lek'tro-lit)—Substances that separate into their component atoms when dissolved in water. They play an important part in maintaining fluid balance and a normal acid-base balance, and in the functions of cells in the body. EXAMPLES: sodium, potassium, calcium, magnesium, chloride, and bicarbonate.

electrophoresis (e-lek"tro-fo-re'sis)—A laboratory method used to diagnose certain diseases by analyzing the plasma protein content.

endoscope (en'do-skōp)—A specially designed instrument made of metal, rubber, or glass that is used for direct visual examination of hollow organs or body cavities. All endoscopes have similar working elements, even though the design will vary according to its specific use. The viewing part (scope) is a hollow tube fitted with a lens system that allows viewing in a variety of directions. Each endoscope has a light source, power cord, and power source; examples include bronchoscope, cystoscope, proctoscope, and sigmoidoscope.

endoscopy (en-dos'ko-pi)—Visual examination of internal cavities of the body with an endoscope, for example, a proctoscope, bronchoscope, cystoscope, gastroscope, and laryngoscope.

enema (en'ĕ-mah)—The introduction of a solution into the rectum; for an x-ray examination of the colon, a radiopaque solution is administered by enema.

enuresis (en"u-re'sis)—The involuntary excretion of urine, especially at night during sleep; bedwetting; most frequently seen in children with either physical or emotional problems.

epinephrine (ep"ĭ-nef'rin)—A hormone produced by the adrenal glands. Epinephrine can be administered parenterally, topically, or by inhalation. It is used as an emergency heart stimulant, to relieve symptoms in allergic conditions, and to counteract the lethal effects of anaphylactic shock.

erythrocytosis (ĕ-rith"ro-si-to'sis)—Increased numbers of red blood cells (erythrocytes).

essential hypertension (idiopathic or primary hypertension)—Hypertension that develops in the absence of kidney disease. Its cause is unknown. About 85% to 90% of the cases of hypertension are in this category.

eupnea (ūp-ne'ah)—Easy or normal respiration.

excisional biopsy—Removal of an entire small lesion.

excreta (ek-skre'tah)—Waste material excreted or eliminated from the body. Feces, urine, perspiration, and also mucus and carbon dioxide (CO_2) can be considered excreta.

excrete—To eliminate useless matter, such as feces and urine.

excretion (ek-skre'shun)—The elimination of waste materials from the body. Ordinarily, what is meant by excretion is the elimination of feces, but it can refer to the material eliminated from any part of the body.

excruciating pain—Torturing, extreme pain, often intractable.

exfoliative cytology—Microscopic examination of cells desquamated (shedding) from a body surface as a means of detecting malignant change.

expectorate—The ejection of sputum and other materials from the air passages.

exquisite pain—Intense pain to which an individual is extremely sensitive.

external auditory meatus (me-a'tus)—The canal or passage leading from the outside opening of the ear to the eardrum. Also called the external acoustic meatus.

external ear—Includes the auricle, or pinna, and the external auditory meatus.

FDA—Food and Drug Administration (a federal government agency).

febrile (feb'rile) **pulse**—A full, bounding pulse at the onset of a fever, becoming feeble and weak when the fever subsides.

feces (fe'sēz)—Body waste excreted from the intestine; also called stool, excreta, or excrement.

fever—Pyrexia, or elevation of body temperature above normal, 98.6° F (Fahrenheit) or 37° C (centigrade or Celsius) registered orally. Some classify it as:

Low   99° to 101° F
             (37.2° to 38.3°C)

Moderate   101° to 103° F
            (38.3° to 39.5°C)
High   103° to 105° F
            (39.5° to 40.6°C)

- **crisis**—Sudden drop of a high temperature to normal or below; generally occurs within 24 hours.
- **intermittent fever**—Variations with alternate rises and falls, with the lowest often dropping below 98.6° F. An intermittent fever reaches the normal line at intervals during the course of an illness, for example, AM 98° F, PM 101° F.
- **onset**—Beginning of a fever.
- **remittent fever**—Variations in temperature but always above 98.6° F (37° C), a persistent fever that has a daytime variation of 2° F (1.2° C) or more, for example AM 100° F, PM 103° F; AM 99° F, PM 102.4° F.

fibrillation (fi"brĭ-la'shun)—A cardiac arrhythmia characterized by rapid, irregular, and ineffective electrical activity in the heart. Ventricular fibrillation is a common cause of cardiac arrest.

fixation of a smear—Spraying with or immersing a slide into a special solution, or drying the slide over a flame, or air drying to harden and preserve the bacteria for future microscopic examination.

flatulence (flat'u-lens)—Excessive formation of gases in the stomach or intestine.

flatus (fla'tus)—Air or gas in the stomach or intestine.

fluoroscope (floo'or-o-skōp")—An instrument that is used during x-ray examinations for visual observation of the internal body structures by means of x-rays. The body part that is to be viewed is placed between the x-ray tube and a fluorescent screen. As x-rays pass through the body, shadowy images of the internal organs are projected on the screen.

fluoroscopy (floo"or-os'ko-pe)—Visual examination by means of a fluoroscope.

forced respiration—Voluntary hyperpnea.

formicant (for'mi-kant') **pulse**—A small, feeble pulse.

frequency—The need to urinate frequently.

fungicide (fun'jĭ-sīd)—A substance that destroys fungi.

gastroscopy (gas'tros'ko-pī)—Internal inspection of the stomach with a gastroscope.

gelatin culture—A culture of bacteria on gelatin.

germicide (jer'mĭ-sīd)—A substance that is capable of destroying pathogens.

glucosuria (gloo"ko-su're-ah) or **glycosuria** (gli"ko-su're-ah)—Abnormally high sugar content in urine.

granulocyte (gran'u-lo-sīt")—A white blood cell having granules in its cytoplasm. These types of WBCs are neutrophils, basophils, and eosinophils.

guaiac (gwī'ak) **test**—The preferred chemical test to determine the presence of occult blood in feces.

guarding—A reflex usually related to abdominal pain; the action of muscles tensing, knees drawn up and/or hand placed over a part to prevent examination and/or protect against increasing pain.

habituation—Emotional dependence on a drug due to repeated use, but without tendencies to increase the amount of the drug.

hanging drop culture—A culture in which the bacteria are inoculated into a drop of fluid on a coverglass, and then mounted into the depression on a concave slide.

health—The state of mental, physical, and social well-being of an individual, and not merely the absence of disease.

hematuria (hem"ah-tu"re-ah)—The presence of blood in urine.

hemoglobin (he"mo-glo'bin)—A protein in an RBC that carries oxygen and carbon dioxide.

The pigment in hemoglobin is what gives the blood its red color. The protein in hemoglobin is globin; the red pigment is heme. For the body to make hemoglobin, it must have iron, which is derived from the food we eat.

hemolysis (he-mol'ĭ-sis)—The destruction of red blood cells with the release of hemoglobin into the plasma.

hemoptysis (he-mop'-tĭ-sis)—Coughing up blood as a result of bleeding from any part of the respiratory tract. The appearance of the secretion in true hemoptysis is bright red and frothy with air bubbles.

HHS—Health and Human Services (a federal government agency).

histology (his-tol'o-je)—The study of the microscopic form and structure of tissue.

hyperbilirubinemia (hī"per-bil"i-roo"bĭ-nē'mē-ah) — Increased or excessive levels of bilirubin in the blood.

hypercalcemia (hī"per-kal-sē'mē-ah)—Increased or excessive levels of calcium in the blood.

hypercholesterolemia (hi'per-kō-les"ter-ol-ē'mē-ah)—Excessive levels of cholesterol in the blood.

hyperchromia (hi'per-kro'me-ah)—An abnormal increase of the hemoglobin levels in red blood cells.

hypercythemia (hy'per-sī-thē'mē-ah)—An excessive number of red blood cells in the circulating blood.

hyperemia (hi'per-ē'mē-ah)—An excessive amount of blood in a part.

hyperglycemia (hī"per-glī-sē'mē-ah)—Excessive amounts of glucose in the blood.

hyperkalemia (hī"per-kah-lē'mē-ah)—An excessive level of potassium in the blood.

hypernatremia (hī'per-na-trē'mē-ah)—An excessive amount of sodium in the blood.

hyperoxemia (hī"per-ok-sē'mē-ah)—A condition in which the blood is excessively acidic.

hyperpnea (hy"perp-ne'ah)—Increase in rate and depth of breathing.

hyperproteinemia (hī"per-prō"tē-ĭ-nē'mē-ah)—An excessive amount of protein in the blood.

hypertension (hi'per-ten'shun)—High blood pressure; a condition in which patient has higher blood pressure than normal for his or her age; for example, systolic pressure consistently above 160 mm Hg and a diastolic pressure above 90 mm Hg.

hyperventilation—Increase of air in the lungs above the normal amount; abnormally prolonged and deep breathing, usually associated with acute anxiety or emotional tensions.

hypo (hī'pō)—A word part meaning an abnormal decrease or deficient amounts. If you replace this word element and definition for the word element "hyper" in all of the preceding terms (except in hyperemia and hyperoxemia), the correct meaning will be defined.

hypotension (hi'po-ten'shun)—A decrease of systolic and diastolic blood pressure to below normal; for example, below 90/50 is considered low blood pressure.

hypothermia (hi'po-ther'me-ah)—Low body temperature.

hypoxemia (hi'pok-se'me-ah)—A deficient amount of oxygen (O_2) in the blood.

hypoxia (hi-pok'se-ah)—Reduced amounts of oxygen to the body tissues.

immunization (im"u-nĭ-za'shun)—The process of rendering a person immune (protected from or not susceptible to a disease) or of becoming immune; frequently called vaccination or inoculation. A process by which a person is artificially prepared to resist infection by a specific pathogen.

immunosuppressive agents—Drugs that inhibit the formation of antibodies to antigens that may be present.

incisional biopsy—Incision into and removal of part of a lesion.

incontinence (in-kon′tĭ-nens)—The inability to refrain from the urge to urinate. This may occur in times of stress, anxiety, anger, postoperatively, or from obstructions that prevent the normal emptying of the urinary bladder, spasms of the bladder, irritation due to injury or inflammation of the urinary tract, damage to the spinal cord or brain, or from the development of a fistula (an abnormal tube-like passage) between the bladder and the vagina or urethra.

incubation (in″ku-ba′shun) **period**—The interval of time between the invasion of a pathogen into the body and the appearance of the first symptoms of disease.

incubation (in-ku-ba′shun)—When pertaining to bacteriology, this term refers to the period of culture development.

induration (in″du-ra′shun)—An abnormally hard spot; a process of hardening.

infection (in-fek′shun)—A condition caused by the multiplication of pathogenic microorganisms that have invaded the body of a susceptible host.
- **acute**—rapid onset, severe symptoms, and usually subsides within a relatively short period of time.
- **chronic**—develops slowly, milder symptoms; lasts for a long period of time.
- **latent**—dormant or concealed; pathogen is ever-present in the host, but symptoms are present only intermittently, often in response to a stimulus. At other times the pathogen is dormant.
- **localized**—restricted to a certain area.
- **generalized**—systemic; involving the whole body.

infectious mononucleosis—Also called glandular fever, is an acute infectious disease, caused by the Epstein-Barr virus.

inoculate (ĭ-nok″ū-lāt)—In microbiology, this refers to introducing infectious matter into a culture medium in an effort to produce growth of the causative organism.

insufflator (in′sŭf-fla-tor)—An instrument, device, or bag used for blowing air, powder, or gas into a cavity.

intermittent pulse—A pulse in which occasional beats are skipped.

intractable—Unmanageable, not controllable with conventional means, that is, rest, heat, medication.

ionizing (i″on-i-zing)—Radiant energy given off by radioactive atoms and x-rays.

irradiate (ĭ-ra′dē-āt)—To treat with radiant energy.

irradiation (i-ra″dē-ā′shun)—Exposure to radiation; the passage of penetrating rays through a substance or object.

irregular pulse—A pulse with variation in force and frequency; an excess of tea, coffee, tobacco, or exercise may cause this.

ischemia (is-kē′mē-ah)—A deficient amount of blood in a body part due to an obstruction or a functional constriction of a blood vessel.

isocytosis (ī″sō-sī-tō′sis)—A state in which cells are equal in size, especially equality of size of red blood cells.

labored breathing—Dyspnea or difficult breathing; respiration that involves active participation of accessory inspiratory and expiratory muscles.

laryngeal (lar-in′je-al) **mirror**—An instrument used to view the pharynx and larynx consisting of a small rounded mirror attached to the end of a slender (metal or chrome plate) handle.

laryngoscope (lar-in′go-skōp)—An endoscope used to examine the larynx. It is equipped with mirrors and a light for illumination of the larynx.

leukemia (lū-kē′mē-ah)—A malignant disease of various types that is classified clinically as acute or chronic, depending on the character and duration of the disease; myeloid, lymphoid, or monocytic, depend-ing on the cells involved. This disease affects the tissues of the lymph nodes, spleen, and/or bone marrow. Symptoms include an uncontrolled increase of white blood cells, accompanied by a decrease in red blood cells and platelets. This results in anemia and an increased tendency to infection and hemorrhage. Other classical symptoms include pain in bones and joints, fever, and swelling of the liver, spleen, and lymph nodes. The precise cause is unknown.

leukocytosis (lū″kō-sī-tō′sis)—An increased number of circulating white blood cells.

leukopenia (lū″kō-pē′nē-ah)—A deficient number of circulating white blood cells.

lienteric stool—Feces containing much undigested food.

ligate (li′gāt)—To apply a ligature.

ligature (lig′ah-tūr)—A suture; material used to tie off blood vessels to prevent bleeding, or to constrict tissues.

light therapy or phototherapy (fo′to-ther′ah-pe)—The use of light rays in the treatment of disease processes. By custom, this includes the use of ultraviolet and infrared or heat rays (radiation).

lysis—Gradual decline of a fever.

macrocyte (mak′rō-sīt)—The largest type of red blood cell; seen in cases of pernicious anemia (vitamin B$_{12}$ deficiency) and folic acid deficiency.

macroscopic (mak-rō-skop′ĭk) **examination**—An examination in which the specimen is large enough to be seen by the naked eye.

malignant (mah-lig′nant) **hypertension**—Hypertension that differs from other types in that it is a rapidly developing hypertension and may prove fatal if not treated immediately after symptoms develop, before damage is done to the blood vessels. This type occurs most often in persons in their twenties or thirties.

Mayo stand (mā′ō)—A stand with a flat metal tray used to hold sterile supplies during an aseptic procedure.

medical microbiology—The study and identification of pathogens, and the development of effective methods for their control or elimination.

melena (mě-lē′nah)—Darkening of stool by blood pigments.

microcyte (mī′krō-sīt)—An abnormally small red blood cell, found in cases of iron deficient anemia and thalassemia.

microorganism (mī-krō-or′gan-ism)—A minute living body not perceptible to the naked eye, especially a bacterium or protozoon; these are viewed using a microscope.

microscopic (mī-krō-skop′ik) **examination**—An examination in which the specimen is visible only with the aid of a microscope.

miotic (mi-ot′ik)—A medication that causes the pupil of the eye to contract.

modality (mo-dal′ĭ-te)—Therapeutic agents used in physical medicine and physical therapy.

mononucleosis (mon″ō-nū″klē-ō′sis)—An abnormal increase of the mononuclear white blood cells in the blood.

mydriatic (mid″rē-at′ik)—A medication that causes the pupil of the eye to dilate.

myocardial infarction (MI) (mi″o-kar′de-al in-fark′shun)—The formation of ischemic necrosis in the heart muscle due to an interference of blood supply to the area.

myocardium (mi″o-kar′de-um)—The heart muscle.

nasal speculum (na′zl spěk′ū-lŭm)—A short, funnel-like instrument used to examine the nasal cavity.

necrosis (ne-kro′-sis)—The death of a cell or a group of cells because of injury or disease.

negative culture—A culture made from suspected material that fails to reveal the suspected microorganism.

normal flora—Microorganisms that normally reside in various body locations such as in the vagina, intestine, urethra, upper respiratory tract, and on the skin. These microorganisms are nonpathogenic and do not cause any harm (they may become pathogenic and cause harm if they are introduced into a body area in which they do not normally reside).

objective symptom—A symptom that is apparent to the observer; also called a sign, for example, rash, swelling.

obstipation (ob′stī-pa′shun)—Extreme constipation due to an obstruction.

occult blood—Obscure or hidden from view.

occult blood test—A microscopic or a chemical test performed on a specimen to determine the presence of blood not otherwise detectable. Stool is tested when intestinal bleeding is suspected, but there is no visible evidence of blood in the stool.

ocular (ok′ū-lar)—Pertaining to the eye.

oliguria (ol″i-gu′rē-ah)—Scanty amounts of urine.

ophthalmic (of-thal′mik)—Pertaining to the eye.

ophthalmology (of″thal-mol′ō-jē)—The study and science of the eye and its diseases.

ophthalmoscope (ŏf-thăl′mō-skōp)—An instrument used for examining the interior parts of the eye. It contains a perforated mirror and lens. When the ophthalmoscope is turned on and brought close to the eye, it sends a narrow, bright beam of light through the lens of the eye. By looking through the lens of the instrument, the physician is then able to examine the interior parts of the eye, including the lens, anterior chamber, retinal structures, and blood vessels, to detect any possible disorders. Many ophthalmoscopes come with an interchangeable otoscope, throat illuminator head, or nasal illuminator head.

oral examination—Examination pertaining to the mouth.

orthopnea (or″thop-ne′ah)—Severe dyspnea in which breathing is possible only when the patient sits or stands in an erect position.

orthostatic (or″tho-stat′ik) **hypotension**—Hypotension occurring when a patient assumes an erect position.

oscilloscope (ŏ-sil′ō-skōp)—An instrument for visualizing the shape or wave form of sound waves, as in ultrasonography; or of electric currents, as when monitoring heart action and other body functions.

otic (ō′tik)—Pertaining to the ear.

otology (ō-tol′ō-je)—The study and science of the ear and its diseases.

otoscope (ō′tō-skōp)—An instrument used for visual examination of the external ear canal and eardrum.

pacemaker (pās′māk-er)—The pacemaker of the heart is the sinoatrial node located in the right atrium.

Papanicolaou smear or test (pap″ah-nik″o-la′oo)—A smear examined microscopically to detect cancer cells from body excretions (urine and feces), secretions (vaginal fluids, sputum or prostatic fluid), or tissue scrapings (as obtained from the stomach or uterus); most commonly done on a cervical scraping to detect abnormal or cancerous cells in the mucus of the uterus and cervix. This test is often referred to as a Pap smear or test.

parasite (par′ah-sīt)—An organism that lives on or in another organism, known as the host, from which it gains its nourishment, for example, fungi, bacteria, and single-celled and multi-celled animals.

pathogen (păth′ō-jěn)—A disease-producing substance or microorganism.

pathogenic (path′o-jěn′ic)—Pertaining to a disease-producing microorganism or substance.

• **pathogenic microorganism**—One that produces disease in the body.

- **PDR**—*Physician's Desk Reference,* a book on drugs.

pelvic examination—Examination of the external and internal female reproductive organs.

percussion (pŭr-kŭsh'ŭn) **hammer**—A small hammer with a triangular-shaped rubber head used for percussion.

pericarditis (per"ĭ-kar-di'tis)—Inflammation of the pericardium, the fibroserous sac enveloping the heart.

phagocytosis (fag"ō-sī-tō'sis)—The process by which white blood cells destroy and engulf or ingest harmful microorganisms.

physical signs—Objective manifestations of disease that are apparent on a physical examination; observable changes representing alterations resulting from a disease or dysfunction in the body (see also sign).

placebo (plah-sē'bō)—An inactive substance resembling and given in place of a medication for its psychological effects to satisfy the patient's need for the drug; it hopefully will produce the same effect as the real medication through psychological means. A placebo may be used experimentally.

poikilocytosis (poi"kĭ-lō-sī-tō'sis)—The presence of red blood cells in the blood that show abnormal variations in their shape.

polycythemia (pol"ē-sī-thē'mē-ah)—An abnormal increased amount of red blood cells or hemoglobin.

polyuria (pol"ē-u'rē'ah)—Excessive excretion of urine.

positive culture—A culture that reveals the suspected microorganism.

positive findings—Evidence of disease or body dysfunction.

postoperative (pōst-op'er-ah-tiv)—Pertaining to the period of time following surgery.

postural hypotension—Hypotension occurring upon suddenly arising from a recumbent position or when standing still for a long period of time.

preoperative (pre-op'er-ah-tiv)—Pertaining to the time preceding surgery.

proctoscope (prŏk'tō-skōp)—A specially designed tubular endoscope that is passed through the anus to permit internal inspection of the lower part of the large intestine.

prodrome—An early symptom, indicating the onset of a disease, such as an achy feeling before having the flu.

prognosis—A statement made by the physician indicating the probable or anticipated outcome of the disease process in a patient; usually stated simply as *good, fair, poor,* or *guarded.*

prophylaxis (prō"fĭ-lak'sis)—Prevention of disease.

proteinuria (pro"te-in-u'rē-ah)—An abnormal increase of protein in urine.

psoriasis (so-ri'ah-sis)—A chronic inflammatory recurrent skin disease characterized by scaly red patches on the body surfaces. The lesions are seen most often on knees, elbows, scalp, and fingernails. Other areas frequently affected are the chest, abdomen, palms of the hands, soles of the feet, and backs of the arms and legs. The cause is unknown, although a hereditary factor is suggested.

pulse deficit—The apical rate is greater than the radial pulse rate.

pulse pressure—The difference between the systolic and the diastolic blood pressure.

EXAMPLE: If BP is 120/80

$$120 = \text{systolic pressure}$$
$$-\ \ 80 = \text{diastolic pressure}$$
$$40 = \text{pulse pressure}$$

A pulse pressure consistently over 50 points or under 30 points is considered abnormal.

pure culture—A culture of a single microorganism.

pure drug—A refined drug; one that has been processed to remove all impurities.

pyuria (pī-u'rē-ah)—The presence of pus in the urine.

qualitative tests—Used for screening purposes. These tests provide an indication as to whether or not a substance is present in a specimen in abnormal quantities. A qualitative test does not determine the exact amount of a substance present in a specimen. Color charts are usually used to interpret qualitative tests. *Sometimes they are called semiquantitative tests.* Results are reported in terms such as trace, small amount, moderate, large amount, or 1+, 2+, 3+, and so on, or simply as positive or negative.

quantitative tests—More precise tests. They determine accurately the amount of a specific substance that is present in a specimen. A high level of skill is required to perform these tests on sophisticated equipment. Results are reported in units such as grams (gm) per 100 milliliters (ml), or milligrams (mg) percent, or milligrams per deciliter (dl).

radiating—Diverting from a common central point; for example, gallbladder pain begins in the right upper quadrant of the abdomen, and it is diverted from that central point to the right flank and right scapular area.

radiation (rā"dē-ā'shun)—Electromagnetic waves of streams of atomic particles capable of penetrating and being absorbed into matter. Examples of electromagnetic waves are x-rays, gamma rays, ultraviolet rays, infrared rays, and rays of visible light. Atomic particles are alpha and beta particles.

radiogram (rā'dē-ō-gram")—A picture of internal body structures produced by the action of gamma rays or x-rays on a special film.

radiograph (rā'dē-ō-graf") or **roentgenograph** (rent'gen-ō-graf) or **roentgenogram** (rent'gen-ō-gram")—The film or photographic record produced by radiography.

radiography (rā"dē-og'rah-fe)—The taking of radiograms.

radioisotope (rā"dē-ō-ī'so-tōp)—A radioactive form of an element consisting of unstable atoms that emit rays of energy or streams of atomic particles. Radioisotopes occur naturally, as in the case of radium, or can be created artificially, as in the case of cobalt.

radiologist (rā″dē-ol′o-jist)—A physician specialist in the study of radiology.

radiolucent (rā″dē-ō-lū-sent)— That which permits the partial or complete passage of radiant energy such as x-rays. Dense objects appear white on the x-ray film because they absorb the radiation. An example of this is bone.

radionuclide (rā″dē-ō-nū′klīd)—A radioactive substance.

radiopaque (rā-dē-ō-pāk′)—That which is impenetrable by x-rays and other forms of radiant energy; matter that obstructs the passage of radiant energy, such as lead which is frequently used as a protective device.

rales (rahls)—An abnormal bubbling sound heard on auscultation of the chest; often classified as either moist or crackling and dry.

rebound tenderness—A sensation of pain felt when pressure applied on a body part is released.

regular pulse—The rhythm of the pulse rate is regular.

renal hypertension—Hypertension resulting from kidney disease.

reservoir (rez′er-vwrar)—The source in which pathogenic microorganisms grow and from which they leave to spread and cause disease.

resistance (re-zis′tans)—The ability of the body to resist disease or infection because of its own defense mechanisms.

reticulocyte (rĕ-tik′ū-lō-sīt)—A nonnucleated immature red blood cell. Generally, of all the red blood cells in the circulating blood, less than 2% are reticulocytes.

rhythm strip—A rhythm strip is an EKG recording of a single lead that is used to determine the *rhythm* of the heartbeat, such as

a fast, slow, regular, or irregular rhythm, and certain types of ventricular fibrillation. It is also used to determine if the patient is in any type of heart block, such as third-degree heart block. The rhythm strip gives a one-dimensional picture of the beating of the heart which determines *only* the rhythm of the heartbeat in contrast to the 12 lead EKG, which can slow damage to the heart and other conditions. Data from the rhythm strip can be a useful "screening" tool because frequent runs of arrhythmias can be more easily observed. The rhythm strip can also be used to confirm the basic assessment made on the 12-lead EKG.

Currently for the rhythm strip most practitioners will record Lead V_1, and possibly Leads V_2 and V_5, although one could record any lead that is desired. Rhythm strips are frequently recorded from a continuous cardiac monitor in intensive care units in the hospital and by paramedics when they are in the field in emergency situations.

roentgenological (rĕnt-gĕn-ōl′ōj-i-cal)—Pertaining to an examination with the use of x-ray film (radiographs).

saliva (sah-li′vah)—The enzyme-containing secretion of the salivary glands in the mouth.

secondary hypertension—Hypertension that is traceable to known causes such as a pheochromocytoma (tumor of the adrenal gland), hardening of the arteries, kidney disease, or obstructions to kidney blood flow. Approximately 10% to 15% of the cases of hypertension are secondary. Patients with **secondary hypertension** can often be cured *if* the underlying cause can be eliminated.

sepsis (sep′sis)—A morbid state or condition resulting from the presence of pathogenic microorganisms.

septicemia (sep″tĭ-sē′mē-ah)—A condition in which there are

bacteria or toxins in the blood.

serological (sē-rō-lŏj′ik-al) **test**—A laboratory test involving the examination and study of blood serum.

serum (se′rum)—The clear, straw-colored liquid portion obtained after blood clots; it consists of plasma minus fibrinogen, which is removed in the process of clotting.

side effect—A response in addition to that for which the drug was used, especially an undesirable result.

• **untoward effect**—an undesirable side effect.

sigmoidoscope (sĭg-moy′dō-skōp)—A tubular endoscope used to examine the interior of the sigmoid colon.

sign—Sometimes called a *physical sign*; any objective evidence (apparent to the observer) representing disease or body dysfunction. Signs may be observed by others or revealed when the physician performs a physical examination; examples include swollen ankles, a distended rigid abdomen, elevated blood pressure, and decreased sensation.

Sims vaginal speculum—A form of bivalve speculum used in the examination of the vagina and cervix.

slow pulse—A pulse between 40 and 60 beats per minute, often found among the aged and among athletes at rest.

smear (smēr)—Material spread thinly across a slide or culture medium with a swab, loop, or another slide in preparation for microscopic study.

smear culture—A culture prepared by smearing the specimen across the surface of the culture medium.

specimen (spec′ĭ-men)—A small part or sample taken to show kind and quality of the whole, as a specimen of urine, blood, or other body excretions, or a small piece of tissue for macroscopic and microscopic examination.

speculum (spĕk′ū-lŭm)—An instrument used for distending or opening a body cavity or orifice to allow visual inspection; a bivalve speculum is one having two parts or valves.

spore (spōr)—A reproductive cell, usually unicellular, produced by plants and some protozoa, and possessing thick walls to withstand unfavorable environmental conditions. Bacterial spores are resistant to heat and must undergo a prolonged exposure to extremely high temperatures to be destroyed.

sprain (sprān)—A joint injury in which some fibers of a supporting ligament are ruptured, but continuity of the ligament remains intact. There may also be damage to the associated muscles, tendons, nerves, and blood vessels.

sputum (spū'-tŭm)—A mucous secretion from the trachea, bronchi, and lungs, ejected through the mouth, in contrast to saliva, which is the secretion of the salivary glands.

stab culture—A bacterial culture made by thrusting a needle inoculated with the microorganisms under examination deep into the culture medium.

stabbing pain—Deep, sharp, intermittent pain.

sterile (ster'il)—Free from all microorganisms.

sterile field—A work area prepared with sterile drapes (coverings) to hold sterile supplies during a sterile procedure.

sterile setup—Specific sterile supplies used in a specific sterile procedure.

stertorous (stĕr'tō-rŭs) **respirations**—Characterized by a deep snoring sound with each inspiration.

stethoscope—An instrument used in auscultation to amplify the sounds produced by the lungs, heart, intestines, and other internal organs; also used when taking a blood pressure reading.

stock supply—A large supply of medications kept in the physician's office or pharmacy.

stool (stōol)—Body waste material discharged from the large intestine; *synonym:* feces, bowel movement.

strain (strān)—An overexertion or overstretching of some part of a muscle.

streak culture—A bacterial culture in which the infectious material is implanted in streaks across the culture media.

subjective symptoms—Symptoms of internal origin that are apparent or perceptible only to the patient; examples include pain, dizziness (vertigo).

suture (soo'cher)—Various types and sizes of absorbable and nonabsorbable materials used to close a wound with stitches.

swab (swŏb)—A small piece of cotton or gauze wrapped around the end of a slender stick used for applying medications, cleansing cavities, or obtaining a piece of tissue or body secretion for bacteriological examination; *synonym:* cotton-tipped applicator.

symmetry (sim'ĕt-ri)—Correspondence in form, size, and arrangement of parts on opposite sides of the body.

symptom—Any subjective evidence of disease or body dysfunction; a change in the physical or mental state of the body that is perceptible or apparent only to the individual; examples include anorexia, nausea, headache, pain, itching.

syndrome—A combination of symptoms resulting from one cause or commonly occurring together to present a distinct clinical picture; an example is the dumping syndrome, which consists of nausea, weakness, varying degrees of syncope, sweating, palpitation, and sometimes diarrhea and a feeling of warmth. This may occur immediately after eating in patients who have had a partial gastrectomy.

tachycardia (tak"y-kar'di-a)—A pulse of 170 or more beats per minute; abnormal rapidity of heart action.

tendinitis (ten'dĭ-ni'tis)—Inflammation of a tendon; one of the most common causes of acute pain in the shoulder.

thready pulse—A pulse that is very fine and scarcely perceptible, as seen in syncope (fainting).

threshold—The level that must be exceeded for an effect to be produced; the level of pain that an individual can tolerate without external intervention. Threshold is unique to each individual, and the overall physiopsychological makeup of an individual must be considered when evaluating pain.

thrombocyte (throm'bō-sīt)—A blood platelet.

thrombocythemia (throm"bō-sī-thē'mē-ah)—An increased number of platelets in the circulating blood.

thrombocytopenia (throm"bo-si"to-pe'ne-ah)—A decreased number of platelets in the circulating blood.

tissue culture—The growing of tissue cells in artificial nutrient media.

tongue blade—A flat, thin, smooth piece of wood or metal with rounded ends approximately 6 inches long; also called a tongue depressor. It is used for pressing tissue down to permit a better view when examining the mouth and throat. In addition, it may be used for application of ointments to the skin.

tonometer (to-nom'ĕ-ter)—An instrument used to measure tension or pressure, especially intraocular pressure.

tourniquet (toor'nĭ-ket)—A constricting device used to compress an artery or vein to stop excessive bleeding or to prevent the spread of snake venom.

toxicity (tok-sis'ĭ-tē)—The nature of exerting harmful effects on a tissue or organism. The level at which a drug becomes toxic to the body. Minor or major damage may result.

toxin (tok'sin)—A poisonous substance produced by pathogenic bacteria and some animals and plants. The toxins produced by bacteria include toxic enzymes, exotoxins, and endotoxins. Toxins in the body cause antitoxins to form, which provide a means for establishing immunity to certain diseases.

transfer forceps—A type of instrument (forcep) that is kept in a chemical disinfectant or germicide and used for transferring or handling sterile supplies and equipment.

transient—Fleeting, brief, passing, coming and going.

tuning fork—A steel, two-pronged, forklike instrument used for testing hearing; the prongs give off a musical note when struck.

tympanic (tim-pan'ik) **membrane**—The eardrum, abbreviated TM; it serves as the membrane that separates the external auditory meatus from the middle ear cavity.

type culture—A culture that is generally agreed to represent microorganisms of a particular species.

unequal pulse—A pulse in which some beats are strong and others are weak; pulse in which rates are different in symmetrical arteries.

unit-dose—A system that supplies prepackaged, premeasured, prelabeled, individual portions of a medication for patient use.

uremia (ū-rē'mē-ah)—A toxic condition in which there are substances in the blood that should normally be eliminated in the urine.

urgency—The need to urinate immediately.

urination (u-"rī-na'shun), **voiding, micturition** (mik"tu-rish'un)—The act of passing urine from the body.

urine (ū'rine)—The fluid containing certain waste products and water that is secreted by the kidneys, stored in the bladder, and excreted through the urethra.

urobilinogen—A colorless compound formed in the intestines by the reduction of bilirubin.

USP-NF—*United States Pharmacopeia-National Formulary,* a drug book listing all official drugs authorized for use in the United States.

vaccination (vak"sī-na'shun)—The introduction of weakened or dead microorganisms (inoculation) into the body to stimulate the production of antibodies and immunity to a specific disease.

venipuncture (vēn"ī-pungk'tūr)—Puncturing a vein to collect a blood specimen or to administer a medication.

venous pulse—A pulse in a vein, especially one of the large veins near the heart such as the internal and external jugular. Venous pulse is undulating and scarcely palpable.

ventricle (ven'trĭ-kl)—One of the lower chambers of the heart. The right ventricle receives deoxygenated blood from the right atrium and pumps this blood through the pulmonary arteries to the lungs; the left ventricle receives oxygenated blood from the left atrium and pumps this blood out through the aorta to all body tissues.

vesicle (ves'ĭ-kl)—A circular, blisterlike elevation on the skin containing fluid.

viable (vī'ah-bl)—Able to maintain an independent existence.

virulence (vir'u-lens)—The degree of ability of a pathogen to produce disease.

vitamin K—A vitamin that is essential for the formation of prothrombin and the normal clotting of blood. A deficiency may result in hemorrhage because of a prolonged prothrombin time.

voltage (vōl-tij)—The electromotive force measured in volts (the units of force for electricity to flow).

wheal (hwēl)—A temporary, more or less round, elevation on the skin that is white in the center and often accompanied by itching.

Suggested Readings

American Medical Association: The wonderful human machine, Chicago, 1976, The Association.

American National Red Cross: Advanced first aid and emergency care, ed. 2, Garden City, N. Y., 1979, Doubleday & Co, Inc.

American Sterilizer Co.: Sterilization aids. Erie, Pa., 1975.

Ames Co.: Modern urine chemistry, a guide to the diagnosis of urinary tract diseases and metabolic disorders, Revised reprint, Elkhart, Ind., 1982.

Ames Co.: Urodynamics: concepts relating to routine urine chemistry, Elkhart, Ind., 1978.

Anthony, C. P., and Thibodeau, G. A.: Textbook of anatomy and physiology, ed. 11, St. Louis, 1983, The C. V. Mosby Co.

Artz, C.: Trauma can be conquered. Emergency Medicine Today pp. 1–6, July 1974.

Asperheim, M.: Pharmacology for practical nurses, ed. 5, Philadelphia, 1981, W. B. Saunders Co.

Bauer, J. D., Ackermann, P. G., and Toro, G.: Clinical laboratory methods, ed. 9, St. Louis, 1982, The C. V. Mosby Co.

Beaumont, E.: Blood pressure equipment, Nursing 75 **5:**56, January, 1975.

Beaumont, E.: Diagnostic kits, Nursing 75 **5:**28, April 1975.

Bergeron, J. D.: First responder, ed. 2. Bowie, Md., 1987, Robert J. Brady Co.

Bergersen, B.: Pharmacology in nursing, ed. 14, St. Louis, 1979, The C. V. Mosby Co.

Bird, B.: Talking with patients, ed. 2, Philadelphia, 1973, J. B. Lippincott Co.

Blainey, C.: Site selection in taking body temperature, Am. J. Nurs. **74:**1859, October 1974.

Bredow, M. and Cooper, M.: The medical assistant, ed. 4, New York, 1978, McGraw-Hill Book Co.

Brunner, L. S., and Suddarth, D. S., and others: The Lippincott manual of nursing practice, ed. 3, Philadelphia, 1982, J. B. Lippincott Co.

Btesh, S., ed.: Disease of the urinary tract and male genital organs, Geneva, Switzerland, 1974, Council for International Organizations for Medical Sciences.

Buckner, J.: Interpersonal skills: necessary conditions for professional helpers, Professional Medical Assistant **9:**17, March/April 1976.

Burdick Corp.: Electrocardiography: a better way, Milton, Wis., 1976.

Chabner, D. E.: The language of medicine, ed. 2, Philadelphia, 1981, W. B. Saunders Co.

Ciuca, R., Bradish J., and Trombly, S.: Passive range-of-motion exercises: a handbook, Nursing 78, **8:**59, July 1978.

Clark, C.: Communicating with hearing impaired elderly adults, Journal of Gerontological Nursing **4** (3):40–44, 1979.

Clarke, W. L., and Pohl, S. L.: New developments in blood glucose monitoring and insulin delivery, Occupational Health Nursing **30:**40, Dec. 1982.

Collen, M. F.: Periodic health examinations, Primary Care **3:**197, 1976.

Conover, M. H.: Understanding electrocardiography: physiological and interpretive concepts, ed. 4, St. Louis, 1984, The C. V. Mosby Co.

Cope, Z.: The early diagnosis of acute abdomen, ed. 15, New York, 1979, Oxford University Press, Inc.

Daleske, E. E., and others: The who, what, and when of tetanus prophylaxis, Patient Care **10:**144–145, August 1976.

DeWeese, D. F., and Saunders, W. H.: Textbook of otolaryngology, ed. 6, St. Louis, 1982, The C. V. Mosby Co.

Dison, N.: Simplified drugs and solutions for nurses, including arithmetic, ed. 8, St. Louis, 1984, The C. V. Mosby Co.

Dison, N.: Clinical nursing techniques, ed. 4, St. Louis, 1979, The C. V. Mosby Co.

Dubay, E. C., and Grubb, R. D.: Infection: prevention and control, ed. 2, St. Louis, 1978, The C. V. Mosby Co.

DuGas, B.: Introduction to patient care, ed. 4, Philadelphia, 1983, W. B. Saunders Co.

Ehrlich, R. A., and Givens, E. M. C.: Patient care in radiography, ed. 2, St. Louis, 1985, The C. V. Mosby Co.

Ethicon, Inc.: Suture use manual, Somerville, New Jersey, 1978.

Fischer, P., Addison, L., Curtis, P., and Mitchell, J.: The office laboratory, Norwalk, CT., 1983, Appleton-Century-Crofts.

Frederick, P., and Kinn, M.: The medical office assistant: administrative and clinical, ed. 5, Philadelphia, 1981, W. B. Saunders Co.

French, R. M.: The nurse's guide to diagnostic procedures, ed. 5, New York, 1981, McGraw-Hill Book Co.

Fowler, N. O.: Inspection and palpation of venous and arterial pulses, New York, 1970, American Heart Association, Inc.

Garb, S.: Laboratory tests in common use, ed. 6, New York, 1976, Springer Publishing Co.

Garfield, S. R., Collen, M. F., Richart, P. H., and others: Evaluation of new ambulatory medical care delivery system, N. Eng. J. Med. **294:**426, 1976.

Geolot, D., and McKinney, N.: Administering parenteral drugs, Am. J. Nurs. **75:**788, May 1975.

Gordon, M.: Initial care of burn victim often a matter of life or death, Occupational Health and Safety, p. 34, Jan. 1984.

Gould, J. A., and Davies, G. J., editors: Orthopaedic and sports physical therapy, St. Louis, 1985, The C. V. Mosby Co.

Govoni, L., and Hayes, J.: Drugs and nursing implications, ed. 4, New York, 1982, Appleton-Century-Crofts.

Guthrie, H. A.: Introductory nutrition, ed. 5, St. Louis, 1983, The C. V. Mosby Co.

Hahn, R. L., Burgess, A., and Oestreich, S. J. K.: Pharmacology in nursing, ed. 15, St. Louis, 1982, The C. V. Mosby Co.

Hammond, C.: ECG's made easier than ever, RN **10:**42, October 1979.

Hammond, C.: ECG's made easier than ever — when the natural pacemakers fail, RN **11:**30, November 1979.

Hammond, C.: ECG's made easier than ever — fast rhythms and early beats, RN **12:**29, December 1979.

Haynes, D. M.: Medical complications during pregnancy, New York, 1969, McGraw-Hill Book Co.

Heidrich, G., and Perry, S.: Helping the patient in pain, Am. J. Nurs. **82:**1828–1833, 1982.

Hicks, D. J., Innes, B. S., and Shores, W. L.: Patient care techniques, Indianapolis, 1975, The Bobbs-Merrill Co.

Hill, G.: Outpatient surgery, ed. 2, Philadelphia, 1980, W. B. Saunders Co.

Hirsh, R.: Can your examining rooms pass this test? Medical Economics, p. 191, June 13, 1977.

Hirsh, R.: Can your office soundproofing pass this test? Medical Economics, p. 131, June 27, 1977.

Hobson, L.: Examination of the patient, New York, 1975, McGraw-Hill Book Co.

Holvey, D. N., and others: The Merck manual of diagnosis and therapy, ed. 12, Rahway, N.J., 1972, Merck, Sharp and Dohme Research Laboratories.

Hughes, E. C., ed.: Obstetric-gynecologic terminology, Philadelphia, 1972, W. B. Saunders Co.

Iorio, J.: Childbirth: family-centered nursing, ed. 3, St. Louis, 1975, The C. V. Mosby Co.

Kent, T. H., Hart, M. N., Shires, T. K.: Introduction to human disease, New York, 1979, Appleton-Century-Crofts.

Kirkindall, W. M., and others: Recommendations for human blood pressure determination by sphygmomanometers, New York, 1979, American Heart Association.

Koren, M. D.: Cancer immunotherapy: what, why, when, how? Nursing 81 **11**(1):34–41, 1981.

Krusen, F. H.: Handbook of physical medicine and rehabilitation, ed. 2, Philadelphia, 1971, W. B. Saunders Co.

Lambert, M.: Drug and diet interactions. Am. J. Nurs. **75:**402, March 1975.

Lancour, J.: How to avoid pitfalls in measuring blood pressure. Am. J. Nurs. **76:**773, May 1976.

Lang, S., Zawacki, A., and Johnson, J.: Reducing discomfort from I.M. injections, Am. J. Nurs. **76:**800, May 1976.

Lee, L. W.: Elementary principles of laboratory instruments, ed. 4, St. Louis, 1978, The C. V. Mosby Co.

Leser, D. R.: Synthetic blood: a future alternative, Am. J. Nurs. **82:**452, March 1982.

Lewis, L.: Fundamental skills in patient care, ed. 3, Philadelphia, 1984, J. B. Lippincott Co.

Littmann, D.: The electrocardiogram, New York, 1973, American Heart Association, Inc.

Loebl, S., Spratto, G., and Wit, A.: The nurse's drug handbook, ed. 3, New York, 1983, John Wiley & Sons.

Long, B. C., and Phipps, W. J.: Essentials of medical-surgical nursing, St. Louis, 1985, The C. V. Mosby Co.

Lynch, J. M.: Helping patients through the recurring nightmare of herpes, Nursing 82 **12**(10):52, 1982.

Malasanos, L., Barkauskas, V., Moss, M., and Allen, K. S.: Health assessment, ed. 2, St. Louis, 1981, The C. V. Mosby Co.

McGucklin, M.: The problems with respiratory tract cultures — and what you can do about them, Nursing 76 **7:**19, February 1976.

McGucklin, M.: Tips for assisting with cultures of CSF and other body fluids, Nursing 76 **7:**17, April 1976.

Mechner, F.: Examination of the eye, part 1, Am. J. Nurs. **74:**2039, November 1974.

Memmler, R. L., and Wood, D. L.: The human body in health and disease, ed. 5, Philadelphia, 1983, J. B. Lippincott Co.

Menard, R. H.: Introduction to arrhythmia recognition. San Francisco, 1968, California Heart Association.

Meschan, I.: Radiographic positioning and related anatomy, ed. 2, Philadelphia, 1978, W. B. Saunders Co.

Meshelany, C. M.: Post-op wound dressing, RN **42:**22, May 1979.

Miller, B., and Keane, C.: Encyclopedia and dictionary of medicine, nursing, and allied health, ed. 3, Philadelphia, 1983, W. B. Saunders Co.

Mueller, C.: Perfecting physical assessment: part 1, Nursing 77 **7:**28, May 1977.

Mueller, C.: Perfecting physical assessment: part 2, Nursing 77 **7:**38, June, 1977.

Mueller, C.: Perfecting physical assessment: part 3, Nursing 77 **7:**44, July 1977.

Mueller, C.: Vital signs — how to take them more accurately and understand them more fully, Nursing 76 **6:**31, April 1976.

National Safety Council: Accident facts, Chicago, 1981.

Nealon, T.: Fundamental skills in surgery, ed. 3, Philadelphia, 1979, W. B. Saunders Co.

Newton, D, and Newton, M.: Needles, syringes and sites for injectable medications, American Pharmaceutical Association Journal, **NS17:**685–687, November 1977.

Nichols, G. A., and Kucha, D. H.: Taking adult temperatures: oral measurement, Am. J. Nurs. **72:**1090, 1972.

Oppenheim, I.: Textbook for laboratory assistants, ed. 3, St. Louis, 1981, The C. V. Mosby Co.

Oppenheim, M.: Suppose you were getting that physical exam, Medical Economics, p. 249, June 13, 1977.

Parcel, G. S.: Basic care of the sick and injured, ed. 2, St. Louis, 1982, The C. V. Mosby Co.

Perkins, J.: Principles and methods of sterilization in health sciences, ed. 2, Springfield, Ill., 1982, Charles C. Thomas, Publisher.

Pfizer Laboratories: How to give an intramuscular injection, New York, 1976.

Phelps, J.: Radiation protection and the medical assistant, Professional Medical Assistant **10:**32, July/August 1977.

Phibbs, B.: The cardiac arrhythmias, ed. 3, St. Louis, 1978, The C. V. Mosby Co.

Phipps, W. J., Long, B. C., and Woods, N. F.: Medical-surgical nursing, St. Louis, 1979, The C. V. Mosby Co.

Pitel, M.: The subcutaneous injection, Am. J. Nurs. **71:**76–79, January 1971.

Potts, A. M., editor: The assessment of visual function, St. Louis, 1972, The C. V. Mosby Co.

Poulos, J.: Diagnostic tests: A guide to patient instruction, Professional Medical Assistant **8:**15, May/June 1975.

Rana, A. N. and Luskin, A.: Immunosuppression, autoimmunity, and hypersensitivity, Heart Lung **9:**655, 1980.

Raphael, S.: Lynch's medical laboratory technology, ed. 4, Philadelphia, 1983, W. B. Saunders Co.

Raus, E., and Raus, M.: Manual of history taking, physical examination and record keeping, Philadelphia, 1974, J. B. Lippincott Co.

Renshaw, D.: Psychiatric first aid in an emergency, Am. J. Nurs. **72:**497, 1972.

Resler, M. M., and Tumutty, G.: Glaucoma update, Am. J. Nurs. **83:**752, 1983.

Saver, G. C.: Manual of skin diseases, ed. 3, Philadelphia, 1973, J. B. Lippincott Co.

Scherer, J.: Introductory clinical pharmacology, ed. 2, Philadelphia, 1982, J. B. Lippincott Co.

Sellars, D.: A basic understanding of immunology for the medical assistant, Professional Medical Assistant **10:**8, July/August 1977.

Shanas, E.: Health status of older people, Am. J. Public Health **64:**261, 1974.

Shuman, D.: Doing it better. Tips for improving urine testing techniques, Nursing 76 **6:**23, February 1976.

Sloboda, S.: Understanding patient behavior, Nursing 77 **7:**74, September 1977.

Smith, A. L.: Microbiology and pathology, ed. 12, St. Louis, 1980, The C. V. Mosby Co.

Soukhanov, A. H., and Haverty, J. R., eds.: Webster's medical office handbook, Springfield, Mass., 1979, G. & C. Merriam Co., Publishers.

Stein, E.: The electrocardiogram: a self-study course in clinical electrocardiography, Philadelphia, 1976, W. B. Saunders Co.

Stephenson, H. E., Jr., editor: Immediate care of the acutely ill and injured, ed. 2, St. Louis, 1978, The C. V. Mosby Co.

Stevens, A. D.: Monitoring blood glucose at home—who should do it, Am. J. Nurs. **81:**2026, Nov. 1981.

Strand, M. M., and Elmer, L. A.: Clinical laboratory tests, ed. 3, St. Louis, 1983, The C. V. Mosby Co.

Thomas, V.: Life sciences for nursing and health technologies, Long Beach, Calif., 1974, Technicourse Inc.

Thompson, D. A.: Teaching the client about anticoagulants, Am. J. Nurs. **82:**78, Feb. 1982.

Thompson, J. M., and Bowers, A. C.: Health assessment—a pocket guide, St. Louis, 1984, The C. V. Mosby Co.

Tilkian, S. M., Conover, M. B., and Tilkian, A. G.: Clinical implications of laboratory tests, ed. 3, St. Louis, 1983, The C. V. Mosby Co.

Ur, A., and Gordon, M.: Origin of korotkoff sounds, Am. J. Physiol. **218:**524, 1970.

U.S. Department of Health, Education, and Welfare: Collection handling and shipment of microbiological specimens, Atlanta, 1973, Center for Disease Control.

U.S. Department of Health, Education, and Welfare: Criteria and techniques for the diagnosis of gonorrhea, Atlanta, 1974, U.S. Public Health Service.

Van Meter, M.: What every nurse should know about EKGs, Nursing 75 **5:**19, April 1975.

Varricchio, C. G.: The patient on radiation therapy, Am. J. Nurs. **81:**334, 1981.

Vaughan-Wrobel, B. C., and Henderson, B.: The problem-oriented system in nursing—a workbook, ed. 2, St. Louis, 1982, The C. V. Mosby Co.

Walter, J. B.: An introduction to the principles of disease, ed. 2, Philadelphia, 1983, W. B. Saunders Co.

Warner, C. G.: Emergency care: assessment and intervention, ed. 3, St. Louis, 1982, The C. V. Mosby Co.

Weed, L. L.: Medical records, medical education, and patient care, Cleveland, 1971, The Press of Case Western Reserve University.

Westfall, E.: Electrical and mechanical events in the cardiac cycle, Am. J. Nurs. **76:**23, February 1976.

Williams, S. R.: Nutrition and diet therapy, ed. 4, St. Louis, 1982, The C. V. Mosby Co.

Williamson, J., and others: Teaching quality assurance and cost containment in health care, San Francisco, 1982, Jossey-Bass Inc., Publishers.

Wood, L., and Rambo, B.: Nursing skills for allied health services, ed. 3, Philadelphia, 1982, W. B. Saunders Co.

Woolley, F., and others: Problem-oriented nursing, New York, 1974, Springer Publishing Co.

Wu, R.: Behavior and illness, Englewood Cliffs, N.J., 1973, Prentice-Hall, Inc.

Wyeth Laboratories: Intramuscular injections, Philadelphia, 1984.

Yates, D. A.: The electrodiagnosis of muscle disorders. Proc. R. Soc. Med. **65:**617, 1972.

Young, C. G., and Barger, J. D.: Introduction to medical science, ed. 3, St. Louis, 1977, The C. V. Mosby Co.

Zimmer, M. J.: Quality assurance for outcomes of patient care, Nurs. Clin. North Am. **9:**305–315, June 1974.

Index

Index